Textbook on High-Risk Pregnancy for Postgraduates

Textbook on
High-Risk Pregnancy
for Postgraduates

Professor Firoza Begum
MBBS FCPS FICS
Founder Chairman and Former Professor
Feto-Maternal Medicine Department
Bangabandhu Sheikh Mujib Medical University
Dhaka, Bangladesh

Foreword
TA Chowdhury

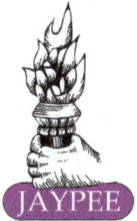

JAYPEE BROTHERS MEDICAL PUBLISHERS
The Health Sciences Publisher
New Delhi | London

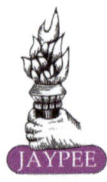

Jaypee Brothers Medical Publishers (P) Ltd

Headquarters
Jaypee Brothers Medical Publishers (P) Ltd
EMCA House, 23/23-B
Ansari Road, Daryaganj
New Delhi 110 002, India
Landline: +91-11-23272143, +91-11-23272703
+91-11-23282021, +91-11-23245672
Email: jaypee@jaypeebrothers.com

Corporate Office
Jaypee Brothers Medical Publishers (P) Ltd
4838/24, Ansari Road, Daryaganj
New Delhi 110 002, India
Phone: +91-11-43574357
Fax: +91-11-43574314
Email: jaypee@jaypeebrothers.com

Overseas Office
JP Medical Ltd
83 Victoria Street, London
SW1H 0HW (UK)
Phone: +44 20 3170 8910
Fax: +44 (0)20 3008 6180
Email: info@jpmedpub.com

Website: www.jaypeebrothers.com
Website: www.jaypeedigital.com

© 2023, Jaypee Brothers Medical Publishers

The views and opinions expressed in this book are solely those of the original contributor(s)/author(s) and do not necessarily represent those of editor(s) or publisher of the book.

All rights reserved. No part of this publication may be reproduced, stored or transmitted in any form or by any means, electronic, mechanical, photocopying, recording or otherwise, without the prior permission in writing of the publishers.

All brand names and product names used in this book are trade names, service marks, trademarks or registered trademarks of their respective owners. The publisher is not associated with any product or vendor mentioned in this book.

Medical knowledge and practice change constantly. This book is designed to provide accurate, authoritative information about the subject matter in question. However, readers are advised to check the most current information available on procedures included and check information from the manufacturer of each product to be administered, to verify the recommended dose, formula, method and duration of administration, adverse effects and contraindications. It is the responsibility of the practitioner to take all appropriate safety precautions. Neither the publisher nor the author(s)/editor(s) assume any liability for any injury and/or damage to persons or property arising from or related to use of material in this book.

This book is sold on the understanding that the publisher is not engaged in providing professional medical services. If such advice or services are required, the services of a competent medical professional should be sought.

Every effort has been made where necessary to contact holders of copyright to obtain permission to reproduce copyright material. If any have been inadvertently overlooked, the publisher will be pleased to make the necessary arrangements at the first opportunity. The **CD/DVD-ROM** (if any) provided in the sealed envelope with this book is complimentary and free of cost. **Not meant for sale**.

Inquiries for bulk sales may be solicited at: jaypee@jaypeebrothers.com

Textbook on High-Risk Pregnancy for Postgraduates

First Edition: **2023**

ISBN: 978-93-5465-858-7

Dedicated to

*My beloved parents, my children, my husband, and
to the memory of my teachers who have encouraged me
and inspired my pursuit of knowledge.*

Foreword

Professor Firoza Begum is an academician and reputed Obstetrician and Gynecologist in Bangladesh. I am happy that she has written a *Textbook on High-Risk Pregnancy for Postgraduates*. I have gone through few chapters of the book.

This book is a fully revised and updated version following all the available literature, guidelines and recent advances on high-risk pregnancies. The aim of this textbook is to provide an up-to-date overview of the care of high-risk pregnancies. It focuses on an evidence-based approach to the available management options, equipping you with the most appropriate strategy for each patient.

Although this book has been written especially for the postgraduates, it should also prove to be useful to the practicing obstetricians involved in the care of women with high-risk pregnancies. This book is written in a clear and concise language and in author's own style, which holds the reader's interest. The readers will enjoy being stimulated by the fascination and intellectual stimulation that comes from the study of feto-maternal medicine.

I hope, this book will be an essential reference for obstetricians, medical students and physicians who are seeking the most up-to-date information and guidance on high-risk pregnancies. This book will create more qualified consultant in feto-maternal medicine who shows skills in application of medical knowledge, clinical skills and professional values in the provision of high-quality and patient-centered care.

TA Chowdhury
MBBS FCPS FRCS FRCP FRCOG
Professor
Department of Obstetrics and Gynecology
BIRDEM, General Hospital, Dhaka
President, GOSB, Infertility Society
Past President, OGSB, SAFOG, BCPS
Former Professor, Department of Obstetrics and Gynecology
Institute of Postgraduate Medical Research (IPGMR)
Dhaka, Bangladesh

Preface

During my journey as an academic, I started teaching feto-maternal medicine to postgraduate students and discovered the challenges faced by students in mastering this topic. The length and complexity of existing textbooks have created real and unnecessary impediments to student learning. At the insistence of my beloved students, I agreed to write a compact, comprehensive, and practical *Textbook on High-Risk Pregnancy for Postgraduates*. This book is the result of combining decades of experience in feto-maternal medicine with extensive research of available literature in the field.

I have attempted to provide comprehensive and updated information in a concise and easy-to-read format to facilitate the learning process. Extensive illustrations and flowcharts have been used to add clarity to the topics and to emphasize the practical nature of the textbook. My extensive experience in high-risk pregnancies helped me identify and synthesize the underlying principles of feto-maternal medicine which are most relevant to students. Although the book has been written especially for postgraduates, it can also serve as a handbook for the undergraduate students focusing on obstetrics. In addition to serving as a textbook, the book is also intended to provide obstetricians with a guide to the most up-to-dated information and evidence-based treatment options for high-risk pregnancies.

A total of 22 chapters are included in this book. The chapters cover the pathophysiology of the disorders of pregnancies, formulation of diagnosis and systematic investigation, and appropriate management of high-risk pregnancies. This book is based on available literature and guidelines up to 2021 on high-risk pregnancies. It is organized in a logical manner so that students can first learn the basics of high-risk pregnancies and then build on their understanding to appreciate the complexities of the topic.

The development of feto-maternal medicine and high-risk pregnancy care is a triumph of modern medicine. Advancements in medical technology and greater understanding of this complex topic have facilitated the management of high-risk pregnancies and reduced maternal mortality rates. I hope this book will provide a wealth of knowledge to both students and practitioners in this field and inspire young doctors to focus on the specialty and contribute to greater advancements in the future.

It is my expectation and hope that high-risk pregnancies in Bangladesh can be both reframed and reformed to achieve the improved outcomes that we know are possible at lower economic cost, leading to substantial benefits for families and communities, as well as for our nation.

I am grateful to all teachers who have taught me, my beloved students, and most of all the patients.

I would like to thank M/s Jaypee Brothers Medical Publishers (P) Ltd, New Delhi, India, with the editorial team for their support in the publication of this textbook.

Professor Firoza Begum

Acknowledgments

I would like to thank all individuals and institutions who contributed to this book's creation and turned my dream of publishing this book into reality.

Firstly, I would like to express my deepest appreciation and gratitude to my respected teachers for their guidance and encouragement to write this book. I thank my mentors, Professors TA Chowdhury, Shahla Khatun and Anwara Begum, for being a source of inspiration.

I owe an enormous debt of gratitude to Professor Tabassum Parveen who was with me from the very beginning of the idea of writing a book for the postgraduate students, who gave me detailed and constructive comments on different chapters, and contributed to writing one chapter for the book. I would also like to express my very profound appreciation to Drs Syeda Sayeeda, Khandaker Shehneela Tasmin, Shanzida Mahmud, Mahfuza Asma, Most Arifa Sharmin, Masuda Sultana, Rajosree Debnath, Tajmira Sultana, Raunak Jahan, Marzia Khanam and Hasina Begum—all of whom contributed to different chapters of the book as well.

I extend my heartfelt thanks to my colleagues Dr Fatima Wahid and Professor Sahana Afroz for the pictorial support; Mr Mijanur Rahman and Professor AN Nashimuddin Ahmed for their valuable and constructive suggestions during the development of this book; and Dr Shamima Nasreen Barsa for giving me mental support while I was editing this book.

I thank my beloved postgraduate students from different medical colleges/institutions for their inspiration in writing a book.

Finally, I would like to acknowledge my family for their love and support along this journey. I would like to thank my parents, whose love and guidance are with me in whatever I pursue. I wish to thank my husband and my two daughters for their unwavering faith in me.

Contents

1. Anemia in Pregnancy 1
2. Thalassemia in Pregnancy 9
3. Hypertensive Disorders in Pregnancy 21
4. HELLP Syndrome 41
5. Fetal Growth Restriction 46
6. Doppler in Obstetrics 61
7. Diabetes in Pregnancy 71
8. Cardiac Diseases in Pregnancy 86
9. Liver Diseases in Pregnancy 101
10. Coagulation Disorders in Pregnancy 115
11. Placenta Previa 131
12. Placenta Accreta Spectrum Disorders 143
13. Thyriod Disorders in Pregnancy 152
14. Systemic Lupus Erythematosus in Pregnancy 163
15. Recurrent Pregnancy Loss 176
16. Multiple Gestation 187
17. Rhesus Alloimmunization 202
18. Preterm Birth 216
19. Premature Rupture of Membranes 229
20. Amniotic Fluid Disorder 237
21. Congenital TORCH Infections 249
22. Fetal Congenital Malformation... 262

Index *293*

Anemia in Pregnancy

INTRODUCTION

Anemia during pregnancy is a public health problem especially in developing countries. The World Health Organization (WHO) has defined anemia in pregnancy as the hemoglobin (Hb) concentration of <11 g/dL. According to WHO (2015 report), about 32.4 million pregnant women suffer from anemia worldwide, of which 0.8 million women are severely anemic. The global prevalence of anemia among pregnant women is 36.5% (WHO, 2019), the prevalence is higher (56%) among women living-in low and middle-income countries (LMIC). The prevalence rate is highest among pregnant women in Sub-Saharan Africa (57%), in South and Southeast Asian countries (52%) and lowest prevalence (24.1%) in South America. In Bangladesh 42.9% women suffer from anemia in pregnancy.

Iron deficiency anemia (IDA) during pregnancy is associated with adverse outcomes in pregnancy, increases the risk of low birth weight (LBW), preterm birth, maternal and perinatal mortality, and poor Apgar score. An estimate by WHO attributes about 591,000 perinatal deaths and 115,000 maternal deaths globally to IDA, directly or indirectly. According to Lone et al., anemic women as compared to nonanemic women are at fourfold higher risk of preterm birth, 1.9 fold increased risk of delivering LBW infants, and 1.8 fold increased risk of having neonates with Apgar score <5 at 1 minute.

ETIOLOGY OF ANEMIA IN PREGNANCY

The causes of anemia are multifactorial, include micronutrient deficiencies of iron, folate, vitamin A and B_{12}, anemia due to parasitic infections such as malaria and hookworm or chronic infections such as tuberculosis (TB) and human immunodeficiency virus (HIV), and anemia resulting from acute blood loss. Contributions of each of the factors vary due to geographical location, dietary practice, and season. According to WHO 50% cases of anemia in pregnancy are attributable to IDA with the rest due to conditions such as folate, vitamin B_{12} or vitamin A deficiency, chronic inflammation, parasitic infections, and inherited disorders (WHO 2015). Most IDA in pregnancy is related to the maternal and fetal demands of pregnancy, although some women start pregnancy with IDA, mainly due to menstrual losses, previous pregnancies, and/or inadequate dietary intake.

HEMATOLOGICAL CHANGES IN PREGNANCY

Pregnancy is associated with normal physiological changes that assist fetal survival and prepares the mother for labor, delivery, and breastfeeding. The changes start as early as 4 weeks of gestation and are largely as a result of progesterone and estrogen. The total blood volume increases steadily from as early as 4 weeks of pregnancy to reach a maximum of 35–45% above the nonpregnant level at 28–32 weeks. The plasma volume increases by 40–45% (1,000 mL). Red blood cell (RBC) mass increases by 30–33% (approximately 300 mg) as a result of the increase in the production of erythropoietin, which reaches approximately 150% of their prepregnancy levels at term **(Fig. 1)**. The greater increase in plasma

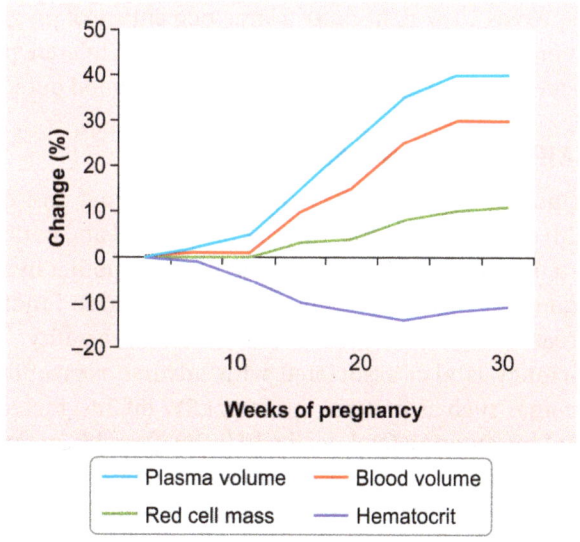

Fig. 1: Changes in plasma volume, blood volume, red cell mass, and hematocrit with pregnancy.
Source: Ezechi Oliver and Kalejaiye Olufunto. Management of Anaemia in Pregnancy. *www.intechopen.com.*

volume than the increase in RBC mass results in a modest reduction in hematocrit; peak hemodilution occurs at 24–26 weeks, resulting in physiological anemia of pregnancy. This dilutional picture is often normochromic and normocytic. Occasionally, physiologic anemia can also be associated with a physiologic macrocytosis, mean corpuscular volume (MCV) increases to 120 fL (average at term is 104 fL).

The physiological demand for iron during pregnancy is three times higher than in nonpregnant women, and increases as pregnancy progresses. The net iron requirements for pregnancy have been calculated as 1,000 mg taking into account the requirements for fetus, placenta, expansion of maternal erythrocyte mass, and losses due to delivery. Though iron requirements decrease during the first trimester, there is an increase of 4–6 mg/day in the second and third trimesters which may reach up to 10 mg/day during the last 6–8 weeks of pregnancy. The iron absorption has been found to decrease during the first trimester of pregnancy, which rises during the second trimester, and this increase lasts the remainder of pregnancy. While the transferrin and total iron binding capacity rises, the serum iron falls. So, women who enter pregnancy in an iron deficient state are unable to meet the demands of pregnancy by diet alone and require supplementation. It takes approximately 2–3 weeks after delivery for these hematologic changes to revert to prepregnancy status.

DEFINITION OF ANEMIA

The World Health Organization defines anemia in pregnancy as a Hb concentration of <11 g/dL. The United States (US) Centers for Disease Control and Prevention (CDC) defines anemia in pregnancy as Hb concentration <11 g/dL in the first and third trimesters and <10.5 g/dL in the second trimester. In most developing countries the lower limit is often accepted as 10 g/dL because a large percentage of pregnant women in this setting with Hb level of 10 g/dL tolerate pregnancy, labor, and delivery very well and with good outcome.

IMPACT OF ANEMIA

Anemia is reported to have negative maternal and child health effect and increases the risk of maternal and perinatal mortality. The negative health effects for the mother include fatigue, poor work capacity, impaired immune function, increased risk of cardiac diseases, and mortality. Iron deficiency is also associated with adverse reproductive outcomes such as preterm delivery, LBW infants, increased risk of intrauterine fetal deaths (IUFDs), possibly placental abruption, and increased peripartum blood loss. Some studies have shown that anemia contributes to 23% of indirect causes of maternal deaths in developing countries. Tissue enzyme malfunction occurs in the early stages of iron deficient erythropoiesis, may contribute to maternal morbidity through effects on immune function with increased susceptibility to or severity of infections, poor work capacity and performance, and disturbances of postpartum cognition and emotions.

The fetus is relatively protected from the effects of iron deficiency by upregulation of placental iron transport. Evidence suggests that maternal iron depletion increases the risk of iron deficiency in the first 3 months of newborn's life and decreased iron stores for the baby, which may lead to impaired development. Impaired psychomotor and/or mental development are well described in infants with IDA, therefore, may negatively contribute to infant's social and emotional behavior and have an association with adult-onset diseases, although this is a controversial area.

CLASSIFICATION OF ANEMIA IN PREGNANCY

Classification Based on Etiology

- *Deficiency anemia:* Iron, vitamin B_{12}, and folic acid deficiency.
- *Blood loss:*
  - Acute [antepartum hemorrhage (APH), intrapartum hemorrhage]
  - Chronic (hookworm infestation, bleeding piles, and peptic ulcer disease)
- *Bone marrow failure:*
  - Aplastic anemia
  - Isolated secondary failure of erythropoiesis
  - Drugs (e.g., chloramphenicol, zidovudine)
- *Hemolytic anemia:*
  - Inherited:
    - *Hemoglobinopathy:* Thalassemia's, sickle cell hemoglobinopathies
    - *Red blood cell membrane defects:* Hereditary spherocytosis, elliptocytosis
    - *Enzyme defect:* Glucose-6-phosphate dehydrogenase (G6PD), pyruvate kinase deficiency
  - Acquired:
    - *Immune hemolytic:* Autoimmune, alloimmune, and drug induced
    - *Nonimmune hemolytic:*
      - Acquired membrane defect (paroxysmal nocturnal hemoglobinuria)
      - *Mechanical damage:* Microangiopathic hemolytic anemia
    - *Secondary to systemic disease:* Renal anemia, anemia due to liver disease
    - *Infection:* Malaria, sepsis, and HIV.

Classification According to Red Cell Morphology

Hypochromic microcytic:
- Iron deficiency
- Thalassemia
- Sideroblastic anemia
- Anemia of chronic disorders
- Lead poisoning

Macrocytic:
- Folic acid deficiency
- Vitamin B_{12} deficiency
- Liver disease
- Myxedema
- Chronic obstructive pulmonary disease
- Myelodysplastic syndrome
- Anemia due to blood loss

Normocytic normochromic (MCV 80–90 fL):
- Autoimmune hemolytic anemia
- Systemic lupus erythomatosis
- Collagen vascular disorders
- Hereditary spherocytosis
- Hemoglobinopathies
- Bone marrow failure
- Malignancies
- Myelodysplasia
- Blood loss anemia
- Anemia of chronic disease

Classification According to Severity

Classification of anemia according to severity		
Degree	**Hb g%**	**Hematocrit (%)**
Mild	10–10.9	31–32%
Moderate	7–9.9	24–30%
Severe	4–6.9	13–23%
Very severe	<4	<13%

IRON-DEFICIENCY ANEMIA

Iron-deficiency anemia is the most common form of anemia in pregnancy. Iron deficiency represents a spectrum ranging from iron depletion to IDA. In iron depletion, the amount of stored iron measured by serum ferritin concentration is reduced (ferritin level 30 μg/L), but the amount of transport and functional iron may not be affected. Those with iron depletion have no iron stores to mobilize if the body requires additional iron. In IDA, the most severe form of iron deficiency, there is shortage of iron stores, transport and functional iron, resulting in reduced Hb in addition to low serum ferritin, low transferrin saturation. The shortage of iron limits RBC production and increased erythrocyte protoporphyrin concentration.

Clinical Features

Clinical symptoms and signs of IDA in pregnancy are usually nonspecific, unless the anemia is severe. The clinical features depend on the rapidity of onset and severity of anemia. In general, symptoms occur with moderate to severe anemia and are more severe when anemia has been rapidly progressive. Fatigue is the most common symptom. Patients may complain of pallor, weakness, light headedness, headache, irritability, palpitations, dizziness, dyspnea or symptoms of angina. IDA may also impair temperature regulation and cause pregnant women to feel colder than normal, rarely a patient may present with heart failure.

Signs: The signs of anemia can be general or specific. General signs of anemia include pallor of the mucous membranes, hyperdynamic circulation with tachycardia, a bounding pulse, cardiomegaly, and an apical systolic flow murmur (hemic murmur). The specific signs are associated with particular types of anemia, e.g., painless glossitis, angular stomatitis, ridged or spoon-shaped nails, unusual dietary cravings for nonfood substances (pica) in iron deficiency.

Investigations

Pregnant women should be offered screening for anemia at booking and at 28 weeks. Women with multiple pregnancies should have an additional full blood count done at 20–24 weeks [Royal College of Obstetricians and Gynaecologists (RCOG)].

National Institute for Health and Care Excellence (NICE) guidelines recommendation: Screen women for anemia at booking and again at 28 weeks. Measuring only Hb is an inadequate screening. Screening should include Hb, MCV, mean corpuscular hemoglobin (MCH), mean cell hemoglobin concentration (MCHC), red cell distribution width (RDW), reticulocyte count, and percent of hypochromic cells along with the examination of various RBC indices. Peripheral blood smear (PBS) evaluation should also be considered as an essential component of evaluating various hematological disorders, examination of blood smear could provide important clues in the diagnosis of anemia.

Full Blood Count

A primary step in the diagnosis of IDA is to consider the complete blood count (CBC). It is simple, inexpensive, rapid to perform, and helpful for early prediction of IDA and may show low Hb, low mean red cell volume (MCV), and low mean cell hemoglobin (MCH). MCV is the most sensitive indicator. Reduced MCV (<75 fL) with normal MCHC is suggestive of hemoglobinopathies. If the MCV <75 fL or MCH is <27 pg, laboratory screening for thalassemia by Hb electrophoresis should be offered (NICE 2008).

Serum Ferritin

Serum ferritin is a stable glycoprotein which accurately reflects iron stores in the absence of inflammatory change. It is a sensitive indicator of IDA in pregnant women, correlates closely with body iron store, generally considered the best single test to assess iron deficiency in pregnancy. Although it is an acute phase reactant and levels will rise when there is active infection or inflammation, it has the advantage of steady concentration even on the recent intake of iron-rich foods. Iron therapy must be discontinued for 24–48 hours before carrying out the test. A concentration <15 µgL (normal range in women 15–300 ug/L, mean 56 ug/L) indicates iron depletion in all stages of pregnancy, has shown specificity of 98% and sensitivity of 75% for iron deficiency. Treatment needs to be initiated when the concentration falls below 30 µg/L, as this indicates early iron depletion which will worsen unless treated.

Red Cell Distribution Width

The RDW is a measure of the change in RBC width and is used in combination with the MCV to distinguish an anemia of mixed cause from that of a single cause. Increased RDW represents variance in the RBC volume distribution, similar to a PBS anisocytosis. In the initial stages of IDA, there is a fall in MCV accompanied with increasing RDW values due to a preponderance of microcytes. Following treatment, marked reticulocytosis occurs in the first 4 weeks, manifested as a sudden increase in RDW, sometimes to over 30%. Thus, falling MCV accompanied by a rising RDW should alert the clinician to the presence of possible IDA which is then confirmed by marked RDW increase occurring early after the initiation of therapy. A few studies have reported sensitivity and specificity of RDW in the diagnosis of IDA in pregnancy, 97.4% and 83.2% respectively.

Serum Iron Profile

Serum Fe and total iron-binding capacity (TIBC) are unreliable indicators of iron stores or availability of iron to the tissues because of wide fluctuation in levels due to recent ingestion of Fe, diurnal rhythm, and other factors such as infection. The TIBC decreases with malnutrition, inflammation, chronic infection, and cancer. Transferrin saturation also fluctuates due to a diurnal variation in serum iron and is affected by the nutritional status. This may lead to a lack of sensitivity and specificity. In IDA, transferrin saturation decreases (≤10%), plasma iron decrease <30 µg/dL (normal 60–180 µg/dL in women), and TIBC increased >400 µg/dL (normal 240–450 µg/dL).

Peripheral Blood Smear

Peripheral blood smear could help in differentiating the IDA from megaloblastic anemia and anemia of chronic disease. Macrocytes, oval-shaped macrocytes, and hypersegmented neutrophils are associated with megaloblastic anemias (folate or cobalamin deficiency); target cells and pencil cells are associated with IDA. Presence of target cells frequently in the smear rules out anemia of chronic diseases. Moreover, poikilocytes (prekeratocytes) are also observed in more numbers in IDA.

Zinc Protoporphyrin

Zinc protoporphyrin (ZPP) increases when iron availability decreases, as zinc, rather than iron, is incorporated into the protoporphyrin ring during the biosynthesis of heme. Short supply of iron as in IDA increases ZPP production and elevates ZPP/heme ratio. Before the onset of anemia, ZPP/heme reflects iron status and detects ID. This test is most accurately reported as the ZPP or ZPP/heme ratio. It is a sensitive test, but with limited specificity, because ZPP increases in the settings of inflammation, lead poisoning, anemia in chronic disease, and hemoglobinopathies. Normal value of ZPP <2.3 micrograms ZPP/g Hb.

Serum Transferrin Receptor

The transferrin receptor (TfR) is a transmembrane protein which transports iron into the cell. Circulating concentrations of soluble transferrin receptor (sTfR) are proportional to cellular expression of the membrane associated TfR and therefore gives an accurate estimate of iron deficiency. Measurement of sTfR is reported to be a sensitive measure of tissue iron supply. There is little change in the early stages of iron store depletion, but once iron deficiency is established, the sTfR concentration increases in direct proportion to total TfR concentration. However, this is an expensive test which restricts its general availability.

Bone Marrow Examination

Bone marrow biopsy should be considered to make a definitive diagnosis of IDA when the diagnosis remains ambiguous even after the analysis of laboratory results. It is indicated when there is no response to treatment after 4 weeks of therapy or to rule out other conditions. The absence of stainable iron is the "gold standard" for diagnosis of IDA.

Other Tests

Urine examination—to see hematuria, stool examination—for occult bleeding, renal function tests (RFT), liver function test (LFT), and sputum examination to exclude TB.

■ MANAGEMENT OF IRON-DEFICIENCY ANEMIA

The aim of management:
- To correct iron deficiency
- To restore iron reserve
- To correct associated complicating factor

At Booking

Women with normal Hb but low MCV should have their ferritin checked and levels below 15 µg/L are diagnostic of established iron deficiency. If ferritin level below 30 µg/L, oral iron should be commenced. Hb <11 g/dL: start 100–200 mg of elemental iron daily. Repeat Hb level 3 weeks later, if Hb <9 g/dL: start 200 mg of oral iron, F/U as above. *If Hb <7 g/dL*: refer to joint obstetric/hematologic clinic to investigate further and make management plan. *Do not give transfusion* before investigation unless acute blood loss.

At 28 Weeks

All women should have their Hb rechecked, if Hb <10.5 g/dL; oral iron dose as above, recheck in 3 weeks. If no response, check serum ferritin and if low, consider total dose iron infusion. If Hb <9 g/dL: start oral iron, 200 mg elemental iron/day, recheck in 3 weeks. If no response, check serum ferritin and if low, consider total dose iron infusion. If <7 g/dL; urgent referral to joint obstetric/hematologic clinic to investigate further and make management plan. No blood transfusion unless symptomatic or currently actively bleeding. Total dose iron infusion can be considered.

Special point: Women with known hemoglobinopathy should have serum ferritin checked and offered oral supplements if their ferritin level is <30 μg/L (British Committee for Standards in Hematology, 2014).

Dietary Advice

The average daily iron intake from food for women in Great Britain is 10.5 mg. An approximately 15% of dietary iron is absorbed. Physiological iron requirements are three times higher in pregnancy than in the menstruating women, with increasing demand as pregnancy advances, 2.5 mg/day in early pregnancy, 5.5 mg/day from 20 to 30 weeks, and 6–8 mg/day from 32 weeks onward. Absorption of iron also increases with advancement of pregnancy, three-fold by the third trimester.

The amount of iron absorption depends upon the amount of iron in the diet, its bioavailability, and physiological requirements. The main sources of dietary heme iron are Hb and myoglobin from red meats, fish, and poultry. Heme iron is absorbed 2–3 fold more readily than nonheme iron. Meat contains organic compounds which promote absorption of iron from other less bioavailable nonheme iron sources. Approximately 95% of dietary iron intake is from nonheme iron sources. Vitamin C (ascorbic acid) significantly enhances iron absorption from nonheme foods. Iron absorption is inhibited by phytic acid (6-phosphoinositol) which is found in whole grains, lentils, and nuts. Germination and fermentation of cereals and legumes improve the bioavailability of nonheme iron by reducing the content of phytate that inhibits iron absorption. Tannins in tea and coffee and red wines inhibit iron absorption. Iron should be taken on an empty stomach, 1 hour before meals, with a source of vitamin C to maximize absorption. Other medications, e.g., calcium or antacids, tea or coffee should not be taken at the same time.

■ MANAGEMENT

All women should have a full blood count at the booking appointment and at 28 weeks (NICE, 2008). This enables selective iron supplementation early in pregnancy and appropriate follow-up to avoid delays in management. The average daily requirement of iron is 4–6 mg/day in the second and third trimesters which increases to 10 mg/day during the last 6–8 weeks of pregnancy. These requirements are unlikely to be met by the diet alone because of poor accessibility, availability, and affordability of diversified food. Once a woman becomes iron deficient regular iron supplementation is necessary to prevent IDA.

Choice of Therapy

- Depends on severity of anemia
- Duration of pregnancy
- Associated complicating factor

Oral Iron Therapy

Women with a Hb <11 g/dL up until 12 weeks or <10.5 g/dL beyond 12 weeks should be offered a trial of therapeutic iron replacement. Oral iron is an effective, cheap, and safe way to replace iron. WHO recommends daily oral iron and folic acid supplementation as part of the antenatal care to reduce the risk of LBW, maternal anemia, and iron deficiency. Universal iron supplementation with 60 mg of elemental iron along with folic acid 400 μg (0.4 mg) daily for 6 months in pregnancy and to continue for 3 months postpartum as *prophylaxis* and daily 120 mg iron + 400 μg folic acid till term as *treatment* (WHO). Folic acid supplementation should begin as early as possible. CDC and ACOG recommends 30 mg of elemental iron daily. Women should be counseled how to take oral iron supplementation correctly. With this treatment store is replenished in 4–6 months.

Available oral iron, ferrous salts, include ferrous fumarate, ferrous sulfate, and ferrous gluconate. There is no significant differences in the efficacy and safety among the different oral iron formulations, though ferric salts are much less well absorbed. The recommended dose of elemental iron for treatment of iron deficiency is 100–200 mg daily. If the ferritin is <30 μg/L, 65 mg elemental iron once a day should be offered. Ferrous sulfate 325 mg contains 57 mg of elemental iron, and is the most efficient form; it is given once or twice daily, ferrous gluconate causes fewer gastrointestinal (GI) symptoms, but it only has 34 mg of elemental iron.

Ferrous fumarate is better tolerated than carbonyl iron as shown by patient global assessment of response to therapy (PGART) score (1.416 vs. 1.750, $p < 0.0001$) and patient global assessment of tolerability to therapy (PGATT) score (1.416 vs. 1.652, $p = 0.002$) scales response. Few studies have found iron polymaltose complex to be more effective and better tolerated than ferrous sulfate in pregnant women.

Daily versus Intermittent Regimen

A recent Cochrane systematic review has shown similar maternal and infant outcomes with both intermittent and daily supplementation. Intermittent supplementation was associated with fewer side effects, although, the risk of mild anemia near term was increased. Intermittent supplementation has been proposed as a feasible alternative to daily supplementation for those pregnant women who are not anemic and have an adequate antenatal care. WHO recommends once a week intermittent iron and folic acid supplementation (120 mg elemental iron and 2.8 mg folic acid) for *nonanemic* pregnant women.

Response to Oral Iron

Response is evidenced by sense of well-being, increased appetite, and improved outlook. To see treatment response hematological examination—Hb and PBS, reticulocyte count should be done. Rise in Hb level is about 0.8 g/dL/week; hematocrit returning to normal and reticulocytosis is observed within 7–10 days. The degree of increase in Hb that can be achieved with iron supplements will depend on the Hb and iron status at the start of supplementation, ongoing losses, iron absorption, and other factors contributing to anemia, such as other micronutrient deficiencies, infections, and renal impairment. A repeat Hb at 2 weeks is required to assess response to treatment. If no significant clinical or hematological improvement within 3 weeks, diagnostic re-evaluation is needed.

Parenteral Iron Therapy

Parenteral iron therapy is indicated when there is absolute noncompliance with or intolerance to oral iron therapy or proven malabsorption (RCOG, 2007) or need rapid restoration of iron stores or if the woman is approaching term and there is insufficient time for oral supplementation to be effective. Parenteral iron may be used from the second trimester and during the postpartum period. It circumvents the natural GI regulatory mechanisms to deliver nonprotein bound iron to the red cells.

Several authors have now reported on their experience with use of parenteral iron therapy for IDA in pregnancy, with faster increases in Hb and better replenishment of iron stores in comparison with oral therapy, particularly for iron sucrose and iron carboxymaltose. A large retrospective study reported fewer postpartum transfusions in the group treated with intravenous iron.

Contraindications to Parenteral Therapy

History of anaphylaxis to parenteral iron therapy, first trimester of pregnancy, active acute/chronic infection, chronic liver diseases, asthma, acute renal failure, active rheumatoid arthritis, and anemia not attributable to iron deficiency and iron overload are the few contraindications to parenteral therapy.

Types of Parenteral Iron Therapy

Parenteral iron is available as intramuscular (IM) and intravenous forms. Preparations include—iron dextran (50 mg/mL), iron sucrose (20 mg/mL), and ferric carboxymaltose (50 mg/mL). *Iron dextran* is given as deep IM injection/total dose infusion. IM injection should not exceed 2 mL daily; side effect includes anaphylactic reaction. *Iron sucrose*—maximum 200 mg iron can be given at a time up to three doses in a week. *Iron carboxymaltose*—a next-generation dextran-free iron preparation and can be administered in high dose up to 1,000 mg of iron during a minimum time of ≤15 minutes **(Table 1)**. It does not release large amounts of reactive iron into the circulation and does not trigger dextran-associated immunological reactions.

TABLE 1: Types of parenteral iron therapy with dose.

Formulation	Ferric carboxymaltose	Iron sucrose	Iron–dextran complex
Product name	Ferinject/Maltofer	Venofer/deferon	CosmoFer
Dose of elemental iron (mg/mL)	50 mg/mL	20 mg/mL	50 mg/mL
Presentation	2 mL (100 mg) or 10 mL (500 mg)	5 mL ampules	5 mL ampules
Maximum dose in a single administration for patients ≥35 kg	1,000 mg (not >1,000 mg/week) (maximum 20 mg iron/kg body weight)	100 mg not more than three times per week Most patients will require a minimum cumulative dose of 1,000 mg	Not to exceed 100 mg/day
Rate of administration	IV infusion: • 100–200 mg 3 minutes • >200–500 mg 6 minutes • >500–1,000 mg 15 minutes IV bolus injection: • 200–500 mg@100 mg/min • >500–1,000 mg over 15 minutes	Intravenous infusion 100 mg over 15 minutes	IV/IM preparation
Total dose single infusion	Yes (up to 20 mg/kg body weight maximum of 1,000 mg/week over 15 minutes)	No	Yes (up to 20 mg/kg body weight over 4–6 hours)

(IM: intramuscular; IV: intravenous)

Calculation of Iron Deficit (Different Formula)

- Required iron dose (mg) = [2.4 × (target Hb – actual Hb) × prepregnancy weight (kg)] + 1,000 mg for replenishment of stores.
- *Simple method:*
  - 250 mg elemental iron for each g of Hb below normal. Another 50% is to be added to replenish the store.
  - *Calculation according to body weight:*

Hb (g/dL)	weight 35 to <70 kg	weight ≥70 kg
<10	1,500 mg	2,000 mg
≥10	1,000 mg	1,500 mg

PLACE OF BLOOD TRANSFUSION

Blood transfusion is indicated if anemia is not responding to either oral or parenteral therapy, to correct anemia due to blood loss and associated infection. Massive obstetric hemorrhage (MOH) is widely recognized as an important cause of morbidity and mortality and requires prompt use of blood and components as part of appropriate management. Severe anemia in last trimester does not permit iron supplementation to completely replenish iron levels, hence, blood transfusion is the treatment of choice for immediate improvement in Hb status. Patients with severe anemia seen in later months of pregnancy, if Hb <6 and gestational age (GA) >37 weeks, consider transfusion for fetal perfusion concerns (ACOG). The RCOG green-top guidelines (RCOG, 2009) suggest multidisciplinary approach, together with the implementation of intraoperative cell salvage in this setting as a transfusion sparing strategy. Outside the massive hemorrhage setting, audits indicate that a high proportion of blood transfusions administered in the postpartum period may be inappropriate, with underutilization of iron supplements.

Clinical assessment and measuring Hb concentration are necessary in postpartum to consider the best method of iron replacement. In healthy, asymptomatic patients there is little evidence of the benefit of blood transfusion, which should be reserved for women with continued bleeding or at risk of further bleeding, imminent cardiac compromise or significant symptoms requiring urgent correction. The recent RCOG blood transfusion guideline recommends blood transfusion in labor or immediate postpartum in the following situations.

Indications of Blood Transfusion (RCOG)

I. *Antepartum period:*
- *Pregnancy <34 weeks:*
  - Hb <5 g/dL with or without signs of cardiac failure or hypoxia
  - Hb 5–7 g/dL—in presence of impending heart failure
- *Pregnancy >34 weeks:*
  - Hb <7 g/dL even without signs of cardiac failure or hypoxia
  - Severe anemia with decompensation

Anemia not due to hematinic deficiency:
- Hemoglobinopathy or bone marrow failure syndromes
- Hematologist should always be consulted.

Acute hemorrhage:
- Always indicated if Hb <6 g/dL
- If the patient becomes hemodynamically unstable due to ongoing hemorrhage

II. *Intrapartum period:*
- Hb <7 g/dL (in labor)
- Decision of blood transfusion depends on medical history or symptoms

III. *Postpartum period:*
- Anemia with signs of shock/acute hemorrhage with signs of hemodynamic instability.
- *Hb <7 g (postpartum):* Decision of blood transfusion depends on medical history or symptoms.

DELIVERY IN WOMEN WITH IRON-DEFICIENCY ANEMIA

Anemic women may require additional precautions for delivery, including delivery in a hospital setting, available intravenous access, blood group-and-save, active management of the third stage of labor, and plans to deal with excessive bleeding. Suggested Hb cut-offs are <10 g/dL for delivery in hospital and <9.5 g/dL for delivery in an obstetrician-led unit (British Committee for Standards in Hematology).

POSTNATAL MANAGEMENT

In the postnatal period anemic women with Hb 8–10 g/dL—if asymptomatic and hemodynamically stable, 200 mg elemental iron/day for 3 months, CBC and serum ferritin checked after 3 months. If Hb <8 g/dL total dose of intravenous iron; CBC and ferritin at 10 days. If Hb <7 g/dL—transfusion and/or total dose of intravenous iron indicated.

SUGGESTED READING

1. American College of Obstetricians and Gynecologists. ACOG Practice Bulletin No. 95: anemia in pregnancy. Obstet Gynecol. 2008;112(1):201-7.
2. Auerbach M, Simpson LL. Anemia in pregnancy. UpToDate, 2021. [online] Available from https://www.uptodate.com/contents/anemia-in-pregnancy [Last accessed April, 2022].
3. Chaparro CM, Suchdev PS. Anemia epidemiology, pathophysiology, and etiology in low- and middle-income countries. Ann NY Acad Sci. 2019;1450(1):15-31
4. FIGO Working Group on Good Clinical Practice in Maternal–Fetal Medicine. Good clinical practice advice: iron deficiency anemia in pregnancy. Int J Gynaecol Obstet. 2019;144(3):322-4.
5. Kriplani A, Aparna KA, Radhika AG, Rizvi ZL, Nair MK, Tank P, et al. FOGSI General Clinical Practice Recommendations. Management of Iron Deficiency Anemia in Pregnancy. 2016.

6. Oliver E, Olufunto K. (2012). Management of Anaemia in Pregnancy. [online] Available from https://www.intechopen.com/chapters/30549 [Last accessed, April 2022].
7. Panicker NK, Hridya A, Prabhu R. Comparison of efficacy and safety profile of oral iron formulations in patients with iron deficiency anemia. Int J Pharm Sci Rev Res. 2016;41(2):248-52.
8. Pavord S, Daru J, Prasannan N, Robinson S, Stanworth S, Girling J. UK guidelines on the management of iron deficiency in pregnancy. Br J Haematol. 2020;188(6):819-30.
9. RCOG. (2015). Blood transfusion in Obstetrics. RCOG Green Top Guideline No. 47. [online] Available from https://www.rcog.org.uk/guidance/browse-all-guidance/green-top-guidelines/blood-transfusions-in-obstetrics-green-top-guideline-no-47/ [Last accessed April, 2022].
10. Stephen G, Mgongo M, Hussein Hashim T, Katanga J, Stray-Pedersen B, Msuya SE. Anaemia in Pregnancy: Prevalence, Risk Factors, and Adverse Perinatal Outcomes in Northern Tanzania. Anemia. 2018;2018:1846280.
11. Sunuwar DR, Singh DR, Chaudhary NK, Pradhan PMS, Rai P, Tiwari K. Prevalence and factors associated with anemia among women of reproductive age in seven South and Southeast Asian countries: evidence from nationally representative surveys. PLoS One. 2020;15(8):e0236449.
12. World Health Organization. (2012). Daily iron and folic acid supplementation in pregnant women. [online] Available from http://apps.who.int/iris/bitstream/handle/10665/77770/9789241501996_eng.pdf?sequence=1 [Last accessed April, 2022].
13. World Health Organization. (2016). WHO recommendations on antenatal care for a positive pregnancy experience. Luxembourg; 2016. [online] Available from https://www.who.int/publications/i/item/9789241549912 [Last accessed April, 2022].
14. World Health Organization. Haemoglobin concentrations for the diagnosis of anaemia and assessment of severity. Geneva: World Health Organization; 2011.

CHAPTER 2

Thalassemia in Pregnancy

INTRODUCTION

Thalassemias are a heterogeneous group of genetic disorder of hemoglobin (Hb) synthesis characterized by a reduction in the synthesis of one or more of the globin chains leading to imbalanced globin-chain synthesis, defective Hb production resulting in anemia. The precise structure of the globin chain is coded by genes on chromosomes 16 (the α-gene cluster, comprising the α- and ζ-globin chains) and chromosome 11 (the β-gene cluster, comprising the globin chains γ, ε, β, and δ). Hb must have the correct structure and be trimmed in such a way that the number of α-chains precisely matches that of the β-chains. Adult Hb consists of approximately 98% HbA ($\alpha_2\beta_2$), <3% HbA$_2$ ($\alpha_2\delta_2$), and traces of HbF ($\alpha_2\gamma_2$).

Thalassemias result from partly or completely suppressed synthesis of one of the two types of polypeptide chains (α or β) as a result of missense/nonsense mutations (single-base substitutions) or frameshift mutations of the genes controlling the structure of the Hb chain in one or both "allelic" globin genes. Depending on the genes affected, the resulting defect, and the corresponding effect on the globin chain, several types of thalassemia have been described, the most common types of clinical importance being α-, β/δ-, and β-thalassemia. A variety of thalassemia phenotypes can result from simultaneous inheritance of two different mutations from each parent or the coinheritance of thalassemia together with structural Hb variants (e.g., HbE-β thalassemia). **Figure 1** shows alpha and Beta globin genes on chromosomes 16 and 11.

The thalassemia syndromes are characterized by a basic defect in the synthesis of one type of globin chains. As a result, there is insufficient Hb content in the resultant red cells resulting in decreased Hb concentration, microcytosis, and anemia. The other type of globin chains whose synthesis is not affected accumulates in the red cells, resulting in defective red cells, which are released into the circulation. These damaged red cells undergo extravascular hemolysis.

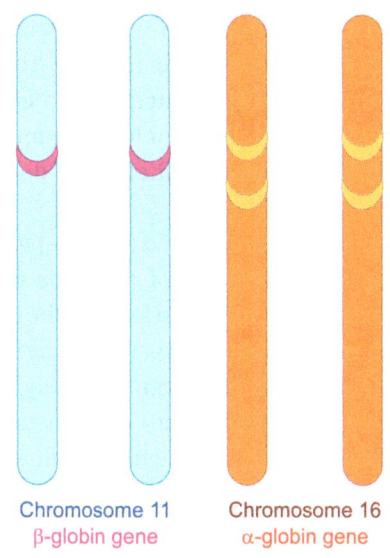

Fig. 1: Alpha- and Beta-globin genes on chromosomes 16 and 11.
Source: Thalassaemia.com

EPIDEMIOLOGY

The term thalassemia is derived from the Greek word "thalassa" for sea, and "hema" for blood. Thalassemias were initially distinctive in the tropics and subtropics but are now commonly found worldwide as a result of population migration. This defect is seen more often in the Indian subcontinent, the Mediterranean region, Southeast Asia, and West Africa. Approximately, 15 million people are globally affected by thalassemia. Alpha-thalassemia is more prevalent among individuals from African and Southeast Asian descent, whereas beta-thalassemia is most common in persons of Mediterranean, African, and Southeast Asian descent. Most children with thalassemia are born to women in the low-income countries. World Health Organization recommends screening and genetic counseling for Hb disorders as an intrinsic part of healthcare system for improvement of survival among children born with thalassemia.

INCIDENCE

Thalassemia is detected in approximately 4% women of reproductive age. More than 70,000 babies are born with thalassemia worldwide each year and there are 100 million individuals who are asymptomatic thalassemia carriers [Royal College of Obstetricians and Gynaecologists (RCOG), Green-top guideline].

GENETIC BASIS OF THALASSEMIAS

Alpha-thalassemia is the most common inherited disorder of Hb and is characterized by reduced or suppressed production of α-globin chains. Almost 5% of the world's population are carriers, and approximately 1,000,000 patients are affected by various α-thalassemia syndromes worldwide. The α-globin chain synthesis begins in fetal life. The responsible genes—four in total—are situated in two genetic loci in chromosome 16. Gene deletion or less commonly mutation results in α-thalassemia, and phenotype depends on the affected gene number.

When all four genes are affected (–/–|–/–) in homozygous α-thalassemia, fetal synthesis of α-chains is impossible, leading to an excess of γ-chains and forming the unstable Bart's Hb (γ_4), which is incapable of oxygen exchange. The affected fetuses sustain severe anemia, cardiomegaly, and hydrops fetalis, and these lead to intrauterine or neonatal death. When three genes are affected ($\alpha^{-/-/-}$), α-chain synthesis is restricted to a minimum. Therefore, β-chains that exist in excess form the unstable HbH (β_4). HbH disease has a phenotypic variability based on mutation type, ranging from mild anemia to a transfusion-dependent one. The existence of two α-genes (α-thalassemia trait) is expressed as a mild hypochromic microcytic anemia. Globin synthesis is still unbalanced, leading to hemolysis and iron overload.

In α^0-thalassemia, the two deleted genes belong to the same allele (–/–|α/α), prevalent among Asian and Eastern Mediterranean populations, while α^+-thalassemia, prevalent among African people, the deleted genes belong to different homologous chromosomes. When only one α-gene is affected (α/–|α/α), the remaining three functional genes are capable of normal Hb production, the individual becomes a "silent" carrier **(Table 1)**.

Beta-thalassemia: The β-gene cluster region located on chromosome 11, regulates the synthesis of β-globin. It is extremely heterogeneous in terms of both genotype and phenotype, depending on the nature of β-gene mutation and the extent of impairment in β-globin chain production. β-thalassemia occurs due to one or more than 250 point mutations. Rarely, it may occur due to the deletion of two genes. β^0 refers to the complete absence of production of β-globin on the affected allele, β^+ refers to alleles with some residual production of β-globin, and β^{++} to a very mild reduction in β-globin production. Decreased production of β-globin chain leads to the excessive production of other chains, e.g., α-globulin chains, γ-globulin chains.

As a rule, heterozygous carriers of β-thalassemia (one-affected allele), are asymptomatic, and have only altered laboratory values. Thalassaemia minor causes mild-to-moderate microcytic anemia with no significant detrimental effect on overall health. In contrast, inheritance of two defective β-globin genes results in a wide phenotype spectrum, ranging from transfusion-dependent [thalassemia major (TM)] to mild or moderate anemia [thalassemia intermedia (TI)].

Thalassemia intermedia represents up to a quarter of β-thalassemia patients with a wide spectrum of genotypes and a clinical phenotype ranging between transfusion-dependent thalassemia and the asymptomatic carrier state. At the severe end of the clinical spectrum

TABLE 1: Thalassemia: Genetics and clinical features.

Alpha-thalassemia	α-, γ-genes	Globin chains	Hemoglobin	Anemia
Normal	αα/αα	$\alpha_2\beta_2$	A	None
Silent carrier	αα/α–	$\alpha_2\beta_2$	A	None
Trait	α–/α– ––/αα	$\alpha_2\beta_2$	A	Mild
HbH disease	––/–α	$\alpha_2\beta_2$, β_4	A, H	Intermediate
Hydrops fetalis	––/––	γ_4, $\zeta_2\gamma_4$	Bart's Portland	Lethal
Beta-thalassemia	**β-genes**	**Globin chains**	**Hemoglobin**	**Anemia**
Normal	β/β	$\alpha_2\beta_2$	A	None
Thalassemia minor	β^+/β β^0/β	$\alpha_2\beta_2$, $\alpha_2\delta_2$, $\alpha_2\gamma_2$	A, A_2, F	Mild
Thalassemia minor	β^+/β^+ β^0/β^0	$\alpha_2\beta_2$, $\alpha_2\delta_2$, $\alpha_2\gamma_2$, $\alpha_2\gamma_2$, $\alpha_2\delta_2$	A, A_2, F, F, A_2	Severe Severe
HPFH	γ/γ	$\alpha_2\gamma_2$	F	Mild

(HPFH: hereditary persistence of fetal hemoglobin)
Source: https://library-g.kau.edu.sa/Files/237/Researches/65509_36921.pdf

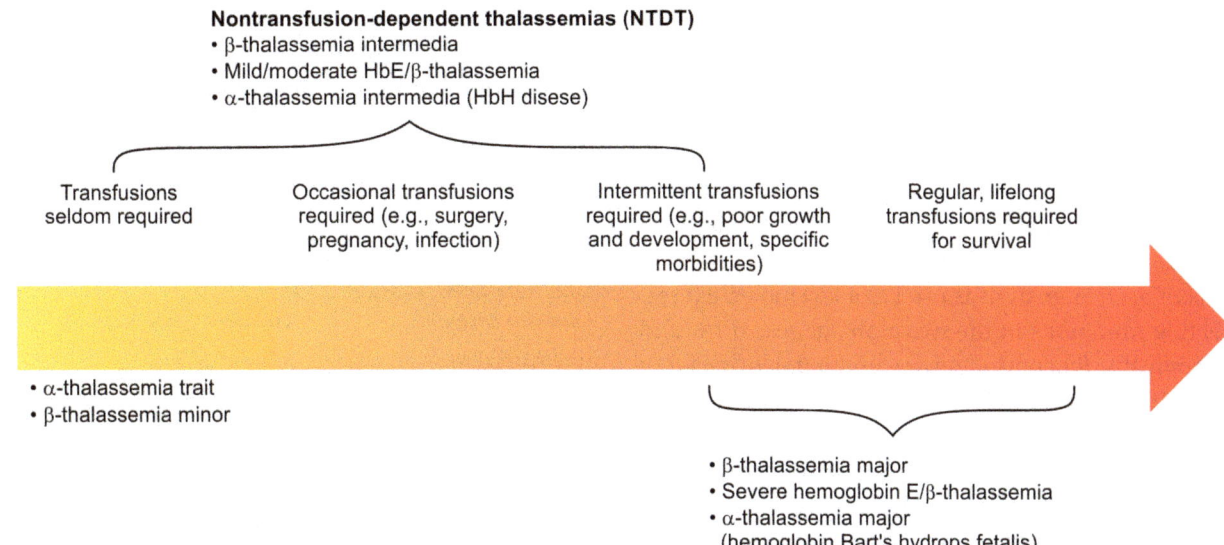

Fig. 2: Tranfusion need in different thalassaemia group.
(HbE: hemoglobin E; HbH: hemoglobin H)
(*Source*: Musallam KM, Rivella S, Vichinsky E, Rachmilewitz EA. Non-transfusion-dependent thalassemias. Haemotologica. 2013;98(6):833-44)

of TI, patients are usually diagnosed between the ages of 2 and 6 years and, although they survive without regular blood transfusions, growth and development are impaired. At the other end of the spectrum, there are patients who are completely asymptomatic until adulthood, when they present with mild anemia and splenomegaly often found by chance during hematological examinations or family studies.

Beta-TM or Cooley's anemia (β^0/β^0 or β^0/β^+) is characterized by severe hypochromic microcytic anemia, which becomes symptomatic at infancy or early childhood. TM (homozygous β-thalassemia) results from the inheritance of a defective β-globin gene from each parent. This results in a severe transfusion-dependent anemia, requiring regular red blood cell (RBC) transfusions for survival. The globin chain-synthesis reduction leads to an unbalanced β/α-globin chain production, where the chains in abundance precipitate, forming erythrocyte inclusions. These cells are destroyed in the bone marrow, giving rise to ineffective erythropoiesis, which is a prominent feature of the disease. This erythropoiesis causes skeletal deformities and bony fractures, megaloblastic anemia due to folate deficiency, and hyperuricemia with gout. Enlarged maxillary sinuses, a maxillary overbite, and "mongoloid" appearance of the face are commonly observed in thalassemic patients.

Peripheral blood smear will show the characteristic features of polychromatic RBCs, microcytosis, poikilocytosis and anisocytosis, basophilic stippling (punctate basophilia), nucleated RBCs (normal, mature RBCs are enucleated), and irregular distribution of Hb (resulting in "target cells" which appear like a bull's eye under the microscope).

Pathophysiology of TM is characterized by damaged RBCs, hemolysis, and erythroid-precursor release in the peripheral circulation, due to ineffective erythropoiesis. The phenotype includes anemia, bone marrow expansion, skeletal deformities, growth restriction, and late sexual maturity. The main clinical features in these patients are hypertrophy of erythroid marrow with medullary and extramedullary hematopoiesis and its complications (osteoporosis, masses of erythropoietic tissue that primarily affect the spleen, liver, lymph nodes, chest and spine, and bone deformities and typical facial changes), gallstones, painful leg ulcers, and an increased predisposition to thrombosis. Advances in care by optimal blood transfusion and iron-chelation therapy have improved patient survival into adulthood, as well as quality of life in recent years. Consequently, concern about favorable reproductive outcome has increased.

DIAGNOSIS OF THALASSEMIA

Hematological Indices

Screening for thalassemia is done by examining the hematological indices and measurement of HbA_2 levels. Thalassemia traits are associated with a reduced mean corpuscular volume (MCV), reduced mean corpuscular hemoglobin (MCH), and a normal to near-normal mean corpuscular hemoglobin concentration (MCHC); low, normal, or slightly subnormal hemoglobin levels. Of all these markers the most accurate is MCH. Additionally, β-thalassemia is associated with elevated HbA_2 levels (>3.5 g%). Deoxyribonucleic acid (DNA) analysis is required to confirm the diagnosis.

Iron Profile Analysis

Various parameters of the iron storage and usage by the body are measured which include serum iron, ferritin, unsaturated iron-binding capacity, total iron-binding capacity (TIBC), and percent saturation of transferrin. Indistinguishable β-thalassemia minor can be well-differentiated from iron deficiency or lead poisoning by using erythrocyte porphyrin tests.

Normal porphyrin levels are observed in case of β-thalassemic patients, while elevated porphyrin levels have been noted in patients suffering from iron-deficiency anemia.

Deoxyribonucleic Acid Analysis

Deoxyribonucleic acid (DNA) analysis is essential after presumptive diagnosis of hemoglobinopathies for defining the mutation or deletion, to determine silent carrier. In α-thalassemia, DNA analysis is used as a key molecular test for detecting mutations in the two alpha genes, HBA_1 and HBA_2, responsible for controlling the production of α-globin chain. In β-thalassemia, analysis or sequencing of Hb β-gene, *HBB*, is done to check the presence of thalassemia-causing mutations. Greater than 250 mutations have been associated with β-thalassemia, presence of any of these mutations in the test will validate the diagnosis of β-thalassemia.

For confirmation, DNA extracted from white blood cells is used in prepregnancy state while amniocytes, or chorionic tissue may be utilized for prenatal diagnosis.

Differentiation of Thalassemia from Iron-deficiency Anemia

Early detection should be part of good medical practice. Diagnosis of thalassemia during pregnancy is difficult as iron deficiency also causes microcytosis, low MCV ≤72 fL is maximally sensitive and specific for presumptive diagnosis of thalassemia, often is the first or only clue. Exclusion of iron deficiency is done by measuring serum iron, TIBC and ferritin, and Hb-electrophoresis in suspicious cases.

Red blood cell count is a useful diagnostic adjunct. Thalassemias produce a microcytic anemia with an associated increase in the RBC number. Iron deficiency and anemia of chronic disease are typically associated with a decrease in the RBC number that is proportional to the degree of decrease in Hb concentration.

Red cell distribution width (RDW) is a measure of the degree of variation in RBC size. Iron deficiency is characterized by an increase in RDW. Thalassemias, in contrast, tend to produce a uniform microcytic red cell population without a concomitant increase in RDW **(Table 2)**.

Iron Study

Iron study is given in **Table 3**.

TABLE 3: Iron study in beta-thalassaemia and Iron deficiency anemia.

Beta-thalassemia	Iron-deficiency anemia
Serum iron level increased	Serum iron-low
Serum ferritin increased	Serum ferritin <12 ng/mL
Transferrin saturation >50%	Transferrin saturation <10%
TIBC—normal	TIBC—increased
Marrow iron store increased	Marrow iron store—very low

(TIBC: total iron-binding capacity)

Fertility in Thalassemia

Hypogonadotropic hypogonadism (HH) is the most frequent endocrinopathy in transfused patients with TM. Almost 51–66% of thalassemic patients with marked hemosiderosis are predisposed to develop pubertal failure, sexual dysfunction, infertility, and short stature. Iron accumulation in the anterior pituitary gland, with high levels of transferrin receptor, results in free radical oxidative stress, impairing gonadotropins, and growth-hormone secretion. TM patients may suffer from iron accumulation in the ovaries or testes, with development of oxidative stress. Infertility results from imbalance between generation of reactive oxygen species (ROS) and the scavenging capacity of antioxidants in the reproductive tract. Furthermore, HH may be related to iron toxicity in adipose tissue, impairing and changing the physiological role of leptin, whose function is acting as a permissive signal allowing puberty—sexual maturation and fertility. Fertility is reduced in transfusion–dependent individuals where suboptimal chelation with iron overload has resulted in damage to the anterior pituitary.

Screening and Genetic Counseling

Identifying high-risk populations for thalassemia is the main step for reducing the incidence. Screening programs differ throughout the world, depending on population needs, culture, and/or ethics, and although antenatal diagnosis remains a personal choice, policies are focused on education and counseling. In Greece, where carriers account for 7.5% of the general population, raising awareness and drawing attention to this inherited disease program has been in place since the 1970s. In Cyprus, prenatal screening and selective termination, has reduced disease from 1 in 158 to almost 0. In Iran, premarital screening is done, where man's red cell indices done. If he has microcytosis (MCH <27 pg,

TABLE 2: Blood parameter of thalassemia trait and iron-deficiency anemia.

Parameter	Beta-thalassemia trait	Iron-deficiency anemia
Hb (g/L)	N/↓	↓
RBC count (× 10^{12}/L)	↑↑	↓
MCV (fL) (<80)	↓	↓
MCH (pg) (<27)	↓	↓↓
MCHC (%)	N	↓
RDW (CV%)	N	↑↑
Hb-electrophoresis	HbA$_2$ and HbF ↑	N

Note: Red cell indices should be interpreted with caution during pregnancy as β-thalassemia may present with concomitant iron-deficiency anemia or a αα/α⁻ thalassemia.
(Hb: hemoglobin; MCH: mean corpuscular hemoglobin; MCHC: mean corpuscular hemoglobin concentration; MCV: mean corpuscular volume; RBC: red blood cell; RDW: red cell distribution width)

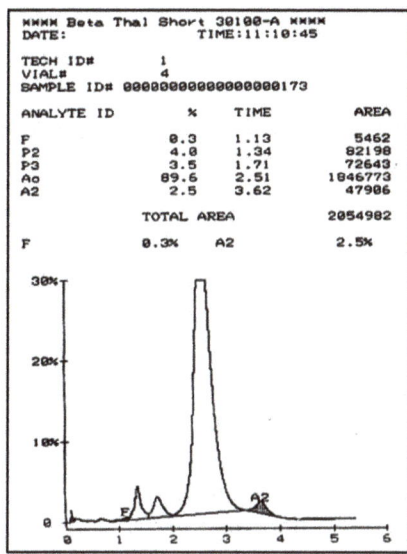

Fig. 3: Electrophoresis in normal individual, HbA$_2$ is 2.5%.

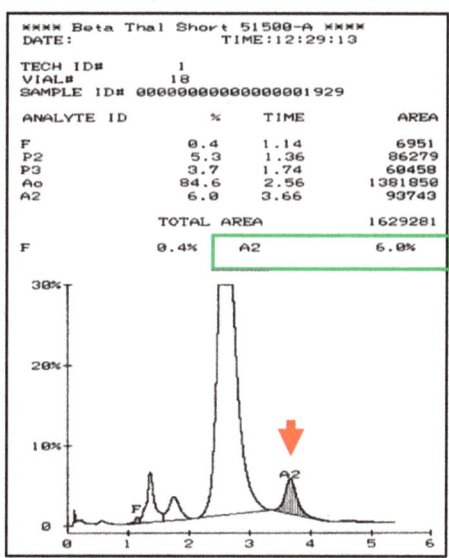

Fig. 4: Beta thalassaemia trait.

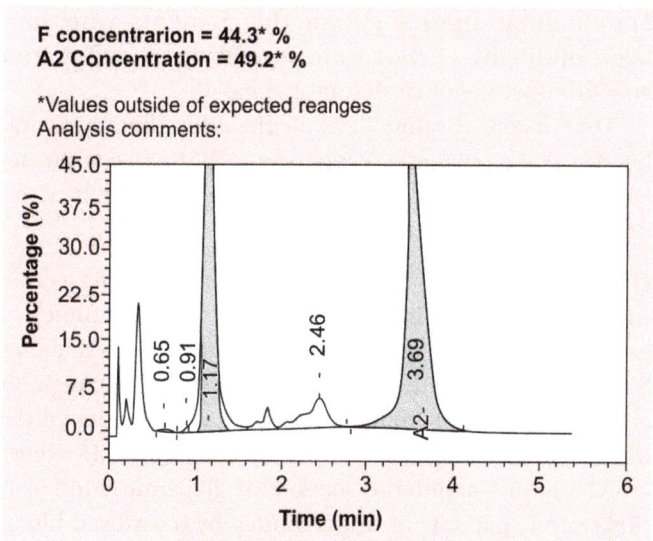

Fig. 5: Beta-thalassaemia major.

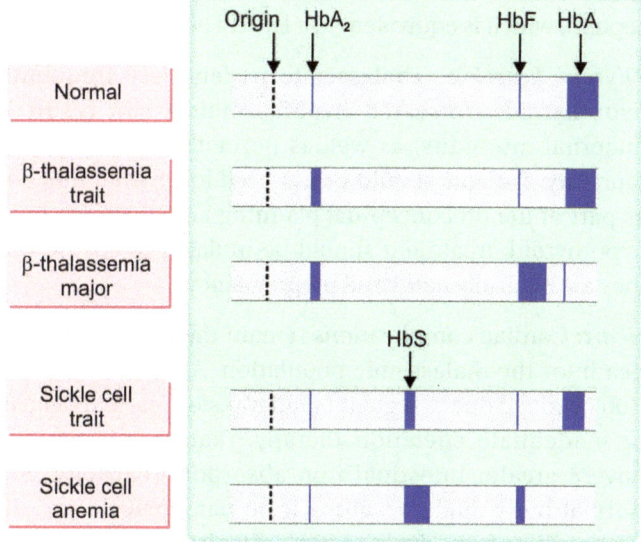

Fig. 6: Capillary eletrophoresis detect HbA, A2, HbF and HbS (HbF: hemoglobin F)

MCV <80 fL), expected wife is tested. If both have microcytosis—HbA$_2$ is measured. If both are thalassemia trait—genetic counseling done.

Hemoglobin electrophoresis remains the gold standard for the diagnosis and classification of thalassemia. Quantitative evaluation of HbA$_2$ can be made by either electrophoresis or by high-pressure liquid chromatography. The latter has the additional advantage of quantifying HbF at the same time. Carriers of the β-thalassemia trait demonstrate increased values of HbA$_2$ and HbF **(Fig. 4)**.

PREVENTION (PRENATAL DIAGNOSIS)

Fetal DNA analysis: Fetal DNA is obtained at 11–12 weeks of gestation by chorionic villus sampling (CVS) or amniocentesis (after 16 weeks). When both parents are carriers of the same trait (α–α or β–β couple), genetic counseling should be performed to achieve prenatal diagnosis. The couple should be informed of the possibility (25%) of a TM fetus and offer prenatal diagnosis. When both parents suffer from a certain hemoglobinopathy, donor gametes screened for hemoglobinopathies may be used.

PRECONCEPTUAL CARE

Thalassemia is associated with an increased risk to both mother and baby. In particular, there are issues surrounding cardiomyopathy in the mother due to iron overload and the increased risk of fetal growth restriction (FGR). Additionally, with around 9 months of little or no chelation, women with TM may develop new endocrinopathies: diabetes mellitus, hypothyroidism, and hypoparathyroidism. Aggressive chelation in the preconception stage can reduce and optimize body iron burden and reduce end-organ damage.

Longitudinal studies shown that patients who have been optimally chelated are less likely to suffer from endocrinopathies or cardiac problems.

Due to lack of safety data, all chelation therapy should be regarded as potentially teratogenic in the first trimester. Desferrioxamine (DFO) is the only chelating agent with a body of evidence for use.

Diabetes mellitus is common in adults with thalassemia. Insulin resistance, iron-induced islet cell insufficiency, genetic factors, and autoimmunity all may lead to diabetes. Similar to women without thalassemia, glycated hemoglobin (HbA1c) <43 mmoL/moL is associated with a reduced risk of congenital abnormalities during pregnancy. However, HbA1c is not a reliable marker of glycemic control in thalassemic patients as this is diluted by transfused blood, may result in underestimation. Serum fructosamine is preferred for monitoring glycemic control, concentrations should be <300 nmoL/L for at least 3 months prior to conception, which is equivalent to a HbA1c of 43 mmoL/moL.

Thyroid function: Thalassemic patients are frequently hypothyroid. Untreated hypothyroidism can result in maternal morbidity, as well as perinatal morbidity, and mortality. Patients should be assessed for thyroid function as part of the preconceptual planning and, if known to be hypothyroid, treatment should be initiated to ensure that they are clinically euthyroid prepregnancy.

Heart: Cardiac complications remain the leading cause of death for the thalassemic population. Apart from cardiac iron overload due to regular blood transfusions and delayed or inadequate chelation therapy, thalassemic patients have a greater intestinal iron-absorption capacity than normal individuals, resulting from paradoxical hepcidin suppression from dyserythropoiesis. Iron stored in cells, including myocytes, in the form of ferritin, hemosiderin, and free iron, is referred as labile cellular iron. The latter form stimulates the formation of free radicals, provoking cellular injury due to peroxidation damage of membrane lipids and proteins. In thalassemic women, iron overload increases the oxidative stress of pregnancy, which peaks by the second trimester of gestation, and can induce great damage to the fetus.

Thalassemic pregnant women with normal resting cardiac performance and intensive pregestational chelation therapy usually carry out gestation and delivery successfully. Cardiac magnetic resonance imaging (MRI) has been proven of high value with regard to preconception cardiac management, can accurately define iron overload. The target is T_2^* ≥20 ms; however, successful pregnancies have been achieved with lower T_2^* levels ≤10 ms, though this level suggests a high risk of developing heart failure. All women should be assessed by a cardiologist with expertise in managing thalassemia and/or iron overload prior to embarking on a pregnancy. It is important to determine the cardiac status, as well as the severity of any iron-related cardiomyopathy. Cardiac arrhythmias are more likely in older patients who have previously had severe myocardial iron overload and are now clear of cardiac iron.

Liver: Women should be assessed for liver iron concentration using a FerriScan® or liver T2*. Ideally, the liver iron should be <7 mg/g [dry weight (dw)]. If liver iron exceeds the target range, a period of intensive preconception chelation is required to optimize liver iron burden. If liver iron exceeds 15 mg/g (dw) prior to conception, the risk of myocardial iron loading increases, so iron chelation with low-dose DFO should be commenced between 20 and 28 weeks under guidance from the hemoglobinopathy team.

Liver and gallbladder (and spleen if present) ultrasound should be used to detect cholelithiasis and evidence of liver cirrhosis due to risk of iron overload or transfusion-related viral hepatitis.

Bone density scan: Most women with thalassemia syndromes are vitamin D deficient and often osteoporotic as well. The pathology is complex, but thought to be due to a variety of factors including underlying thalassemic bone disease, chelation of calcium by chelation drugs, hypogonadism, and vitamin D deficiency. All women should be offered a bone density scan to document pre-existing osteoporosis. Serum vitamin D concentrations should be optimized before pregnancy with supplements if necessary and maintained in the normal range.

Infection: Iron overload is considered to be the main etiologic factor that disturb the immune balance. Apart from this, transfusion-transmitted viral infections can be a great risk. All women with thalassemia should be tested for hepatitis B virus (HBV), HCV, HIV, cytomegalovirus, and human parvovirus B19. The majority of women with TM are immunized against hepatitis B, if already not vaccinated should be vaccinated against hepatitis B. Hepatitis C is a common and often asymptomatic virus, so all women who are transfused require hepatitis C antibody testing. If she has a positive hepatitis C test, RNA titer should be determined with referral to a hepatologist.

Splenectomized women should take penicillin prophylaxis and should be vaccinated for pneumococcus and *Haemophilus influenzae* type b if this has not been done before. HIV-positive women should be advised to commence highly active antiretroviral therapy, deliver by cesarean section (CS), and avoid breast-feeding, whereas HCV-positive women should start appropriate therapy so as to eliminate HCV ribonucleic acid (RNA).

Medication Review

Before contemplating pregnancy potentially teratogenic medication needs to be reviewed, including oral

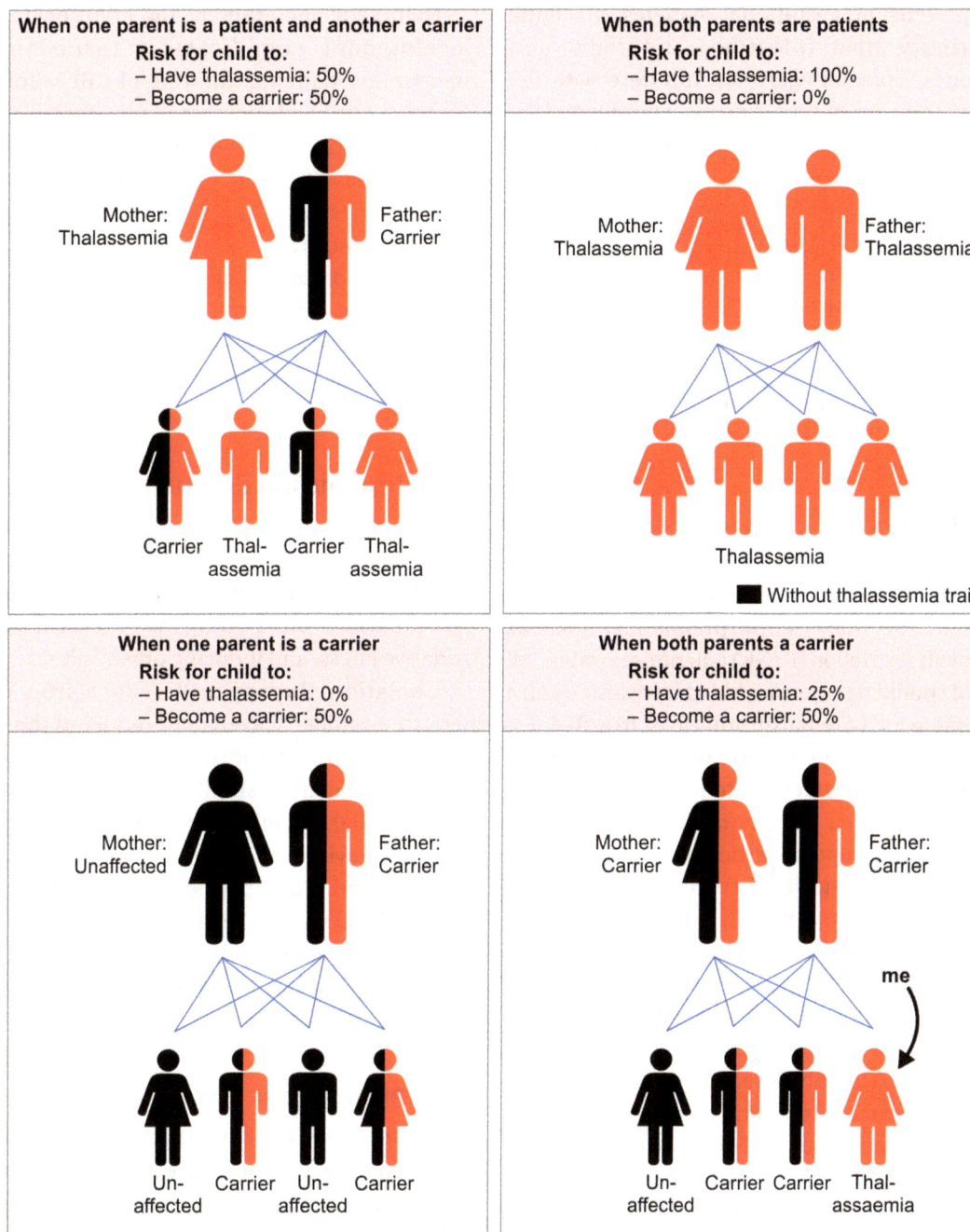

Fig. 7: How thalassaemia is inherited?
Source: blogspot.com. Interesting facts about Thalassemia Carriers. Dr Sharon Lim by Dr Khoo Yoong Khean, November 10, 2014.

hypoglycemic agents, bisphosphonates, and angiotensin-converting enzyme (ACE) inhibitors. Women on oral chelators [deferasirox (DFX) or deferiprone] are recommended to switch to DFO prior to induction of ovulation/spermatogenesis. Medications that should be discontinued at least 6 months prior to fertility treatment include interferon, ribavirin, and hydroxyurea. Hypothyroid patients receiving thyroid-replacement therapy should receive increased doses to ensure they are euthyroid. Folate demand in pregnancy is normally increased, and all thalassemic women are advised to receive folic acid supplementation at a dose of 5 mg/day, in order to prevent fetal neural tube defects, as well as a significant increase in predelivery hemoglobin level, and in heterozygous cases to prevent superimposed megaloblastic anemia.

Antepartum Management

Pregnant women must be reviewed monthly until the 28th gestational week and every 2 weeks thereafter. A multidisciplinary team should provide routine as well as specialist antenatal care. Preterm birth related to poor maternal condition, fetal distress, multiple-pregnancies, and placental ischemic disease can complicate pregnancy. Other commonly met obstetric complications include gestational hypertension, gestational diabetes, placental abruption, urinary tract infection, and renal and gallbladder stones. Splenomegaly can interfere with the enlargement of the uterus and can be complicated by hypersplenism, necessitating splenectomy during gestation or after delivery.

Women should be screened for diabetes at first prenatal visit, and if normal this should be repeated again at 28 weeks. Diabetic women should have monthly assessment of serum fructosamine concentrations and review in the specialist diabetic pregnancy clinic. All women with TM should undergo specialist cardiac assessment at 28 weeks of gestation and thereafter as appropriate. Thyroid function should be monitored during pregnancy in hypothyroid patients.

Maternal Transfusion

Thalassemia per se in combination with gestational anemia (secondary to hemodilution) accounts partly for different complications of the thalassemic pregnancy, such as intrauterine growth restriction (IUGR) and preterm labor. All women with TM should be receiving blood transfusions on a regular basis aiming for a pretransfusion Hb of 10 g/dL.

Thalassemia major patients already be established on transfusion regimens generally remain stable during pregnancy. In cases where lower pretransfusion thresholds have been used preconceptually, the aim is to achieve a pretransfusion Hb of >10 g/dL. If there is worsening of maternal anemia or evidence of FGR, regular transfusions should be started aiming for maintenance of pretransfusion Hb concentration above 10 g/dL. Initially, 2-3 units transfusion should be administered with additional top-up transfusion, if necessary, in the following week until the Hb reaches 12 g/dL. The Hb should be monitored after 2-3 weeks and a 2-unit transfusion administered if the Hb has fallen below 10 g/dL. Each woman's Hb falls at different rates after transfusion, so, close surveillance of pretransfusion Hb concentrations is required. Nontransfused women with Hb ≥8 g/dL at the 36th week of gestation should be advised not to initiate blood-transfusion, erythropoietin administration could be an alternative.

In pregnancy with TI, 60-80% of the patients need transfusions during pregnancy, although 30% of them have never had a transfusion before. Women with TI who have never previously received a blood transfusion or have received a minimal quantity of blood are at risk of severe alloimmune anemia, if transfusion is necessary, extended genotype and antibody screening should be performed and fully phenotyped matched blood given. The major fear of blood transfusions during pregnancy is the developing of alloantibodies, which can stimulate anemia aggravation and patient may develop severe hemolytic anemia along with viral transmissions.

Hemolytic alloantibody and erythrocyte-autoantibody development complicates transfusion therapy in thalassemia patients; the rate of RBC alloimmunization following one single unit blood transfusion is 1-1.6%, while the rate in patients receiving regular blood transfusions may be as high as 60%. Alloantibodies can cross the placenta and may cause fetal and/or neonatal hemolytic anemia. If fetal/neonatal transfusion is necessary, fully phenotyped matched blood should be given. Referral to a fetal medicine specialist for consideration of invasive treatment if the middle cerebral artery peak systolic velocity rises above 1.5-fold the median threshold or if there are other signs of fetal anemia.

Chelation during Pregnancy

Acceptable levels of maternal Hb should be maintained throughout pregnancy to minimize hypoxia. Intensive transfusion treatment can aggravate hemosiderosis in patients with a pre-existing iron-overload status, elevating oxidative stress, and inducing organ failure.

Chelation therapy will reduce iron overload and help free radical scavenging, reducing the inflammatory process. As DFO fetotoxicity has not yet been definitely assessed, chelation should be restricted for cases where the potential benefit outweighs the risk. Iron chelators should be reviewed and deferasirox and deferiprone ideally discontinued 3 months before conception. According to experts, DFO should be avoided during the first trimester, but subcutaneous administration may be considered in the second and third trimesters for patients with a strong indication for treatment.

Thromboembolic Risks

Thalassemic women have an increased risk for thrombosis, risk as high as 29% in splenectomized and nontransfused TI patients. Inherent red-cell defects activate endothelial cells, creating a procoagulant state, along with platelet abnormalities, deficiency of coagulation inhibitors, cardiac and liver dysfunction, and hormonal deficiencies, which seem to comprise the pathophysiology.

Thromboprophylaxis might be essential during pregnancy and the postpartum period in cases of nontransfused TI. According to recent data, low-dose aspirin, frequently administered to splenectomized β-thalassemia patients, seems to be effective in preventing pre-eclampsia, preterm birth, and IUGR without posing a major safety risk to mothers or fetuses. Splenectomized women or those with a serum platelet count above $600 \times 10^9/L$ should begin or continue taking aspirin at a dose of 75 mg/day, those with a platelet count above $600 \times 10^9/L$ should additionally be offered low-molecular-weight heparin.

Diet

Iron overload leading to oxidative damage is the center of all complications. Iron-rich foods, e.g., meat and nonmeat iron should be avoided. Antioxidants, e.g., vitamin C, E, vegetable oil, carotenoids (carrots, corn, tomato, and papaya), and flavonoids (tea) are encouraged. Iron chelators bind with zinc and excreted in urine. Zinc-rich foods, e.g., dairy products such as milk, cheese, yogurt, egg, and whole meal cereal are encouraged. Milk, a rich source of calcium-1 pint/day to prevent osteoporosis.

Fetal Assessment

Women should be offered an early scan at 7-9 weeks of gestation to determine viability as well as the presence of a multiple pregnancy. In addition to the routine first trimester scan (11-14 weeks of gestation) and a detailed anomaly scan at 18-20^{+6} weeks of gestation, women should be offered serial fetal biometry scans every 4 weeks from 24 weeks of gestation.

Intrapartum Care

Timing of delivery should be in line with national guidance. Senior midwifery, obstetric, anesthetic, and hematology staff should be informed as soon as the woman is admitted in the labor room.

In the presence of red cell antibodies, blood should be cross-matched for delivery since this may delay the availability of blood. Prolonged labor with acidosis may increase the risk of cardiac decompensation, low-dose intravenous DFO 2 g over 24 hours should be administered for the duration of labor. Continuous intrapartum electronic fetal monitoring should be instituted. Thalassemia in itself is not an indication for CS. Active management of the third-stage of labor is recommended to minimize blood loss.

There is a high risk of venous thromboembolism due to the presence of abnormal red cells in the circulation. Women should receive low-molecular-weight heparin prophylaxis while in hospital. In addition, low-molecular-weight heparin should be administered for 7 days postdischarge following vaginal delivery or for 6 weeks following CS. Breastfeeding is safe and should be encouraged.

Peripartum chelation therapy is recommended. Women with TM who plan to breastfeed should restart DFO as soon as the initial 24-hour infusion of intravenous DFO finishes after delivery. DFO is secreted in breast milk but is not orally absorbed and therefore not harmful to the newborn. There is minimal safety data on other iron chelators.

CONCLUSION

Healthy pregnancy outcomes have become the expectation in women with thalassemia and provided that a multidisciplinary team is available, gestation can be completely safe for both mother and child. Advances in chelation treatment along with regular transfusions have introduced a new era for the thalassemic population, increasing the average life span and rendering the perspective of reproductive capacity attainment and creation of a family.

Pregnancy in TM and TI should be considered high risk and should always be preceded by a complete preconception assessment. In patients with severe myocardial or liver iron overload, conception should be delayed until after a period of intensive chelation. During pregnancy, a close follow-up of maternal disorders, as well as that of fetus status, is recommended.

HEMOGLOBIN E DISEASE

Hemoglobin E (HbE) is the most common abnormal Hb in South East Asia, (Thailand, Myanmar, Cambodia, Laos, and Vietnam), Sri Lanka, Northeast India, and Bangladesh with a carrier frequency of >50% in some regions. HbE accounts for approximately 13–17% of the population of Thailand, especially in the Thai-Laos-Cambodian boundary or "Hb E triangle" where more than 32–60% of the people carry *HbE* gene. In Bangladesh, the estimated prevalence of β-thalassemia carriers is in the range of 3–6%, and HbE carrier is 3–4%.

Genetics: HbE is a β-hemoglobin variant, which results from a single nucleotide mutation of the β-globin gene, glutamic acid being substituted by lysin at position 26 (GAG-AAG)—a mutation that produces a structurally abnormal Hb as well as activates a cryptic splice site, resulting in abnormal messenger RNA (mRNA) processing. The level of normally spliced mRNA $β^E$, is reduced and, because a new stop codon is generated, the abnormally spliced mRNA is nonfunctional. Hence, HbE is synthesized at a reduced rate, resulting in the clinical phenotype of a mild form of β-thalassemia (**Fig. 1**).

Hemoglobin E disease is inherited in an autosomal recessive manner and is caused by a mutation in the *HBB* gene. HbE disease results when the offspring inherits the gene for HbE from both parents (two abnormal alleles). Heterozygous AE occurs when the gene for HbE is inherited from one parent and the gene for HbA from the other. HbE can be detected on electrophoresis.

■ CLINICAL SYMPTOMS

Heterozygotes for *HbE* are clinically normal and manifest with 25–30% of HbE on electrophoresis and 75% HbA, and with only minimal changes in RBC indices. Homozygotes for HbE are clinically silent and may be only mildly anemic. On microscopic examination, the peripheral blood smear demonstrates microcytosis with 20–80% of target red cells, while Hb electrophoresis shows 85–95% of HbE and 5–10% of HbF. **Figure 2** shows Hb electrophoresis in Hb E trait.

■ TREATMENT

Treatment for HbE disease is typically not needed. Folic acid supplements may be prescribed to help to produce normal RBCs if mild anemia causes symptoms. Most people do not have any symptoms. People with HbE disease can be expected to lead a normal life.

1	2	3	4	5	6	7	8	9	10	11	12	13	14	15
Val	His	Leu	Thr	Pro	Glu	Glu	Lys	Ser	Ala	Val	Thr	Ala	Leu	Try
16	17	18	19	20	21	22	23	24	25	26	27	28	29	30
Gly	Lys	Val	Asp	Val	Asp	Glu	Val	Gly	Gly	Glu	Ala	Leu	Gly	Arg
1	2	3	4	5	6	7	8	9	10	11	12	13	14	15
Val	His	Leu	Thr	Pro	Glu	Glu	Lys	Ser	Ala	Val	Thr	Ala	Leu	Try
16	17	18	19	20	21	22	23	24	25	26	27	28	29	30
Gly	Lys	Val	Asp	Val	Asp	Glu	Val	Gly	Gly	Lys	Ala	Leu	Gly	Arg

Fig. 1: Genetics of HbE disease.
Source: Wikipedia, the free encyclopedia

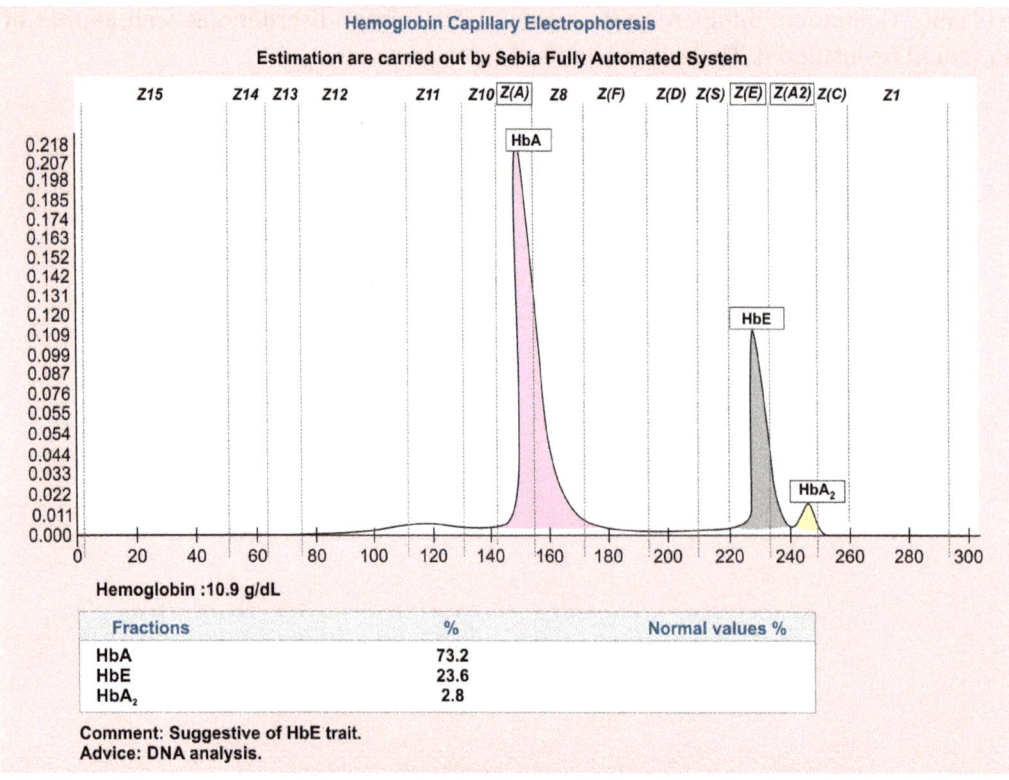

Fig. 2: Electrophoresis in Hemoglobin E trait.

HEMOGLOBIN E/BETA-THALASSEMIA

EPIDEMIOLOGY

Hemoglobin E/β-thalassemia constitutes the most common combination of β-thalassemia with a structural variant HbE. The highest frequencies are observed in India, Bangladesh, and throughout Southeast Asia, particularly in Thailand, Laos, and Cambodia owing to the high prevalence of both HbE and β-thalassemia genetic mutations. In Thailand about 3,000 affected children are born annually. HbE/β-thalassemia is also common in Indonesia and Sri Lanka, and while previously rarely diagnosed in North America or Europe, has recently become the most common form of β-thalassemia identified by many newborn screening program.

PATHOPHYSIOLOGY

Hemoglobin E/β-thalassemia results from coinheritance of a β-thalassemia allele from one parent and the structural variant HbE from the other. The βE mutation affects β-gene expression creating an alternate splicing site in the mRNA at codons 25–27 of the β-globin gene. Through this mechanism, there is a mild deficiency in normal β mRNA and production of small amounts of anomalous β mRNA. The reduced synthesis of β chain may cause features of β-thalassemia. Also, this Hb variant has a weak union between α- and β-globin, resulting in globin chain imbalance.

The pathophysiology of HbE/β-thalassemia reflects both the reduced output of HbE together with the added globin-chain imbalance consequent on the coinheritance of β-thalassemia. There is ineffective erythropoiesis, apoptosis, oxidative damage, and shortened red cell survival. It appears that the recognized instability of HbE is a minor factor in the overall pathophysiology of HbE/β-thalassemia, except during intercurrent febrile illnesses during which such instability may result in accelerated hemolysis. Like other forms of severe β-thalassemia, there is marked expansion of the erythroid bone marrow with ineffective erythropoiesis. Using a combination of electron-microscopic and immunocytochemical studies, Wickramasinghe and Lee (1997) demonstrated that the erythroblast inclusions in the bone marrow of patients with this condition consist entirely of precipitated α chains; there is no evidence of coprecipitation of $β^E$ chains. Therefore, the mechanisms of damage to red cells and their precursors are similar to those in other forms of β-thalassemia.

CLINICAL PRESENTATION

Hemoglobin HbE/β-thalassemia is a form of β-thalassemia that results in clinical presentation ranging from those characterizing TI to severe transfusion-dependent TM, requiring transfusions from infancy. At birth, infants with severe HbE/β-thalassemia are asymptomatic because HbF levels are high. As HbF production decreases and is replaced by HbE at 6–12 months of age, anemia with splenomegaly develops. Signs of impaired growth appear during the first decade of life. The initial complaints vary from patient to patient, most common are the development of pallor. With time and without transfusions, anemia, jaundice, hepatosplenomegaly, growth retardation, and thalassemic facies evolve. Absence of secondary sexual development is common and chronic leg ulcers are sometimes observed. These manifestations, secondary to decreased oxygen delivery to tissue, ineffective erythropoiesis, and iron overload, resemble those of β-TM. Mild and moderate HbE-β-thalassemias (a Hb concentration of 9–12 g/dL and 6–7 g/dL respectively) are classified and managed as nontransfusion-dependent thalassemia.

Patients with the milder forms of HbE/β-thalassemia tend to grow and develop reasonably well during early childhood and are fully active. There may be some delay in the pubertal growth spurt and in the appearance of secondary sexual characteristics but they usually attain a reasonable height and sexual maturation.

LABORATORY FINDINGS

The red-cell indices and morphological changes are similar to those described in other forms of severe β thalassemia. Compound heterozygotes for HbE and $β^+$ thalassemia usually have a milder disorder and produce variable amounts of HbA, with the mildest phenotype resulting from mild $β^+$ type mutations such as –28 (A → G) and codon 19 (G → A), although some patients with severe $β^+$ type mutations such as IVS I-5 (G → C) and IVS II 654 (C → T) can produce symptoms as severe as HbE/$β^0$-thalassemia. In the severest form individual usually have about 50–70% HbF, the remainder being HbE. Severe HbE-β-thalassemia manifests a Hb concentration ranging from 4 to 5 g/dL, extensive erythropoiesis found in the liver, spleen, bone marrow, and in extramedullary sites.

MANAGEMENT

A number of factors, both genetic and environmental, appear to modify the severity of HbE/β-thalassemia. The remarkable variation, and the instability of the clinical phenotype of HbE/β-thalassemia suggests that there may be changes in adaptation to anemia and, possibly, attenuation of the erythropoietin response over time. Therefore, careful tailoring of treatment is required for each patient, and that therapeutic approaches should be reassessed over-time, periodic reassessment for the need for transfusion therapy is recommended.

It is generally appreciated that no patient with HbE/β-thalassemia should be placed on a regimen of regular transfusions without an extended period of monitoring (at least 3–6 months without intercurrent illness) in which growth, pubertal development if applicable, quality of life,

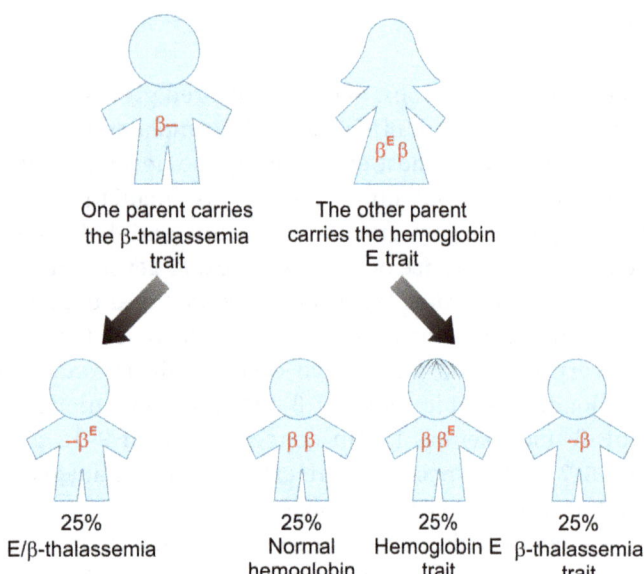

Fig. 1: Inheritance of HbE/β-thalassemia.
Source: Wikipedia

and symptoms and signs of anemia including changes in spleen size, are monitored. Intermittent transfusion therapy may now be explored as an approach in this disorder.

■ SUGGESTED READING

1. David R, Reed EP. Hemoglobinopathies and Thalassemias. Emery and Rimoin's Principles and Practice of Medical Genetics. Netherlands: Elsevier Science & Technology; 2013.
2. Fucharoen S, Weatherall DJ. The Hemoglobin E thalassemias. Cold Spring Harb Perspect Med. 2012;2(8):a011734.
3. Hoffbrand AV, Moss PAH. Hoffbrand's Essential Haematology, 7th Edition. Hoboken, NJ: John Wiley & Sons; 2016.
4. Keohane EM, Otto C, Walenga J. Rodak's Hematology: clinical principles and applications, 6th edition. St Louis, Missouri: Elsevier; 2020.
5. NIH. Hemoglobin E disease. [online] Available from https://rarediseases.info.nih.gov/diseases/2641/hemoglobin-e-disease. [Last accessed April, 2022].
6. Old JM. Screening and genetic diagnosis of haemoglobin disorders. Blood Rev. 2003;17(1):43-53.
7. Olivieri NF, Pakbaz Z, Vichinsky E. Hb E/beta-thalassaemia: a common & clinically diverse disorder. Indian J Med Res. 2011;134(4):522-31.
8. Origa R, Comitini F. Pregnancy in Thalassemia. Mediterr J Hematol Infect Dis. 2019;11(1):e2019019.
9. Petrakos G, Andriopoulos P, Tsironi M. Pregnancy in women with thalassemia: challenges and solutions. Int J Womens Health. 2016;8:441-51.
10. RCOG. Management of Beta Thalassaemia in pregnancy, RCOG Green-top Guideline No 55, March 2014.
11. Ryan K, Bain BJ, Worthington D, James J, Plews D, Mason A, et al. Significant haemoglobinopathies: guidelines for screening and diagnosis. Br J Haematol. 2010;149(1):35-49.
12. Saxena R, Banerjee T, Aniyery RB. Thalassemia and its Management during Pregnancy. World J Anemia. 2017;1(1):5-17.
13. University of Rochester Medical Center. Hemoglobin E Trait. [online] Available from https://www.urmc.rochester.edu/encyclopedia/content.aspx?ContentTypeID=160&ContentID=12. [Last accessed April, 2022].
14. Vichinsky E. Hemoglobin E syndromes. Hematology Am Soc Hematol Educ Program. 2007;79-83.
15. Weatherall DJ. The definition and epidemiology of non-transfusion-dependent thalassemia. Blood Rev. 2012;26 (Suppl 1): S3-6.

CHAPTER 3

Hypertensive Disorders in Pregnancy

INTRODUCTION

Hypertensive disorders are the most common medical disorders encountered during pregnancy, complicates 8-10% of all pregnancies and is a leading cause of maternal and perinatal morbidity and mortality worldwide. With a heavier burden of global maternal and fetal mortality and morbidity, preeclampsia (PE) affects 5-7% of all pregnant women and is responsible for over 70,000 maternal deaths and 500,000 fetal deaths worldwide every year (Circulation Research, 2019). In the United States, the rate of PE has increased by 25% in last two decades and is a leading cause of maternal death, severe maternal morbidity, maternal intensive care admissions, cesarean section, and prematurity (March of Dimes, 2019). Maternal mortality from PE/eclampsia is highest in lower-middle income countries (LMICs). Because of lack of equivalent resources PE accounts for nearly 30% of all maternal deaths in LMIC, which is >200 times higher than the mortality specific rate of 0.03% in the United Kingdom (UK). In addition, for every maternal death there is 50-100 "near miss". In Latin America and the Caribbean, hypertensive disorders are responsible for almost 26% of maternal deaths, whereas in Africa and Asia they contribute to 9% of deaths.

Delivery can resolve most signs and symptoms; however, PE can persist after delivery and, in some cases, can develop de novo in the postpartum period. De novo or persistent postpartum PE has emerged as an important risk factor for peripartum morbidity in the United States. Hypertensive disorders of pregnancy particularly preterm PE is associated with substantial risk for cardiovascular disease (CVD) and cerebrovascular disease in the long-term. Alongside the risks to the fetus during pregnancy, there is also growing evidence that PE has long-term adverse effects on the offspring, particularly hypertension (HTN) and altered vascular function.

CLASSIFICATION AND DEFINITION OF HYPERTENSIVE DISORDERS IN PREGNANCY

The National High Blood Pressure Education Program Working Group on High Blood Pressure in Pregnancy and the International Society for the Study of Hypertension in Pregnancy (ISSHP) have classified hypertensive disorders into four categories: (1) chronic HTN, (2) gestational HTN, (3) PE-eclampsia, and (4) PE superimposed on chronic HTN.

DEFINITION OF HYPERTENTION IN PREGNANCY

Hypertension in pregnancy is defined as systolic blood pressure (SBP) ≥140 mm Hg and/or diastolic blood pressure (DBP) ≥90 mm Hg (Korotkoff 5). Severe HTN is defined as SBP ≥160 mm Hg or DBP ≥110 mm Hg. Severe HTN requiring urgent treatment is defined as a SBP ≥170 mm Hg with or without DBP ≥110 mm Hg. This represents a level of BP above which the risk of maternal morbidity and mortality is increased [Society of Obstetric Medicine of Australia and New Zealand (SOMANZ)].

Measurement of Blood Pressure in Pregnancy

To appropriately measure BP women should be seated, without crossed legs, with feet touching the floor, and the back completely resting on the chair; lying or supine or side position can underestimate the pressure value. Women must refrain from talking, reading, consulting the telephone or watching television. The arm should not be stretched and should be at heart level. If not, a pillow can be used. The first measurement must be taken after at least 5 minutes of sitting position at rest. An appropriately sized cuff should be used, length 1.5 times the circumference of arm. The cuff should not be placed over clothes and should be of the right size. The length should cover two-thirds of the distance between the shoulder and the elbow; the lower edge of the cuff should be 1-2 cm above the fold of the elbow. The width must be such that the inflatable part of the cuff should be around 80% of the woman's arm which will avoid overestimating the pressure if it is too tight (the error can be as much as 7-13 mm Hg for SBP and 5-10 mm Hg for DBP).

Blood pressure should be measured several times by the sphygmomanometer (the gold standard device remains the mercury sphygmomanometer), the first measurement must be discarded, and the average value of the two successive measurements should be considered. By automatic devices, the average of two successive measurements 1 minute apart must be considered. Kortkoff 5th sound is the silence as the cuff pressure falls below the diastolic pressure.

Measurement of Proteinuria

There are various methods for measuring proteinuria (on spot samples: urinary dipstick testing, heat coagulation test, and urinary protein/creatinine ratio), urinary albumin/creatinine ratio and 24-hour collection.

The two most reliable methods are: (1) 24-hour sample and (2) spot sample to measure the urinary protein/creatinine ratio. The 24-hour collection is the gold standard method (threshold 300 mg/24 hours) but it is time-consuming and cumbersome. When quantitative methods are not available or rapid decisions are required, a urine protein dipstick reading can be substituted. However, dipstick urinalysis has high false-positive and false-negative test results. A test result of 1+ proteinuria is false-positive in 71% of cases compared with the 300 mg cutoff on 24-hour urine collection, and even 3+ proteinuria test results may be false-positive in 7% of cases. Using the same 24-hour urine collection standard, the false-negative rate for dipstick urinalysis is 9%. If urinalysis is the only available means of assessing proteinuria, then overall accuracy is better using 2+ as the discriminant value [American College of Obstetricians and Gynecologists (ACOG)].

If using protein/creatinine ratio to quantify proteinuria, use 30 mg/mmoL as a threshold for significant proteinuria; if the result is 30 mg/mmoL or above but there is still uncertainty about the diagnosis of PE, consider retesting on a new sample, alongside clinical review. If using albumin/creatinine ratio as an alternative to protein/creatinine ratio, use 8 mg/mmoL as a diagnostic threshold; if the result is 8 mg/mmoL or above and there is still uncertainty about the diagnosis of PE, consider retesting on a new sample, alongside clinical review National Institute for Health and Clinical Excellence (NICE, 2019).

■ CHRONIC HYPERTENSION IN PREGNANCY

Chronic HTN is present in approximately 1% of woman in pregnancy and is defined either when SBP is ≥140 mm Hg and/or DBP ≥90 mm Hg before the 20th weeks of gestation or persisting 12th weeks postpartum. ACOG, Society of Obstetricians and Gynaecologists of Canada (SOGC), Royal College of Obstetricians and Gynaecologists (RCOG), and Society of Obstetric Medicine of Australia and New Zealand (SOMANZ), in line with ISSHP, describe chronic HTN as HTN detected before 20 weeks of gestation.

Etiology

May be primary (essential HTN) or secondary.

- *Primary (essential familial) HTN:* About 90–95% of cases of chronic HTN are primary, defined as high BP due to nonspecific lifestyle and genetic factors. Lifestyle factors that increase the risk include excess salt in the diet, excess body weight, smoking, and alcohol use.
- *Secondary HTN:* The remaining 5–10% of cases are categorized as secondary high BP. The underlying causes includes:
  - *Arterial abnormality:* Renovascular HTN, coarctation of aorta
  - *Adrenal disease:* Pheochromocytoma, Cushing syndrome, and primary aldosteronism
  - *Endocrine abnormalities:* Diabetes mellitus and thyrotoxicosis
  - *Renal:* Glomerulonephritis (acute and chronic), chronic renal insufficiency, polycystic kidney disease, and acute renal failure
  - *Connective-tissue disease:* Lupus erythematosus, scleroderma, and periarteritis nodosa
  - Birth control pills.

Maternal and Fetal Risks

Maternal Risks

Chronic HTN is associated with increased incidence of:
- Accelerated maternal HTN
- Abruptio placentae
- Superimposed PE.

Fetal Risks

- Fetal growth restriction (FGR)
- *Small for gestational age (SGA):* Incidence of SGA in mild chronic HTN is 8–15.5% and in severe HTN may be as high as 40%
- Increased perinatal mortality.

Prognosis

Stage 1 essential HTN without target organ damage has excellent prognosis. Although at increased risk for superimposed PE, many will experience a physiological lowering of BP during pregnancy and a reduced requirement for antihypertensive. Superimposed PE complicates 25% of pregnancies. Chronic HTN with superimposed PE is more likely to develop severe HTN requiring multiple antihypertensive medications.

Prepregnancy evaluation permits—determination of severity, hemodynamic characteristics, and evidence of secondary HTN or end-organ damage.

Laboratory Evaluation for Chronic Hypertension

Majority of women do not require extensive testing; tests are directed to help defining the extent of end-organ damage. ISSHP recommends that all women with chronic HTN

in pregnancy have the following tests performed at first diagnosis. This will provide a baseline reference should suspicion arise later in pregnancy of superimposed PE (which will complicate up to 25% of these pregnancies).
- A full blood count (hemoglobin and platelet count)
- Liver enzymes [aspartate aminotransferase (AST), alanine aminotransferase (ALT), and lactate dehydrogenase (LDH)] and function tests [international normalized ratio (INR), serum bilirubin, and serum albumin].
- Serum creatinine, electrolytes, and uric acid (serum uric acid is not a diagnostic criterion for PE, but elevated gestation-corrected uric acid levels are associated with worse maternal and fetal outcomes and should prompt a detailed assessment of fetal growth, even in women with gestational HTN. However, uric acid should not be used to determine the timing of delivery).
- Urinalysis and microscopy, as well as protein–creatinine ratio (PCr) or albumin-creatinine ratio.
- Renal ultrasound (USG) if serum creatinine or any of the urine testing is abnormal.
- Women with severe HTN or proteinuria should have antinuclear antibody (ANA) testing and serum compliment studies.
- Electrocardiogram or echocardiogram as appropriate.

Management of Chronic Hypertension

Prepregnancy advice: Preconception counseling include risks explanation and *advice on:*
- Weight management
- Exercise
- Healthy eating
- Lowering the amount of salt in their diet
- *Medication:* Women who take angiotensin converting enzyme (ACE) inhibitors or angiotensin receptor blockers (ARBs), should be counseled that there is an increased risk of congenital abnormalities if these drugs are taken during pregnancy and alternative treatment discussed.

Women taking ACE inhibitors or ARBs should stop these medications *preferably within 2 working days of notification of pregnancy* and alternative medications adviced. Atenolol should be discontinued after diagnosis of pregnancy. Women who take thiazide or thiazide-like diuretics, should be advised regarding an increased risk of congenital abnormalities if these drugs are taken during pregnancy.

Antihypertensive Treatment

Continue existing antihypertensive if safe in pregnancy, or switch to an alternative treatment, unless sustained SBP <110 mm Hg *or* sustained DBP <70 mm Hg *or* the woman has symptomatic HTN.

Antihypertensives: If sustained SBP 140 mm Hg or higher *or* sustained DBP of 90 mm Hg or higher, aim for a target BP of 135/85 mm Hg. Consider labetalol to treat HTN, consider nifedipine in whom labetalol not suitable, or methyldopa if both labetalol and nifedipine are not suitable.

The CHIPS trial (Control of Hypertension in Pregnancy Study) enrolled mostly chronic HTN women; targeting a DBP of 85 mm Hg, was associated with reduced likelihood of developing accelerated maternal HTN and no demonstrable adverse outcome for babies compared with targeting higher DBP. Perinatal mortality rises with DPBs above 90 mm Hg. Therefore, current evidence supports controlling BP to these levels.

Aspirin

Offer pregnant women with chronic HTN aspirin 75–150 mg once daily from 12 weeks till delivery.

Antenatal Visit

Weekly appointments if HTN is poorly controlled. Appointments every 2–4 weeks if HTN is controlled. Women with organ damage should be seen every 2–4 weeks in first two trimesters, then weekly *(NICE, 2020)*.

Fetal Surveillance

For women with underlying medical condition that affects fetal outcome or evidence of FGR or superimposed PE:
- Ultrasound for FGR and amniotic fluid volume (AFV) assessment is recommended. The timing and frequency based on clinical scenario, prior obstetric history, severity of HTN, and coexisting comorbidity.
- Umbilical arterial (UA) Doppler at 28, 32, and 36 weeks in conjunction with antenatal testing [nonstress test (NST), biophysical profile (BPP) or modified BPP] used to determine optimum timing for delivery.
- Cardiotocography (CTG) if clinically indicated.

Timing of Delivery

Do not offer planned early birth before 37 weeks if BP <160/110 mm Hg, with or without antihypertensive treatment, unless there are other medical indications. If BP <160/110 mm Hg after 37 weeks, with or without antihypertensive treatment, timing of birth and maternal and fetal indications for delivery discussed between patient and senior obstetrician. If planned early birth is necessary, offer a course of antenatal corticosteroids and magnesium sulfate if indicated.

Postnatal Investigation, Monitoring, and Treatment

After birth measure BP daily for the first 2 days and at least once between day 3 and 5, aim is to keep BP lower than 140/90 mm Hg. Continue antihypertensive treatment, if required. If she was on methyldopa, stop within 2 days after the birth and change to an alternative antihypertensive treatment. A medical review with specialist between 6 and 8 weeks after birth recommended.

Preeclampsia Superimposed on Chronic Hypertension

About 25% of women with chronic HTN will develop superimposed PE. The rate may be higher in women with underlying renal disease. The diagnosis is made when women with chronic essential HTN develops any of the maternal organ dysfunction consistent with PE.

Rise in BP per se is not sufficient enough to diagnose superimposed PE as such rises are difficult to distinguish from usual rise in BP after 20 weeks. Similarly, in women with proteinuric renal disease an increase in proteinuria is not sufficient per se to diagnose superimposed PE. FGR may also be a part of chronic HTN per se and cannot be used as a diagnostic criteria for superimposed PE. If women with chronic HTN are suspected of developing PE, offer placental growth factor (PlGF)-based testing to help to rule out PE between 20 weeks and up to 35 weeks of pregnancy.

■ GESTATIONAL HYPERTENSION

Gestational HTN (GH), occurs in above 3% of pregnancy, is defined as the *de novo* presence of HTN, with SBP of 140 mm Hg or more or a DBP of 90 mm Hg or more, or both, on two occasions at least 4 hours apart after 20 weeks of gestation in a woman with a previously normal BP and without the characteristics that define PE, BP returns to normal in the postpartum period. SOMANZ and SOGC take into consideration the absence of proteinuria and or fetal features of PE to define GH. GH is considered severe when the systolic level reaches 160 mm Hg or the diastolic level reaches 110 mm Hg, or both.

Outcomes in women with GH are usually good. Up to 50% of women with GH will eventually develop proteinuria or other end-organ dysfunction consistent with the diagnosis of PE and this progression is more likely when the HTN is diagnosed before 32 weeks of gestation. Women with GH who present with severe-range BPs should be managed with the same approach as for women with severe PE. GH and PE may be undistinguishable in terms of long-term cardiovascular risks, including chronic HTN.

Management of Gestational Hypertension

The aim of management is safety of mother and the fetus, to deliver a mature baby who will not require intensive or prolonged neonatal care.

Initial Evaluation for all Women
- Ask about the symptoms
- *Laboratory investigation:* All women should have:
  - Complete blood count (CBC) with platelet count
  - Serum creatinine, uric acid
  - *Liver enzymes:* Bilirubin, AST, ALT, and LDH.

Management of Pregnancy with Gestational Hypertension (NICE, 2020)

Management of pregnancy with gestational hypertension according to NICE, 2020 is shown in **Table 1**.

Consider labetalol to treat GH. Consider nifedipine for women in whom labetalol is not suitable, and methyldopa if labetalol or nifedipine is not suitable. Base the choice on side-effect profiles, risk (including fetal effects), and the woman's preferences.

TABLE 1: Management of pregnancy with gestational hypertension (NICE, 2020).

	Hypertension: BP of 140/90–159/109 mm Hg	*Severe hypertension: BP of 160/110 mm Hg or more*
Admission to hospital	Do not routinely admit to hospital	Admit, but if BP falls below 160/110 mm Hg then manage as for hypertension
Antihypertensive treatment	Treatment if BP remains above 140/90 mm Hg	Offer treatment to all women
Target blood pressure (BP) on antihypertensive treatment	Aim for BP of 135/85 mm Hg or less	Aim for BP of 135/85 mm Hg or less
Blood pressure measurement	Once or twice a week (depending on BP) until BP is ≤135/85 mm Hg	Every 15–30 minutes until BP is <160/110 mm Hg
Dipstick proteinuria testing	Once or twice a week (with BP measurement)	Daily while admitted
Blood tests	Measure full blood count, liver function and renal function at presentation and then weekly	Measure full blood count, liver function and renal function at presentation and then weekly
PlGF-based testing	Carry out PlGF-based testing on 1 occasion between 20 and 35 weeks if there is suspicion of preeclampsia	Carry out PlGF-based testing on 1 occasion between 20 and 35 weeks if there is suspicion of preeclampsia

(PlGF: placental growth factor)

Fetal Monitoring

Women with BP 140/90–159/109 mm Hg

Fetal heart auscultation at every antenatal appointment. Carry out USG for fetal growth at diagnosis and, if normal, repeat every 2–4 weeks. Doppler velocimetry at diagnosis and if normal repeat every 2–4 weeks, if clinically indicated. Carry out a CTG only if clinically indicated.

Women with Severe Gestational Hypertension: BP 160/110 mm Hg

Fetal heart auscultation at every antenatal appointment. Carry out USG assessment of the fetus at diagnosis and, if normal, repeat every 2 weeks, and AFV assessment at least once weekly, if clinically indicated. In addition, an antenatal test one-to-two times per week. Carry out a CTG at diagnosis and then only if clinically indicated.

Timing of Birth

Among women with GH expectant management up to $37^{0/7}$ weeks is recommended, during which frequent fetal and maternal evaluation is recommended. GH whose BP <160/110 mm Hg after 37 weeks, timing of birth, and maternal and fetal indications for birth should be agreed between patient and senior obstetrician. If planned early birth is necessary, a course of antenatal corticosteroids and magnesium sulfate offered (if indicated) (NICE, 2019).

Postnatal Investigation, Monitoring, and Treatment

Measure BP daily for first 2 days and at least once between day 3 and 5. Continue antihypertensive if required and reduce if BP falls below 130/80 mm Hg. In women on methyldopa, stop methyldopa within 2 days after delivery and change to an alternative treatment. In women who did not take antihypertensive treatment, start antihypertensive if their BP is 150/100 mm Hg or higher and conduct medical review after 2 weeks. Offer all women who had GH a medical review with specialist 6–8 weeks after the birth (NICE, 2019).

PREECLAMPSIA

Definition

The American College of Obstetrics and Gynecology (ACOG) defines PE as the presence of HTN and proteinuria occurring after 20 weeks of gestation in a previously normotensive patient. However, a significant proportion of women develop systemic manifestations of PE—such as low platelets or elevated liver enzymes—before the hallmark of proteinuria is detectable, resulting in delayed diagnoses. This has led to ACOG's HTN 2013 task force to revise the definition of PE to include the presence of severe features with or without proteinuria and to exclude degree of proteinuria as a criterion of severe features.

Classically, PE is defined as a new-onset HTN with SBP of 140 mm Hg or more or DBP of 90 mm Hg or more on two occasions at least 4 hours apart after 20 weeks of gestation in a previously normotensive woman, along with proteinuria 300 mg or more per 24 hours urine collection or protein/creatinine ratio of 0.3 mg/mg or more or dipstick reading of 2+ (used only if other quantitative methods not available).

In the absence of proteinuria, new-onset HTN with the new onset of any of the following features:

- Thrombocytopenia (platelet count <100,000 µL), disseminated intravascular coagulation (DIC) or hemolysis.
- Impaired liver function as indicated by abnormally elevated liver enzymes (twice the upper limit of normal concentration), severe persistent right upper quadrant, or epigastric pain not accounted for by alternative diagnosis.
- Renal insufficiency (serum creatinine concentration >1.1 mg/dL or a doubling of the serum creatinine concentration in the absence of other renal disease)
- Pulmonary edema
- Neurological complications such as eclampsia, altered mental status, blindness, stroke, clonus, persistent visual scotomata not accounted for by alternative diagnosis or new-onset headache unresponsive to acetaminophen.
- Uteroplacental dysfunction evidenced by FGR, abnormal UA Doppler waveform or stillbirth.

The American College of Obstetrics and Gynecology definition of PE takes into consideration the presence of proteinuria (>300 mg/day) or target organ damage but the criteria of platelet (PLT) count are <100,000/µL while *ISSHP* use a cut-off of 150,000/µL. *RCOG* considers PE the presence of HTN with proteinuria and eclampsia a convulsive condition associated with PE or hemolysis, elevated liver enzymes, and low PLT count syndrome.

Following the initial documentation of proteinuria and the establishment of the diagnosis of PE, additional quantifications of proteinuria are no longer necessary. Although the amount of proteinuria is expected to increase over time with expectant management, this change is not predictive of perinatal outcome and should not influence the management of PE.

Epidemiology

The complexities of defining PE affect the accuracy of determining its incidence, especially across different countries. A global estimate derived from data of nearly 39 million pregnancies suggests an incidence of PE 4.6% with wide regional differences. As estimated by World Health Organization (WHO) occurrence of PE is seven times higher in developing countries compared to developed countries.

The prevalence of PE ranges between 1.8 and 16.7% in developing countries. The reported incidence is as low as 0.4% in Vietnam; the condition is especially common in women indigenous to, or with ancestry from, sub-Saharan Africa. The incidence was 2.8% reported from a study in Israel, 5.8% reported from Scotland, 14.1% reported from Australia, and 5% reported from Seattle. The overall prevalence of PE was similar in Sweden and China, 2.9% and 2.3% respectively from a study among 555,446 Swedish pregnancies and 79,243 Chinese pregnancies. The incidence of eclampsia is lower but quite variable, ranging from 0.015% in Finland to an estimated 2.9% in some parts of Africa. Pregnancy-related HTN disorders comprise 2.9% of live births in Bangladesh. Eclampsia-related conditions are the second leading direct cause of obstetric deaths and lead to 24% of all maternal deaths in Bangladesh.

Risk Factors

Risk factors for the development of PE have been studied extensively. The NICE, 2019 guidelines classify a woman at high risk of PE as those with preexisting HTN, chronic kidney disease, insulin-dependent diabetics, women with previous early-onset PE, and autoimmune diseases [systemic lupus erythematosus (SLE), antiphospholipid syndrome (APS)]. Women are at *moderate risk* if they are nulliparous, ≥40 years of age, have a body mass index (BMI) ≥35 kg/m^2, a family history of PE, a multifetal pregnancy, or a pregnancy interval of >10 years. Women with one major risk factor or with ≥2 moderate risk factors are likely to develop PE (NICE, 2019).

Risk of PE is high in women with diabetes [risk ratio (RR): 3.56, 95% confidence interval (CI): 2.54-4.99], preexisting HTN (RR: 1.38, 95% CI: 1.01-1.87), women suffering from medical conditions such as APS (RR: 9.72, 95% CI: 4.34-21.75), and those with a family history of PE (RR: 2.90, 95% CI: 1.70-4.93). According to the WHO, among women who have had PE, about 20-40% of their daughters and 11-37% of their sisters also will get the disorder.

Preeclampsia is more common in primigravida women (~4%), and the greater the interpregnancy interval, the risk of PE increases. Prepregnancy obesity and age >40 years increases risk (RR: 2.47, 95% CI: 1.66-3.67 and RR: 1.96, 95% CI: 1.34-2.87) respectively, as does a previous history of PE (RR: 7.19, 95% CI: 5.85-8.83). With previous PE the risk of recurrence was found ~15% after one preeclamptic pregnancy and ~32% after two pregnancies in a cohort of nearly 800,000 pregnancies in Sweden, with some confounding effect from a longer interbirth interval. Women who become pregnant with donor eggs, embryo donation, or donor insemination are other risk factors. It appears that various paternal factors including changed paternity can increase the risk of a pregnancy being complicated by PE.

Symptoms of Preeclampsia

Preeclampsia is usually symptomless, making the syndrome hard to predict. Pregnant women are advised to consult immediately with healthcare professional if she experiences symptoms including:
- Persistent severe headache
- Problems with vision, such as blurring of vision or flushing before the eye
- Severe pain just below the ribs (epigastric or right upper quadrant)
- Persistent nausea and vomiting
- Sudden swelling of face, hands, or feet
- Shortness of breath.

Etiopathology of Preeclampsia

Preeclampsia is a disorder unique to pregnancy characterized by poor perfusion of many vital organs. It is described as a pregnancy-specific systemic disorder of unknown etiology and a potentially serious disease with symptoms related to a generalized vascular endothelial activation. The pathogenesis of PE is poorly understood but is believed to be multifactorial limiting therapeutic interventions. Placenta seems to be a crucial component in the pathophysiology of the disease. PE is a two-stage disorder, *primary stage* involves abnormal trophoblastic invasion resulting in uteroplacental malperfusion secondary to defective remodeling of the uterine spiral arteries, the *second stage* involves "maternal syndrome" (in late second and third trimesters) characterized by an excess of antiangiogenic factors associated with exaggerated endothelial cell activation and a generalized inflammatory response. Placental stress leads to dysfunction of maternal peripheral endothelial cells and the clinical syndrome of PE. Blood flow to maternal organs is reduced, physiological assessment indicates vasospasm, activation of the coagulation cascade, and reduced plasma volume before clinical disease (**Flowcharts 1 to 3**). The exact response to abnormal placentation is influenced by genetic, metabolic, and behavioral factors, resulting in biological variation of the disease.

Proposed mechanisms of PE include:
- Chronic uteroplacental ischemia
- Immune maladaptation
- Increased trophoblast apoptosis or necrosis
- An exaggerated maternal inflammatory response to deported trophoblasts
- *Imbalances of angiogenic and antiangiogenic factors*
- Genetic imprinting

It is possible that a combination of some of these purported mechanisms may be responsible.

Normal and abnormal placentation in pregnancy: Normal and abnormal placentations are shown in **Figure 1**.

Abnormal placentation, trophoblast invasion in PE: In normal pregnancy the uterine arteries are resilient and elastic. In preeclamptic pregnancy, there is increased uterine arterial resistance and higher sensitivity to vasoconstrictors leading to chronic placental ischemia and oxidative stress. The cytotrophoblasts fail to transform from the proliferative epithelial subtype to the invasive endothelial subtype in PE resulting in incomplete remodeling of the spiral artery. Inadequate spiral arteriolar remodeling leads to narrow maternal vessels, and relative placental ischemia. The narrow spiral arteries are prone to atherosis—characterized by the presence of lipid-laden macrophages within the lumen, fibrinoid necrosis of the arterial wall, and a mononuclear perivascular infiltrate, leading to further compromise in placental flow.

Oxidative stress: Inadequate trophoblast activity in the spiral arteries leads to poor placentation with reduced placental perfusion and thus chronic placental ischemia and oxidative stress. While low oxygen tension followed by maternal blood flow oxygenation results in normal placentation, intermittent

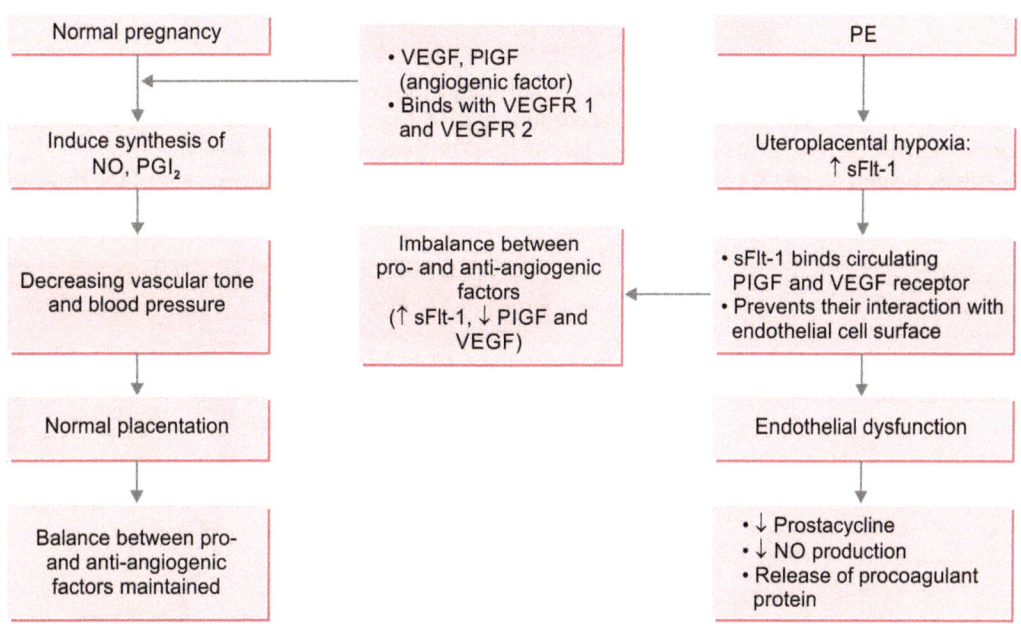

Flowchart 1: Pathophysiology—normal pregnancy and pre-eclampsia.

(NO: nitric oxide; PE: preeclampsia; PlGF: placental growth factor; sFlt-1: soluble fms-like tyrosine kinase 1; VEGF: vascular endothelial growth factor)

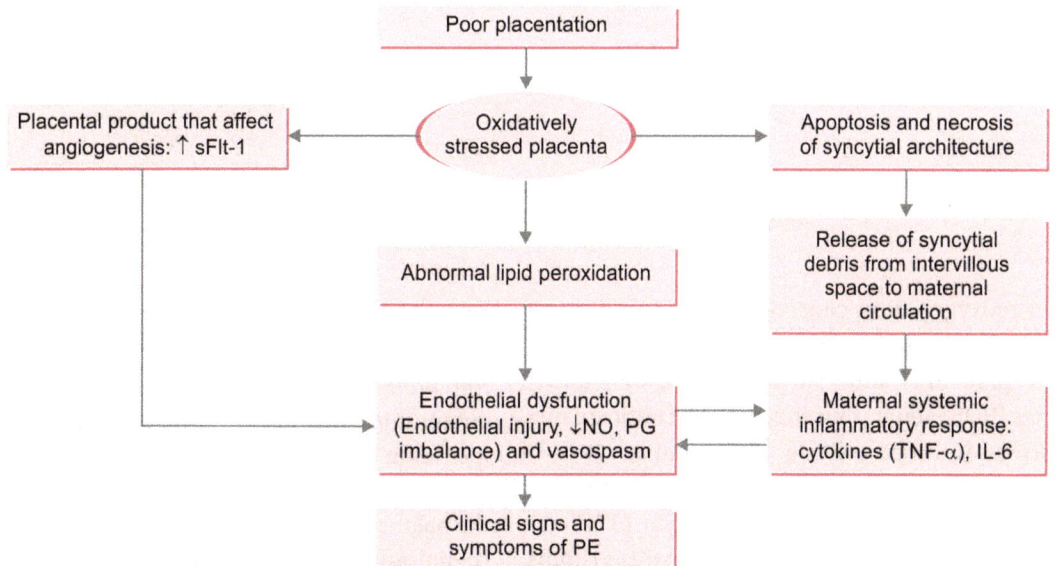

Flowchart 2: PE (2nd stage) from placental stress to maternal syndrome.

(IL-6: interleukin-6; PE: preeclampsia; NO: nitric oxide; PG: prostaglandins; sFlt-1: soluble fms-like tyrosine kinase 1; TNF-α: tumor necrosis factor-alpha)

Flowchart 3: Maternal syndrome in PE.

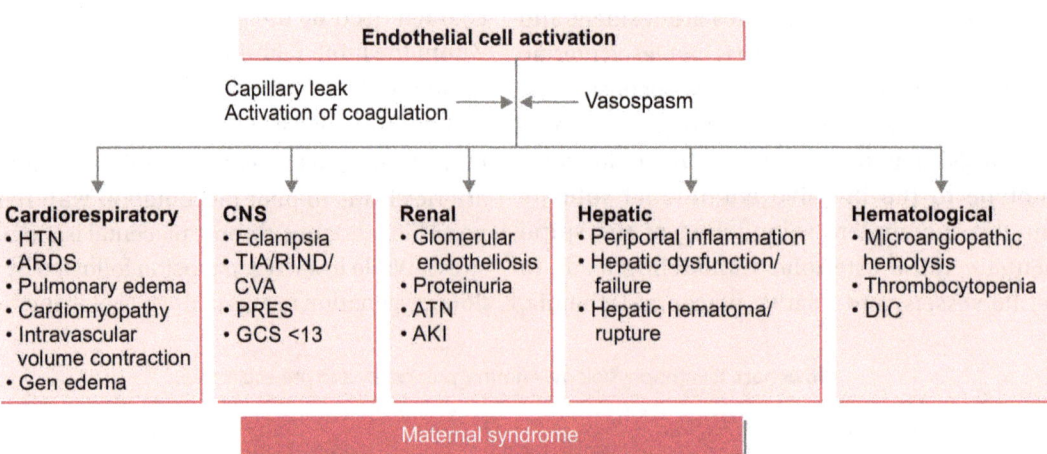

(AKI: acute kidney injury; ARDS: acute respiratory distress syndrome; ATN: acute tubular necrosis; CNS: central nervous system; CVA: cerebrovascular accident; DIC: disseminated intravascular coagulation; GCS: Glasgow coma scale; HTN: hypertension; PRES: postreversible encephalopathy syndrome; RIND: reversible ischemic neurological deficit; TIA: transient ischemic attack)
Source: Magee LA, Pels A, Helewa M, Rey E, von Dadelszen P. Diagnosis, evaluation, and management of the hypertensive disorders of pregnancy: executive summary. J Obstet Gynaecol Can. 2014;36(5):416-41.

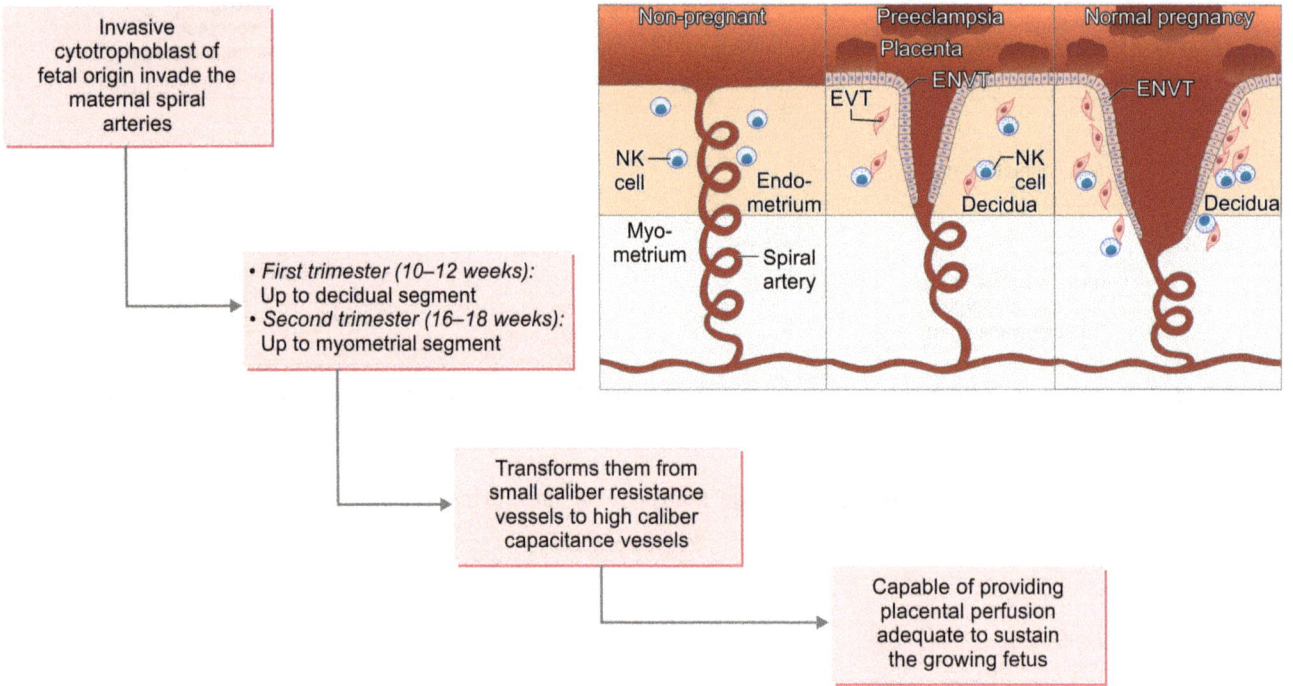

Fig. 1: Placentation in normal pregnancy and pre-eclampsia.
(ENVT: endovascular trophoblast; EVT: extravillous trophoblast)

hypoxia, and reoxygenation caused by poor spiral artery invasion may cause oxidative stress. At the molecular level, preeclamptic placentas show an imbalance of reactive oxygen species (ROS) generating enzymes and antioxidants. Oxidative stress induces release of a complex mix of substances into the maternal circulation. Proinflammatory cytokines [tumor necrosis factor-alpha (TNF-α), interleukin-6 (IL-6)], exosomes, free radicals, oxidized lipids, and cell-free fetal DNA. These disrupt maternal endothelial function resulting in a systemic inflammatory response, with vascular hyperpermeability, thrombophilia, and HTN, the clinical syndrome of PE **(Flowcharts 2 and 3)**.

Imbalance in circulating angiogenic factors: Several factors emanating from the placenta into the systemic circulation including the angiogenic as well as biochemical markers are considered to result in the maternal syndrome of PE. In PE, the balance between angiogenic factors [PlGF; vascular endothelial growth factor (VEGF)] and antiangiogenic factors [soluble fms-like tyrosine kinase 1 (sFlt-1), soluble endoglin (sEng)] are lost in favor of antiangiogenic factors **(Fig. 2)**.

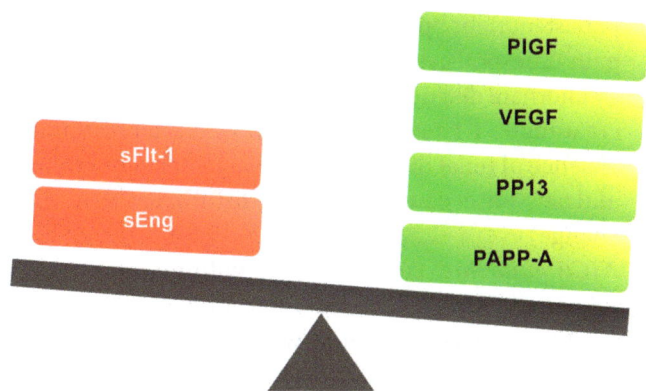

Fig. 2: Loss of balance of angiogenic and antiangiogenic factors in PE. (PAPP-A: pregnancy-associated plasma protein A; PE: preeclampsia; PlGF: placental growth factor; PP13: placental protein 13; sFlt-1: soluble fms-like tyrosine kinase 1; sEng: soluble endoglin; VEGF: vascular endothelial growth factor)

Vascular endothelial growth factor is important for the maintenance of endothelial cell function, especially in fenestrated endothelium, found in the brain, liver, and glomeruli, the primary organs affected by PE. PlGF, a member of the VEGF family whose main source is placental trophoblast, is important in angiogenesis.

Soluble Flt-1 is an antiangiogenic factor, binds the angiogenic factors VEGF and PlGF, preventing their interaction with endothelial receptors on the cell surface, and subsequently induces endothelial dysfunction. Elevated concentration of sFlt-1 has been seen as early as 5 weeks before the diagnosis of PE and abnormally high levels correlates with severity of disease. Another antiangiogenic protein that has also been extensively studied in PE is sEng, an endogenous transforming growth factor-β1 (TGF-$β_1$) inhibitor. sEng is elevated in the sera of preeclamptic women 2 months before the onset of clinical signs of PE, correlates with disease severity, and falls after delivery. It appears to potentiate the vascular effects of sFlt-1 to induce a severe PE-like state, including the development of thrombocytopenia and FGR and in combination with sFlt-1, appears to induce cerebral edema resembling the reversible posterior leukoencephalopathy seen in patients with eclampsia.

Increased trophoblast apoptosis or necrosis: It is well-established that PE is a proinflammatory state. Syncytial knots are allogenic nano to microvesicles, shed from apoptotic or activated trophoblasts that have been identified in the lungs and plasma of normal pregnancies, which is shed in increased amounts in PE. Rich in sFlt-1 and endoglin, syncytiotrophoblast microvesicles and exosomes may instigate an inflammatory response. Shedding of placental microparticles is greater in early-onset PE than in the late-onset form, while levels of exosomes in maternal serum are increased in early-onset but not in late-onset PE compared with age-matched controls.

Endothelial dysfunction: Diffuse endothelial dysfunction possibly secondary to impaired trophoblast invasion of spiral arteries is associated with alterations in maternal serum concentration of VEGF and PlGF and their receptors. The balance is important for effective vasculogenesis, angiogenesis, and placental development. There is mounting evidence that VEGF and TGF-β1 are required to maintain endothelial health in several tissues including the kidney and perhaps the placenta. During normal pregnancy, vascular homeostasis is maintained by physiological levels of VEGF and TGF-β1 signaling in the vasculature. In PE, excess placental secretion of sFlt-1 and sEng (two endogenous circulating antiangiogenic proteins) inhibits VEGF and TGF-β1 signaling, respectively in the vasculature. This results in endothelial cell dysfunction, including decreased prostacyclin and nitric oxide (NO) production, and release of procoagulant proteins.

Decidual vasculopathy (DV) is a lesion common to disorders of placental insufficiency, including intrauterine growth restriction and PE. Within PE phenotypes, the presence of DV is associated with worse clinical outcome, higher DBP, worse renal function, and perinatal fetal death. Histologically, normal third-trimester decidual vessels are characterized by flat endothelium and a loss of medial smooth muscle, while preeclamptic decidua shows signs of loose, edematous endothelium, hypertrophy of the vessel media, and loss of smooth muscle modifications (as seen in atherosclerosis), characterizing DV. There is significant evidence that decidual vessels demonstrate secondary atherosclerotic changes in PE.

Increased pressor response: In normal pregnancy, there is vascular refractoriness to angiotensin II, whereas in PE there is increased vascular reactivity to angiotensin II and norepinephrine. Several studies have shown enhanced angiotensin II sensitivity during and before the onset of PE despite reduced circulating renin and angiotensin II compared to normal pregnancy.

Nitric oxide and prostaglandin imbalance: Synthesis of NO (a potent vasodilator, produced by endothelium) is decreased in PE due to reduced endothelial NO synthesis expression. There is decreased PGI_2 and increased thromboxane A2 leading to increased sensitivity to vasopressor response.

Immune maladaptation: Pregnancy involves an interaction between maternal and fetal genes, which may explain the lack of success in finding genes associated with PE from studying maternal genomes alone. The uterine natural killer (uNK) may play a role in the abnormal placentation observed in PE. Unlike peripheral NKs, uNK is not cytotoxic, rather it regulates the depth of placentation, spiral artery remodeling, and trophoblastic invasion. uNK cells cluster around the spiral arteries, and it is presumed their activation causes the release of cytokines and proteases that stimulate the remodeling process, although evidence is still limited for how they function in normal and abnormal pregnancies.

As the main immunologic player interacting at the allogenic maternal-fetal cell interface, uNKs recognize self-major histocompatibility complexes (MHCs) derived from the maternal contribution and nonself-allogenic MHCs from the paternal genotype. uNK express KIR (killer cell Ig-like receptors), while fetal invasive extravillous trophoblasts (EVTs) express the main KIR ligand, polymorphic HLA-C (human leukocyte antigen-C) MHCs. KIR expressed by uNK cells bind to HLA-C molecules on EVT. Because of independent segregation of maternal KIR and HLA loci and the paternal contribution to EVT HLA-C, every pregnancy result in a unique combination of KIR (maternal) and HLA-C (fetal) which may affect the success of placentation.

Genetic factors: The hereditary predisposition to PE is the result of multiple genes inherited from both maternal and paternal sides. Fetal genes have a role in defective placentation and development of subsequent PE. Pregnant women who have a monozygotic twin show no concordance, pointing to the role of maternal–fetal gene interactions. That paternal genes are important is seen from the change of partner effect, and the increased risk with fathers born of an affected pregnancy or who previously fathered a preeclamptic pregnancy with another woman. The influence of the mother, dominates the variance of heritability is estimated as 35% maternal, 20% fetal, 13% to a couple effect, and the rest to other effects.

Classification of Preeclampsia

Preeclampsia may be classified as early onset, occurring before 34 weeks and late-onset appearing after 34 weeks. Early-onset PE arises owing to defective placentation, while late-onset PE center around interactions between normal senescence of the placenta and a maternal genetic predisposition to cardiovascular and metabolic disease.

Preeclampsia is classified as those without severe features and PE with severe features. *Progression* from PE without severe feature to that with severe feature may be slow or rapid andmay take hours to days to weeks. The finding of SBP ≥160 mm Hg or diastolic ≥110 mm Hg, HTN can be confirmed immediately within a short interval (may be within seconds) to facilitate timely antihypertensive therapy. *ACOG recommends elimination of the use of the term "mild PE".*

Criteria for Severe Preeclampsia

- *ACOG task force, 2019:* A woman with PE is defined to have severe PE if she shows any of the following features: SBP ≥160 mm Hg *or* DBP ≥110 mm Hg *on two occasions at least 4 hours* apart while she is in bed rest, thrombocytopenia (platelet count <100,000 mL), elevated liver transaminase to twice normal, severe persistent right upper quadrant (RUQ) pain or epigastric pain unresponsive to medication and not accounted for by alternate diagnosis, progressive renal disease—serum creatinine >1.1 mg/dL or doubling serum creatinine in absence of renal disease, pulmonary edema or cyanosis, and new-onset cerebral or visual disturbance (HA, vision change).
- *NICE guideline, 2019:* NICE guideline defines severe PE as—PE with severe HTN that does not respond to treatment or is associated with ongoing or recurring severe headaches, visual scotomata, nausea or vomiting, epigastric pain, oliguria and severe HTN, as well as progressive deterioration in laboratory blood tests such as rising creatinine or liver transaminases or falling platelet count below $100 \times 10^9/L$, or failure of fetal growth or abnormal Doppler findings, and hemolysis, elevated liver enzymes, and low platelets (HELLP) syndrome.

Prediction of Pre-eclampsia

Many clinical, ultrasonographic, and laboratory parameters have been explored during early pregnancy as tools for predicting who will later develop PE as well as to detect disease severity, e.g.:

- Uterine artery Doppler studies
- Measurement of angiogenic factors (such as sEng, PlGF, sFlt-1, and sFlt-1/PlGF ratio)
- Numerous other biochemical markers, such as pregnancy-associated plasma protein A, placental protein 13, homocysteine, asymmetrical dimethylarginine, uric acid and leptin, and urinary albumin, or calcium.

The ACOG committee opinion issued in 2015 and reaffirmed in 2017 does not recommend screening to predict PE beyond obtaining an appropriate medical history. The current guideline from the NICE recommends that, at the booking visit, a woman is identified to be preecplamptic if she has one major risk factor or more than one moderate risk factor for PE. Performance of current screening using history alone or from risk factors is poor and identifies only about 35% of PE. Extensive studies in the last decade have established that the best performance for early prediction of PE can be achieved by using a novel *"Bayes theorem-based method"* that combines maternal characteristics and medical history together with measurements of mean arterial pressure (MAP), uterine artery pulsatility index (UtA-PI), PlGF and pregnancy-associated plasma protein-A (PAPP-A) at 11–13 weeks' of gestation. This forms the "combined test", which could be simplified to the "mini-combined test" when only maternal factors, MAP, and PAPP-A are taken into consideration.

A 2017 head-to-head comparison of the *"Fetal Medicine Foundation algorithm"*-based screening method (a combination of maternal factors, MAP, UtA-PI, and PlGF) demonstrated superiority to the screening methods currently recommended by NICE and ACOG. The recently published *"Federation of Gynecology and Obstetrics (FIGO) initiative on PE"* suggests the use of a combination of biochemical (PlGF and PAPP-A), anamnestic factors (age, BMI, MAP, ethnicity, obstetric history, interpregnancy interval, family history of PE, method of conception, history of chronic HTN or diabetes or SLE or APS, and smoking habit), and clinical parameters (MAP and uterine PI) to obtain a reliable estimation of risk. Evidence is based on three studies on >120,000 pregnancies at 11–13 weeks of gestation. With use of this tool the detection rate of early-PE, preterm-PE, and all-PE was about 90%, 75%, and 50%, respectively at the screen-positive rate of 10%.

Maternal factors as predictor of PE: Several authorities have identified maternal risk factors based on maternal demographic characteristics and medical history as predictor of PE (shown below in **Table 2**). However, the detection rate with the risk factors alone was proven to be very low (39% for preterm PE and 34% for term PE) with a quite high risk of false-positive rate (FPR) (10.3%).

Uterine artery Doppler: UtA Doppler (11^+–13^{+6} weeks) is a noninvasive method for assessment of uteroplacental circulation. With advanced gestation there is significant loss of resistance of spiral arteries **(Figs. 3A and B)**. Resistance is measured as increased PI and resistance index (RI). A persistently raised PI >95th centile is associated with greater risk of adverse outcome with PE. However, UtA Doppler alone has low predictive value for the development of early-onset PE, even lower value for late-onset PE. *Combined assessment* including maternal factors (MFs) + first trimester UtA Doppler velocimetry + biochemical markers improves detection rate of early-onset PE over 90% with 10% FPR.

Biochemical markers: Several studies have evaluated the role of biochemical markers or a combination of biochemical and biophysical markers in the prediction of PE in the first and second trimesters of pregnancy. Perhaps the most promising screening methods is the use during the second trimester of combined biomarkers—such as sFlt-1, sEng, and PlGF—for prediction of early-onset PE. In May 2016, the

TABLE 2: Risk factors for PE according to ISSHP, NICE, ACOG and FIGO.

ISSHP	NICE: One high-risk or two moderate-risk factors	ACOG: Any risk factor	FIGO
• Prior preeclampsia • Chronic hypertension • Multiple gestation • Pregestational diabetes • Maternal BMI >30 kg/m² • Antiphospholipid syndrome • Assisted reproduction therapy	*High-risk factor:* • Hypertensive disease in previous pregnancy • Chronic hypertension • Chronic renal disease • Diabetes mellitus, or autoimmune disease *Moderate-risk factors:* • Nulliparity • Age ≥40 years • BMI ≥35 kg/m² • Family history of PE • Interpregnancy interval >10 years	• Conception by IVF • Age ≥40 first pregnancy • BMI ≥30 kg/m² • F/H/O of PE • Previous PE • Diabetes mellitus • Chronic HTN • SLE or thrombophilia • Chronic renal disease	• *Age:* 35 years • Nulliparity • History of PE in previous pregnancy (second pregnancy—14.7% and 31.9% who had PE in the previous two pregnancies) • ART-Double the risk • Family history of PE • Obesity (BMI ≥30 kg/m²) • Race and ethnicity (PE is also higher in women of South Asian origin)

(ACOG: American College of Obstetricians and Gynaecologists; BMI: body mass index; ISSHP: International Society for the Study of Hypertension in Pregnancy; FIGO: Federation of Gynecology and Obstetrics; IVF: in vitro fertilization; NICE: National Institute for Health and Care Excellence; PE: preeclampsia; SLE: systemic lupus erythematosus)

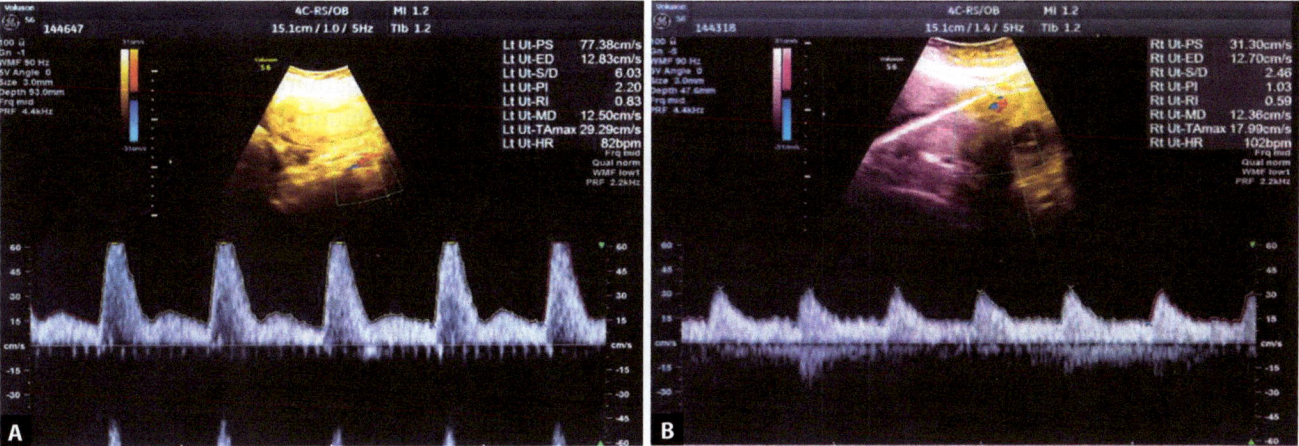

Figs. 3A and B: (A) Uterine artery Doppler in early pregnancy showing diastolic notch; (B) Uterine artery Doppler in mid-pregnancy.

NICE published NICE Diagnostics guidance [DG23; (https://www.nice.org.uk/guidance/dg23)] recommending that the Elecsys immunoassay for the sFlt-1/PlGF ratio, or the Triage PlGF test, be used with standard clinical assessment to help to rule out proteinuric PE or PE requiring delivery within the next 7 (for the sFlt-1/PlGF ratio) or 14 days (for Triage PlGF) in women with suspected PE between 20 and 34^{+6} weeks' of gestation.

In normal pregnancy, there is a balance between angiogenic and antiangiogenic factors, in PE the concentration of antiangiogenic factor sFlt-1 is high and angiogenic factor PlGF is low. An alteration in concentration of these biomarkers precede clinical onset of PE by several weeks to months. PlGF begins to decrease 9–11 weeks before the onset of PE, correlate with disease severity, and normalize after delivery. PlGFs measured in the first trimester have the highest detection rate and perform better in predicting early-onset PE than late-onset PE (sensitivity 40%, specificity 90%).

Soluble Flt is altered 4–5 weeks before onset of clinical symptoms of PE, again, higher the sFlt concentration, more predictive it is of early-onset PE. Combination of these biomarkers has high sensitivity and specificity for early diagnosis and prognosis of PE. In a study of over 600 women undergoing initial evaluation of PE, presenting <34 weeks gestation, a sFlt-1/PlGF ratio ≥85 correlated with diagnosis of PE and predicted adverse outcomes and delivery within 2 weeks.

The PROGNOSIS study (prediction of short-term outcome in pregnant women with suspected PE): shed new lights on usefulness of sFlt-1/PlGF ratio for prediction of absence or presence of PE for women with suspected PE. This was a prospective multicentric study conducted on 1,050 women between 24^{+0} and 36^{+6} weeks of gestation with suspected PE; ruled out PE within 1 week using sFlt-1/PlGF ratio with a single cut-off value of 38. The negative predictive value (NPV) in this study was 99.9%. A follow-up study from the same cohort showed a NPV of 95% within 4 weeks. Single sFlt-1/PlGF ratio cut-off <38 in third trimester also rule out late-onset PE and FGR, with a sensitivity 84.4%, specificity 93%.

Algorithm for prediction of PE: No single test can reliably predict PE. Fetal Medicine Foundation screening method includes combination of low maternal serum concentrations of PlGF, high UtA-PI, and other maternal parameters in the first trimester, identified 93.1% of patients who would develop PE requiring delivery before 34 weeks of gestation. This algorithm demonstrated superiority to the screening methods currently recommended by NICE and ACOG **(Fig. 4)**.

Prediction of Adverse Outcome

Uric acid: Uric acid clearance usually decreases before a measurable decrease in glomerular filtration rate (GFR). It is associated with poor perinatal outcomes but not with adverse maternal outcomes. Elevated concentration

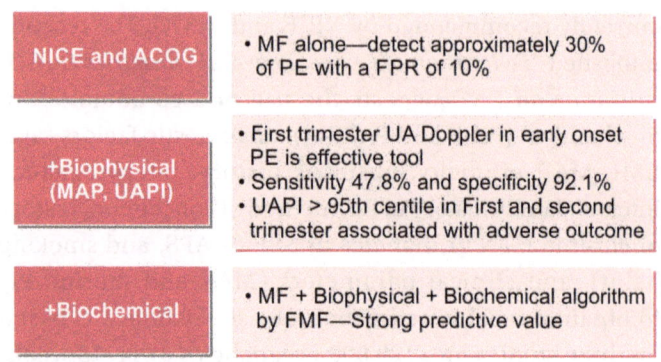

Fig. 4: Algorithm for prediction of PE.
(ACOG: American College of Obstetricians and Gynaecologists; FPR: false-positive rate; NICE: National Institute for Health and Care Excellence; PE: preeclampsia; MAP: mean arterial pressure; MF: maternal factor; UAPI: uterine artery-pulsatility index)

has been suggested as useful in identifying women with gestational HTN who may progress to PE, develop adverse maternal fetal outcome or both.

Full preeclampsia integrated estimate of risk (fullPIERS or PREP-S): The PREP collaborative network (Prediction of Complications in Early-onset Preeclampsia) published prognostic models that assist in predicting the overall risk of women with established PE to experience a complication using logistic regression (PREP-L) and for predicting the time to adverse maternal outcome using a survival model (PREP-S). The PREP-S model included maternal age, gestation, medical history, SBP, deep tendon reflexes, urine protein creatinine ratio, platelets, serum alanine aminotransaminase, urea, creatinine, oxygen saturation, and treatment with antihypertensives or $MgSO_4$. The PREP-L model included the above except deep tendon reflexes, serum alanine aminotransaminase, and creatinine. (*http://stg.pocketapp.co.uk/qmul/#home*).

NICE guideline, 2019, recommended consider using either the fullPIERS or PREP-S validated risk prediction models to help decisions about the most appropriate place of care (such as the need for in utero transfer) and thresholds for intervention. The pre-eclampsia integrated estimation of risk, a clinical predictive model, can predict the likelihood of a composite severe adverse maternal outcome using the following variables gathered from 0 to 48 hours after admission with PE—gestational age, chest pain or dyspnea, oxygen saturation, platelet count, serum creatinine, and AST. ISSHP recommends this as a useful adjunct in the initial assessment of women with PE.

Note:
- fullPIERS is intended for use at any time during pregnancy
- PREP-S is intended for use only up to 34 weeks of pregnancy
- fullPIERS and PREP-S models do not predict outcomes for babies.

Prevention of Preeclampsia

Role of aspirin: Alteration in systemic prostacycline–thromboxane balance contributes to PE. Inflammation is increased in PE. Low-dose aspirin has been studied in large randomized controlled trial (RCT) both in low and high-risk women. A Cochrane review of low dose aspirin on PE found overall 17% reduction in risk, with significant risk reduction in high-risk women. Low-dose aspirin prophylaxis may be considered for primary prevention of PE in high-risk women.

In a recent multicenter, double blind, placebo-controlled trial, pregnant women at increased risk of preterm PE (<37 weeks of gestation) were randomly assigned to receive aspirin, at a higher dose (150 mg/day), or placebo from 11 to 14 weeks of gestation until 36 weeks of gestation. Preterm PE occurred in 1.6% of the participants in the aspirin group, as compared with 4.3% in the placebo group (odds ratio, 0.38; 95% CI, 0.2020.74; P5.004). The authors reported that there were no significant differences in the incidence of neonatal adverse outcomes between groups. The authors concluded that low-dose aspirin in women at high risk of PE was associated with a lower incidence for preterm PE (ACOG, 2020). Pharmacological prevention of PE with low-dose aspirin is based on analysis of risk factors from maternal demographic characteristics and medical history. Factors to be considered for assuming low-dose aspirin are hypertensive disease in previous pregnancy, chronic HTN, chronic renal disease, diabetes mellitus, autoimmune disease or any two of the moderate-risk factors (nulliparity, age ≥40 years, BMI ≥35 kg/m^2, family history of PE, or interpregnancy interval >10 years).

International Society for the Study of Hypertension in Pregnancy recommends that women with established strong clinical risk factors for PE be treated, ideally before 16 weeks but definitely before 20 weeks, with low-dose aspirin (defined as 75–162 mg/day). Low-molecular-weight heparin is not indicated to prevent PE, even with a history of prior early-onset PE. Pregnant women at high risk of PE to take 75–150 mg of aspirin daily from 12 weeks until the birth of the baby (NICE). Pregnant women with moderate to high risk for developing PE should receive 81 mg of aspirin, and ideally, it should be started between 12 and 16 weeks of gestation and continue till 36 weeks (ACOG).

Calcium supplementation: To date, no intervention has been proved unequivocally effective at eliminating the risk of PE. With regard to nutritional interventions, evidence is insufficient to demonstrate effectiveness for vitamins C and E, fish oil, garlic supplementation as well as vitamin D, folic acid or sodium restriction for reducing the risk of PE. A meta-analysis of 13 trials (15,730 women) reported a significant reduction in PE with calcium supplementation, with the greatest effect among women with low-baseline calcium intake. Women considered at increased risk for PE, in addition to aspirin, should receive supplemental calcium (1.2–2.5 g/day) if their intake is likely to be low (<600 mg/day). When intake cannot be assessed or predicted, it is reasonable to give calcium. Calcium at a dose of at least 1 g/day has been shown to reduce the likelihood of PE in women with low calcium intake. The WHO currently recommends this therapy for women in settings with low calcium intake.

Antioxidant therapy: The central role of placental oxidative stress in the pathophysiology provided a rationale for the administration of antioxidant vitamins. But clinical trials of antioxidant vitamins (C and E) have proved to be ineffective in several large interventional studies.

Vitamin D: Deficiency has been suggested as a factor contributing to PE, however whether supplementation is helpful or not is unknown.

Exercise: Women should exercise during pregnancy to maintain health, appropriate body weight, and reduce the likelihood of HTN.

MANAGEMENT OF PREGNANCY WITH PREECLAMPSIA

Timely delivery of the fetus and placenta remains the only definitive cure for PE. The principle aim of management is to prolong pregnancy as long as it is considered safe for mother and fetus. Plan of management is done meticulously according to degree of HTN.

Delivery versus expectant management (ACOG, 2020): Continued monitoring of women with PE without severe features at the initial evaluation, consists of a complete blood count with platelet estimate, serum creatinine, LDH, AST, ALT, and testing for proteinuria obtained in parallel with a comprehensive clinical maternal and fetal evaluation. In the settings of diagnostic dilemmas, such as in the evaluation of possible PE superimposed upon chronic HTN, a uric acid test may be considered. Fetal evaluation includes sonographic evaluation for estimated fetal weight and amount of amniotic fluid, as well as antepartum fetal testing. The frequency of these tests may be modified based on clinical findings and patient's symptoms. Subsequent management will depend on the results of the evaluation and gestational age. The decision to deliver must balance the maternal and fetal risks. In women with gestational HTN without severe features, when there is progression to PE with severe features, this progression usually takes 1–3 weeks after diagnosis, whereas in women with PE without severe features, the progression to severe PE could happen within days. Women should be advised to immediately report any persistent, concerning, or unusual symptoms.

Continued observation is appropriate for a woman with a preterm fetus if she has PE without severe features. There are no RCTs in this population, but retrospective data suggest that without severe features, the balance should be in favor of continued monitoring until delivery at $37^{0/7}$ weeks of gestation in the absence of abnormal antepartum testing, preterm labor, preterm prelabor rupture of membranes or vaginal bleeding for neonatal benefit. The risks associated with expectant management in the late preterm period include the development of severe HTN, eclampsia, HELLP syndrome, placental abruption, FGR, and fetal death; however, these risks are small and counterbalanced by the increased rates of admission to the neonatal intensive care unit, neonatal respiratory complications, and neonatal death that would be associated with delivery before $37^{0/7}$ weeks of gestation.

Inpatient versus outpatient management: Ambulatory management at home is an option only for women with PE without severe features and requires frequent fetal and maternal evaluation. Hospitalization is appropriate for women with severe features and for women in whom adherence to frequent monitoring is a concern.

Offer admission—if uncontrolled severe-range BPs (persistent SBP 160 mm Hg or more or DBP 110 mm Hg or more), not responsive to antihypertensive medication, any maternal biochemical or hematological investigations that cause concern, sign of severe features/other signs of severe PE—persistent headaches, refractory to treatment, epigastric pain or RUQ pain unresponsive to repeat analgesics, visual disturbances, motor deficit or altered sensorium, new or worsening renal dysfunction (serum creatinine >1.1 mg/dL or twice baseline), impending pulmonary edema, suspected acute placental abruption or vaginal bleeding in the absence of placenta previa, suspected fetal compromise, abnormal fetal testing, fetus without expectation for survival at the time of maternal diagnosis (e.g., lethal anomaly, extreme prematurity), fetal death, persistent reversed end-diastolic flow in the umbilical artery or any other clinical signs that cause concern, stroke, myocardial infarction, and HELLP syndrome *(ACOG, 2020).*

MANAGEMENT OF PREECLAMPSIA (NICE, 2020)

Management of PE (NICE, 2020) is given in **Table 3**.

Laboratory tests: Laboratory tests are done, for monitoring and to assess severity of the condition **(Table 4)**.

Fetal Assessment

Fetal assessment is given in **Table 5**.

Ultrasonography in women with previous PE: USG for fetal growth and AFV assessment and UA Doppler starting

TABLE 3: Management of preeclampsia (NICE, 2020).

	Hypertension: BP 140/90–159/109 mm Hg	*Severe hypertension: BP 160/110 mm Hg or more*
Admission to hospital	Admit if any clinical concerns for the well-being of the woman or baby or if high risk of adverse events suggested by the fullPIERS or PREP-S risk prediction models	Admit, but if BP falls below 160/110 mm Hg, manage as for hypertension
Antihypertensive pharmacological treatment	Offer antihypertensive if BP remains above 140/90 mm Hg	Offer treatment to all women
Target BP on antihypertensive treatment	Aim for BP of 135/85 mm Hg or less	Aim for BP of 135/85 mm Hg or less
BP measurement	At least every 48 hours, and more frequently if the woman is admitted to hospital	Every 15–30 minutes until BP is <160/110 mm Hg, then at least four times daily while the woman is an inpatient, depending on clinical circumstances

(BP: blood pressure; fullPIERS: full preeclampsia integrated estimate of risk)

TABLE 4: Laboratory tests in PE (NICE).

Laboratory tests	*BP 140/90–159/109 mm Hg*	*BP ≥160/110 mm Hg*
Dipstick proteinuria testing	Only repeat if clinically indicated, e.g., if new symptoms and signs develop or if there is uncertainty over diagnosis	Only repeat if clinically indicated, e.g., if new symptoms and signs develop or if there is uncertainty over diagnosis
Blood tests	Measure full blood count, liver function, and renal function twice a week	Measure full blood count, liver function, and renal function three times a week

(BP: blood pressure)

TABLE 5: Fetal assessment in PE (NICE).	
BP 140/90–159/109 mm Hg	**BP ≥160/110 mm Hg**
• Offer fetal heart auscultation at every antenatal appointment • Carry out ultrasound assessment of the fetus at diagnosis and, if normal, repeat every 2 weeks • Carry out a CTG at diagnosis and then only if clinically indicated	• Offer fetal heart auscultation at every antenatal appointment • Carry out ultrasound assessment of the fetus at diagnosis and, if normal, repeat every 2 weeks • Carry out a CTG at diagnosis and then only if clinically indicated; change in fetal movement, vaginal bleeding, abdominal pain, and deterioration in maternal condition

(BP: blood pressure; CTG: cardiotocography)

between 28 and 30 weeks (or at least 2 weeks before previous gestational age of onset if earlier than 28 weeks) and repeating every 4 weeks in women with previous severe PE, PE that resulted in birth before 34 weeks, PE with a baby whose birth weight was less than 10th centile, intrauterine death, and placental abruption.

Control of HTN: BP consistently at or >140/90 mm Hg in clinic or office (or ≥135/85 mm Hg at home) should be treated, aiming for a target DBP of 85 mm Hg in the office (and SBP of 110–140 mm Hg) to reduce the likelihood of developing severe maternal HTN (ISSHP). As antihypertensive offer labetalol in pregnant women with PE. Offer nifedipine for women in whom labetalol is not suitable, and methyldopa if labetalol or nifedipine is not suitable.

Timing of Birth

The clinical course of PE with severe features is characterized by progressive deterioration of maternal and fetal condition. Therefore, delivery is recommended when PE with severe features is diagnosed at or beyond $34^{0/7}$ weeks of gestation, after maternal stabilization or with labor or prelabor rupture of membranes. Delivery should not be delayed for the administration of steroids in the late preterm period. In women with PE with severe features at $<34^{0/7}$ weeks of gestation, with stable maternal and fetal condition, expectant management may be considered. If delivery is indicated at $<34^{0/7}$ weeks of gestation, administration of corticosteroids for fetal lung maturation is recommended; however, delaying delivery for optimal corticosteroid exposure may not always be advisable.

Planned early birth before 37 weeks include the followings: Inability to control maternal BP despite using three or more classes of antihypertensives in appropriate doses, maternal pulse oximetry <90%, progressive deterioration in liver function, renal function, hemolysis, or platelet count, ongoing neurological features, e.g., severe intractable headache, repeated visual scotomata, or eclampsia, placental abruption, reversed end-diastolic flow in the umbilical artery Doppler velocimetry, and a nonreassuring cardiotocograph or stillbirth.

In addition to appropriate management of labor and delivery, the two main goals of management of women with PE during labor and delivery are: (1) prevention of seizures and (2) control of HTN.

INTRAPARTUM MANAGEMENT OF SEVERE PREECLAMPSIA

Blood pressure: During labor, BP has to measure hourly. Every 15–30 minutes until BP is <160/110 mm Hg in women with severe HTN. Continue antenatal antihypertensive treatment during labor.

Hematological and biochemical tests have to done during labor if not done previously.

Route of delivery: Delivery is typically done by the vaginal route. Cesarean delivery reserved for the usual obstetric indications. The decision to expedite delivery in the setting of severe PE does not mandate immediate cesarean section. Cervical ripening agents may be used if the cervix is not favorable before induction. But avoidance of prolong induction in the setting of intrauterine growth retardation (IUGR) or oligohydramnios.

Management of second stage of labor: If BP is controlled, there is no need to routinely limit the duration of second stage of labor. In severe HTN not responding to treatment, consideration of operative or assisted birth in second stage of labor. Continuous electronic fetal monitoring is recommended in labor. Oxytocin may be used in third stage of labor, ergometrine is contraindicated.

Fluid Management

To avoid fluid overload careful fluid balance is necessary. Do not preload with intravenous (IV) fluid before epidural spinal analgesia. In severe PE, total input (IV and oral) should be restricted to 80 mL/hour. Oxytocin if needed should be used at high concentration. Volume expanders should be avoided [increased risk of neonatal complications, e.g., artificial ventilation and patent ductus arteriosus (PDA)]. Urine output should be recorded hourly (>80 mL in 4 hours). If total input is >750 mL in excess of output in 24 hours, 20 mg of IV frusemide should be given.

Regional versus General Anesthesia

Epidural is preferred in a severely preeclamptic patient in a nonurgent setting, for urgent cases spinal is also safe. Epidural allows to avoid general anesthesia (GA) with potential for encountering a swollen, difficult airway, and/or labile HTN; which may cause stroke secondary to increased systemic and intracranial pressures during intubation and extubation. Neuraxial anesthesia and analgesia are contraindicated in the presence of a coagulopathy. Thrombocytopenia also increases the risk of epidural hematoma. Prior to placing regional block, it is recommended to check the platelet count (> 70,000/microliter of blood), any clinical evidence of DIC would contraindicate regional anesthesia.

Maternal and Fetal Consequences of Preeclampsia

Maternal outcome: PE with severe features can result in acute and long-term complications for the woman and her newborn. Maternal complications include pulmonary edema, myocardial infarction, stroke, acute respiratory distress syndrome, coagulopathy, renal failure, and retinal injury. These complications are more likely to occur in the presence of preexistent medical disorders.

Fetal outcome: Because of impaired uteroplacental blood flow secondary to failure of physiologic transformation of the spiral arteries or placental vascular insults, or both, manifestations of PE may also be seen in the fetal–placental unit. Clinical manifestations that follow uteroplacental ischemia include FGR, oligohydramnios, placental abruption, and nonreassuring fetal status demonstrated on antepartum surveillance. Consequently, fetuses of women with PE are at increased risk of spontaneous or indicated preterm delivery or even stillbirth.

Postnatal Investigation, Monitoring, and Treatment

Delivery does not immediately reverse the pathophysiologic changes of PE, and it is necessary to continue palliative therapy for various periods. Approximately 20-30% of eclampsia and 30% HELLP occurs in the postpartum period, mostly within 24 hours and almost all within 48 hours, although there are rare exceptions. Therefore, more vigilance is needed to identify fatal or life-threatening complications within 48 hours.

Antihypertensive Treatment during Postnatal Period, including Breastfeeding

Most antihypertensive drugs can pass into breast milk, monitor babies, especially those preterm, for drowsiness, lethargy, pallor, cold peripheries or poor feeding.

Recommended Antihypertensives in Postpartum Period (NICE, 2019)

Offer enalapril during postnatal period, with appropriate monitoring of maternal renal function and serum potassium. If BP is not controlled with a single medicine, consider a combination of nifedipine (or amlodipine) and enalapril. If this combination is not tolerated or is ineffective, consider either: adding *atenolol or labetalol to the combination* treatment *or* swapping one of the medicines already being used for atenolol or labetalol. Use medicines that are taken once daily whenever possible, avoid using diuretics or ARBs who are breastfeeding.

Hematological and biochemical monitoring: In women who have PE with mild-to-moderate HTN or step down from critical care, measure platelet count, transaminase, and serum creatinine 48–72 hours after birth or step down. Do not repeat if normal at 48–72 hours. If biochemical and hematological indices are outside the reference range, repeat platelet count, transaminases, and serum creatinine measurements as clinically indicated until normal. A urinary reagent strip test 6–8 weeks after delivery. If still have proteinuria 1+ or more, a further review at 3 months after delivery to assess kidney function. If abnormal referred to nephrologist.

POSTNATAL MANAGEMENT

Antihypertensive treatment has to continue, consider reducing the dose if BP falls below 140/90 mm Hg and reduce dose if BP is below 130/80 mm Hg. If methyldopa was used antenatally—stop within 2 days after birth and change to alternative treatment if necessary. Transfer to community care if there are no symptoms of PE, BP with or without treatment 150/100 mm Hg or less, and blood test results are stable or improving. Review within 1 week if still requiring antihypertensives at discharge from hospital, should be reviewed at 3 months postpartum to ensure that BP, urinalysis, and any laboratory abnormalities have normalized. If proteinuria or HTN persists, then appropriate referral for further investigations should be initiated.

Nonsteroidal anti-inflammatory drugs (NSAIDs) for postpartum analgesia should be avoided unless other analgesics are not working; avoid especially, if they have known renal disease, or is associated with placental abruption, acute kidney injury (AKI), or other known risk factors for AKI (e.g., sepsis, postpartum hemorrhage).

Long-term Prognosis of Preeclampsia

The overall risk of recurrence in future pregnancies is approximately 20% (1 in 5). With severe disease (birth between 28 and 34 weeks), recurrence is approximately 33% (1 in 3 women). If birth takes place between 34 and

37 weeks, recurrence is approximately 23% (1 in 4 women). HELLP recurs in about 5% cases. Long-term risk of CVD approximately 2–3 times. There is increased risk of chronic HTN and undiagnosed renal disease, and risk of FGR in subsequent pregnancy.

Counseling

Avoid smoking, maintain a healthy lifestyle, and maintain a healthy weight before being pregnant again (BMI before next pregnancy 18.5–24.9 kg/m^2).

ANTIHYPERTENSIVE THERAPY IN HYPERTENSIVE DISORDERS OF PREGNANCY

Offer antihypertensive treatment if BP remains >140/90 mm Hg, target BP is 135/85 mm Hg or less. Aim of antihypertensive is to—lower BP and lower the risk of maternal cerebrovascular accidents without compromising uterine blood flow and compromising the fetus. There is evidence that anti-hypertensives may be useful in preventing eclamptic seizures. Antihypertensives lower perfusion pressure and prevents vasogenic edema, inhibits cerebral arterial vasospasm that causes tissue ischemia, and pericapillary bleeding.

Suitable Antihypertensives in Pregnancy

- Labetalol (first line) to treat HTN
- Nifedipine in whom labetalol is not suitable
- Alpha-methyldopa if labetalol or nifedipine is not suitable

Acute:
- Labetalol (oral or IV)
- Oral nifedipine
- Intravenous hydralazine

Long-term:
- Labetalol (oral 100, 200 mg)
- Nifedipine (oral 10, 20 mg)
- Methyldopa (250 mg)
- Second or third-line agent: Hydralazine and prazosin.

Dose, Mode of Action, and Side Effects

Labetalol: Is a dual alpha (α1) and beta-(β1/β2) adrenergic receptor blocker, *highly selective* for postsynaptic α1-adrenergic, and nonselective for β-adrenergic receptors. The amount of α to β blockade depends on whether administered orally or IV. Orally, the ratio of α to β blockade is 1:3, intravenously α to β blockade ratio is 1:7; thus, labetalol can be thought to be a β-blocker with some alpha-blocking effects.

It is a partial agonist at β2-receptors located in the vascular smooth muscle. Labetalol relaxes vascular smooth muscle by a combination of this partial β2-agonism and through α1-blockade. Overall, this vasodilatory effect can result in decreased peripheral vascular resistance (PVR), decrease BP, without significant alteration of heart rate or cardiac output. Can cause rapid lowering of BP without causing hypotension. No adverse effect on uteroplacental blood flow. Labetalol is considered as medication of choice because of its effectiveness, low side effects, and availability of oral and parenteral preparation. Labetalol is the medication of choice in acute severe HTN as well as maintenance treatment.

Oral: The initial dose is 100 mg twice daily, may be increased up to 200–400 mg 2/3 times daily, to a maximum of 2.4 g.

Side effects include fatigue, lethargy, and exercise intolerance.

Contraindication: In patients with asthma (cause bronchospasm), heart disease or congestive cardiac disease.

Nefidipine

Nifedipine, a calcium-channel blocker, achieves treatment success in most women. An excellent peripheral vasodilator, lowers BP by inhibiting intracellular influx of calcium into cardiac and vascular smooth muscle and by decreasing PVR. Nifedipine is rapidly absorbed after oral administration and reaches peak level in 30 minutes, plasma half-life is approximately 2 hours.

Side effects: Very few (<2%) experiences hypotension, may observe reflex tachycardia, palpitation, headache, facial flushing, and peripheral edema. It has no deleterious effect on uteroplacental blood flow. No adverse maternal or fetal outcomes.

Dose: In less acute condition 30–120 mg/day, slow-release preparation.

Methyldopa

Methyldopa has been the most widely used antihypertensive in pregnancy. A centrally acting α-2 adrenergic receptor agonist. Methyldopa lowers BP by synthesis of α *methyl norepinephrine* which stimulates α2 receptors and decreases sympathetic outflow from the central nervous system. Effect of methyldopa is mainly on PVR with little effect on CO. Causes dilation of both arterial circulation and capacitance vessels, allowing expansion of intravascular volume. Renal blood flow is maintained during treatment.

Maximum effect is achieved 4–6 hours after oral administration. A single dose at bed time is usually effective for BP control, to obtain maximum therapeutic effect 2–3 times daily dose required.

Dose: Initial dose is 250 mg thrice daily, may be increased up to 2 g/day, requires 24 hours to achieve therapeutic levels. Long-term administration causes salt and water retention, may cause rebound HTN.

Side effects include fatigue, depression, poor sleep, and decreased salivation. Not suitable for patients with renal impairment as it is maximally excreted in urine, should be avoided in postpartum period as it causes depression.

Beta-blockers

Safe in pregnancy, lowers BP by competing with endogenous catecholamines for β-adrenergic receptors, leaving α-mediated vasoconstriction unopposed. May be the first drug of choice in patients with chronic HTN as majority of these patients has increased CO and hyperkinetic circulation. Beta-blockers are called cardioselective when they bind to β1 receptors only and noncardioselective when they bind to both β1 and β2 receptors.

Propranolol: Propranolol inhibits the sympathetic nervous system by blocking the beta-receptors on the nerves. It is a competitive antagonist of β-1-adrenergic receptors in the heart. Competes with sympathomimetic neurotransmitters for binding to receptors, which inhibits sympathetic stimulation of the heart, reduces the force of contraction of heart muscle, and thereby lowers BP. Propranolol is indicated in the management of essential HTN.

Propranolol is noncardioselective, reduces CO 15–30%, and suppress renin-production by 60%. Other action includes diminution of tonic sympathetic outflow from the vasomotor center in the brain, restoration of defective vascular relaxation, and inhibition of presynaptic β-receptors. There is also drop of PVR, this makes it ideal drug for majority patients with chronic HTN. Half-life is 3–6 hours but can be given once or twice daily.

Dose: Initial dose 40–60 mg twice daily, may be increased up to 480–640 mg/day.

Side effects include bronchospasm and blunted response to hypoglycemia, making it unsuitable for asthmatics and brittle diabetics.

Atenolol: Selective β1 receptor blocker, does not cause bronchospasm and has prolonged duration of action. It has been associated with increased incidence of fetal growth retardation and not suitable in pregnancy. Classified as Food and Drug Administration (FDA) class D drug.

Prazosin (minipress): Postsynaptic α-blockers, lowers BP by relaxing veins and arteries. There is abrupt loss of venous tone with peripheral pooling—may cause severe hypotension. Prazosin in combination with a diuretic is highly effective for treatment of severe HTN refractory to treatment to other medication. Considered as a second-line agent by SOMANZ, dose 2–4 mg twice daily, initial dose 1 mg at bed-time to avoid postural HTN.

Hydralazine: Peripherally-acting antihypertensive. Acts directly on arteriolar smooth muscle and reduce PVR. Increase CO and plasma volume by vasodilatation and reflex stimulation of the renin-angiotensin system. Resistance to treatment or treatment failure is common. Cause rapid lowering of BP if given IV, not suitable for long-term use during pregnancy.

Adverse effects include headache, nausea, flushing, and palpitation. Higher or frequent dose associated with maternal hypotension, or fetal distress due to lowering of uteroplacental circulation. May be used with diuretics and β-blockers.

Treatment of Severe Hypertension

Acute severe HTN: HTN with acute onset, severe systolic HTN, and severe diastolic HTN or both require urgent antihypertensive therapy. With severe HTN who are in critical care during pregnancy or after birth, treatment has to start immediately with one of the following.

Labetalol

Injection labetalol 20, 40, and 80 mg boluses, slowly over a 2 minutes period at interval of 10 minutes. Monitor BP before, at 5 and 10 minutes after each injection, and maximum dose 220 mg. Maximum effect is reached within 5 minutes after injection, half-life 5–8 hours.

Contraindications: Asthma, cardiac failure, severe bradycardia, metabolic acidosis, and more than first degree heart block.

Hydralazine

Injection hydralazine: 5–10 mg boluses every 20–30 minutes (maximum dose 25 mg). It is a direct vasodilator. Onset of action is 20 minutes. The goal of IV therapy is not to normalize BP, but to achieve a range of 140–150/90–100 mm Hg. Once the aforementioned BP threshold is achieved, repeat BP measurement every 10 minutes for 1 hour, then every 15 minutes for 1 hour, then every 30 minutes for 1 hour, and then every 1 hour for 4 hours. Then shift to oral administration of labetalol and nifedipine.

Contraindications: Idiopathic SLE, severe tachycardia, high-output heart failure, myocardial insufficiency with mechanical obstruction, and acute porphyria.

Nifedipine

Commenced at a dose of 10–20 mg initially, repeat in 30 minutes if needed; then 10–20 mg every 2–6 hours, can be increased to 120 mg/day orally. Onset of action: immediate-release capsule—10–20 minutes. Oral long-acting tablet—30–45 minutes. Immediate-release capsule should be administered orally, not punctured or otherwise administered sublingually (ACOG, 2019). The oral form is not absorbed through buccal mucosa but rapidly absorbed through gastrointestinal tract (GIT). Sublingual use may cause precipitate fall in BP and lead to fetal distress.

Contraindication: Aortic stenosis.

Thromboprophylaxis: PE is considered a major risk factor for venous thromboembolism (VTE) and pharmacological prophylaxis is indicated in a woman who has 2 major or 1 major and 2 minor risk factors as recommended in the Australian guidelines, unless there are surgical contraindications.

Management of Severe Fulminating Preeclampsia and Impending Eclampsia

- *Intravenous antihypertensive:*
  - Hydralazine/labetalol—IV infusion, titration rapidly against changes in the BP *or,*
  - Oral nifedipine—sustained release tablet
- *Anticonvulsant therapy*

Magnesium sulfate (ACOG, 2019): Women with PE who have proteinuria and severe HTN, or HTN with neurological signs or symptoms, should receive magnesium sulfate ($MgSO_4$) for convulsion prophylaxis. $MgSO_4$ is the anticonvulsant of choice as treatment for eclampsia. A systematic review that included the Magpie study and five other studies found $MgSO_4$ reduced the risk of fits to half, reduced the risk of placental abruption, and reduced the risk of maternal mortality albeit nonsignificantly. $MgSO_4$ should be used for the prevention and treatment of seizures in women with GH and PE with severe features, eclampsia, and HELLP syndrome. $MgSO_4$ is not recommended as an antihypertensive agent. It remains the drug of choice for seizure prophylaxis for women with acute-onset of severe HTN in pregnancy and the postpartum period. Starting of $MgSO_4$ should not be delayed in the setting of acute severe HTN.

Dose: Administration of a 4-6 g loading dose over 20-30 minutes, followed by a maintenance dose of 1-2 g/hour maintained for 24 hours (in case of eclampsia after the last seizure). For recurrent seizure—a further dose of 2-4 g IV over 5 minutes. For women requiring cesarean delivery (before onset of labor), the infusion should ideally begin before surgery and continue during surgery, as well as for 24 hours afterward. For women who deliver vaginally, the infusion should continue for 24 hours after delivery.

Check BP, respiratory rate, oxygen saturation, deep tendon reflexes-at least every 30 minutes, and urine output every hour.

Serum magnesium levels must be monitored frequently either clinically (patellar reflexes, urinary output) or by checking serum levels 6-8 hours.
- *Therapeutic level:* 4-7 mEq/L
- *Patellar reflexes lost:* 8-10 mEq/L
- *Respiratory depression:* 10-15 mEq/L
- *Respiratory paralysis:* 12-15 mEq/L
- *Cardiac arrest:* 25-30 mEq/L.

TABLE 6: Antihypertensives to avoid in pregnancy and preconception.

Antihypertensive	Advice	Potential adverse effects
ACE inhibitors	Contraindicated	Teratogenic *First trimester:* Fetal renal dysfunction *Second and third trimester:* Oligohydramnios and skull hypoplasia
ARB blockers	Contraindicated	Teratogenic *First trimester:* Fetal renal dysfunction and second and third trimester—oligohydramnios
Diuretics	Avoid	Fetal electrolyte disturbances, reduction in maternal blood volume
Beta-blockers (except labetalol and oxprenolol)	Avoid	Fetal bradycardia, long-term use of atenolol associated with fetal growth restriction
Calcium-channel blocker (except nifedipine)	Avoid	Maternal hypotension and fetal hypoxia

(ACE: angiotensin-converting enzyme; ARB: angiotensin receptor blocker)
Source: Australian Prescriber

Treatment of Magnesium Toxicity

If magnesium toxicity is suspected, the infusion should be discontinued immediately. Calcium gluconate, the antidote for $MgSO_4$, may also be ordered (10 mL of a 10% solution, or 1 g), given by slow IV push (usually by the physician) over at least 3 minutes to avoid undesirable reactions such as arrhythmias, bradycardia, and ventricular fibrillation.

Potential adverse effects of $MgSO_4$: Include toxicity from overdose (respiratory, cardiac), decreased uterine contractility-causing increased bleeding and hypotension from hemorrhage. Because $MgSO_4$ is also a tocolytic agent, its use may increase the duration of labor. A preeclamptic woman receiving $MgSO_4$ may need augmentation with oxytocin during labor. The amount of oxytocin needed to stimulate labor may be more than that needed for a woman who is not on $MgSO_4$.

ANTIHYPERTENSIVES TO AVOID IN PREGNANCY AND PRECONCEPTION

Antihypertensives to avoid in pregnancy and preconception is given in **Table 6**.

SUGGESTED READING

1. Abalos E, Cuesta C, Grosso AL, Chou D, Say L. Global and regional estimates of preeclampsia and eclampsia: a systematic review. Eur J Obstet Gynecol Reprod Biol. 2013;170(1):1-7.

2. Altman D, Carroli G, Duley L, Farrell B, Moodley J, Neilson J, et al. Do women with preeclampsia, and their babies, benefit from magnesium sulphate? The Magpie Trial: a randomised placebo-controlled trial. Lancet. 2002;359(9321):1877-90.
3. Arias F, Bhide AG, Arulkumaran S, Damania K, Daftary S. Arias's practical guide to high-risk pregnancy and delivery. A South Asian Perspective, 5th Edition. [online] Available from https://www.amazon.in/Arias-Practical-High-Risk-Pregnancy-Delivery-ebook/dp/B07ZZ5JS24 [Last accessed April, 2022].
4. Bartsch E, Medcalf KE, Park AL, Ray JG. Clinical risk factors for pre-eclampsia determined in early pregnancy: systematic review and meta-analysis of large cohort studies. BMJ. 2016;353:i1753.
5. Bartsch E, Medcalf KE, Park AL, Ray JG. High Risk of Pre-eclampsia Identification Group. Clinical risk factors for pre-eclampsia determined in early pregnancy: systematic review and meta-analysis of large cohort studies. BMJ. 2016;353:i1753.
6. Bernstein PS, Martin JN Jr, Barton JR, Shields LE, Druzin ML, Scavone BM, et al. National Partnership for Maternal Safety: consensus bundle on severe hypertension during pregnancy and the postpartum period. Obstet Gynecol. 2017;130(2):347-57.
7. Brosens I, Pijnenborg R, Vercruysse L, Romero R. The "Great Obstetrical Syndromes" are associated with disorders of deep placentation. Am J Obstet Gynecol. 2011;204(3):193-201.
8. Brown MA, Magee LA, Kenny LC, Karumanchi SA, McCarthy FP, Saito S, et al. Hypertensive Disorders of Pregnancy ISSHP Classification, Diagnosis, and Management Recommendations for International Practice. Hypertension. 2018;72:24-43.
9. Burton GJ, Jauniaux E. The cytotrophoblastic shell and complications of pregnancy. Placenta. 2017;60:134-9.
10. Burton GJ, Redman CW, Roberts JM, Moffett A. Preeclampsia: Pathophysiology and clinical implications. BMJ. 2019;366:l2381.
11. Cade TJ, Gilbert SA, Polyakov A, Hotchin A. The accuracy of spot urinary protein-to-creatinine ratio in confirming proteinuria in pre-eclampsia. Aust N Z J Obstet Gynaecol. 2012;52(2):179-82.
12. Di Lorenzo G, Ceccarello M, Cecotti V, Ronfani L, Monasta L, Vecchi Brumatti L, et al. First trimester maternal serum PlGF, free β-hCG, PAPP-A, PP-13, uterine artery Doppler and maternal history for the prediction of preeclampsia. Placenta. 2012;33(6):495-501.
13. Duckitt K, Harrington D. Risk factors for pre-eclampsia at antenatal booking: systematic review of controlled studies. BMJ. 2005;330(7491):565.
14. English FA, Kenny LC, McCarthy FP. Risk factors and effective management of preeclampsia. Integr Blood Press Control. 2015;8:7-12.
15. Fox R, Kitt J, Leeson P, Aye CYL, Lewandowski AJ. Preeclampsia: risk factors, diagnosis, management, and the cardiovascular impact on the offspring. J Clin Med. 2019;8(10):1625.
16. Gestational Hypertension and Preeclampsia: ACOG Practice Bulletin, Number 222. Obstet Gynecol. 2020;135(6):e241.
17. Gillon TE, Pels A, von Dadelszen P, MacDonell K, Magee LA. Hypertensive disorders of pregnancy: a systematic review of International Clinical Practice Guidelines. PLoS One. 2014;9(12):e113715.
18. Kleinrouweler CE, Wiegerinck MM, Ris-Stalpers C, Bossuyt PM, van der Post JA, von Dadelszen P, et al. Accuracy of circulating placental growth factor, vascular endothelial growth factor, soluble fms-like tyrosine kinase 1 and soluble endoglin in the prediction of pre-eclampsia: a systematic review and meta-analysis. BJOG. 2012;119(7):778-87.
19. Lowe SA, Bowyer L, Lust K, McMahon LP, Morton M, North RA, et al. SOMANZ (Society of Obstetric Medicine of Australia and New Zealand). Guidelines for the management of hypertensive disorders of pregnancy 2014. Aust N Z J Obstet Gynaecol. 2015;55(5):e1-29.
20. McLaughlin K, Zhang J, Lye SJ, Parker JD, Kingdom JC. Phenotypes of pregnant women who subsequently develop hypertension in pregnancy. J Am Heart Assoc. 2018;7(14):e009595.
21. Morris RK, Riley RD, Doug M, Deeks JJ, Kilby MD. Diagnostic accuracy of spot urinary protein and albumin to creatinine ratios for detection of significant proteinuria or adverse pregnancy outcome in patients with suspected pre-eclampsia: systematic review and meta-analysis. BMJ. 2012;345:e4342.
22. NICE. NICE guideline. (2019). Hypertension in pregnancy: diagnosis and management. [online] Available from www.nice.org.uk/guidance/ng133 [Last accessed April, 2022].
23. Nicolaides KH. Aspirin versus placebo in pregnancies at high risk for preterm preeclampsia. N Engl J Med. 2017;377(24):2400.
24. Rana S, Lemoine E, Granger JP, Karumanchi SA. Preeclampsia: Pathophysiology, Challenges, and Perspectives. Circ Res. 2019;124(7):1094-112.
25. Report of the National High Blood Pressure Education Program Working Group on High Blood Pressure in Pregnancy. Am J Obstet Gynecol. 2000;183(1):S1-22.
26. Sibai BM. Diagnosis, prevention, and management of eclampsia. Obstet Gynecol. 2005;105(2):402-10.
27. SOGC Clinical Practice Guideline. Diagnosis, Evaluation, and Management of the Hypertensive Disorders of Pregnancy: Executive Summary No. 307. 2014. [online] Available from https://www.jogc.com/article/S1701-2163(15)30588-0/pdf [Last accessed April, 2022].
28. Tagetti A, Fava C. Diagnosis of hypertensive disorders in pregnancy: an update. JLPM. 2020;5.
29. Tan MY, Koutoulas L, Wright D, Nicolaides KH, Poon LCY. Protocol for the prospective validation study: Screening programme for pre-eclampsia (SPREE). Ultrasound Obstet Gynecol. 2017;50(2):175-9.
30. Tranquilli AL, Brown MA, Zeeman GG, Dekker G, Sibai BM. The definition of severe and early-onset preeclampsia. Statements from the International Society for the Study of Hypertension in Pregnancy (ISSHP). Pregnancy Hypertens. 2013;3(1):44-7.
31. Tranquilli AL, Dekker G, Magee L, Roberts J, Sibai BM, Steyn W, et al. The classification, diagnosis and management of the hypertensive disorders of pregnancy: a revised statement from the ISSHP. Pregnancy Hypertens. 2014;4(2):97-104.
32. von Dadelszen P, Payne B, Li J, Ansermino JM, Broughton Pipkin F, Cote AM, et al. Prediction of adverse maternal outcomes in pre-eclampsia: development and validation of the fullPIERS model. Lancet. 2011;377(9761):219-27.

CHAPTER 4

HELLP Syndrome

■ INTRODUCTION

Hemolysis, elevated liver enzymes, and low platelets (HELLP) is an acronym that refers to a syndrome in pregnant and postpartum women characterized by hemolysis with a microangiopathic blood smear, elevated liver enzymes, and a low platelet count. It probably represents a severe form of preeclampsia, but the relationship between the two disorders remains controversial because as many as 15-20% of patients with HELLP syndrome do not have antecedent hypertension or proteinuria. Although different diagnostic benchmarks have been proposed, many clinicians use the following criteria to make the diagnosis: lactate dehydrogenase (LDH) elevated to 600 IU/L or more, aspartate aminotransferase (AST), and alanine aminotransferase (ALT) elevated more than twice the upper limit of normal, and the platelets count <100,000mm^3.

Hemolysis, elevated liver enzymes, and low platelets syndrome may have an insidious and atypical onset, with up to 15% of the patients lacking either hypertension or proteinuria. The main presenting symptoms are right upper quadrant (RUQ) pain and generalized malaise in up to 90% of cases and nausea and vomiting in 50% of cases. Some patients may present without these signs/symptoms when first evaluated for unexplained thrombocytopenia. The diagnosis of HELLP syndrome should be considered in any pregnant patient presenting in the second half of gestation or immediate postpartum with significant new-onset epigastric/RUQ pain until proven otherwise.

■ INCIDENCE

Hemolysis, elevated liver enzymes, and low platelets syndrome occurs in approximately 0.2-0.6% of all pregnancies. In pregnancies complicated by preeclampsia, laboratory findings of HELLP are present in 2-20% of cases; in those complicated by eclampsia, HELLP syndrome is present in 10-30% of cases. About 70% of cases occur in the third trimester of pregnancy, and the remainder occurs within 48 hours of delivery.

■ RISK FACTORS

A variety of genetic variants associated with an increased risk for HELLP syndrome has been reported, but they have no role in clinical management. A prior pregnancy with preeclampsia with or without HELLP syndrome is a risk factor for HELLP syndrome. In contrast to preeclampsia, nulliparity is not a risk factor for HELLP syndrome. Key risk factors include white ethnicity, advanced maternal age >35 years, multiparity, obesity, chronic hypertension, diabetes mellitus, autoimmune disorders, and abnormal placentation (e.g., molar pregnancy).

■ PATHOGENESIS

The pathogenesis of HELLP syndrome is not well understood. The findings of this multisystem disease are attributed to abnormal vascular tone, vasospasm, and coagulation defects. To date, no common precipitating factor has been found. The syndrome seems to be the final manifestation of some insult that leads to microvascular endothelial damage and intravascular platelet activation. With platelet activation, thromboxane A and serotonin are released, causing vasospasm, platelet agglutination and aggregation, and further endothelial damage. Dysfunction in the complement system via excessive activation or defective regulation for a given amount of endothelial injury has been proposed to cause damage to hepatic vessels in HELLP. In <2% of patients with HELLP syndrome, the underlying etiology appears to be related to fetal long-chain 3-hydroxyacyl-CoA dehydrogenase (LCHAD) deficiency.

■ PATHOPHYSIOLOGICAL CHANGES

The hemolysis in HELLP syndrome is a microangiopathic hemolytic anemia. Red blood cells become fragmented as they pass through small blood vessels with endothelial damage and fibrin deposits. The peripheral smear may reveal spherocytes, schistocytes, triangular cells, and burr cells. The elevated liver enzyme levels in the syndrome are thought to be secondary to obstruction of hepatic blood flow by fibrin deposits in the sinusoids. This obstruction leads to periportal necrosis and, in severe cases, intrahepatic hemorrhage, subcapsular hematoma formation, or hepatic rupture. The thrombocytopenia has been attributed to increased consumption and/or destruction of platelets.

Although some investigators speculate that disseminated intravascular coagulopathy (DIC) is the primary process in HELLP syndrome, most patients show no abnormalities on coagulation studies except those with well-developed HELLP syndrome who shows features of coagulopathy.

■ DIAGNOSIS

Clinical Presentation

The syndrome generally presents in the third trimester of pregnancy, although it occurs in <27 weeks of gestation in an estimated 11% of patients. HELLP syndrome occurs in 69% of patients in the antepartum and in 31% of patients in the postpartum period. With postpartum presentation, the onset is typically within the first 48 hours after delivery; however, signs and symptoms may not become apparent until as long as 7 days after delivery.

The vague nature of the presenting complaints can make the diagnosis difficult. Approximately 90% of patients present with generalized malaise, 65% with epigastric pain, 30% with nausea and vomiting, and 31% with headache. Because early diagnosis of this syndrome is critical, any pregnant woman who presents with malaise or a viral-type illness in the third trimester should be evaluated with a complete blood cell count and liver function tests (LFTs).

The physical examination may be normal. On physical examination, two-thirds patients manifest edema and hypertension; RUQ tenderness is present in as many as 90% of affected women as are brisk reflexes. Jaundice and bleeding manifestations, such as hematuria may rarely be present.

The differential diagnosis of HELLP syndrome includes acute fatty liver (AFP) of pregnancy, thrombotic thrombocytopenic purpura (TTP), and hemolytic uremic syndrome. Because of the variable nature of the clinical presentation, the diagnosis of HELLP syndrome is generally delayed for an average of 8 days. Many woman with this syndrome are initially misdiagnosed with other disorders, such as cholecystitis, esophagitis, gastritis, hepatitis, or idiopathic thrombocytopenia.

Laboratory Criteria for Diagnosis

The following laboratory criteria should be met for diagnosis of HELLP syndrome:
- *Hemolysis:* One of the features of HELLP syndrome is microangiopathic hemolytic anemia. Schistocytes or helmet cells, burr cells, and polychromasia present on a peripheral blood smear are diagnostic of microangiopathic hemolytic anemia, making peripheral smears useful in the workup for HELLP syndrome **(Fig. 1)**.
- Elevated LDH (>600 IU/L or twice the upper limit of normal concentration)

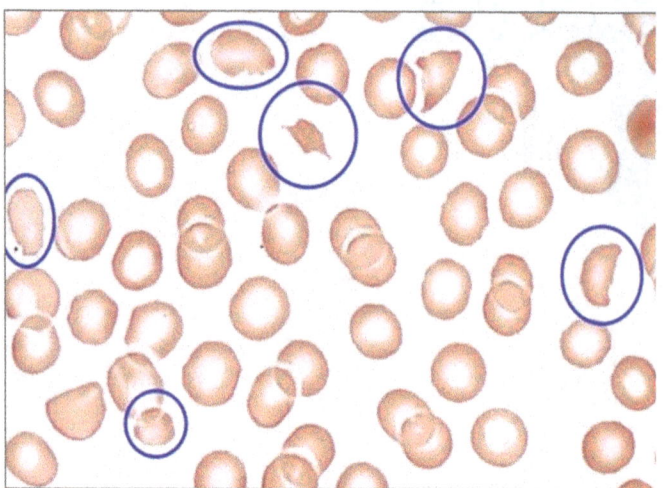

Fig. 1: Schistocytes.
Source: GP online (Photograph: D Roberts and J Burthem)

- Elevated total and indirect (unconjugated) bilirubin (total bilirubin 1.2 mg/dL or more)
- *Elevated liver transaminases:* AST and/or ALT >70 IU/L, or twice the upper limit of normal concentration
- *Thrombocytopenia:* Platelets <100,000/mm^3.
- Low serum haptoglobin (≤25 mg/dL)

In HELLP syndrome, an elevated LDH level is a nonspecific marker that can be associated with severe hemolysis, acute hepatocellular injury, or both. The total bilirubin level is increased as a result of an increase in the indirect (unconjugated) fraction from hemolysis. Haptoglobin level is a specific marker of hemolysis: 25 mg/dL provides the best cutoff between hemolytic and nonhemolytic disorders.

■ CLASSIFICATION

Two classification systems are used for HELLP syndrome. "The Tennessee classification" is based on the number of abnormalities that are present. Patients are classified as having partial HELLP syndrome when one or two abnormalities are present or full HELLP syndrome when all three abnormalities are present. Women with full HELLP syndrome are at higher risk for complications, including DIC, than women with the partial syndrome.

"Mississippi classification" measures the severity of the syndrome using the lowest observed platelet count along with the other two main clinical criteria (LDH and AST). Class I is the more severe, with a relatively high risk of morbidity and mortality, compared to the other two classes.
- *Class 1, severe thrombocytopenia:* Platelet count ≤50,000/mm^3, LDH ≥600 IU/L, AST, and/or ALT ≥70 IU/L (major maternal morbidity 40–60%)
- *Class 2, moderate thrombocytopenia:* Platelet >50,000 to ≤100,000/mm^3, LDH ≥600 IU/L, and AST and/or ALT ≥70 IU/L (major maternal morbidity 20–40%)
- *Class 3, mild thrombocytopenia:* Platelet >100,000 to ≤150,000/mm^3, LDH ≥600 IU/L, and AST ≥40 IU/L (major maternal morbidity 20%).

LABORATORY STUDIES

Initial laboratory studies in all patients with clinical features suspicious for severe preeclampsia or HELLP syndrome should include:
- Complete blood count (CBC)
- Liver function tests (AST, bilirubin, and LDH)
- Peripheral blood smear
- Uric acid, fibrinogen, and prothrombin time/partial thromboplastin time. These are undertaken in the patient with severe disease who might have evidence of advanced renal compromise, placental abruption, or the suspicion of a similar disorder.
- Optional studies include serum electrolytes, serum creatinine, and serum glucose.
- Patients with HELLP syndrome who complain of severe RUQ pain, neck pain, or shoulder pain should be considered for hepatic imaging, [computed tomography/magnetic resonance imaging (CT/MRI)] of liver in addition to ultrasound (USG) regardless of the severity of the laboratory abnormalities, to assess for subcapsular hematoma or rupture.

While hemolytic anemia is part of the pathology, patients with HELLP syndrome are frequently hemoconcentrated at baseline, a situation that may mask the hemolysis, at least until later stages of the disease. A urinalysis should be performed in all patients, and proteinuria, caused by increased renal tubular permeability, is found in 66–100% of patients. Uric acid level should be performed in patients with severe disease who might have evidence of advanced renal compromise, placental abruption, or the suspicion of an imitator disorder. Prolonged prothrombin time/partial thromboplastin time or reduced fibrinogen levels (<100 mg/dL) in addition to thrombocytopenia is indicative of progression to DIC. A positive D-dimer test in the setting of preeclampsia has recently been reported to be predictive of patients who will develop HELLP syndrome. The *D-dimer* is a more sensitive indicator of subclinical coagulopathy and may be positive before coagulation studies are abnormal.

HISTOPATHOLOGY

In the liver, intravascular fibrin deposits give rise to sinusoidal obstruction, intrahepatic vascular congestion, and increased hepatic pressures leading to hepatic necrosis. This may eventually result in intraparenchymal or subcapsular hemorrhage and capsular rupture.

DIFFERENTIAL DIAGNOSIS

Hemolysis, elevated liver enzymes, and low platelets syndrome should be differentiated from other disorders of pregnancy with similar features **(Table 1)**:
- *Preeclampsia:* Usually normal/slightly high liver enzymes, with normal platelet count. Schistocytes (fragmented red cells) are also absent.
- *Acute fatty liver of pregnancy:* Hypoglycemia is present in AFL but absent in HELLP syndrome.
- *Thrombotic thrombocytopenic purpura:* Usually manifests in second or third trimester, and liver abnormalities are not as elevated as in HELLP syndrome. Patients are typically normotensive and have undetectable ADAMTS 13 activity.
- *Hemolytic-uremic syndrome (HUS):* HUS has the same findings as TTP except that its incidence is higher in the postpartum period, and patients have signs of renal failure.
- *Lupus flare:* Liver pathology is absent in lupus.
- *Antiphospholipid syndrome (APS):* Dominant features of APS are arterial/venous thrombosis and repeated pregnancy loss. Lupus anticoagulant, cardiolipin

TABLE 1: Differentiating features.

Findings	HELLP syndrome	AFLP	TTP	HUS
Jaundice (%)	5–10	40–90	Rare	Rare
Urine findings	Proteinuria and evidence of hemolysis	Occasional proteinuria with conjugated bilirubin	Proteinuria with blood	Proteinuria
Thrombocytopenia	Present	Present	Present	Present
Hemolysis (%)	50–100	15–20	100	100
Anemia	Sometimes	No	Yes	Yes
DIC (%)	<20	50–100	Uncommon	Uncommon
Hypoglycemia	No	Common	No	No
Elevated ammonia	Rare	Sometimes	No	No
Elevated transaminases	High	High	Usually mild	Usually mild
Elevated bilirubin	Sometimes	Always	Always	Always
Impaired renal function (%)	50	90–100	30	100

Source: Sibai BM. Imitators of severe preeclampsia. Obstet Gynecol. 2007;109(4):956-66.
(AFLP: acute fatty liver of pregnancy; DIC: disseminated intravascular coagulopathy; HELLP: hemolysis, elevated liver enzymes, and low platelets; HUS: hemolytic-uremic syndrome; TTP: thrombotic thrombocytopenic purpura)

antibodies, beta-glycoprotein antibodies, prothrombin time, and an activated partial thromboplastin time (aPTT) should be checked to confirm the diagnosis.

- *Other:* Viral hepatitis, cholecystitis, cholangitis, gastritis, gastric ulcer, acute pancreatitis, and upper urinary tract infection (UTI).

■ MANAGEMENT

Although the disorder is considered to be a severe form of preeclampsia, not all patients affected by HELLP syndrome meet the presenting diagnostic criteria for severe preeclampsia. In independent studies, severe hypertension was initially absent in 12–18% of patients and in another 15% blood pressure was normal, and 4–14% of patients had no proteinuria. So, all women suspected of preeclampsia, including those with nonspecific symptoms such as nausea, vomiting, or malaise, should be evaluated for possible HELLP syndrome.

Hemolysis, elevated liver enzymes, and low platelets syndrome is a serious condition characterized by progressive and sometimes rapid maternal and fetal deterioration. Prompt recognition of HELLP syndrome and timely initiation of therapy are vital to ensure the best outcome for mother and the fetus. Recent research suggests that morbidity and mortality do not increase when patients with HELLP are treated conservatively. The treatment approach should be based on the estimated gestational age and the condition of the mother and fetus. Once, the diagnosis of HELLP syndrome has been established, the best markers to follow are the LDH level and the platelet count.

Antenatal administration of dexamethasone in a high dosage of 10 mg intravenously every 12 hours has been shown to markedly improve the laboratory abnormalities associated with HELLP syndrome. Other expected outcomes include less progression to class 1 HELLP syndrome, infrequent need for antihypertensive therapy, less transfusion, a lower incidence of new major maternal morbidity after starting therapy, increased latency between diagnosis and delivery to enable vaginal delivery, facilitating maternal transfer to a tertiary care center, and postnatal maturity of fetal lungs. In these studies, dexamethasone is administered intravenously until delivery for any patient with class 1 or class 2 HELLP syndrome regardless of gestational age or any patient with class 3 HELLP syndrome regardless of gestational age who also has eclampsia, severe epigastric pain, severe hypertension, or any major organ system morbidity shown improvement in clinical and laboratory features. Dexamethasone was initiated for antepartum and/or first detected postpartum disease, following delivery and with evidence of resolving laboratory and clinical parameters of disease the dose of dexamethasone was reduced for at least 2 doses and then stopped.

The two largest, randomized, double-blind, placebo-controlled trials evaluating the use of dexamethasone to improve maternal outcome in patients with HELLP syndrome did not establish a benefit in contrast to initial observational studies and small randomized trials that suggested more rapid improvement in maternal laboratory and clinical parameters.

Patients with HELLP syndrome should be treated prophylactically with magnesium sulfate to prevent seizures, whether hypertension is present or not. A bolus of 4–6 g of magnesium sulfate as a 20% solution is given initially. This dose is followed by a maintenance infusion of 2 g/hour. The infusion should be titrated to urine output and serum magnesium level.

Antihypertensive therapy should be initiated if blood pressure is consistently >160/110 mm Hg to reduce the risk of maternal cerebral hemorrhage, placental abruption, and seizure. The goal is to maintain diastolic blood pressure between 90 and 100 mm Hg. The most commonly used antihypertensive agent is hydralazine (apresolin) given intravenously in small incremental doses of 2.5–5 mg (with 5 mg as the initial dose) every 15–20 minutes until the desired blood pressure is achieved. Labetalol and nifedipine are also used. A hypertensive crisis may be treated with a continuous infusion of nitroglycerin or sodium nitroprusside (nipride).

Between 38 and 93% of patients with HELLP syndrome receive some form of blood product. Patients with a platelet count >40,000/mm^3 (40×10^9/L) are unlikely to bleed. These patients do not require transfusion unless the platelet count drops to <20,000/mm^3 (20×10^9/L). Actively bleeding patients with thrombocytopenia should be transfused with platelets. Patients who undergo cesarean section should be transfused if their platelet count is <50,000/mm^3 (50×10^9/L). Effect of platelet transfusion is only transient as consumption occurs rapidly. One unit of platelets is expected to increase the platelet count by 5,000. Prophylactic transfusion of platelets at delivery does not reduce the incidence of postpartum hemorrhage or hasten normalization of the platelet count and therefore use is controversial.

Fibrinogen replacement is necessary at levels <100 mg/dL. To increase the serum level of fibrinogen by 25 mg, 1 g of exogenous fibrinogen has to be administered. This amount is provided by 1 unit of fresh frozen plasma or 6 units of cryoprecipitate. Those having DIC should be given fresh frozen plasma and packed red blood cells.

The laboratory abnormalities in HELLP syndrome typically worsen after delivery and then begin to resolve by 3–4 days postpartum. Plasmapheresis has been successful in patients with severe laboratory abnormalities (i.e., a platelet count of <30,000/mm^3 (30×10^9/L) and continued elevation of liver function values], who require repeated transfusions to maintain their hematocrit at 72 hours postpartum. In these patients, plasmapheresis has resulted in an increase in the platelet count and a decrease in the LDH level.

Candidates for prompt delivery: The cornerstone of therapy for HELLP occurring during pregnancy is delivery, which is the only effective treatment. There is consensus among experts that prompt delivery is indicated after maternal stabilization for any of the following conditions:

- Pregnancies ≥34 weeks of gestation.
- Pregnancies that have not reached a stage of fetal maturity that ensures a reasonable chance of extrauterine survival.
- Fetal demise.
- Abruptio placentae.

In the absence of any of these scenarios *DIC, pulmonary edema, or acute kidney injury* or urgent clinical scenarios patient should be stabilized and delivered, delivery may be delayed until a course of corticosteroids has been administered. For this group of patients, recommendation is to give corticosteroids (betamethasone 12 mg intramuscularly every 12 hours for 2 doses or dexamethasone 12 mg intravenously every 12 hours for 4 doses) then deliver 24 hours after the last dose. Steroid administration is not only beneficial to the fetus for lung maturity but also for improvement of laboratory values in patients, particularly in elevating platelet counts. Maternal-fetal monitoring should be performed throughout each step of management.

In the past, delivery in patients with HELLP syndrome was routinely accomplished by cesarean section. Patients with severe HELLP syndrome, superimposed DIC, or a gestation of <32 weeks should be delivered by cesarean section. A trial of labor is appropriate in patients with mild to moderate HELLP syndrome who are stable, have a favorable cervix, and are at 32 weeks of gestation or greater.

ANESTHESIA

Pain relief with intravenous narcotics and local anesthesia is acceptable. Thrombocytopenia and coagulation abnormalities may preclude use of neuraxial anesthesia for labor and delivery. The minimum platelet count that is necessary to safely perform neuraxial anesthesia is unknown, and practice varies. Insertion of an epidural catheter is generally safe in patients with a platelet count >80,000/mm^3 (80×10^9/L), normal coagulation studies, and a normal bleeding time. General anesthesia can be used when regional anesthesia is considered unsafe.

PROGNOSIS

Hemolysis, elevated liver enzymes, and low platelets syndrome is a life-threatening condition. The mortality rate of women with HELLP syndrome is 0–24%, with a perinatal death rate of up to 37%. Maternal death most commonly occurs due to DIC, placental abruption, postpartum hemorrhage, acute renal failure, adult respiratory distress syndrome, subcapsular hematoma, and hepatic rupture. DIC occurs in 15–62.5% of the cases. Placental abruption occurs in 11–25% of the cases, postpartum hemorrhage occurs in 12.5–40%, and acute renal failure in 36–50% of the cases. Poor perinatal prognosis is because of placental abruption, intrauterine hypoxia and asphyxia, prematurity, and low birth weight.

Patients with HELLP syndrome have a 19–27% risk of developing HELLP syndrome in subsequent pregnancies. Class 1 HELLP syndrome has the highest recurrence rate. Recurrent cases occur in the latter part of the gestation period and are less severe after two episodes.

SUGGESTED READING

1. BMJ Best Practice. (2021). HELLP Syndrome. [online] Available from https://bestpractice.bmj.com/topics/en-us/1000 [Last accessed April, 2022].
2. Dusse LM, Alpoim PN, Silva JT, Rios DR, Brandão AH, Cabral AC. Revisiting HELLP syndrome. Clin Chim Acta. 2015;451(Pt B):117-20.
3. Fitzpatrick KE, Hinshaw K, Kurinczuk JJ, Knight M. Risk factors, management, and outcomes of hemolysis, elevated liver enzymes, and low platelets syndrome and elevated liver enzymes, low platelets syndrome. Obstet Gynecol. 2014;123(3):618-27.
4. Gestational Hypertension and Preeclampsia: ACOG Practice Bulletin, Number 222. Obstet Gynecol. 2020;135(6):e237-60.
5. Hypertension in pregnancy. Report of the American College of Obstetricians and Gynecologists' Task Force on Hypertension in Pregnancy. Obstet Gynecol. 2013;122(5):1122-31.
6. Katz L, de Amorim MM, Figueiroa JN, Pinto e Silva JL. Postpartum dexamethasone for women with hemolysis, elevated liver enzymes, and low platelets (HELLP) syndrome: a double-blind, placebo-controlled, randomized clinical trial. Am J Obstet Gynecol. 2008;198(3):283.e1-8.
7. Khalid F, Tonismae T. HELLP syndrome. NCBI, StatPearls [Internet]. 2021.
8. Kirkpatrick CA. The HELLP syndrome. Acta Clin Belg. 2010;65(2):91-7.
9. Lam MTC, Dierking E. Intensive care unit issues in eclampsia and HELLP syndrome. Int J Crit Illn Inj Sci. 2017;7(3):136-41.
10. Mao M, Chen C. Corticosteroid therapy for management of hemolysis, elevated liver enzymes, and low platelet count (HELLP) syndrome: A Meta-Analysis. Med Sci Monit. 2015;21:3777-83.
11. Martin JN Jr, Rose CH, Briery CM. Understanding and managing HELLP syndrome: the integral role of aggressive glucocorticoids for mother and child. Am J Obstet Gynecol. 2006;195(4):914-34.
12. Padden MO. HELLP syndrome: recognition and perinatal management. Am Fam Physician. 1999;60(3):829-36.
13. Sibai BM. Diagnosis, controversies, and management of the syndrome of hemolysis, elevated liver enzymes, and low platelet count. Obstet Gynecol. 2004;103(5 Pt 1):981-91.
14. Sibai BM. HELLP syndrome (hemolysis, elevated liver enzymes, and low platelets). UpTo Date. [online] Available from https://www.uptodate.com/contents/hellp-syndrome-hemolysis-elevated-liver-enzymes-and-low-platelets [Last accessed April, 2022].

CHAPTER 5

Fetal Growth Restriction

■ INTRODUCTION

Fetal growth restriction (FGR) is a complex obstetrical problem, complicates 10% of all pregnancies, and is a leading cause of stillbirth, neonatal mortality, and short- and long-term morbidity. FGR fetuses have a higher risk of preterm delivery, induction of labor, fetal compromise in labor, and cesarean delivery. FGR represents the second most common cause of perinatal mortality related to an increased risk of perinatal complications such as *hypoxemia*, *low Apgar scores*, and *cord blood acidemia*, with possible negative effects for neonatal outcomes. In addition to its significant perinatal impact, FGR also has an impact on the long-term health outcomes. It has been associated with metabolic programming that increases the risk of future development of metabolic syndrome, consequent cardiovascular diseases, and endocrine disease. Overall, growth-restricted fetuses experience worse neurodevelopmental outcomes and are at an increased risk of noncommunicable diseases in adulthood, such as hypertension (HTN), metabolic syndrome, insulin resistance, Type-2 diabetes mellitus, coronary artery disease, and stroke. Perinatal outcomes are largely dependent on the severity of FGR, with the worst outcomes noted in fetuses with estimated fetal weights (EFWs) at less than the 3rd percentile or in association with abnormal fetal Doppler. Prenatal recognition of FGR is a major factor identified in strategies aimed at preventing stillbirth, in which up to 30% of cases are associated with FGR.

■ TERMINOLOGY AND DEFINITIONS

There is no internationally recognized, integrated definition for the term "fetal growth restriction." The definition, diagnosis, and optimal management of FGR have generated controversy as clinicians strive for more harmonized care. FGR is defined as the failure of the fetus to meet its genetic potential for growth due to a pathological factor, most commonly placental dysfunction. FGR is commonly defined as an *ultrasonographic EFW* below the 10th percentile while *small for gestational age (SGA)* is used to describe a newborn whose birth weight is less than the 10th centile for a population for gestational age. FGR has considerable overlap with SGA but is more difficult to define in practice, as not all FGR infants have a birth weight <10th centile. A significant challenge in the prenatal management of FGR is differentiating the constitutionally small fetus from one who is pathologically growth restricted and at a risk for postnatal complications. Of all fetuses diagnosed as FGR 18–22% will be constitutionally small but healthy at birth with a normal outcome.

Growth restriction implies a pathological restriction of the growth potential, as a result, growth-restricted fetuses may manifest evidence of fetal compromise (abnormal Doppler studies, reduced liquor volume). SGA includes both normal healthy fetuses as well as those who are small because of pathological causes. About 50–70% of SGA fetuses are constitutionally small, with fetal growth appropriate for maternal size and ethnicity, the likelihood of FGR is higher in severe SGA infants. Historically SGA birth has been defined using population centiles. Use of customized centiles for maternal characteristics (maternal height, weight, parity, and ethnic group) as well as gestational age at delivery and infant sex, identifies small babies at higher risk of morbidity and mortality than those identified by population centiles. It has become increasingly apparent that many infants whose weight is less than the 10th centile are completely normal and are constitutionally small. Conversely, adverse perinatal outcomes are observed in infants whose birth weight lies between 10 and 20th centile, who have not achieved their growth potential. This has led investigators to recommend the use of customized chart.

The stillbirth rate of fetuses with weight <10th percentile at all gestational ages is approximately 1.5%, which is twice than that of a normal growth fetus; with fetal weight <5th percentile, the stillbirth rate can be as high as 2.5%. Important new information related to definition of FGR has been obtained from the Prospective Observational Trial to Optimize Pediatric Health (PORTO) study which included over 1,100 pregnancies with nonanomalous fetuses with EFW < 10th percentile on ultrasound examination, among these only 2% of fetuses between the 3rd and 10th percentile

(5/254) experienced adverse perinatal outcomes, while 6.2% of those <3rd percentile (51/826) had an adverse outcome and all eight mortalities were in this group. The investigators also observed a significant association with adverse outcomes and abnormal umbilical artery (UA) Doppler regardless of the EFW. The presence of oligohydramnios was important when associated with a weight less than the 3rd centile. These observations suggest that an appropriate definition of FGR should include a fetal weight less than the 3rd percentile with abnormal fetal growth velocity and the UA Doppler flow. Fetuses with a normal growth velocity and Doppler flow particularly EFW greater than the 3rd percentile are more likely constitutionally small normal fetuses.

The Royal College of Obstetricians and Gynaecologists (RCOG) has defined FGR as EFW <10th customized centile, or AC <10th population centile and high-risk FGR when EFW <3rd centile. International Federation of Gynaecology and Obstetrics (FIGO) has defined FGR based on fetal size percentile with Doppler abnormalities and have used the term SGA when EFW or birth weight lies below the 10th percentile. The Society for Maternal Fetal Medicine has defined FGR as ultrasound EFW or AC below the 10th percentile for gestational age. ACOG has defined SGA as an infant with a birth weight <10th centile for a population or customized standard **(Fig. 1)**.

The major member societies of FIGO follow a definition using the 10th percentile as a means of diagnosing an SGA fetus, which then leads to further testing, assessment, and follow-up. To decrease the likelihood of a false-positive and false-negative diagnoses of FGR, a consensus-based definition for placenta-mediated FGR has been proposed via a Delphi procedure. The consensus definition was based on a combination of measures of fetal size (fetal weight estimation and abdominal circumference) and abnormal Doppler findings in the umbilical, uterine, and middle cerebral arteries (MCA).

■ DEFINITION USED IN DIFFERENT COUNTRIES

Table 1 shows the definition used in different countries.

■ EARLY- VERSUS LATE-ONSET FGR

It has been suggested that FGR should be broadly classified, based on gestational age at the time of diagnosis, into early-onset FGR (<32 weeks) and late-onset FGR (≥32 weeks). The rationale underlying this classification is based on differences between these two phenotypes in severity, natural history, Doppler findings, and association with hypertensive complications, placental findings, and management.

Early-onset FGR

It has a prevalence of 0.5–1%, is usually more severe, and is more likely to be associated with abnormal UA Doppler than late-onset FGR. The underlying placental pathology is frequently similar to that observed in cases of early-onset preeclampsia (maternal vascular malperfusion), which explains the strong association of early-onset FGR with preeclampsia. Early-onset FGR is usually easier to detect, and the natural history tends to follow a predictable sequence of Doppler changes in the UA and ductus venosus. The main challenge in cases of early-onset FGR is management (i.e., timing of delivery), determined by balancing between the opposing risks of stillbirth and prematurity.

Late-onset FGR

It is more common than early-onset FGR with a prevalence of 5–10%. In contrast to early-onset FGR, it is usually milder, is less likely to be associated with preeclampsia, and is usually associated with normal UA Doppler. Therefore, the main challenge with regard to late-onset FGR is diagnosis, while management (i.e., delivery) is relatively simple given that the diagnosis is commonly made during the late-preterm or term periods, where the risks associated with delivery are relatively small. The diagnosis of late-onset FGR mainly relies on adaptive changes in the cerebral circulation "redistribution" or "brain-sparing effect", which is reflected by low resistance to flow in the MCA thereby generating a low cerebroplacental ratio (CPR). Given that the UA and ductus venosus Doppler studies are usually normal in cases of late-onset FGR, the natural history in these cases is less predictable and there is a risk of sudden decompensation and stillbirth.

■ EARLY- VERSUS LATE-ONSET GROWTH RESTRICTION (INTERNATIONAL FEDERATION OF GYNAECOLOGY AND OBSTETRICS)

Table 2 lists the early versus late-onset growth restriction.

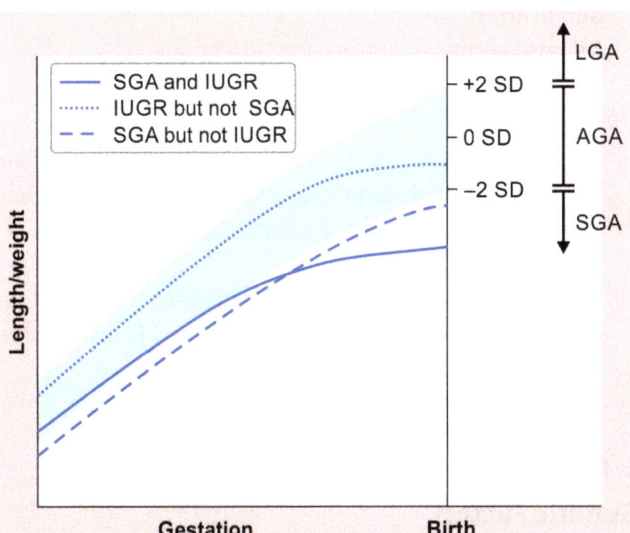

Fig. 1: Growth Chart in FGR, SGA and in both SGA and IUGR. (EFW: estimated fetal weight; FGR: fetal growth restriction; IUGR: intrauterine growth restriction; SGA: small for gestational age)
Source: Researchgate

Fetal Growth Restriction

TABLE 1: Definition used in different countries.

Country	United Kingdom	New Zealand	Canada	Ireland	United States of America	France
SGA	Birth weight <10th customized centile	EFW or birth weight <10th customized centile	EFW <10th population centile	EFW <10th customized centile	Birth weight <10th population centile	EFW or birth weight <10th population centile
FGR	EFW <10th customized centile, or AC <10th population centile	EFW <10th customized centile or AC 5th population centile	EFW <10th or AC <10th population centiles	EFW <10th customized centile	EFW <10th population centile	EFW <10th customized centile
Definition of high-risk FGR/IUGR	EFW <3rd centile	EFW <3rd centile, abnormal UA, uterine artery, MCA or CPR Doppler	Not specified	EFW <3rd, abnormal UA Doppler, oligohydramnios, or reduced interval growth	Not specified	Evidence of reduced/arresting of growth with or without abnormal UA or cerebral Doppler, oligohydramnios

(AC: abdominal circumference; CPR: cerebroplacental ratio; EFW: estimated fetal weight; FGR: fetal growth restriction; IUGR: intrauterine growth restriction; MCA: middle cerebral artery; SGA: small for gestational age; UA: umbilical artery)

TABLE 2: Early versus late-onset growth restriction.

Early-onset FGR (<32 weeks)	Late-onset FGR (≥3 weeks)

• EFW or AC <3rd percentile or
• UA with AREDV or
• EFW or AC <10th percentile, combined with one or more of the following:
  – UA-PI >95th percentile
  – UtA-PI >95th percentile
	• EFW or AC <3rd percentile or
	• ≥2 of the following three criteria:
	  1. EFW or AC <10th percentile
	  2. EFW or AC crossing percentiles >2 quartiles on growth percentiles
	  3. CPR <5th percentile or UA-PI >95th percentile

(AC: abdominal circumference; AREDV: absent or reversed end-diastolic velocity; CPR: cerebroplacental ratio; EFW: estimation of fetal weight; FGR: fetal growth restriction; UA-PI: umbilical artery pulsatility index; UtA-PI: mean uterine arteries pulsatility index)
Source: FIGO (International Federation of Gynecology and Obstetrics) initiative on fetal growth: best practice advice for screening, diagnosis, and management of fetal growth restriction

■ RISK FACTORS

The genetically predetermined growth potential of the fetus can be impaired by maternal, placental, and fetal factors that interfere with the normal mechanisms regulating fetal growth.

Maternal Factors

- Hypoxemia (chronic lung disease, high altitude)
- Anemia
- Smoking, substance abuse (cocaine, methamphetamine)
- Malabsorption, poor weight gain
- Environmental toxins—air pollution, heavy metals (lead, mercury).

Placental Factors

- Maternal vascular malperfusion pathology (infarction, fibrin deposition, chronic abruption)
- Fetal vascular malperfusion pathology
- Chronic placental inflammation, e.g., villitis of unknown etiology
- Confined placental mosaicism.

Umbilical Cord Factors

- Increased coiling
- Increased cord length
- True knot
- Single artery
- Marginal or velamentous cord insertion.

Fetal Disorders

- Genetic disorders (chromosome microdeletion/duplication, single gene mutation, epigenetic disorders)
- Structural anomaly (congenital heart disease, gastroschisis)
- Congenital infections [toxoplasmosis, rubella *Cytomegalovirus*, herpes simplex, and HIV (TORCH) infection, syphilis, *Zika virus*, malaria]
- Teratogen exposure (drugs, toxins).

■ ETIOLOGY

Genetic Factor

Chromosomal abnormality has been suggested to contribute to up to 5% of FGR cases; triploidy, trisomy 13 and 18 are important considerations in early-onset FGR. Aneuploidy is responsible for 2–5% of FGR and the

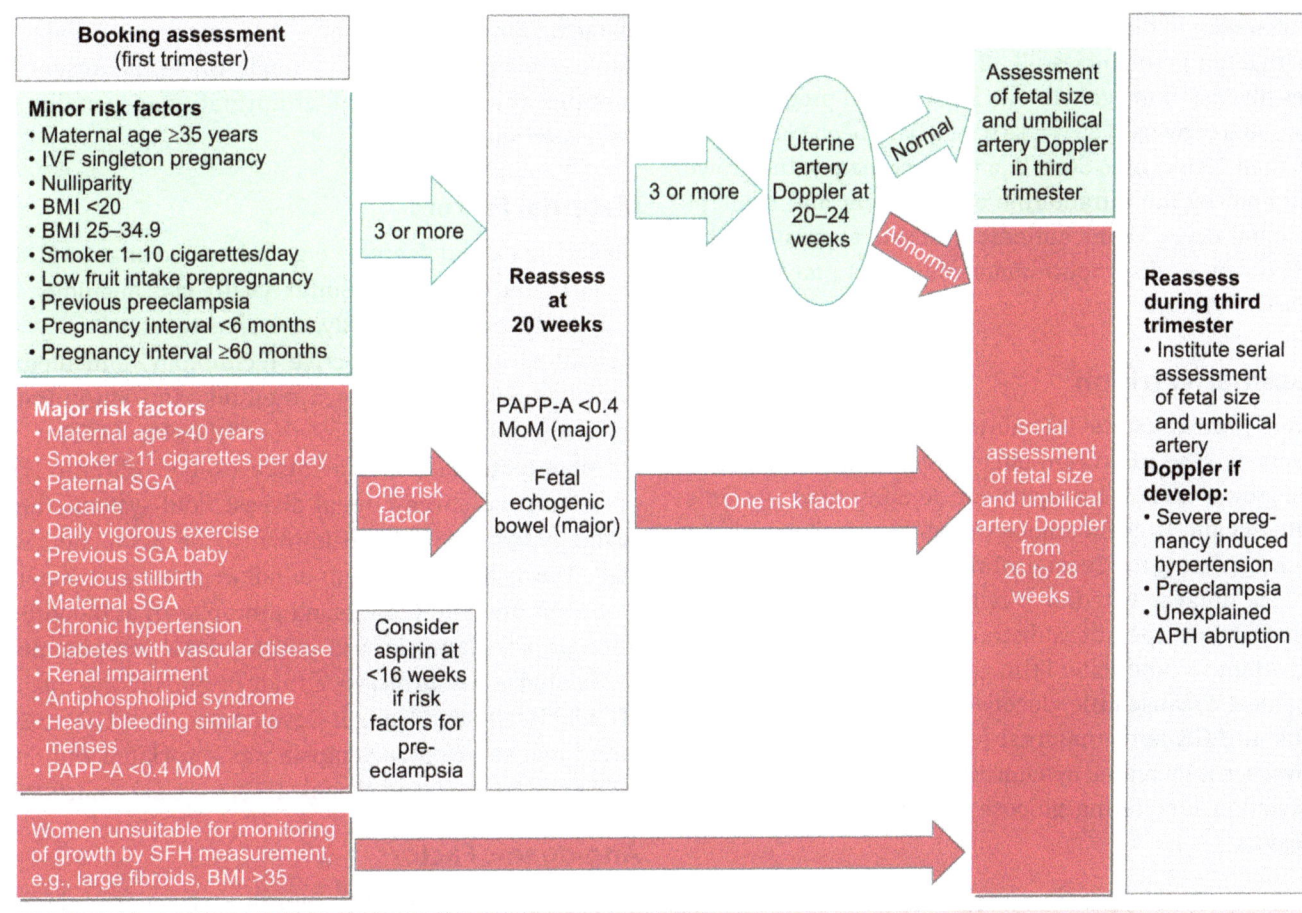

Fig. 2: Screening for small for gestational age (SGA) fetus and management.
(APH: antepartum hemorrhage; BMI: body mass index; IVF: in vitro fertilization; MoM: multiple of the median; PAPP-A: pregnancy-associated plasma protein A; SFH: symphysis fundal height)
Source: RCOG guideline.

incidence increases to 20% if growth restriction is detected in the first-half of pregnancy. Any pregnancy noted to have symmetric intrauterine growth restriction (IUGR) before 24 weeks should be considered as a suspect for aneuploidy. In 1-6% cases of FGR with normal karyotype submicroscopic deletion or duplication can be found using chromosomal microarray (CMA) analysis even when FGR is an apparently isolated finding.

Structural Abnormality

Fetal growth restriction is more prevalent in fetuses with structural malformations, and the risk increases with multiple anomalies. Many types of structural abnormalities are associated with FGR without any specific *genetic aberration*. Fetuses with congenital heart defects are far more likely to be growth restricted compared with normal fetuses as are fetuses with gastroschisis. Although fetuses with a single UA may be of low birth weight, this is not generally a result of FGR.

Infectious Disease

There is ample evidence for a casual relationship between infectious disease and FGR for rubella and *Cytomegalovirus*, there is also some relationship with varicella, toxoplasmosis, human immunodeficiency virus, and *Zika* virus. Malaria is known to be a common cause of FGR in the underdeveloped countries. The main mechanism involved in the pathogenesis of FGR in these cases is a decline in the cell population. Although no bacterial infection is known to cause FGR, histological *chorioamnionitis* is strongly associated with symmetric IUGR between 28 and 36 weeks of gestation and with asymmetric IUGR after 36 weeks. Fetal infection accounts for 5-10% of FGR.

Multiple Gestation

These are associated with a progressive decrease in fetal and placental weight as the number of offspring increases. The increase in fetal weight in *singleton pregnancy* is linear from approximately 22-24 weeks until approximately

32–36 weeks. In dichorionic twin growth trajectory is similar to singleton pregnancies till 32 weeks after which growth rates diverge. If the growth rate for singleton pregnancies is used, 38% of twins at 35 weeks would have been classified as less than 10th centile SGA. In a twin pregnancy, the growth is limited by the intrauterine environment and available placental mass. Monochorionic twins are at greater risk of FGR owing to disproportionate sharing of placentas and *twin-twin transfusion*.

Maternal Nutrition

Severe protein-calorie malnutrition can affect fetal growth adversely. The important effect of maternal nutrition on fetal growth and birth weight were demonstrated by studies in Russia and Holland among women who had inadequate nutrition during the Second World War.

It is unclear whether it is generalized calorie intake reduction or specific substrate limitation or both are important in producing FGR. Glucose uptake by the fetus is critical because little gluconeogenesis occurs in normal fetus. In FGR fetus maternal-fetal glucose concentration difference is increased as a function of the severity of growth restriction facilitating glucose transfer across the small placenta.

Environmental Toxins and Teratogens

Maternal cigarette smoking reduces birth weight by approximately 135–300 g in a dose response manner and the fetus is symmetrically small. If smoking is stopped before the third trimester, the adverse effect on birth weight is reduced. Reduction in birth weight occurs with maternal intake of alcohol as little as one or two drinks/day. Cocaine and heroin use similarly reduces birth weight, reduction in head circumference is more pronounced than the reduction in birth weight. Some prescribed medications, e.g., antiepileptic drugs (hydantoin, valproic acid), warfarin, and antineoplastic agents (cyclophosphamide) also has been implicated in FGR. Finally, maternal exposure to teratogens such as radiation is another important etiology of FGR.

Placental Factors

Adequate trophoblast invasion of decidua and resultant alteration in uterine blood flow is necessary for the initial establishment and adherence of the pregnancy and also for an adequate supply of nutrients to the fetus. In FGR particularly early-onset FGR the depth of invasion of trophoblast is shallow and the endovascular invasion is rudimentary resulting in suboptimal uteroplacental perfusion. The terminal villi are maldeveloped, absent end diastolic flow indicates that these morphological changes are associated with increased vascular impedance. Velamentous insertion of cord, abruptio placenta, and placenta previa are also associated with FGR. A single UA in the absence of aneuploidy or structural abnormality is usually not associated with FGR.

Maternal Factors

Several maternal factors, e.g., advanced maternal age, racial/ethnic origin (e.g., South Asian), consanguinity, low body mass index, nulliparity, use of recreational drugs and alcohol-assisted reproductive technology, and medical disorders, such as diabetes mellitus, and autoimmune conditions influence fetal growth and the risk of FGR.

Most maternal vascular diseases, e.g., chronic HTN, preeclampsia, chronic renal disease, and systemic lupus erythematosus (SLE) are known to be associated with FGR. This is likely the result of failure to expand maternal blood volume and diminished uteroplacental blood flow. Though preeclampsia and chronic HTN are commonly considered as *causal factors*, a study by the National Institute of Child Health and Human Development (NICHD) in 2019 found that severe preeclampsia was associated with FGR, mild preeclampsia, and chronic HTN were not associated.

Angiogenic Factors

Angiogenic factors play a key role in the regulation of placental vascular development. Low first-trimester placental growth factor (PlGF) levels have been shown to be associated with adverse pregnancy outcomes including preeclampsia and SGA. Elevated level of soluble fms-like tyrosine kinase-1 (sFlt1) and endoglin, and decreased concentration of PlGF have been reported in both preeclampsia and FGR. A multicenter screening study found detection rate of a combined screening using maternal factors, fetal biometry, and serum PlGF and *alpha-fetoprotein* at 19–24 weeks for the delivery of SGA infants below the fifth percentile at <32, 32–36, and ≥37 weeks of gestation 100%, 76%, and 38%, respectively, at a false-positive rate of 10%.

■ EVALUATION AND MANAGEMENT

Diagnosis

Evaluation and management of suspected FGR involve:
- Adequate history taking to identify the risk factors and correction of remediable causes.
- Accurate determination of gestational age and confirming the diagnosis.
- Distinguishing between the constitutionally small and the growth-restricted fetus.
- Monitoring fetal weight trajectories.
- Managing maternal comorbidities.
- Serial assessment of fetal well-being.
- Preterm delivery when indicated.

History

A detailed maternal and family history is essential to correctly identify the etiology of FGR. This should include information on maternal age, racial/ethnic group, height, and weight, nutritional status, socioeconomic status, medications, cigarette smoking, and use of recreational drugs. In addition, history of any chronic medical conditions, personal or family history suggestive of thrombophilia, genetic disorders or consanguinity, obstetric history including birth weight of previous children should be included.

Detailed Anatomy Scan

Detailed anatomy scan should be routinely performed when FGR is suspected, especially in cases of early-onset severe FGR. The presence of major structural anomalies, soft sonographic markers, or disorders of amniotic fluid (e.g., polyhydramnios) may raise the possibility of chromosomal, subchromosomal, or single gene abnormalities as the cause of FGR. Confirmation of gestational age based on first-trimester ultrasound (when available) should be the first step when FGR is suspected; the earliest scan with a crown-rump length of at least 10 mm should be used.

Women who have a major risk factor [odds ratio (OR) >2.0] should be referred for serial ultrasound measurement of fetal size and assessment of well-being with umbilical artery Doppler from 26 to 28 weeks of pregnancy. Women who have three or more minor risk factors should be referred for uterine artery (UtA) Doppler at 20–24 weeks of gestation.

Abdominal Palpation

Abdominal palpation has limited accuracy for the prediction of SGA neonates. Serial measurement of symphysis fundal height (SFH) is recommended at each antenatal appointment from 24 weeks of pregnancy. SFH should be plotted on a customized chart rather than a population-based chart as this may improve prediction of SGA. Women with a single SFH which plots below the 10th centile or serial measurements which demonstrate slow or static growth by crossing centiles should be referred for ultrasound measurement of fetal size.

In a meta-analysis of 34 observational studies, SFH was reported to have a sensitivity of 58% and a specificity of 87% for predicting birth weight below the 10th percentile but there was marked heterogeneity between the studies, mainly due to the use of different SFH charts. A single SFH between 32 and 34 weeks has been reported to be approximately 65–85% sensitive and 96% specific for detecting FGR. It is important to acknowledge that factors such as maternal obesity, uterine leiomyomas, and polyhydramnios may further limit the accuracy of SFH as a screening tool.

Confirm the Diagnosis

An estimated fetal weight <10th percentile or abdominal circumference <10th percentile signifies a SGA fetus. It is then the clinician's task to distinguish between the constitutionally small fetus that achieves its normal growth potential and not at increased risk of adverse outcomes from the similarly small fetus whose growth potential is restricted (FGR) and is at increased risk of perinatal morbidity and mortality.

Sonographic fetal biometry is the cornerstone for detection of fetal growth disorders. The diagnosis of FGR is based on discrepancies between actual and expected sonographic biometric measurements for a given gestational age. In customized charts, fetal weight and growth are adjusted for variables known to impact fetal size, including maternal height, weight, age, parity, ethnicity, and fetal sex. Adjustment for these variables is suggested to allow for better identification of SGA fetuses at risk of perinatal complications. When a fetus <10th percentile weight for gestational age is identified, monitoring fetal growth and fetal physiology over the time is required. Normal fetal anatomy, normal growth trajectory, normal Doppler velocimetry of the UA and/or MCA, and normal amniotic fluid volume suggest a constitutionally small fetus or a fetus that is minimally impacted from uteroplacental insufficiency or other pathologic factors that impair fetal growth. Using a lower thresh hold (between 5th and 10th centile) to define FGR, may help distinguishing between a small fetus at an increased risk of adverse outcomes from a small fetus at a low risk.

Characteristics of Constitutionally Small Fetus

- Modest smallness (estimated weight between 5th and 10th centile)
- Normal growth velocity across gestation
- Normal physiology [normal amniotic fluid volume (AFV), UA Doppler]
- Abdominal circumference growth velocity above 10th centile
- Appropriate size in relation to maternal characteristics (height, weight, race/ethnicity).

Maternal Characteristics

The maternal characteristics have a major influence on fetal growth potential; race and ethnicity should be taken into account when diagnosing a case of FGR. Overdiagnosis of SGA among non-white population using a white reference have been reported in fetal growth studies by the Eunice Kennedy Shriver National Institute of Child Health and Human Development (NICHD) in the United States. The study included low-risk pregnancies between 4 ethnic groups and illustrated that the 5th percentiles of growth for White, Hispanic, Black, and Asian women are different. Recent publication of World Health Organization (WHO) on fetal growth charts in low-risk pregnancies from 10 countries in Africa, Asia, Europe, and South America also showed considerable variation in both fetal ultrasound parameters and birth weight between countries and described these differences as "adaptive," or physiological.

Fetal Survey

A detailed fetal anatomic survey should be performed in all cases since 10% of FGR are accompanied by congenital anomalies and 20–60% of malformed infants are SGA. Anomalies associated with FGR include omphalocele, gastroschisis, diaphragmatic hernia, skeletal dysplasia, and a congenital heart defect. Fetal echocardiography is indicated if any suspicion arises after a level II ultrasound sonography (USG).

Indications of Fetal Genetic Studies

- Early-onset FGR (<24 weeks)
- Severe FGR (<5th centile)
- Symmetric growth restriction
- FGR with major structural anomaly
- FGR with soft ultrasound markers associated with an increased risk of aneuploidy, such as thickened nuchal fold/choroid plexus cyst, and abnormal hand positioning.

The evaluation of the fetal karyotype/microarray is indicated if FGR is associated with structural anomalies, ultrasound markers of aneuploidy, or severe early-onset of FGR (<5th percentile before 24 weeks of gestation). The combination of FGR with a fetal malformation or polyhydramnios should prompt genetic counseling.

Although chromosome abnormalities are more frequent in FGR with structural anomalies a systematic review that included fetuses with no structural malformations found mean rate of chromosomal abnormalities as 6.4%. RCOG suggests karyotyping in severely SGA fetuses with structural anomalies and in those detected before 23 weeks of gestation, especially if UA Doppler is normal. The American College of Obstetricians and Gynecologists suggest genetic counseling and offering diagnostic testing by CMA for patients with diagnosis of FGR before 32 weeks or FGR in combination with polyhydramnios or fetal malformation. FGR with a normal microarray could be due to a single gene disorder, particularly if FGR is severe (<1st percentile) and/or associated with additional ultrasound findings (e.g., short-long bones, microcephaly, cardiac defects, relative macrocephaly, abnormalities of the face, hands, and/or genitalia).

Work-up for Infection

Infections associated with FGR include *Cytomegalovirus*, toxoplasmosis, rubella, and varicella. Sonographic markers for fetal infection are often nonspecific but include echogenicity and calcification of the brain and/or liver and hydrops. Maternal serum should be examined for seropositivity when an infection is suspected clinically because of maternal history, physical examination, or fetal ultrasound findings and also if evidence of acute infection is present. Serological screening for congenital *Cytomegalovirus* and toxoplasma infection should be offered in severely SGA fetuses (RCOG).

Work-up for Antiphospholipid Syndrome

Although early-onset placental insufficiency is one of the clinical criteria for the diagnosis of antiphospholipid syndrome by expert consensus, a link between antiphospholipid antibodies alone and FGR has not been established, and there is insufficient evidence to support screening all women with FGR for these antibodies.

Management

Fetal growth restriction can result from a variety of maternal, fetal, and placental conditions. Although the primary underlying mechanisms for FGR are varied, they often share the same final common pathway of suboptimal fetal nutrition and uteroplacental perfusion. Chromosomal disorders and congenital malformations are responsible for approximately 20% of cases; suboptimal perfusion of maternal and placental circulation is the most common cause of FGR and accounts for 25–30% of all cases.

The management is based on early diagnosis, determining the cause and severity of FGR, counseling the parents, optimal fetal surveillance, and timely delivery to reduce perinatal mortality and minimize short- and long-term morbidity. There is currently no consensus on the best approach to the management of FGR, despite a large body of literature on the subject. Accumulating evidence suggests a benefit to the use of UA Doppler in the surveillance of FGR.

The management depends on the specific abnormality, FGR resulting from intrinsic risk factors, e.g., aneuploidy, congenital malformation, or infection often cannot be improved with any intervention. FGR related to uteroplacental insufficiency has a better prognosis, but the risk of adverse outcomes remains high.

The optimal management of pregnancy with suspected growth restriction related to uteroplacental insufficiency consists of serial USG to see the following:

- Fetal growth velocity
- Fetal behavior biophysical profile (BPP)
- Impedance to blood flow in fetal arterial and venous system (Doppler velocimetry)

Fetal Growth Velocity

Ultrasound estimated fetal weight is plotted on a population-based or customized growth curve to monitor growth velocity. Persistent growth deficiency in multiple examinations over many weeks strengthens the likelihood of FGR. Conversely, normal growth velocity in a small fetus suggests a constitutionally small fetus. To ascertain the growth velocity serial sonograms are generally obtained at 3–4 weeks intervals in fetuses with mild FGR (e.g., EFW near the 10th percentile, normal amniotic fluid volume, normal Doppler findings); and a shorter 2–3 weeks interval is appropriate for the fetus with features of moderate or severe disease (e.g., EFW ≤5th percentile, oligohydramnios, abnormal Doppler findings).

Doppler Velocimetry

The rationale behind the application of Doppler velocimetry in fetal growth assessment is that it can identify uteroplacental function through evaluation of the uterine and umbilical arteries. Doppler of the ductus venosus and MCA, as well as other fetal vessels, may also provide information about the fetal hemodynamic status.

Uterine Artery Doppler

In high-risk population, UtA Doppler at 20–24 weeks of pregnancy has a moderate predictive value for a severely SGA neonate. Women with an abnormal UtA Doppler at 20–24 weeks [defined as a pulsatility index (PI) >95th centile] and/or notching should be referred for serial ultrasound measurement of fetal size and assessment of well-being with UA Doppler commencing at 26–28 weeks of pregnancy **(Figs. 3A and B)**.

Umbilical Artery Doppler

Umbilical artery Doppler is an excellent tool for the assessment in FGR when the etiology is placental dysfunction related to progressive obliteration of the villus vasculature. Doppler velocimetry of the UA is the primary surveillance tool for monitoring pregnancies with suspected FGR. Normal diastolic flow is infrequently associated with significant perinatal morbidity or mortality and is strong evidence of fetal well-being; this finding provides support for delaying delivery when it is important to achieve further fetal maturity. When 30% of the villous vasculature ceases to function, an increase in UA resistance leading to reduced end-diastolic flow is consistently seen and is a weak predictor of adverse outcomes. When 60–70% of the villous vasculature is obliterated, UA diastolic flow is absent or reversed, and the fetal prognosis is poor. Reversed diastolic flow is associated with poorer neonatal outcomes than absent diastolic flow. In a study of 143 FGR pregnancies with either reversed or absent UA flow, mortality was over fivefold higher with the reversed flow.

After the diagnosis of FGR weekly Doppler velocimetry of the UA is indicated. If consecutive Doppler results are normal, the frequency of Doppler examination can be decreased to 2 weeks intervals. The 2 weeks interval is reasonable for the fetus with EFW ≥5th percentile, normal growth velocity, normal amniotic fluid volume, and no maternal risk factors for placental dysfunction. If UA diastolic flow is present but decreased, pulsatility index (UAPI) >95th percentile, weekly Doppler evaluation is recommended to look for progression to absent or reversed flow **(Figs. 4A to D)**.

Absent or reversed end-diastolic flow in the UA can be a sign of impending fetal cardiovascular and metabolic deterioration. If either of these abnormal patterns is identified, delivery should be considered. The decision to deliver in this setting is based on gestational age as long as daily nonstress test (NST) or BPP testing is normal. The absence of abnormal flow patterns in the ductus venosus has been used to support the decision to extend such a pregnancy and may enable the pregnancy to be prolonged for as long as 2 weeks; however, clinical use of this test is controversial.

Middle Cerebral Artery

Doppler's interrogation of the MCA also provides information about the hemodynamic status of the fetus. The fetal brain in uncomplicated pregnancies has a high resistance circulation. With progressive hypoxia, the blood flow increases to compensate for the decrease in available oxygen (brain-sparing effect). This result in a reduction in

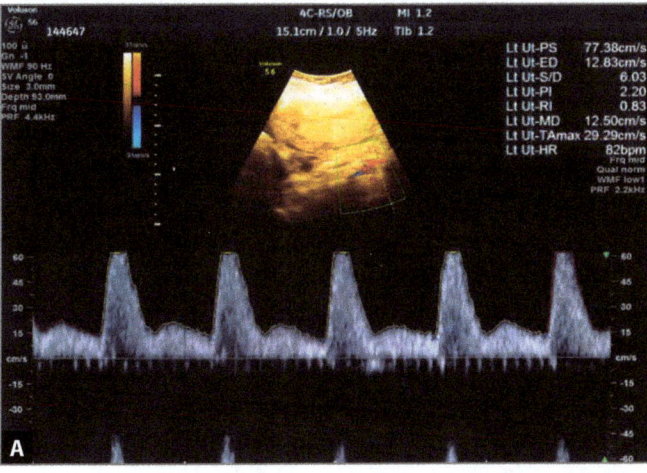 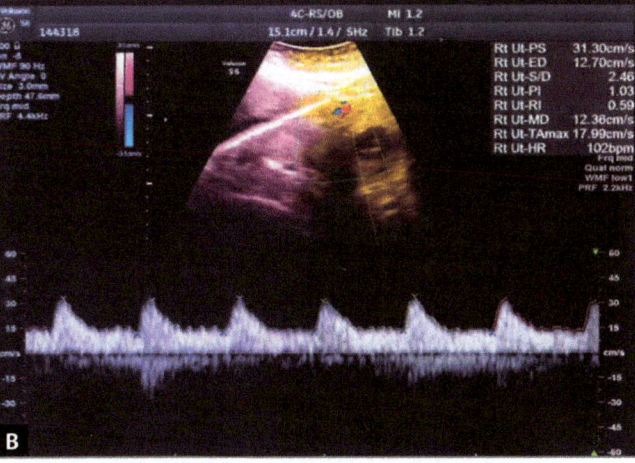

Figs. 3A and B: (A) Uterine artery Doppler in early pregnancy showing diastolic notch; (B) Uterine artery Doppler in mid-pregnancy good blood flow in diastole.

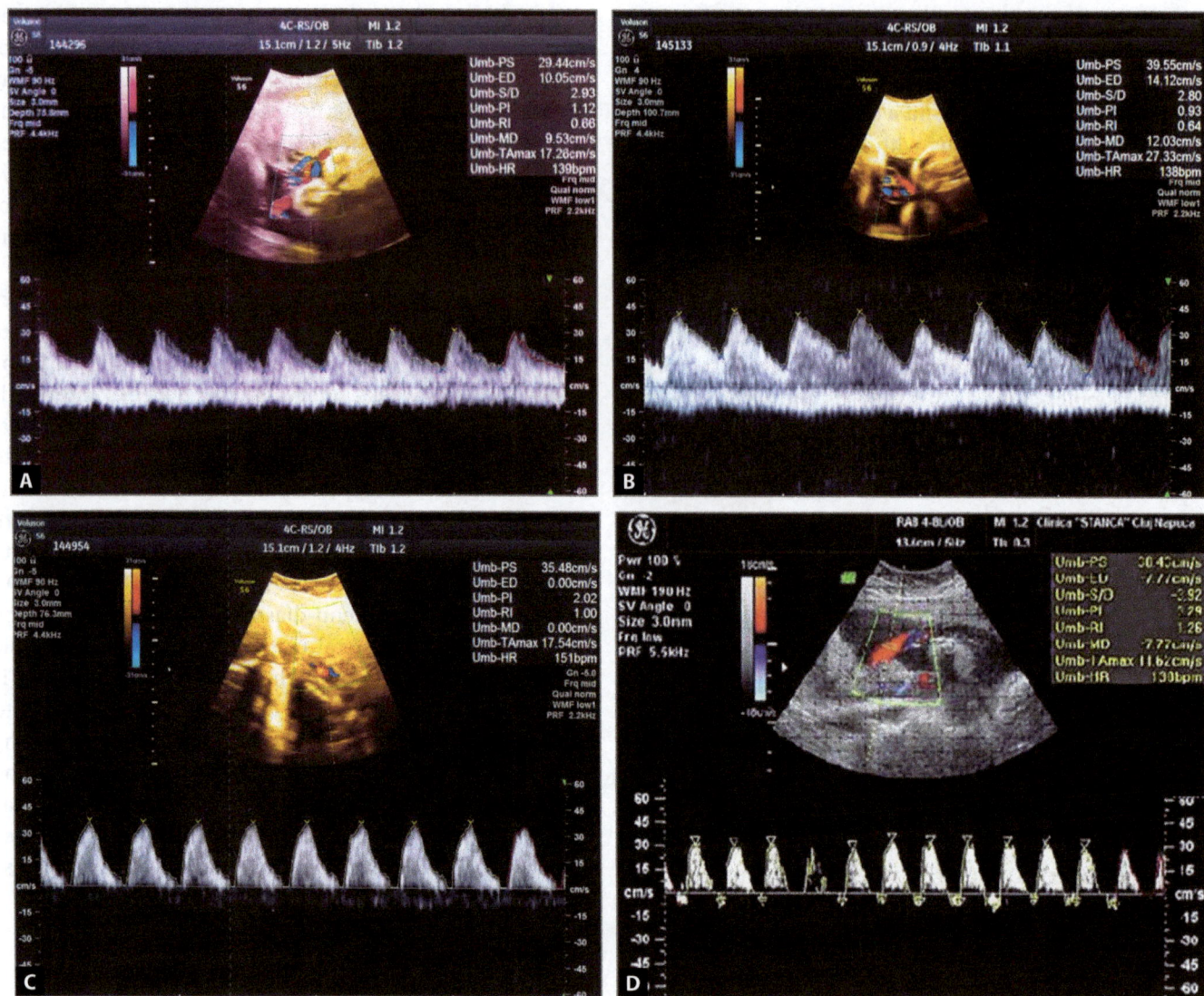

Figs. 4A to D: (A) Normal S/D ratio of UA at 30 weeks; (B) UA Doppler at 36 weeks showing reduced S/D ratio; (C) UA absent diastolic flow; (D) Reverse flow in UA.

the Doppler parameters used to assess blood flow through the MCA, the systolic/diastolic (S/D) ratio, resistance index, and pulsatility index decreases. Subsequent normalization of the indices may occur when the autoregulatory response becomes dysfunctional. There is no convincing evidence that interrogation of the MCA Doppler alone is useful in guiding clinical decisions about the timing of delivery, although MCA Doppler alterations may be useful as an adjunct to UA Doppler interrogation for assessing the severity of hypoxia and predicting neonatal outcomes **(Figs. 5A and B)**.

Cerebroplacental Ratio

The cerebroplacental Doppler ratio is the middle cerebral artery pulsatility index (MCA-PI), or (resistance index) divided by the UA-PI (or resistance index); a low CPR indicates fetal blood flow redistribution (brain sparing). CPR was initially described for detecting FGR fetuses. Following a few initial studies, it was abandoned because it did not appear to provide more information than the UA alone. In the last 10 years, many additional studies measured this ratio to predict the perinatal outcome in FGR pregnancies and reported widely variable estimates of its accuracy. Several threshold values for CPR (<1, <1.05, ≤1.08, <5th percentile) have been proposed for predicting adverse outcomes **(Fig. 6)**.

Ductus Venosus Doppler

Doppler's interrogation of the ductus venosus provides information about the hemodynamic status of the fetus. Flow in the venous circulation is forward and uniform in normal fetuses. Changes in the venous circulation in the growth-restricted fetus, including absent or reversed flow in the ductus venosus (absent or reversed a-wave) or pulsatile umbilical venous flow are late findings, generally occurring approximately two weeks after changes are observed in the arterial circulation.

With progressively increasing umbilical arterial resistance, fetal cardiac performance can become impaired, and central

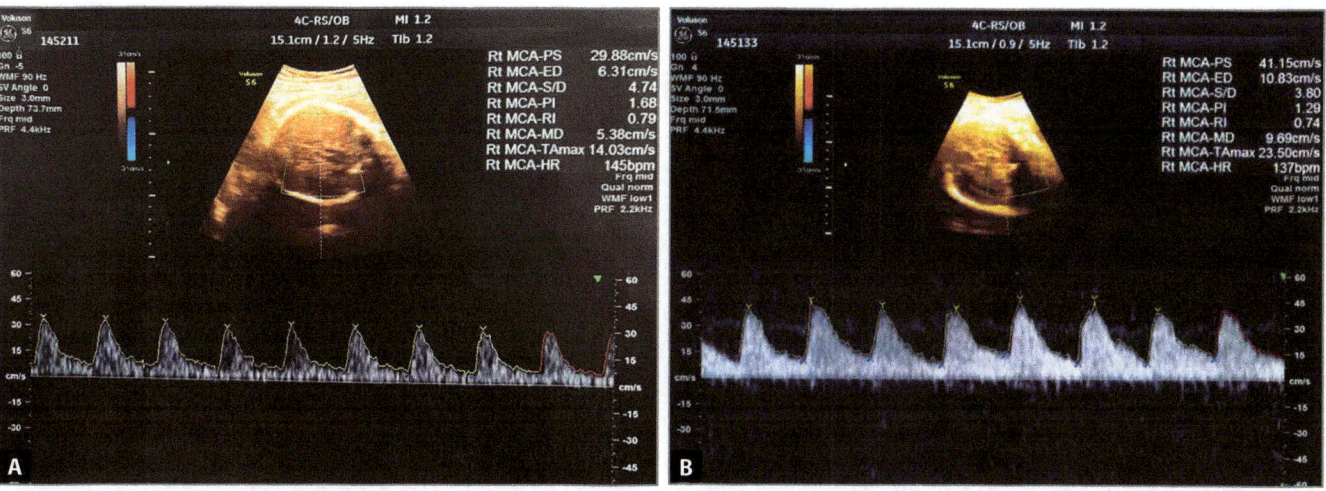

Figs. 5A and B: (A) Middle cerebral artery (MCA) Doppler showing resistance diastolic flow; (B) MCA Doppler shows brain-sparing effect.

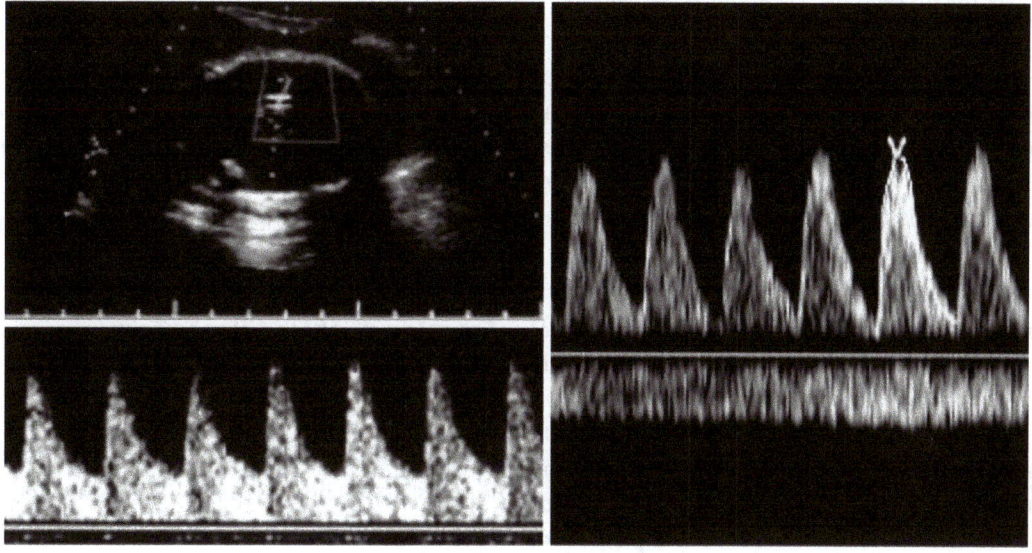

Fig. 6: Altered cerebroplacental ratio.
Source: Researchgate, RNSA.

venous pressure increases, resulting in reduced diastolic flow in the ductus venosus and other large veins. Vasodilatation of the ductus venosus diverts nutrient and oxygen-rich blood to the heart but enhances retrograde transmission of atrial pressure. The ductus venosus resistance index increases, ultimately with loss of the a-wave. An absent or reversed ductus venous a-wave indicates cardiovascular instability and can be a sign of impending acidemia and fetal death **(Figs. 7A and B)**.

Although the use of venous Doppler interrogation remains largely investigational, an increasing number of maternal-fetal medicine specialists are using this tool to avoid very preterm delivery in fetuses with absent or reversed end-diastolic arterial flow in the UA with reassuring antepartum fetal testing [nonstress test (NST) and biophysical profile (BPP)]. In these pregnancies, the absence of abnormal flow patterns in the ductus venosus is used to support the decision to extend the pregnancy to 32–34 weeks, if the NST and BPP remain reassuring. *Trial of Randomized Umbilical and Fetal Flow in Europe (TRUFFLE)* demonstrated no immediate neonatal benefit from delaying delivery until ductus venosus monitoring showed significant abnormalities (absent or reversed flow) and only a possible marginal benefit in neurodevelopment at 2 years of age.

Nonstress Test and Biophysical Profile

Either the NST with amniotic fluid volume determination or the BPP or a combination of both tests is reasonable for monitoring of fetal well-being. Observational studies have indicated that an abnormal BPP is a late manifestation of placental disease that appears to become abnormal 48–72 hours after ductus venosus Doppler abnormalities in 90% of cases. More recent studies have questioned the value of BPP in fetal surveillance in high-risk pregnancies, including

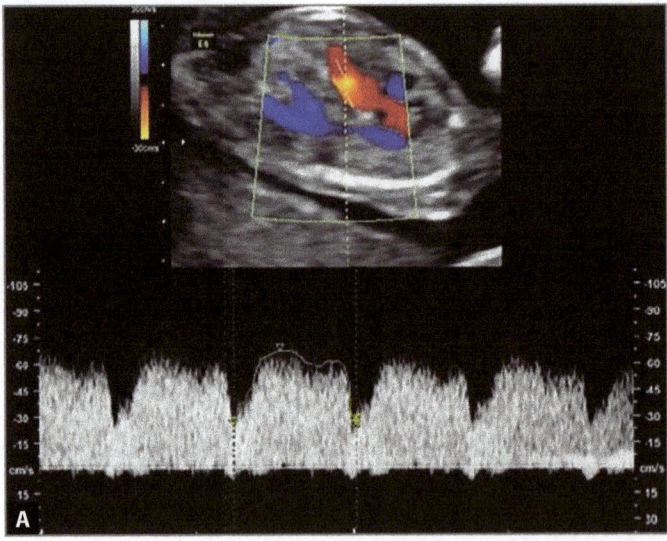 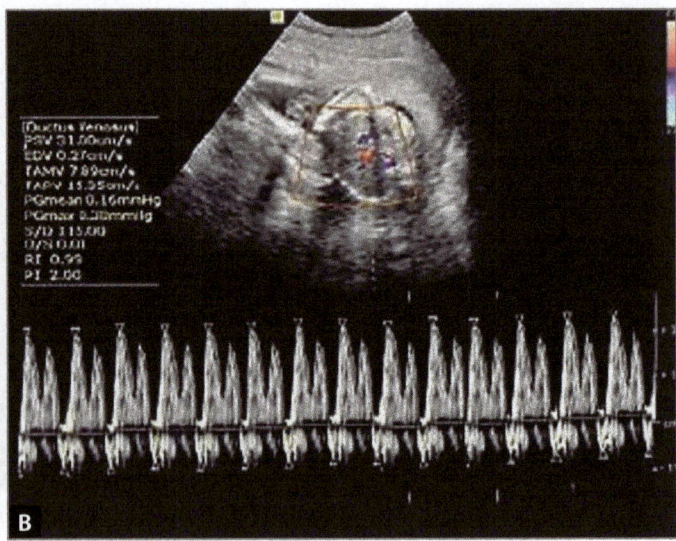

Figs. 7A and B: (A) DV Doppler with normal flow; (B) Reversed flow in DV in FGR.
(DV: ductus venosus; EDV: end-diastolic velocity; FGR: fetal growth restriction; PSV: Peak systolic velocity)

early-onset severe FGR, because of a high prevalence of false-positive and false-negative results. A Cochrane review concluded that available evidence from randomized controlled trials does not support the use of BPP as a test of fetal well-being in high-risk pregnancies.

Amniotic Fluid Volume

Oligohydramnios is defined as a single deepest vertical pocket of amniotic fluid of <2 cm. The PORTO study (a Multicenter Prospective Observational Trial to Optimize Pediatric Health in IUGR), which included >1,100 pregnancies with FGR, noted that amniotic fluid volume abnormalities did not independently increase the risk for adverse outcomes in FGR. There is currently a paucity of data on the role of amniotic fluid volume measurement in FGR management and delivery. Current guidelines on medically indicated late-preterm and early-term deliveries suggest delivery at 34 0/7 to 37 6/7 weeks of gestation for FGR associated with oligohydramnios.

Cardiotocography

Cardiotocography (CTG) is currently accepted as the primary method for fetal surveillance in high-risk pregnancies in the United States. Despite the absence of large prospective studies on the role of CTG in the management of FGR, a normal CTG in pregnancies with FGR is more likely to be associated with a normal perinatal outcome, and the presence of spontaneous repetitive late decelerations is accepted as an indication for delivery in viable pregnancies with FGR, irrespective of Doppler findings. Society for Maternal-Fetal Medicine (SMFM) suggests weekly CTG testing after viability in FGR without absent end-diastolic velocity (AEDV)/reversed end-diastolic velocity (REDV) and that the frequency should be increased when FGR is complicated by AEDV/REDV or other comorbid conditions or risk factors. Royal College of Obstetricians and Gynaecologists suggests that CTG should not be used as the only form of surveillance in SGA fetuses. Interpretation of the CTG should be based on short-term fetal heart rate variation from the computerized analysis.

Frequency of Nonstress Test and Biophysical Profile

Pregnancies with mild FGR (estimated weight 5th to <10th centile), normal growth velocity, and normal Doppler indices, do not need NSTs or BPPs. Normal Dopplers provide strong evidence of fetal well-being, especially in the absence of risk factors for or signs of uteroplacental insufficiency. For pregnancies with FGR that is severe (<5th centile) or with oligohydramnios, preeclampsia, decelerating growth velocity, increasing UA Doppler index, or other concerning findings, testing should be performed twice per week (e.g., two BPPs, two NSTs, or one NST and one BPP). For pregnancies with FGR and absent or reversed diastolic flow, perform daily testing because these fetuses can deteriorate rapidly. Monitor FGR pregnancies <32 weeks that have either absent or reversed flow of the UA with a combination of an NST every 12 hours and a daily BPP until delivery (UpToDate).

The general sequence of Doppler and biophysical changes in FGR are summarized below:

- A reduction in umbilical venous flow is the initial hemodynamic change. Venous flow is redistributed away from fetal liver towards the heart. Liver size decreases, causing a lag in abdominal circumference, which is the first biometric sign of FGR.

- UA Doppler indices increases (diminished end diastolic flow) due to increased resistance in placental vasculature.
- MCA Doppler index PI decreases (increased end diastolic flow), preferential perfusion of the brain (brain sparing effect).
- Increasing placental vascular resistance results in absent and then reversed end diastolic flow in the UA.
- MCA peak systolic velocity increases secondary to an increase in the PCO_2 and decrease in PO_2 in blood delivered to the brain.
- MCA PI normalizes or abnormally increases as diastolic flow falls due to loss of brain sparing hemodynamic changes.
- As cardiac performance deteriorates due to chronic hypoxemia and nutritional deprivation, absent or reversed end diastolic flow in the ductus venosus, pulsatile ductus venosus may develop.
- Lastly, tricuspid regurgitation and reversed flow at aortic arch develops, which is a preterminal event.

Near the end of this sequence, biophysical changes usually become apparent: The NST becomes nonreactive, the BPP score falls, and late decelerations accompany contractions. Cardiovascular Doppler and behavioral BPP manifestations of fetal deterioration in FGR fetuses can occur largely independent of each other, resulting in discordant Doppler and BPP findings. Progression through the entire sequence does not always occur before delivery; Doppler abnormalities in some growth-restricted fetuses progress slowly or not at all or along a different pathway, for example, FGR due to preeclampsia will have a distinct clinical course that is different from idiopathic FGR. The sequence is most likely to progress when FGR and Doppler abnormalities are identified in the second trimester and the Doppler indices worsen within the first 2 weeks of Doppler monitoring.

Antenatal Corticosteroids

Ideally, a course of antenatal betamethasone is given to pregnancies <34 + 0 weeks of gestation in the week before preterm delivery is anticipated. Administration at 34 + 0 to 36 + 6 weeks does not appear to decrease the need for respiratory support and increases the rate of neonatal hypoglycemia but is recommended by some guidelines (UpToDate).

Maternal Interventions

There is no convincing evidence that any intervention in healthy women improves the growth of growth-restricted fetuses. Numerous approaches have been tried in small randomized trials, including maternal nutritional supplementation, oxygen therapy, and interventions to improve blood flow to the placenta, such as plasma volume expansion, low-dose aspirin, bed rest, and anticoagulation. Use of a phosphodiesterase-5 enzyme inhibitor (e.g., tadalafil, sildenafil) or a statin appeared promising and is under investigation. A multicenter Dutch trial of sildenafil for treatment of early-onset growth restriction was halted early because of higher-than expected rate of pulmonary HTN in the intervention group with no benefit in the primary outcome (perinatal mortality or major neonatal morbidity). A concurrent trial in Australia and New Zealand reported sildenafil had no effect on fetal growth velocity after diagnosis of growth restriction before 30 weeks but no adverse effects on newborns were found.

■ DELIVERY

In pregnancies with FGR, delivery decisions require balancing the risk of prematurity against that of stillbirth. There is little consensus about the optimum time to deliver the growth-restricted fetus. Timing is based on multiple factors, including the severity of FGR, Doppler findings, comorbid conditions, and rate of deterioration in fetal status and patient preference. The goal is to maximize fetal maturity and growth while minimizing the risks of fetal or neonatal mortality and short and long-term morbidity. The greatest challenge related to timing of delivery is in the preterm fetus <32 weeks of gestation. Morbidity and mortality related to preterm delivery is relatively high before 32 weeks, and between 26 and 29 weeks of gestation each day gained in utero has been estimated to improve survival by 1-2%.

In cases of early-onset FGR the main goal is to prolong pregnancy and maximize fetal maturation by means of expectant management under close monitoring until there is an evidence of late Doppler change in the UA (AEDV or REDV), ductus venosus alterations, or fetal heart rate (FHR) abnormalities. Therefore, at the point when delivery is indicated in cases of severe early-onset FGR, the fetus might already be experiencing some degree of hypoxia or acidosis in which case the likelihood of the fetus tolerating labor is low. Primary cesarean section is, therefore, the preferred option and has been reported to be >80%. In contrast, late-onset FGR is usually less severe and fetal hypoxia or acidosis is less likely to be present at the time when delivery is indicated. Indeed, in the DIGITAT trial (Disproportionate Intrauterine Growth Intervention Trial at Term), the rate of vaginal delivery was >80% in pregnancies induced for SGA with normal UA Doppler after 36 weeks of gestation. In the SGA fetus with UA AREDV delivery by cesarean section is recommended (RCOG). In the SGA fetus with normal UA Doppler or with abnormal UA PI but end–diastolic velocities present, induction of labor can be offered but rates of emergency cesarean sections are increased.

Timing of Delivery

Deliver immediately in the following conditions:

- Persistent reversed a-wave of the ductus venosus Doppler, gestational age ≥30 weeks. Before 30 weeks, individualize the decision of delivery.

- Umbilical artery reversed diastolic flow and gestational age ≥32 weeks.
- Umbilical artery absent diastolic flow and gestational age ≥34 weeks.

Normal Umbilical Artery Doppler

It provides strong evidence of fetal well-being, especially in the absence of risk factors for or signs of uteroplacental insufficiency, deliver these fetuses at 39–40 weeks of gestation.

Umbilical Artery Decreased Diastolic Flow (Persistent Pulsatility Index >95th Percentile)

This is a weak predictor of fetal death, perform BPP two times per week and deliver these fetuses at 37 weeks or when the BPP becomes abnormal. Delivery at 34–37 weeks is reasonable if UA flow is decreased and risk factors for, or signs of uteroplacental insufficiency are present, such as oligohydramnios, preeclampsia or HTN, renal insufficiency, fetal growth arrest, estimated weight <5th percentile, or prior birth of a SGA infant.

Umbilical Artery Absent or Reversed Diastolic Flow

The gestational age <34 weeks regardless of the presence or absence of oligohydramnios, perform NSTs every 12 hours and daily BPPs in an attempt to delay delivery until 32 weeks (if reversed flow) or 34 weeks (if absent flow), as long as the NST does not suggest fetal compromise and the BPP remains normal. If the BPP and NST become abnormal, deliver immediately. If a course of antenatal betamethasone has not been administered yet, it is given upon diagnosis of reversed or absent diastolic flow **(Flowchart 1)**.

■ INTRAPARTUM MANAGEMENT

Fetal growth restriction is a state of mild-to-moderate chronic oxygen and substrate deprivation. If antenatal testing (NST or BPP) is normal, a trial of labor with continuous intrapartum monitoring is reasonable. An unfavorable cervix is not a reason to avoid induction. Mechanical ripening methods (insertion of a balloon catheter or laminaria)/prostaglandins can be used for cervical ripening. If the Bishop score is >6, administer oxytocin without mechanical ripening.

Potential consequences include antepartum or intrapartum FHR abnormalities, passage of meconium with risk of aspiration, and neonatal polycythemia, impaired thermoregulation, hypoglycemia, and other metabolic abnormalities. Continuous intrapartum fetal monitoring should be done to detect nonreassuring FHR patterns suggestive of progressive hypoxia during labor, and provide skilled neonatal care in the delivery room. Umbilical cord blood analysis should be considered as a component of establishing baseline neonatal status. For fetuses <32 weeks of gestation, magnesium sulfate is given before delivery for neuroprotection.

■ RECURRENCE RISK

There is a tendency to repeat SGA deliveries in successive pregnancies. A prospective national cohort study from Netherlands reported that the risk of a nonanomalous SGA birth (<5th percentile) in the second pregnancy of women whose first delivery was "SGA" versus "not SGA" was 23% and 3%, respectively.

■ PREVENTION OF FGR

There are currently no preventative strategies or treatments for FGR that have been proven to be effective. No consistent evidence that nutritional and dietary supplements or bed rest prevents FGR or reduces the incidence of SGA. Ideally, all women should plan their pregnancies, adopting a healthy lifestyle and optimizing any medical conditions and their body mass index. In subsequent pregnancies, address any potentially treatable causes of FGR (e.g., cessation of smoking and alcohol intake, chemoprophylaxis, and mosquito avoidance in areas where malaria is prevalent, balanced energy/protein supplementation in women with significant nutritional deficiencies). Avoiding a short or long interpregnancy interval may also be beneficial.

The use of low dose aspirin was shown to provide a modest risk reduction in FGR and SGA in two meta-analyses. However, this finding was not confirmed in the Aspirin for Evidence Based on Preeclampsia Prevention (ASPRE) trial, which was primarily designed for preterm preeclampsia. Low-dose aspirin may be effective when FGR is secondary to preeclampsia since aspirin appears to reduce the risk of developing preeclampsia in women at moderate to high risk of developing the disorder. Due to the conflicting evidence, the American College of Obstetricians and Gynecologists recommends against the use of low-dose aspirin for the sole indication of FGR. Royal College of Obstetricians and Gynaecologists recommends the use of antiplatelet agents in women at high risk of preeclampsia, which should be commenced at, or before, 16 weeks of pregnancy. In a recent meta-analysis of 45 trials that included 20,909 women at high risk of preeclampsia, the administration of aspirin starting at ≤16 weeks of pregnancy reduced the risk of FGR by nearly half [relative risk (RR) 0.56; 95% CI, 0.44–0.70], with higher dosages of aspirin associated with a greater reduction, favoring a dose of 100–150 mg.

Anticoagulation with unfractionated heparin or low molecular weight heparin (LMWH) does not reduce the risk of recurrent placenta-mediated late pregnancy complications, such as growth restriction and is not recommended. In a 2016 meta-analysis using individual patient data from randomized trials of LMWH therapy versus no LMWH for women with any prior placenta-mediated pregnancy complications, the intervention did not significantly reduce the incidence of the primary

Flowchart 1: Algorithm for Management of FGR (SMFM).

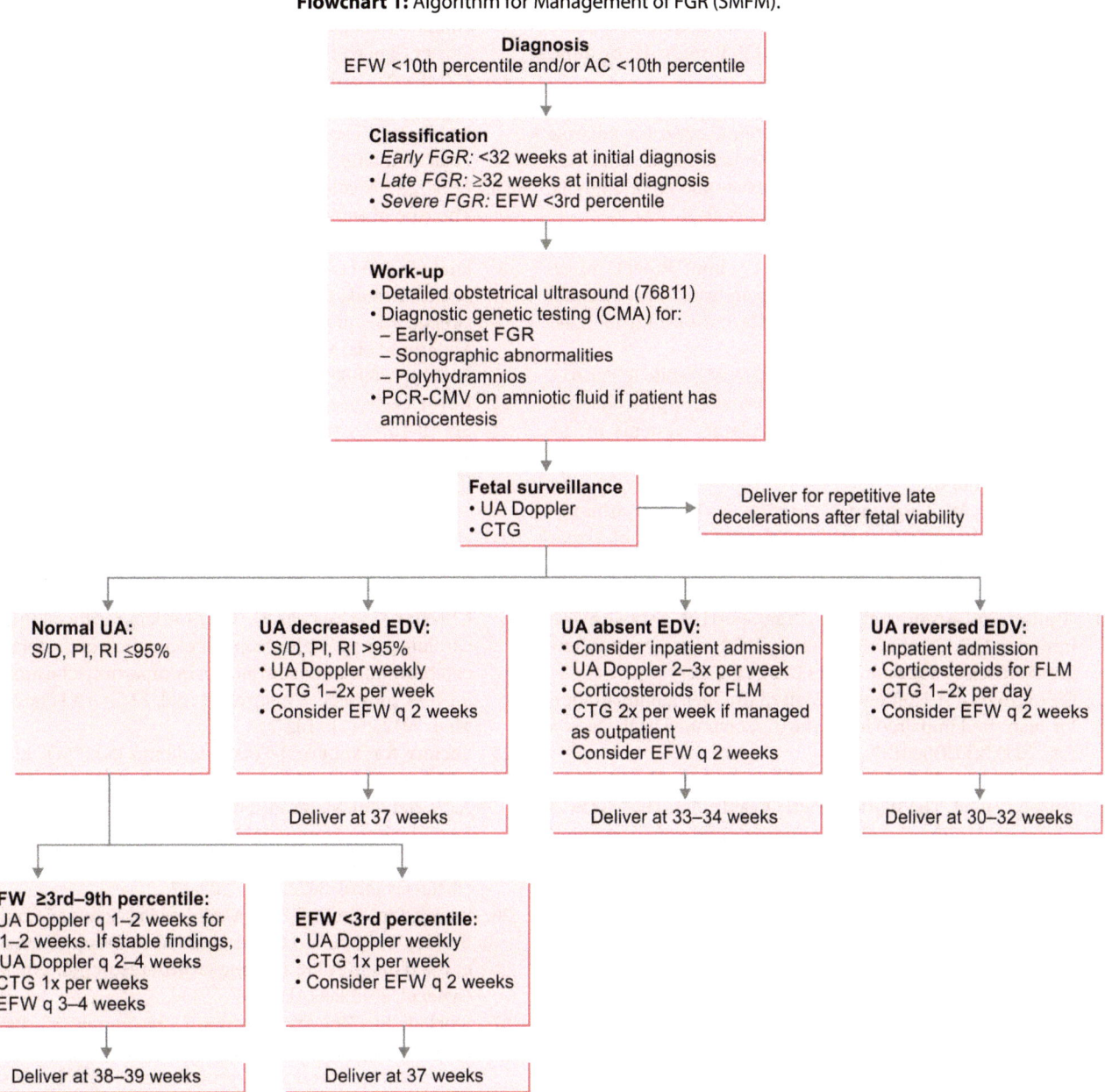

(CTG: cardiotocography; CMA: chromosome microarray; EDV: end-diastolic velocity; EFW: estimate of fetal weight; FGR: fetal growth restriction; SMFM: Society for Maternal-Fetal Medicine; UA: umbilical artery)

composite outcome (early-onset or severe preeclampsia, SGA <5th percentile, abruption, pregnancy loss ≥20 weeks of gestation) [RR 0.64, 95% CI 0.36–1.11].

■ CONCLUSION

Fetal growth restriction is an important cause of stillbirth, neonatal mortality, and short- and long-term neonatal morbidity. Early prediction and preventive strategies, timely diagnosis, and management using a standardized protocol to determine the proper monitoring and timing of delivery can decrease the risk of stillbirth and improve the perinatal outcomes.

■ SUGGESTED READING

1. Alfirevic Z, Stampalija T, Dowswell T. Fetal and umbilical Doppler ultrasound in high-risk pregnancies. Cochrane Database Syst Rev. 2017;6(6):CD007529.
2. American College of Obstetricians and Gynecologists. ACOG Committee Opinion No. 743: Low-Dose Aspirin Use During Pregnancy. Obstet Gynecol. 2018;132(1):e44-52.
3. American College of Obstetricians and Gynecologists. Fetal Growth Restriction: ACOG Practice Bulletin, Number 227. Obstet Gynecol. 2021;137(2):e16-28.
4. Baschat AA, Weiner CP. Umbilical artery Doppler screening for detection of the small fetus in need of antepartum surveillance. Am J Obstet Gynecol. 2000;182(1 Pt 1):154-8.

5. Bilardo CM, Hecher K, Papageorghiou AT, Marlow N, Thilaganathan B, et al. Severe fetal growth restriction at 26-32 weeks: key messages from the TRUFFLE study. Ultrasound Obstet Gynecol. 2017;50(3):285-90.
6. Conde-Agudelo A, Villar J, Kennedy SH, Papageorghiou AT. Predictive accuracy of cerebroplacental ratio for adverse perinatal and neurodevelopmental outcomes in suspected fetal growth restriction: systematic review and meta-analysis. Ultrasound Obstet Gynecol. 2018;52(4):430-41.
7. Eunice Kennedy Shriver National Institute of Child Health and Human Development. (2018). About Preeclampsia and Eclampsia. [online] Available from https://www.nichd.nih.gov/health/topics/preeclampsia/conditioninfo [Last accessed April, 2022].
8. Ferrazzi E, Bozzo M, Rigano S, Bellotti M, Morabito A, Pardi G, et al. Temporal sequence of abnormal Doppler changes in the peripheral and central circulatory systems of the severely growth-restricted fetus. Ultrasound Obstet Gynecol. 2002;19(2):140-6.
9. Ganzevoort W, Thornton JG, Marlow N, Thilaganathan B, Arabin B, Prefumo F, et al. Comparative analysis of 2-year outcomes in GRIT and TRUFFLE trials. Ultrasound Obstet Gynecol. 2020;55(1):68-74.
10. Giuliano N, Annunziata ML, Tagliaferri S, Esposito FG, Imperato OC, Campanile M, et al. IUGR management: new perspectives. J Pregnancy. 2014;2014:620976.
11. Gülmezoglu AM, Hofmeyr GJ. Maternal oxygen administration for suspected impaired fetal growth. Cochrane Database Syst Rev. 2000;(2):CD000137.
12. Kiserud T, Piaggio G, Carroli G, Widmer M, Carvalho J, Neerup Jensen L, et al. The World Health Organization Fetal Growth Charts: A Multinational Longitudinal Study of Ultrasound Biometric Measurements and Estimated Fetal Weight. PLOS Med. 2017;14(1):e1002220.
13. Lausman A, Kingdom J, Maternal Fetal Medicine Committee. Intrauterine Growth Restriction: Screening, Diagnosis, and Management. J Obstet Gynaecol Can. 2013;35(8):741-8.
14. Lees CC, Stampalija T, Baschat A, da Silva Costa F, Ferrazzi E, Figueras F, et al. ISUOG Practice Guidelines: diagnosis and management of small-for-gestational-age fetus and fetal growth restriction. Ultrasound Obstet Gynecol. 2020;56(2):298-312.
15. Maggio L, Dahlke JD, Mendez-Figueroa H, Albright CM, Chauhan SP, Wenstrom KD. Perinatal outcomes with normal compared with elevated umbilical artery systolic-to-diastolic ratios in fetal growth restriction. Obstet Gynecol. 2015;125(4):863-9.
16. McCowan LM, Figueras F, Anderson NH. Evidence-based national guidelines for the management of suspected fetal growth restriction: comparison, consensus, and controversy. Am J Obstet Gynecol. 2018;218(2S):S855-68.
17. Melamed N, Baschat A, Yinon Y, Athanasiadis A, Mecacci F, Figueras F, et al. FIGO (International Federation of Gynecology and Obstetrics) initiative on fetal growth: Best practice advice for screening, diagnosis, and management of fetal growth restriction. Int J Gynecol Obstet. 2021;152(Suppl 1):3-57.
18. Mlynarczyk M, Chouhan SP, Baydoun HA, Wilkes CM, Earhart KR, Zhao Y, Goodier C, et al. The clinical significance of an estimated fetal weight below the 10th percentile: a comparison of outcomes of <5th vs 5th-9th percentile. Am J Obstet Gynecol. 2017(2);198.e1-198.e11.
19. NZMFMN. Guideline for the Management of Suspected Small for Gestational Age Singleton Pregnancies and Infants after 34 Weeks' Gestation. New Zealand: New Zealand Maternal Fetal Medicine Network; 2014.
20. Roberge S, Nicolaides K, Demers S, Hyett J, Chaillet N, Bujold E. The role of aspirin dose on the prevention of preeclampsia and fetal growth restriction: systematic review and meta-analysis. Am J Obstet Gynecol. 2017;216(2):110-20.e6.
21. Robert Resnik, Creasy RK, Iams JD, Lockwood CJ, Moore T, Greene MF. Intrauterine growth restriction. Creasy & Resnik's Maternal-Fetal Medicine, 8th edition. Philadelphia: Saunders; 2019. pp. 789-809.
22. Royal College of Obstetricians & Gynaecologists. (2013). Small-for-Gestational-Age Fetus, Investigation and Management (Green-top Guideline No. 31). [online] available from https://www.rcog.org.uk/en/guidelines-research-services/guidelines/gtg31/ [Last Accessed April, 2022].
23. Sankaran S, Kyle PM. Aetiology and Pathogenesis of IUGR. Best Pract Res Clin Obstet Gynaecol. 2009;23(6):765-77.
24. Siristatidis C, Kassanos D, Salamalekis G, Creatsa M, Chrelias C, Creatsas G. Cardiotocography alone versus cardiotocography plus Doppler evaluation of the fetal middle cerebral and umbilical artery for intrapartum fetal monitoring: a Greek prospective controlled trial. J Matern Fetal Neonatal Med. 2012;25(7):1183-7.
25. Society for Maternal-Fetal Medicine (SMFM). Electronic address: pubs@smfm.org, Martins JG, Biggio JR, Abuhamad A. Society for Maternal-Fetal Medicine Consult Series #52: Diagnosis and management of fetal growth restriction: (Replaces Clinical Guideline Number 3, April 2012). Am J Obstet Gynecol. 2020;223(4):B2-17.
26. Society for Maternal-Fetal Medicine Publications Committee, Berkley E, Chauhan SP, Abuhamad A. Doppler assessment of the fetus with intrauterine growth restriction. Am J Obstet Gynecol. 2012;206(4):300-8.
27. Stockley EL, Ting JY, Kingdom JC, McDonald SD, Barrett JF, Synnes AR, et al. Intrapartum magnesium sulfate is associated with neuroprotection in growth-restricted fetuses. Am J Obstet Gynecol. 2018;219(6):606.e1-606.e8.
28. Unterscheider J, Daly S, Geary MP, Kennelly MM, McAuliffe FM, O'Donoghue K, et al. Optimizing the definition of intrauterine growth restriction: the multicenter prospective PORTO Study. Am J Obstet Gynecol. 2013;208(4):290.e1-6.
29. UpToDate. (2022). Fetal growth restriction: Evaluation and management (Resnik R). [online] Available from https://www.uptodate.com/contents/fetal-growth-restriction-evaluation-and-management#:~:text=When%20ultrasound%20examination%20suggests%20fetal,determining%20the%20optimal%20time%20for. [Last accessed April, 2022].
30. Zhu H, Lin S, Huang L, He Z, Huang X, Zhou Y, et al. Application of chromosomal microarray analysis in prenatal diagnosis of fetal growth restriction. Prenat Diagn. 2016;36(7):686-92.

CHAPTER 6

Doppler in Obstetrics

INTRODUCTION

Doppler ultrasonography has proven to be an invaluable obstetric tool for more than 30 years. Doppler ultrasound (US) was first used in obstetrics when continuous-wave Doppler US allowed the examiner to hear flow in the umbilical cord. With the advent of B-mode US and pulsed-wave Doppler US, it has become possible to see specific vessels and to sample waveforms, providing a window into the fetoplacental circulation.

The Doppler effect is based on the physical phenomenon that the frequency of sound waves reflected by a static object is identical to that before being reflected. On the other hand, change in frequency of sound waves when it is reflected by moving objects, e.g., blood; frequency is proportional to the velocity of moving objects. Thus, blood velocity and resistance to flow can be evaluated using Doppler effects. The frequency increases constantly as the sound source moves closer to the receiver or declines as the source moves further away from it.

Doppler US provides a unique window to the fetoplacental circulation, allowing assessment of fetal well-being. The vessels sampled to assess the fetoplacental unit include the umbilical artery (UA), umbilical vein (UV), ductus venosus (DV), middle cerebral artery (MCA) and the uterine artery. In the first trimester, the focus of Doppler US is: (1) detection of aneuploidy and an increased risk for congenital heart disease with evaluation of the DV waveform, and (2) screening for women more likely to develop preeclampsia by evaluation of the uterine artery waveform. In the second and third trimesters, use of Doppler US is targeted toward risk assessment in growth-restricted fetuses, detection of those with high-output conditions, detection of complications of monochorionic twinning and non-invasive detection of fetal anemia. The vessels interrogated include UA, MCA, UV, and DV. More recently, MCA Doppler has revolutionized the management of pregnancies complicated by alloimmunization and twin-to-twin transfusion syndrome (TTTS).

DOPPLER METHODS OF ANALYSIS

Doppler allows to understand fetoplacental blood flow and fetal hemodynamic events. The method of analysis includes systolic over diastolic ratio (S/D ratio), pulsatility index (PI), and resistance index (RI) **(Fig. 1)**.

- *S/D ratio = peak systolic velocity/end diastolic velocity:* The most commonly used S/D ratio is the UA systolic/diastolic ratio. Doppler index provides information on *resistance to flow in fetal side of placenta.*
- *PI (PSV-EDV/TAPV) (Time-averaged peak velocity):*
  - PI is a measure of the variability of blood velocity in a vessel, equal to difference between the peak systolic and minimum diastolic velocities divided by the mean velocity during the cardiac cycle.
  - With PI, it is possible to obtain a *numerical value even when diastolic flow is absent or reverse*
- *RI (PSV-EDV/PSV):*
  - The RI is altered not by vascular resistance alone but by the combination of vascular resistance and vascular compliance.
  - 0—continuous flow
  - 1—systolic flow, but no diastolic flow
  - >1—reversed diastolic flow

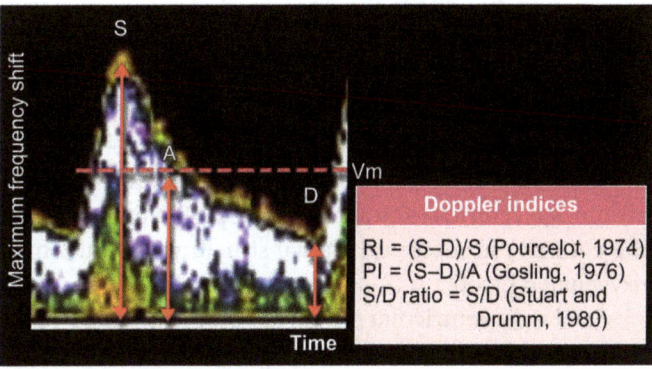

Fig. 1: Doppler interpretation in pregnancy.
(S: systolic peak (max. velocity); D: end diastolic flow; Vm: mean velocity; A: Temporal average frequency over 1 cardiac cycle)

PLACENTAL REMODELING IN PREGNANCY

Implantation and trophoblastic invasion of the placenta plays a crucial role in its development as an organ for the transport of nutrients and oxygen to the fetus. Placental remodeling occurs in two stages. In the first stage, between 8 and 12 weeks' gestation, trophoblastic cells invade the intradecidual portion of the spiral arteries. This is followed by deeper trophoblastic invasion into the myometrial segments of the spiral arteries from 14 weeks' gestation. The loss of smooth muscle and elastic coat from the spiral arteries converts the uteroplacental circulation into a low resistance, high capacitance system. Placental remodeling is completed by 16–18 weeks' gestation. Defective placental implantation leads to hypoperfusion, hypoxic reperfusion injury, and oxidative stress. A derangement in trophoblastic differentiation is thought to underlie the pathophysiology of gestational hypertension, preeclampsia, and fetal growth restriction (FGR). Defective implantation may also play a causative role in preterm labor, placental abruption, and second-trimester miscarriages. Recent studies indicate that poor placentation is associated with an imbalance of circulating vasoactive factors [placental growth factor (PlGF), pregnancy-associated plasma protein-A (PAPP-A), soluble fms-like tyrosine kinase 1 (sFlt-1), soluble endoglin (sEng), activin-A, and inhibin-A] and, in turn, leads to maternal vascular maladaptation with associated systemic endothelial dysfunction. Levels of these biochemical markers reflect the pathophysiology of defective placentation, and are playing an increasing role in early gestation screening tests for later pregnancy complications.

Fetoplacental Circulation

In the fetus, deoxygenated blood is carried to the placenta by the umbilical arteries, which arise from the internal iliac arteries. The UV carries the oxygenated blood from the placenta through the umbilicus, along the free edge of the falciform ligament to the left portal vein. Inside fetal liver the UV becomes the portal sinus, that is, the origin of the portal veins and DV. Some of this blood goes to the liver, but a portion is directed to the upper part of the inferior vena cava (IVC) by the DV **(Fig. 2)**.

This highly O_2 blood (70% O_2) does not mix with blood from lower extremity. DV, a trumpet-shaped vessel, produces a defined stream of this oxygenated blood that preferentially flows through the foramen ovale to the left atrium, left ventricle, and aorta, thence preferentially perfuse the coronary arteries and cranial structures with the most oxygenated blood.

Fetal right ventricular output largely bypasses the lungs, is diverted by way of the ductus arteriosus to the descending aorta to perfuse fetal lower part of the body. The umbilical arteries are responsible for carrying deoxygenated fetal blood to the placenta. When placental resistance

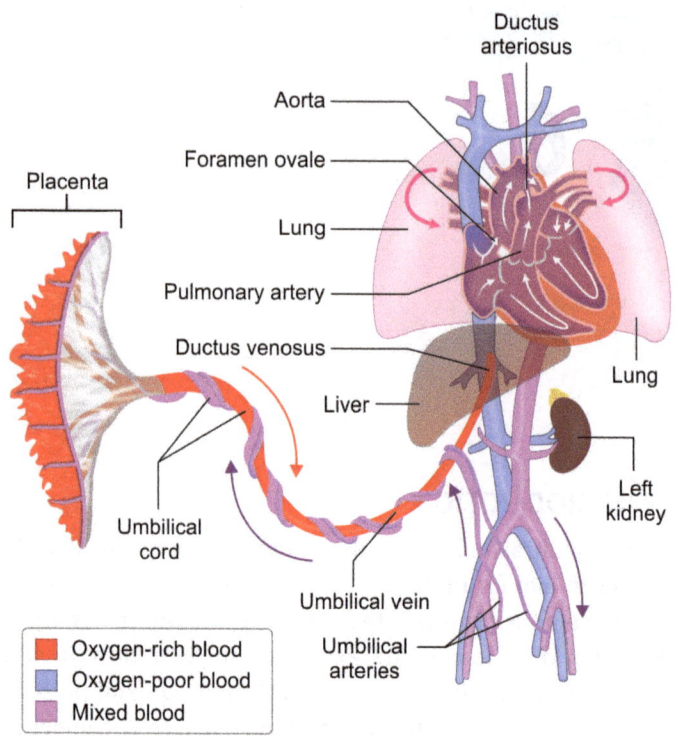

Fig. 2: Fetoplacental circulation.

increases, the abnormal pressures produce increased afterload, which can impair right ventricular function. The right ventricle accounts for >50% of the cardiac output in the fetus; thus, any process that has a negative effect on right ventricular function adversely influences fetal well-being.

MATERNAL AND FETAL DOPPLER INDICATIONS
Maternal Conditions at Risk of Chronic Hypoxemia

- Hypertensive disorders of pregnancy
- Chronic renal disease
- Maternal diabetes
- Antiphospholipid syndrome and related autoimmune disease
- Cyanotic heart disease.

Fetal Indications

- Fetal growth restriction
- Reduced fetal movement
- Previous history of intrauterine death (IUD), stillbirth, intrauterine growth restriction (IUGR), and oligohydramnios
- Raised serum alpha fetoprotein.

FIRST TRIMESTER DOPPLER IN FETAL ANEUPLOIDY SCREENING
Ductus Venosus Doppler

Traditional method of screening for aneuploidies was based on maternal age and gestational age of the fetus. This led to

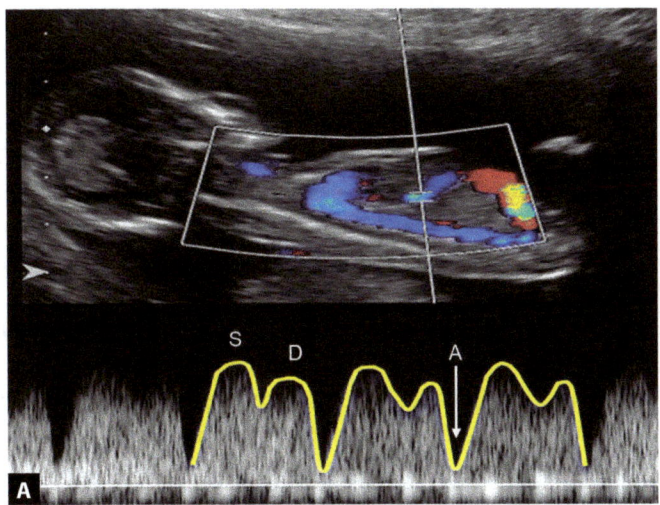
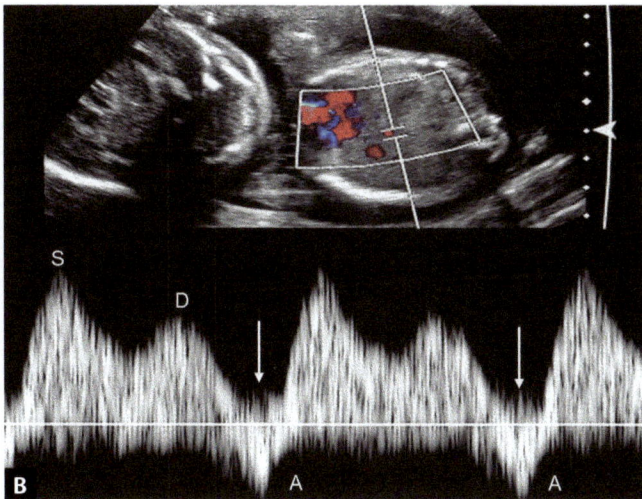

Figs. 3A and B: (A) Normal ductus venosus (DV); (B) Reversed a wave in DV.

increased invasive testing with associated risk of miscarriage and ineffective identification of aneuploidy. For this, noninvasive methods including serum markers and fetal blood flow pattern came into use in prenatal screening.

Ductus venosus Doppler is a useful tool in the first trimester prenatal diagnosis as it can optimize the sensitivity and specificity of first-trimester fetal aneuploidy screening **(Figs. 3A and B)**. There is clear association between abnormal flow in the DV between 11 and 13^{+6} weeks of gestation and the presence of fetal aneuploidy or congenital cardiac defects. DV flow provides an independent contribution in the prediction of chromosomal abnormalities when combined with nuchal translucency (NT) and maternal serum markers [(PAPP-A) and free beta-human chorionic gonadotropin (βhCG)], increasing the detection rate of aneuploidy to 96% at a false-positive rate of 2.6%.

In a cohort of about 20,000 singleton pregnancies, Maiz et al. performed a combined first-trimester screening test, comprising maternal age, fetal NT thickness, fetal heart rate, serum free beta-chorionic gonadotropin, PAPP-A, and the DV Doppler. The a-wave was reversed in 66–75% of aneuploid, but in only 3.2% of euploid fetuses. Universal inclusion of the first-trimester DV Doppler would detect 96%, 92%, 100%, and 100% of trisomy 21, 18, and 13, and Turner syndrome, respectively, at a false-positive rate of 3%.

Ductus venosus Doppler waveforms reflect fetal central hemodynamics, especially that of the right heart. Functional and anatomical abnormalities are expected to alter this waveform. This prompted many to explore its screening potential for the early detection of fetal cardiac disease. In a study involving over 41,000 euploid fetuses, reversal of DV a-wave was observed in about 28% of the fetuses with cardiac anomalies and in about 2% of the fetuses with no cardiac anomalies. Matias et al. performed Doppler velocimetry of the DV in 200 singleton fetuses with increased NT, at 10–14 weeks' gestation, immediately before fetal karyotyping. The results suggested that in euploid fetuses with increased NT, the presence of abnormal DV blood flow recognized those with major cardiac defects. In twin pregnancies, abnormal DV flow is associated with chromosomal abnormalities and cardiac defects. In monochorionic twins, abnormal flow in the DV in at least one of the fetuses increases the risk of developing TTTS.

Tricuspid Flow Pattern

Tricuspid regurgitation (TR) is a common sonographic finding during the fetal life. It has been reported in 7% of normal fetuses, it may be associated with aneuploidy and with both cardiac and extracardiac defects. Assessment for TR has been reported to have prognostic value in predicting perinatal outcome in FGR. When assessing the atrioventricular valves, the Doppler waveform for both mitral and tricuspid valves has a characteristic dual-peak pattern: an E-wave corresponding to ventricular filling and an A-wave corresponding with atrial contraction. The A-wave is typically taller than the E-wave in normal fetuses. However, in those affected by FGR, the E/A ratio increases and in more severe cases there is mitral or TR where a reversed jet can be seen within the right atrium on color flow Doppler. TR in combination with other markers is the strongest predictor for aneuploidy. TR, as an isolated parameter, is a poor screening tool both for all and for each individual chromosomal abnormality and congenital cardiac defects.

FIRST-TRIMESTER PREDICTION OF PREECLAMPSIA AND FETAL GROWTH RESTRICTION

The concept of the "inverted pyramid of care" has received increasing attention in the recent time. This proposes that disorders such as preeclampsia and FGR can be screened for in early gestation by a combination of history, placental biomarkers, mean arterial blood pressure, and uterine artery Doppler measurements.

Uterine Artery Doppler

The uterine artery is a branch of the internal iliac artery that runs anteriorly in the pelvis to enter the myometrium at the cervicoisthmic junction. In the nonpregnant state, the waveform is high resistance with early diastolic notching. A diastolic notch is defined as a reduction in forward flow at the start of diastole and represents abnormal uteroplacental flow during pregnancy. Notch indicates increased impedance to flow and corresponds to sharp decrease on velocity at the beginning of diastole with a nadir smaller than PDV. Early diastolic notching of uterine artery characterizes an abnormal uterine circulation and should disappear by 13 weeks of gestation. A low-resistance flow should be established by 20 weeks at the latest with progressive decrease in impedance with advancing gestation. Persistent early diastolic notching in pregnancies after 20 weeks is thought to reflect abnormal maternal vascular tone.

The maternal side of the fetoplacental circulatory unit is represented by the uterine artery Doppler. Remodeling of the uterine artery branches is essential for successful placentation. Normal trophoblastic invasion of the maternal spiral arteries causes maximum vessel dilatation and impairs sympathetic and parasympathetic responses to ensure arterial dilatation and increased blood flow to the pregnant uterus.

In a prospective cross-sectional study, Gómez et al. has shown the mean uterine artery PI continued to fall in the third trimester until 34 weeks. Doppler of uterine artery is increasingly used in screening for preeclampsia and FGR. Defective trophoblastic invasion leads to increase in RI, PI values. Uterine artery Doppler thus can be used to help distinguish placental causes of growth restriction from other causes of growth restriction. If the PI values of both uterine arteries are normal, the patient can be informed that she most likely will not develop preeclampsia or an IUGR fetus (>99% negative predictive value). High-risk pregnancy with abnormal Doppler is an indication for close prenatal follow-up, high risk pregnancy with normal Doppler is reassuring.

The use of Doppler interrogation of this vessel in the first trimester has gained momentum in recent years, assessment is performed between 11 and 13^{+6} weeks' of gestation via a transabdominal or transvaginal approach. The transabdominal approach is the preferred method as it is less invasive with good interobserver reproducibility. Various impedance indices have been used to evaluate the relationship between uterine artery Doppler velocimetry and adverse pregnancy outcomes, including FGR, maternal preeclampsia, increased risk of preterm delivery, and fetal distress in labor. Depth of protodiastolic notch is an index of severity of FGR **(Figs. 4A and B)**.

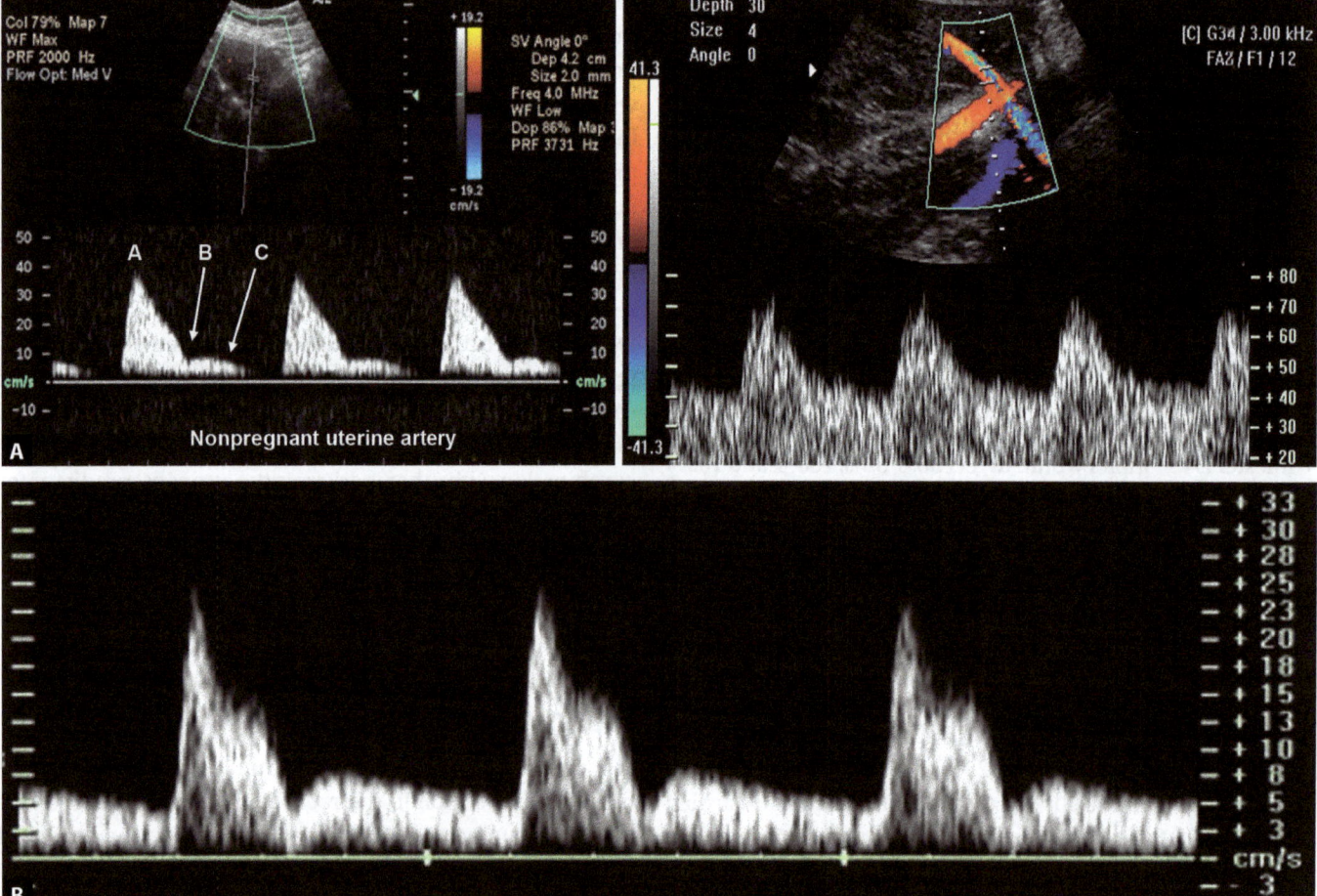

Figs. 4A and B: (A) Normal uterine artery Doppler; (B) Pulsatile flow waveform with low diastolic velocities, indicative of high distal resistance.

Overall, first-trimester Doppler interrogation of the uterine artery performs better in the prediction of early-onset than late-onset preeclampsia. As an isolated marker of future disease, its sensitivity in predicting preeclampsia and FGR in low-risk pregnant women is moderate, at 40–70%. The sensitivities and specificities for the prediction of preeclampsia in low-risk population vary between 34–76% and 83–93%, respectively. In the first trimester, uterine artery Doppler can apparently predict 81% of women with early-onset preeclampsia, 45% with late-onset preeclampsia, and 50% with gestational hypertension, with a false-positive rate of 10%. With the addition of biomarkers, mean arterial blood pressure, and maternal history this detection rate increases to 96% for early-onset preeclampsia and to 54% for all preeclampsia, with a false-positive rate of 10%. In a low-risk population, uterine artery Doppler has limited accuracy in predicting a small-for-gestational-age (SGA). In high-risk women, uterine artery Doppler has a moderate predictive value for a SGA neonate and hence the Royal College of Obstetricians and Gynaecologists (RCOG) guideline recommends its use in this population. The benefit of performing such an assessment is that it allows the provision of aspirin prior to 16 weeks of gestation in high-risk women. Low-dose aspirin has been demonstrated to reduce the risk of preeclampsia by 17% in at-risk pregnancies.

Crovetto et al. used a two-tier model to screen for early SGA: serum PAPP-A and free β-hCG at 8–10 weeks in combination with uterine artery PI at $11–13^{+6}$ weeks; maternal priori risk factors, including mean arterial pressure (MAP), were included in the assessment. In the cohort of 4,970 women, the prevalence of early and late SGA was 0.6% and 7.9%, respectively. Sixty-seven percent of women with early SGA later developed superimposed preeclampsia compared to 8% in the late SGA group. The overall detection rate for early SGA in the study was 75% (FPR 10%), but the detection rate was only 30% in the absence of preeclampsia. The detection rate for late SGA was 31.3% and 22.3% for cases with and without preeclampsia.

DOPPLER ULTRASOUND IN THE SECOND AND THIRD TRIMESTERS

In the second and third trimesters, Doppler US is used to assess fetal well-being and to noninvasively monitor the fetoplacental unit. The UA and MCA are the most important vessels sampled; supplemental information may be obtained from evaluation of the DV and the UVs.

Umbilical Artery Doppler

The umbilical arterial circulation is normally a low impedance circulation, with an increase in the amount of end-diastolic flow with advancing gestation. Umbilical arterial Doppler waveforms reflect the status of the placental circulation, and the increase in end-diastolic flow that is seen with advancing gestation is a direct result of an increase in the number of tertiary stem villi that takes place with placental maturation. Flow increases as pregnancy progresses, so the S/D ratio in the UA decreases with advancing gestational age. The 50th percentile for the S/D ratio at 20 weeks is 4, at 30 weeks 2.83; and at 40 weeks it is 2.18. Diseases that obliterate small muscular arteries in placental tertiary stem villi result in a progressive decrease in end-diastolic flow in the umbilical arterial Doppler waveforms until absent and then reverse flow during diastole. Reversed diastolic flow in the umbilical arterial circulation represents an advanced stage of placental compromise and is associated with >70% of placental arterial obliteration. Absent or reverse diastolic flow indicates extreme downstream resistance, placental dysfunction, and fetal compromise with chances of growth restriction.

Umbilical artery Doppler remains the most extensively studied fetal surveillance tool. In clinical practice, S/D ratio and the presence of absent or reversed end-diastolic flow (REDF) are used to manage FGR and to stage the twin-twin transfusion syndrome. In most clinical settings, Doppler US of the UA is not performed until viability (24 weeks); but in the twin-twin transfusion syndrome, Doppler US of the UA is part of the staging system. Therefore, it is performed whenever that diagnosis is suspected, regardless of gestational age. The RCOG guideline advises that in terms of surveillance, women who are at high risk of having a baby affected by FGR (such as a previously SGA baby, smoking, and advancing maternal age) should undergo serial UA Doppler assessment fortnightly from 26 to 28 weeks of gestation.

Resistance to flow in the umbilical arteries varies along the length of the umbilical cord. Resistance is highest at the abdominal site of insertion of the umbilical cord, is intermediate in free-floating loops, and is lowest at the placental site of cord insertion. In 2012, the Society for Maternal-Fetal Medicine recommended sampling at the abdominal site of umbilical cord insertion, but this site can be challenging in later gestation when it may be obscured by the fetal lower extremities or when there is oligohydramnios limiting acoustic access (as often occurs in association with FGR). In multiple gestations, it is essential to sample at, or as close as possible to, the abdominal site of umbilical cord insertion of each fetus to ensure appropriate comparisons in the same fetus over time. In 2013, the guidelines of the International Society of Ultrasound in Obstetrics and Gynecology for obstetric Doppler US recommended sampling the vessels in free-floating loops of umbilical cord in singletons. Ideally, during Doppler examination, the fetus should be at rest and not breathing, because movement and breathing cause variations in the spectral waveform. Measure the S/D ratio, and compare the value to nomograms for flow at specific gestational ages. Also note whether there is of absent end-diastolic flow or REDF and whether it is intermittent or sustained.

CHANGES IN UMBILICAL ARTERY IN PLACENTAL INSUFFICIENCY

In IUGR because of defective trophoblast invasion of spiral artery there is increased placental vascular resistance resulting in decreased forward flow in UA and decreased diastolic flow resulting in increase in S/D, PI, and RI. With further increase in placental vascular resistance eventually diastolic flow reaches zero or absent, further increase in placental vascular resistance causes flow reversal in diastole = REDF. Fetuses with reversed umbilical artery end diastolic flow are acidotic and need prompt delivery **(Figs. 5A and B)**.

In 2020, the Society for Maternal-Fetal Medicine published a clinical guideline for Doppler US assessment of the fetus with growth restriction; the guideline recommends weekly Doppler US of the UA. If the results of Doppler US remain normal, delivery is recommended at 38–39 weeks. When these results are abnormal, management is determined by the severity of the finding. With decreased diastolic flow, antenatal testing (e.g., nonstress tests, amniotic fluid measurement, and biophysical profile) is increased in frequency, Doppler US is performed weekly, and delivery is considered after 37 weeks. When absent end-diastolic flow or REDF is present, corticosteroid is given in anticipation of preterm delivery, and Doppler US is performed two to three times per week, in addition to standard antenatal tests of fetal well-being. Goal of gestational ages for delivery is at 33–34 weeks with absent end-diastolic flow and 30–32 weeks with REDF.

Ductus Venosus Doppler

The DV is an intrahepatic end-part of the UV. It is a small trumpet-shaped connection between the umbilical/portal system and the IVC. Its shape effectively funnels the oxygen-rich blood returning from the placenta directly into the right atrium, with flow dynamics that then facilitate flow across the foramen ovale into the left atrium. The DV has a characteristic waveform and sound. The latter has been likened to the sound of a washing machine. DV waveforms include, A = A wave (atrial contraction), D = D wave (ventricular diastole), S = S wave (ventricular systole). DV gives information about venous side of fetal circulation. The S-wave reflects the pressure gradient between the peripheral venous vessels and the right atrium, occurs during ventricular systole which results in the highest blood flow velocities toward the fetal heart during that part of the cardiac cycle, D-wave represents the opening of the atrial ventricular valves and passive early filling of the ventricles. Between the S and the D wave is a period of isovolumetric relaxation (IVR) during late diastole when atrial pressure and waning systolic ejection pressure are comparable **(Fig. 6)**. With increasing myocardial hypoxia and acidosis, the cardiac muscle is less compliant and IVR decreases, may become absent or even reversed.

Abnormal findings in DV flow include the absence or reversal of the A wave. An evaluation of IVR and the A-wave (atrial contraction) is a more accurate predictor of fetal outcome than reversed A-wave alone.

Doppler US of the DV in the second and third trimesters is used to assess cardiac function in fetuses with high-output conditions and to assess cardiac strain in fetuses with FGR attributed to abnormal placentation. The fetus should be at rest and not breathing during DV sampling.

CHANGES IN DUCTUS VENOSUS DOPPLER WITH CARDIAC STRAIN

The DV is the only venous vessel with forward flow during all phases of the cardiac cycle. In contrast to its role in screening fetal aneuploidy and congenital heart disease in the first trimester, DV Doppler is used to assess cardiac strain in the second and third trimesters.

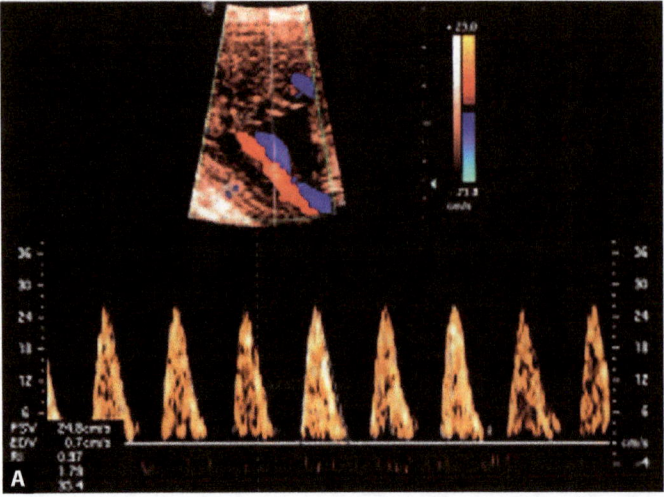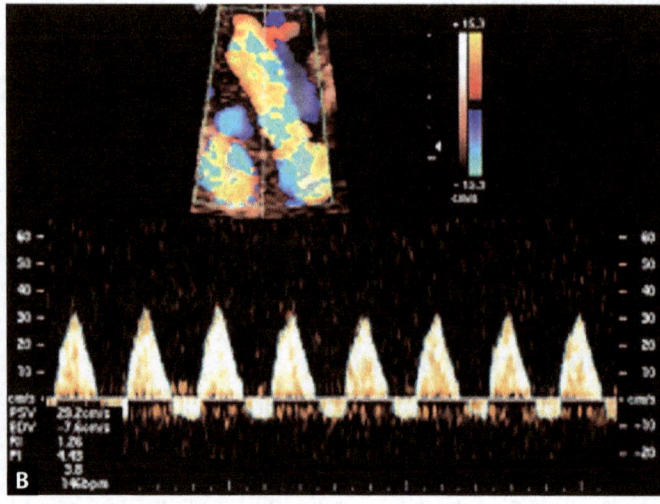

Figs. 5A and B: (A) Umbilical artery (UA) absent flow; (B) UA reversed flow.

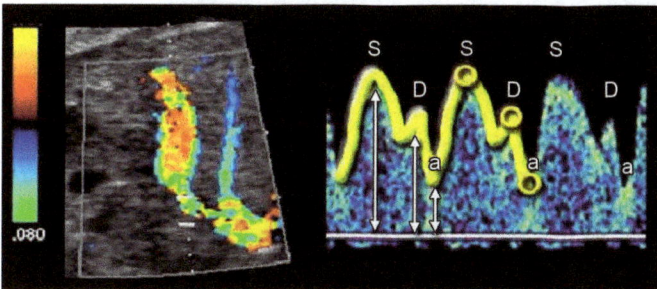

Fig. 6: Normal ductus venosus waveform.
(S: ventricular systole; D: early diastole; a: atrial contraction)

Normally, with advancing gestation cardiac compliance increases and placental resistance falls. As a result, DV-PI declines with advancing gestation. An increase in cardiac afterload or decreased cardiac compliance will result in a decrease in forward flow and an increased PI. Parameters that influence cardiac function include afterload (e.g., increased placental resistance), myocardial performance (e.g., cardiomyopathy), and preload (e.g., the recipient twin in the twin-twin transfusion syndrome). Decreased forward flow during atrial systole (i.e., diminished or reversed A-wave) is the most sensitive and ubiquitous finding when any one of these parameters are affected.

Effect of Hypoxemia on Ductus Venosus Flow

Hypoxemia increases the umbilical venous flow through the DV and a reduction in hepatic blood flow. Normal ductal flow suggests continued fetal compensation. O_2 deficiency and acidosis affects fetal cardiac function, with progressive hypoxemia, there is interrupted forward flow in DV, markedly increased PI, and subsequently absent or reversed flow during atrial contraction. This indicates the failure of compensatory mechanism and the beginning of right heart failure. An absent or reversed A-wave in the DV is used as a sign of substantial cardiac compromise and has been shown to be a strong predictor of stillbirth. The DV Doppler acts as a marker of cardiovascular deterioration in response to FGR, specifically in cases of early-onset FGR, where the DV typically becomes abnormal after an elevation of the PI in the UA. It is currently recommended by RCOG ("good practice point" evidence) that DV Doppler should be used for the surveillance and timing of delivery of the preterm growth-restricted fetus with an abnormal UA Doppler, provided that the fetus is viable.

Middle Cerebral Artery

The MCA is the most accessible cerebral vessel to US imaging in the fetus, and it carries >80% of cerebral blood flow. The cerebral circulation is normally a high-impedance circulation with continuous forward flow throughout the cardiac cycle. MCA Doppler waveforms, obtained from the proximal portion of the vessel, immediately after its origin from the circle of Willis, have shown the best reproducibility.

Doppler of the MCA is used in two situations: (1) noninvasive assessment of fetal anemia, and (2) calculation of the cerebroplacental ratio (CPR) as a measure of fetal brain sparing in FGR. The assessment of fetal anemia by using Doppler US of the MCA can start as early as 18 weeks. The CPR compares fetal brain perfusion to that of the placenta. CPR is a ratio MCA-PI/UA-PI. The CPR has a greater sensitivity than assessing the MCA or UA Doppler PI in isolation, with a low or abnormal result associated with adverse perinatal outcome.

In normal circumstances, flow in the MCA is fairly high resistance, and flow in the UA should be low resistance, with continuous antegrade flow and a continuous increase in the diastolic flow as the pregnancy progresses. Studies found a significant increase in perinatal morbidity and mortality in fetuses with growth restriction who had an abnormal CPR less than the 5th percentile for gestational age—but this applies only until 34 weeks of gestation, thereafter, the correlation was lost. Hence, the stance of the RCOG guideline is that MCA Doppler should not be used to time delivery in the preterm growth-restricted fetus. There does appear to be a role for MCA, however, in the prediction of outcome in late-onset FGR. RCOG guideline recommends SGA fetus with a normal umbilical artery Doppler (UAD), an abnormal MCA Doppler should be used to time delivery.

Changes in Hypoxia

In response to hypoxia, the fetus diverts blood flow to the brain, (the head-sparing effect) increasing the MCA diastolic flow, thereby decreasing the PI, and altering the CPR. This redistribution of blood flow in hypoxemic fetuses may be transient, vasodilatation ability is exhausted with worsening hypoxemia. With the onset of hypercapnia, vasodilatation is suppressed by cerebral edema and the resistance starts increasing again; PI may increase and diastolic flow may be reversed resulting in a "normalization" of the MCA.

The reversal of adaptation in a growth-restricted fetus is considered as a poor prognostic sign. Middle cerebral artery-peak systolic velocity (PSV) is elevated as a late finding in severe IUGR prior to a nonreassuring heart rate tracing, i.e., continuous late decelerations or biophysical profile score <4. When abnormal, it should lead to interaction of other Doppler in the fetal circulation to evaluate the degree of compromise and better timing of delivery. Delivery should be considered when there is a 20–30% increase in the MCA-PI/day for 2 days (trend toward normalization).

Fetal Anemia

In fetal anemia, flow in the MCA increases for several reasons. Fluids move faster through a fixed-diameter tube

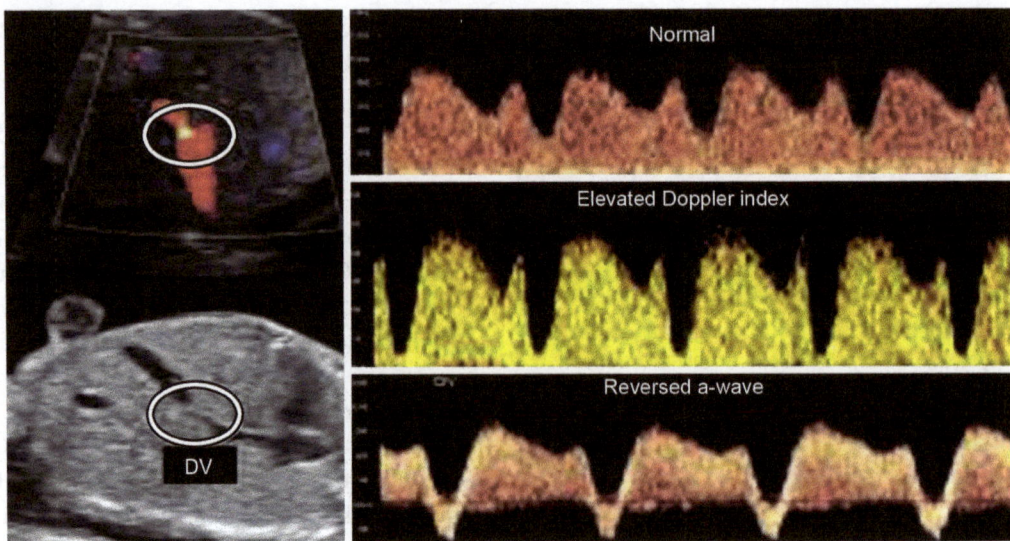

Fig. 7: Ductus venosus (DV) Doppler.

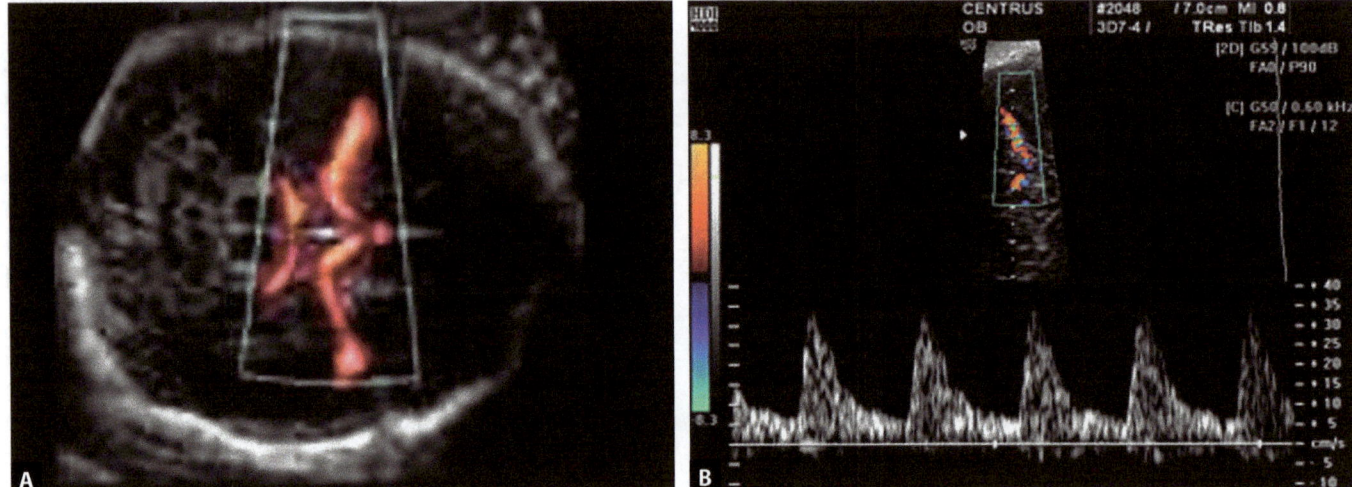

Figs. 8A and B: Normal middle cerebral artery Doppler.

as viscosity decreases; so, as the fetal hematocrit decreases, MCA flow velocity increases. In addition, in a compromised fetus, cerebral vasodilatation diverts blood flow to the brain; because flow velocity in a pipe is proportional to the fourth power of the radius, a small increase of the MCA diameter results in a considerable increase in flow velocity (Poiseuille law).

Red blood cell (RBC) alloimmunized fetuses are at risk of anemia. Other causes include parvovirus infections, fetomaternal hemorrhage, nonimmune hydrops, and twin-twin transfusion. The MCA PSV can predict the existence of moderate-to-severe fetal anemia with a sensitivity of 100% and a false-positive rate of 12%. The velocity of blood flow within the fetal arterial circulation is inversely proportional to the degree of anemia due to increased fetal cardiac output which is secondary to reduced blood viscosity. The risk of anemia is high in fetuses with MCA PSV of 1.5 MoM or higher and may prompt time to perform cordocentesis and intrauterine transfusion. A multicenter study assessed both the MCA PSV and amniocentesis in Rh isoimmunized fetuses undergoing cordocentesis, reported that for the detection of severe anemia the sensitivity of MCA PSV was better than that of amniocentesis. MCA PSV was effective for accurate diagnosis of fetal anemia and can avoid 70% of invasive procedures.

Umbilical Venous Doppler

Umbilical vein returns oxygenated blood from the placenta to the fetus. Normal flow in the UV is monophasic, continuous nonpulsatile flow after first trimester in uncomplicated pregnancy. Fetal breathing is a common observation in

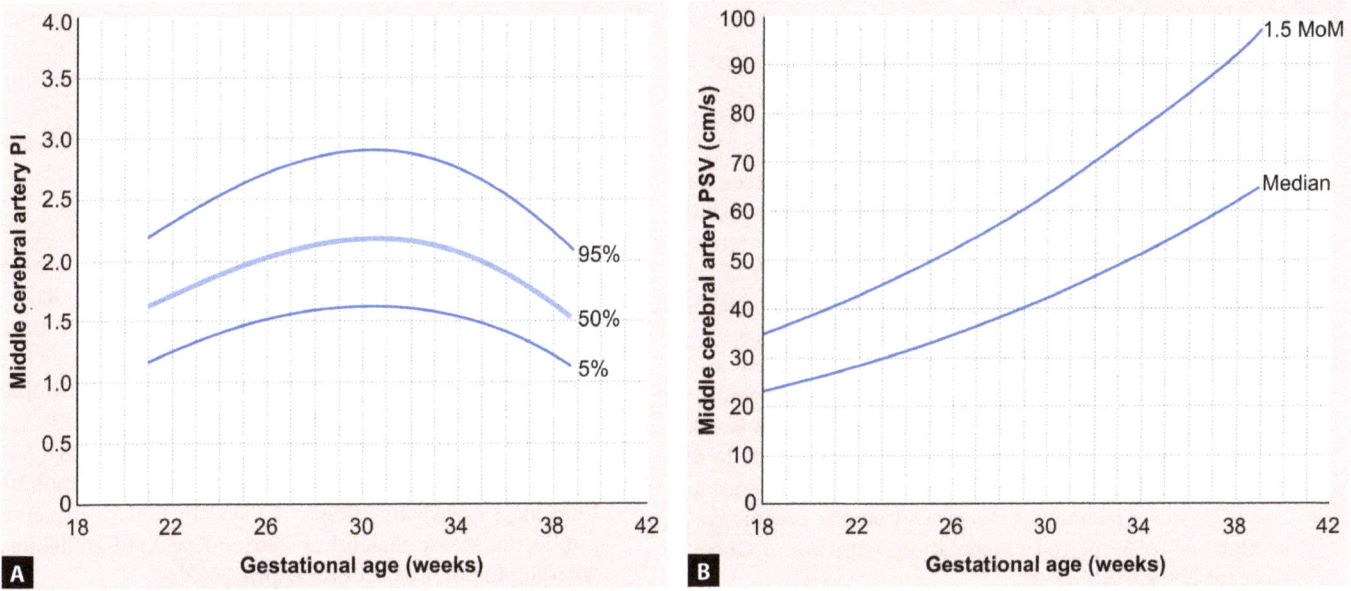

Figs. 9A and B: (A) Normal middle cerebral artery (MCA) Doppler; (B) MCA doppler in fetal hypoxia
(PI: pulsatility index; PSV: peak systolic velocity)

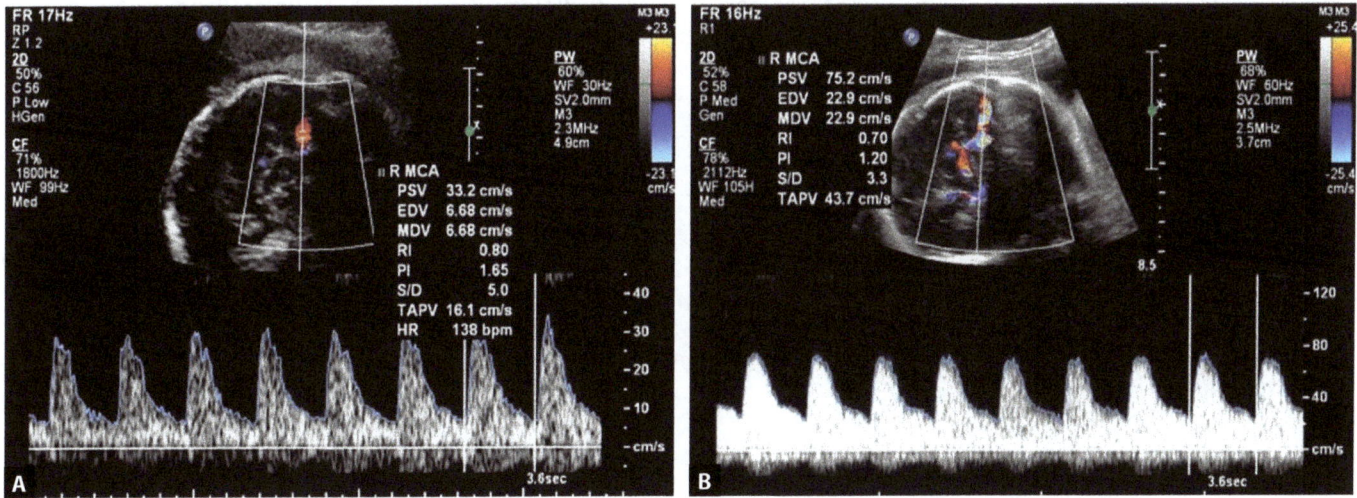

Figs. 10A and B: (A) Normal middle cerebral artery (MCA) Doppler; (B) Abnormal MCA Doppler.

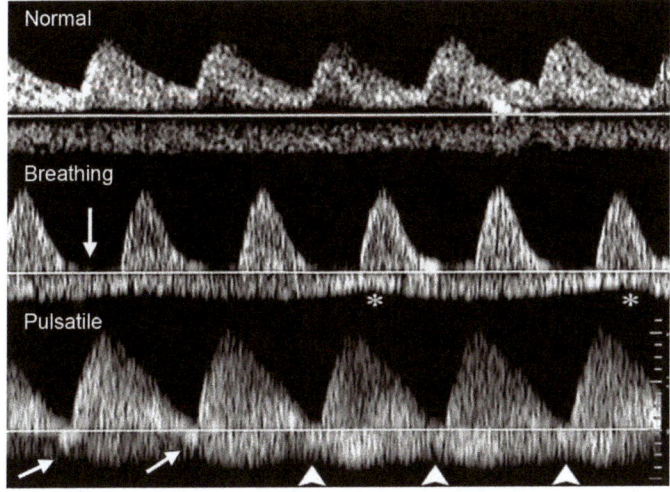

Fig. 11: Umbilical vein Doppler flow.

the third trimester. The changes in intrathoracic pressure alter flow dynamics in the vein to produce undulations in the UV waveform that are not linked to the cardiac cycle. Pulsatile flow in the UV is an ominous finding. When present, it indicates that the abnormal placental pressures have compromised right heart function such that there is back pressure through the right ventricle to the right atrium, back out the DV (which will show a decreased or reversed A-wave) all the way into the UV, where forward flow decreases during diastole. This process causes a pulsatile waveform with diminished forward flow in the UV during ventricular diastole. Fetuses with pulsations in the free-floating UV in the second and third trimester have a higher morbidity and mortality, even in the setting of normal UA blood flow.

SUGGESTED READING

1. Bennasar M, Eixarch E, Martinez JM, Gratacós E. Selective intrauterine growth restriction in monochorionic diamniotic twin pregnancies. Semin Fetal Neonatal Med. 2017;22(6):376-82.
2. Crovetto F, Crispi F, Scazzocchio E. First-trimester screening for early and late small-for-gestational-age neonates using maternal serum biochemistry, blood pressure and uterine artery Doppler. Ultrasound Obstet Gynecol. 2014;43(1):34-40.
3. Figueras F, Gratacos E. Stage-based approach to the management of fetal growth restriction. Prenat Diagn. 2014;34:655-9.
4. Figueras F, Gratacos E. Update on the diagnosis and classification of fetal growth restriction and proposal of a stage-based management protocol. Fetal Diagn Ther. 2014;36:86-98.
5. Herraiz I, López-Jiménez EA, García-Burguillo A. Role of uterine artery Doppler in interpreting low PAPP-A values in first-trimester screening for Down syndrome in pregnancies at high risk of impaired placentation. Ultrasound Obstet Gynecol. 2009;33(5):518-23.
6. Jones J. Fetal middle cerebral arterial Doppler assessment. Radiopaedia. 2021:1-5.
7. Kagan KO, Valencia C, Livanos P, Wright D, Nicolaides KH. Tricuspid regurgitation in screening for trisomies 21, 18 and 13 and Turner syndrome at 11^{+0} to 13^{+6} weeks of gestation. Ultrasound Obstet Gynecol. 2009;33(1):18-22.
8. Kennedy AM, Woodward PJ. A Radiologist's Guide to the Performance and Interpretation of Obstetric Doppler US. Radiographics. 2019;39:3.
9. Khong SL, Kane SC, Brennecke SP, da Silva Costa F. First-trimester uterine artery doppler analysis in the prediction of later pregnancy complications. Dis Markers. 2015;2015:679730.
10. Maiz N, Nicolaides KH. Ductus venosus in the first trimester: contribution to screening of chromosomal, cardiac defects and monochorionic twin complications. Fetal Diagn Ther. 2010;28(2):65-71.
11. Maiz N, Valencia C, Emmanuel EE. Screening for adverse pregnancy outcome by ductus venosus Doppler at $11-13^{+6}$ weeks of gestation. Obstet Gynecol. 2008;112:598-605.
12. Martins JG, Biggio JR. Society for Maternal-Fetal Medicine Consult Series #52: Diagnosis and management of fetal growth restriction. Am J Obstet Gynaecol. 2020;223(4):B1.
13. Maulik D, Bennett TL. Doppler Sonography in Early Pregnancy. New York: Springer; 2016. pp. 195-212.
14. Mone F, McAuliffe FM. The clinical application of Doppler ultrasound in obstetrics. Obstet Gynecol. 2015;17:13-19.
15. New Zealand Maternal Fetal Medicine Network. (2014). New Zealand Obstetric Doppler Guideline. [online] Available from https://www.health.govt.nz/system/files/documents/publications/new-zealand-obstetric-ultrasound-guidelines-2019-dec19.pdf [Last accessed April, 2022].
16. Nicolaides K, Rizzo G, Hecher K. Doppler in Obstetrics. Diploma in Fetal Medicine and ISUOG Educational Series. London: The Fetal Medicine Foundation; 2002.
17. Radiology Key. (2017). Doppler Sonography in Early Pregnancy. [online] Available from https://radiologykey.com/doppler-sonography-in-early-pregnancy. [Last accessed April, 2022].
18. Royal College of Obstetricians and Gynaecologists. Green-Top Guideline 31. In: The Investigation and Management of the Small-for-Gestational-Age Fetus, 2nd edition. London: RCOG; 2013.
19. Thummalakunta P, Panditi S. Approach to Screening for Aneuploidy in First Trimester. J Fetal Med. 2015;1:175-9.

CHAPTER 7

Diabetes in Pregnancy

■ INTRODUCTION

Diabetes is one of the most common medical disorder complicating pregnancy. It is a group of metabolic disorder caused by defects in insulin secretion, insulin action or both which leads to abnormalities of carbohydrate, protein, and lipid metabolism. The prevalence of diabetes in pregnancy has been increasing in parallel with the worldwide epidemic of obesity. Not only is the prevalence of type 1 diabetes and type 2 diabetes increasing in women of reproductive age, but with the rapid socioeconomic and life-style transformation, the prevalence of gestational diabetes mellitus (GDM) has risen dramatically.

Diabetes confers significantly greater maternal and fetal risk largely related to the degree of hyperglycemia but also related to chronic complications and comorbidities of diabetes. Uncontrolled blood glucose (BG) at the time of conception increases spontaneous abortion, risk of birth defect increases 3–4 times; fetal and neonatal mortality increases 3–4 folds compared to normoglycemic population. Risk of serious birth injury doubled, the likelihood of cesarean section (CS) tripled, and the incidence of neonatal intensive care admission is quadrupled. In addition, diabetes in pregnancy increases the risk of obesity, hypertension, and type 2 diabetes in the offspring later in life; women with type 1 DM may progress to nephropathy and retinopathy, as well as diabetic ketoacidosis (DKA).

Programming of Vascular Dysfunction in the Intrauterine Milieu of Diabetic Pregnancies

Mechanisms linking gestational diabetes mellitus (GDM) to vascular dysfunction in the offspring shown in **Figure 1**. Maternal hyperglycaemia exposes the fetus to high levels of glucose. Deleterious effects of hyperglycemia are mediated largely through inflammation and oxidative stress. Highly inter-related pathways of inflammatory and redox signaling are persistently dysregulated after transient hyperglycemia due to transcriptional programming by DNA or histone methylation. Studies in endothelial colony forming cells (ECFC) and human umbilical vein endothelial cells (HUVEC) collected from GDM pregnancies suggest that intrauterine hyperglycemia directly programs vascular dysfunction by modulating methylation patterns and increasing oxidant load and inflammation. Chronic oxidative stress and inflammation lead to endothelial dysfunction characterized by decreased endothelium-derived dilators (NO) and increased contractile mediators (COX-2 prostanoids).

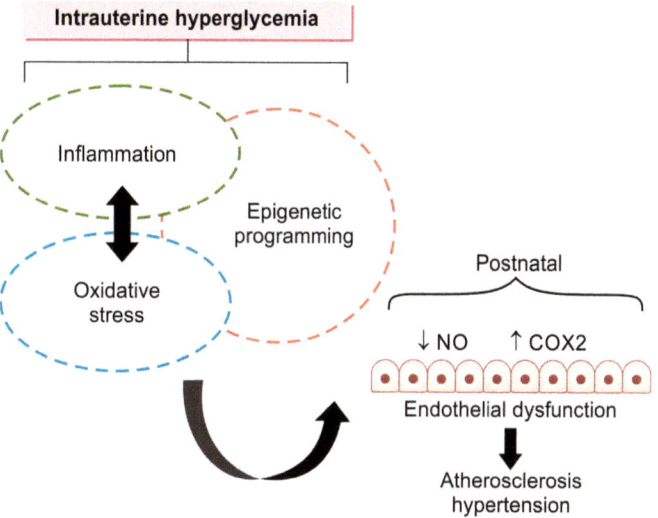

Fig. 1: Intrauterine hyperglycemia and long-term fetal risk. (COX2: cyclooxygenase 2; NO: nitiric oxide)
Source: Int J Mol Sci. 2018; 19(11): 3665; https://doi.org/10.3390/ijms19113665.

■ INCIDENCE

Approximately 90% of women with diabetes during pregnancy are affected by gestational diabetes, 8% have preexisting type 2 diabetes, and the remainder have another form of diabetes, e.g., genetic diabetes. In the United States, about 1–2% of pregnant women have type 1 or type 2 diabetes and about 6–9% of pregnant women develop gestational diabetes. Study revealed South East Asian region has the highest prevalence of diabetes, with 27% of the pregnancies affected by GDM while the lowest prevalence was seen in Africa at 10.5% [Centers for Disease Control and Prevention (CDC)].

ETIOLOGICAL CLASSIFICATION OF DIABETES IN PREGNANCY (AMERICAN DIABETES ASSOCIATION CLASSIFICATION)

- Insulin-dependent type 1 DM
- Insulin-dependent type 2 DM
- Gestational DM
- Other specific types—example:
  - Genetic defect in beta-cell function or insulin action—neonatal diabetes and maturity-onset diabetes of the young (MODY)
  - Disease of pancreas (cystic fibrosis, chronic pancreatitis)
  - Drug- or chemical-induced [Rx of human immuno-deficiency virus (HIV), acquired immunodeficiency syndrome (AIDS), and organ transplantation].

PATHOPHYSIOLOGY OF DIABETES

The pathophysiology of all types of diabetes is related to the hormone insulin. In type 1 diabetes, the pancreas cannot synthesize enough amounts of insulin as required by the body. The pathophysiology of type 1 DM suggests that it is an autoimmune disease, wherein the body's own immune system attack the β-cells of the pancreas resulting in *absolute insulin deficiency*. The pancreas secretes *little or no insulin*. Type 1 diabetes is more common among children and young adults (around 20 years).

Type 2 diabetes mellitus (T2DM) is one of the most common metabolic disorders worldwide. In T2DM there is *relative rather than absolute insulin deficiency*. Its development is primarily caused by a combination of two primary factors: (1) defective insulin secretion by pancreatic β-cells and (2) the inability of insulin-sensitive tissues to respond appropriately to insulin.

Regarding the pathophysiology of the disease, a malfunction of the feedback loops between insulin action and insulin secretion results in abnormally high glucose levels in blood. In case of β-cell dysfunction, insulin secretion is reduced, limiting the body's capacity to maintain physiological glucose levels. On the other hand, insulin resistance (IR) [fasting blood glucose (FBG) (mg/dL): insulin (μIU/L) <4.5] contributes to increased glucose production in the liver and decreased glucose uptake both in the muscle, liver, and adipose tissue; β-cell dysfunction is usually more severe than IR. However, when both β-cell dysfunction and IR are present, hyperglycemia is amplified leading to the progression of T2DM. With persistent IR, there is loss of compensatory β-cell activity, exhaustion, and minimal insulin production, with increased duration type 2 diabetes behaves like type 1. There is unrestrained glucose production by the liver and poor utilization in the muscles and adipose tissue. Since endogenous insulin production is not completely prohibited, DKA (diabetic keto-acidosis) is rare.

Gestational diabetes: Over here, high level of BG is caused by *hormonal fluctuations* during pregnancy. During early gestation, insulin sensitivity increases (probably due to high estrogen), promoting uptake of glucose into adipose stores in preparation for the energy demands of later pregnancy, BG is slightly elevated, and this glucose is readily transported across the placenta to fuel the growth of the fetus **(Flowchart 1)**.

As pregnancy advances, local and placental hormones—estrogen, progesterone, leptin, cortisol, human placental

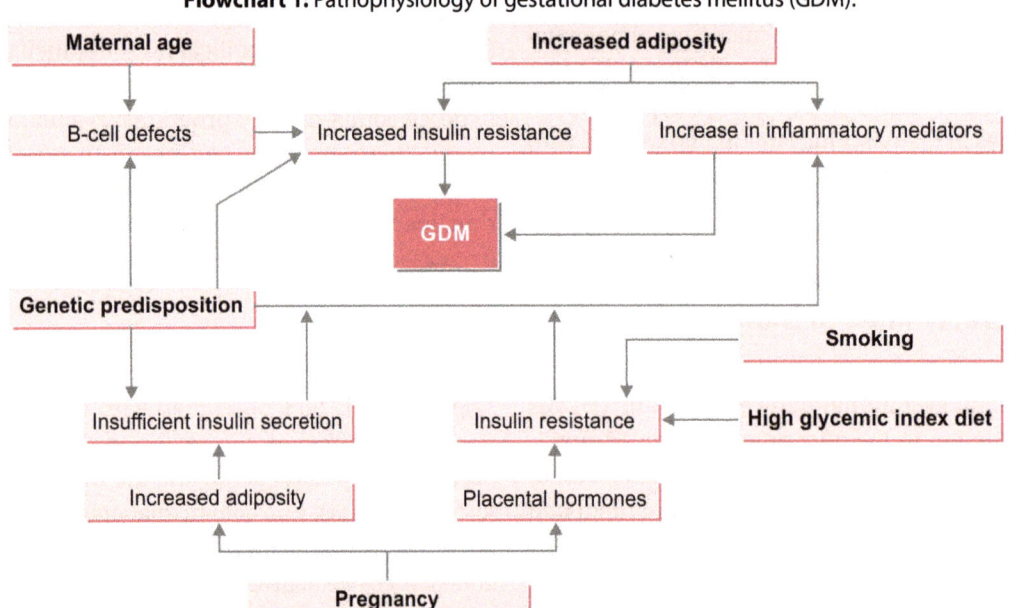

Flowchart 1: Pathophysiology of gestational diabetes mellitus (GDM).

Source: Expert Rev Endocrinol Metab ©2012 Expert Reviews Ltd.

lactogen (HPL), and placental growth hormone together promote a state of IR. Insulinase produced by the placenta causes accelerated insulin catabolism and increased insulin requirements. In order to maintain glucose homeostasis, pregnant women compensate for these changes through hypertrophy and hyperplasia of pancreatic β-cells, as well as increased glucose-stimulated insulin secretion (GSIS). β-cells become exhausted over time due to excessive insulin production in response to excess energy consumption and IR develops, resembling T2DM.

GESTATIONAL DIABETES MELLITUS

INTRODUCTION

Gestational diabetes mellitus is one of the most common medical disorder complicating pregnancies. According to the most recent International Diabetes Federation (IDF, 2017) estimates, GDM affects approximately 14% of pregnancies worldwide, representing approximately 18 million births annually. Almost 90% of cases of hyperglycemia in pregnancy occurs in low- and middle-income countries, where access to maternal healthcare is limited. Even within-countries, GDM prevalence varies depending on race/ethnicity and socioeconomic status. Aboriginal Australians, Middle Easterners, and Pacific Islanders are the most at-risk groups for GDM. In the United States, Native Americans, Hispanics, Asians, and African-American women are at a higher risk of GDM than Caucasian women.

DEFINITION

Gestational diabetes mellitus is defined as hyperglycemia identified at any time during pregnancy in a woman who is not known to have preexisting diabetes. In the majority of women, it resolves after pregnancy, however it may be the first presentation of type 1, type 2 or genetic diabetes. The American College of Obstetricians and Gynecologists (ACOG) has defined gestational diabetes as "any degree of glucose intolerance that either commences or first diagnosed during pregnancy". The definition applies whether insulin or only diet modification is used for treatment and whether or not the condition persists after pregnancy. It does not exclude the possibility that unrecognized glucose intolerance may have antedated or begun concomitantly with pregnancy. Because this definition includes misdiagnosed preexisting diabetes, the American Diabetes Association (ADA) have changed the definition to "first onset of diabetes in the second or third trimester of pregnancy that is not clearly overt diabetes prior to gestation".

According to International Association of Diabetes and Pregnancy study group *(IADPSG)* diabetes first recognized in pregnancy can be classified as either "overt diabetes" or "gestational diabetes mellitus". GDM is defined as diabetes diagnosed during pregnancy that is not clearly overt diabetes. The World Health Organization *(WHO)* (2012) proposed slightly different terminology—according to WHO hyperglycemia first detected at any time during pregnancy should be classified as either:

- Gestational diabetes mellitus or
- Diabetes mellitus in pregnancy

World Health Organization criteria: *Gestational diabetes mellitus* should be diagnosed at any time in pregnancy if one or more of the following criteria are met:

- Fasting plasma glucose (FPG) 5.1-6.9 mmoL/L (92-125 mg/dL)
- 1-hour plasma glucose ≥10.0 mmoL/L (180 mg/dL) following a 75 g oral glucose load*
- 2-hour plasma glucose 8.5-11.0 mmoL/L (153-199 mg/dL) following a 75 g oral glucose load.

Diabetes in pregnancy should be diagnosed (by the 2006 WHO criteria for diabetes) if one or more of the following criteria are met:

- Fasting plasma glucose ≥7.0 mmoL/L (126 mg/dL)
- 2-hour plasma glucose ≥11.1 mmoL/L (200 mg/dL) following a 75 g oral glucose load
- Random plasma glucose ≥11.1 mmoL/L (200 mg/ dL) in the presence of diabetes symptoms.

TABLE 1: IADPSG criteria for diagnosis of diabetes in pregnancy: based on HbA1c or FPG or RPG.		
Overt diabetes	*GDM*	*Normal*
A1c >6.5% or FPG ≥7 mmoL/L or RPG ≥1.1 mmoL/L (confirmed later by fasting glucose or glycosylated Hb)	• A1c 5.7–6.4% or • FPG ≥5.1–6.9 mmoL/L • 2 hours after 75 g glucose: ≥8.5 mmoL/L–11 mmoL/L	A1c <5.7% or FPG <5.1 mmoL/L
One of these must be met to identify patient as having over diabetic	One or more of these values must be equaled or exceeded for the diagnosis of GDM	OGTT at 24–28 weeks if abnormal GDM

Note: The new IADPSG criteria has been adopted globally widely and in the US by the ADA but not endorsed by ACOG.
(ACOG: The American College of Obstetricians and Gynecologists; ADA: the American Diabetes Association; FPG: fasting plasma glucose; GDM: gestational diabetes mellitus; HbA1c: hemoglobin A1c; IADPSG: International Association of Diabetes and Pregnancy study group; OGTT: oral glucose tolerance testing; RPG: random plasma glucose)

■ RISK FACTORS FOR GESTATIONAL DIABETES

There are several risk factors for GDM including overweight/obesity, excessive gestational weight gain, westernized diet, ethnicity, genetic polymorphisms, advanced maternal age, intrauterine environment (low or high birth weight), family and personal history of GDM, and other diseases of IR, such as polycystic ovarian syndrome (PCOS). Each of these risk factors are either directly or indirectly associated with impaired β-cell function and/or insulin sensitivity.

Diets that are high in saturated fats, refined sugars, and red and processed meats are consistently associated with an increased risk of GDM, while diets high in fiber, micronutrients, and polyunsaturated fats are associated with a reduced risk of GDM. Saturated fats directly interfere with insulin signaling, and can also induce inflammation and endothelial dysfunction—both are pathogenic factors in GDM, on the other hand, polyunsaturated fatty acids derived from fish and seafood, have anti-inflammatory properties.

Low and high birth weight are likely risk factors for GDM because of their association with IR. It is believed that the fetus compensates for undernutrition in the womb by epigenetically altering the expression of genes that are involved in fat storage, energy utilization, and appetite regulation. Animal studies suggest that undernutrition in utero is associated with reduced β-cell number. These alterations persist after birth—a phenomenon referred to as "developmental programming". While potentially beneficial in times of famine, once born can contribute to the development of obesity and metabolic disease. On the opposite end of the spectrum, overnutrition in the womb—such as can occur in GDM—can result in fetal overgrowth. These individuals are more likely to have experienced hyperglycemia and β-cell fatigue even before birth, predisposing them to hyperglycemia during times of later metabolic stress, such as during pregnancy.

■ SCREENING AND DIAGNOSIS OF GESTATIONAL DIABETES MELLITUS

Universal recommendation for ideal approach for screening and diagnosis of GDM is still controversial because of the differences in population risk, cost-effectiveness, and lack of evidence to support large national screening program. Opinions differ—whether there should be:
- Selective or universal screening
- When and how screening should be done.

The American Diabetes Association recommends risk assessment for GDM should be undertaken at the first prenatal visit. Women with clinical characteristics consistent with a *high risk* of GDM (marked obesity, personal history of GDM, glycosuria, or a strong family history of diabetes) should undergo glucose testing as soon as feasible. If they are found not to have GDM at that initial screening, they should be retested between 24 and 28 weeks of gestation. Women of average risk should have testing undertaken at 24–28 weeks of gestation. Low-risk status requires no glucose testing, this category includes women meeting all of the following characteristics: Age <25 years, weight normal before pregnancy, member of an ethnic group with a low prevalence of GDM, no known diabetes in first-degree relatives, no history of abnormal glucose tolerance, and no history of poor obstetric outcome.

The American College of Obstetricians and Gynecologists guidance on screening for diabetes and prediabetes, consider early screening in pregnancy if:

Patient is overweight with body mass index (BMI) of 25 (23 in Asian Americans), *and* one of the following:
- Decreased physical inactivity
- Known impaired glucose metabolism
- Previous pregnancy history of:
  - GDM
  - Macrosomia (≥4,000 g)
  - Stillbirth
- Hypertension (140/90 mm Hg or being treated for hypertension)
- High-density lipoprotein (HDL) cholesterol ≤35 mg/dL (0.90 mmoL/L)
- Fasting triglyceride ≥250 mg/dL (2.82 mmoL/L)
- Polycystic ovary syndrome, acanthosis nigricans, nonalcoholic steatohepatitis, morbid obesity, and other conditions associated with IR
- HbA1c ≥5.7%, impaired glucose tolerance (IGT) or impaired fasting glucose. If A1c >6.5%, diagnosis of pregestational diabetes is met and glucose challenge test/glucose tolerance test (GCT/GTT) not needed
- Cardiovascular disease (CVD)
- *Family history of diabetes:* First degree relative (parent or sibling)
- Ethnicity of African American, American Indian, Asian American, Hispanic, Latina, or Pacific Islander.

Protocol for Screening

In 2010, *IADPSG recommended* criteria for the diagnosis of GDM based on hyperglycemia and adverse pregnancy outcome (HAPO) study. At first prenatal visit measure FPG, HbA1c, or random plasma glucose on all or only high-risk women. If result indicates overt diabetes—treat and follow up as preexisting diabetes. *If FPG <5.1 mmoL/L, test for GDM between 24 and 28 weeks*, perform 2 hours 75 g oral glucose tolerance testing (OGTT) after overnight fasting (8–14 hours).

The American Diabetes Association protocol involves: *Early screening* for women with *high risk* for pregestational diabetes. The ADA recommends the use of either the one- or two-step approach at 24–28 weeks of gestation in women not previously known to have diabetes. The one-step approach involves performing a 75-g OGTT, after an overnight fast of 8-14 hours and testing at 1 and 2 hours. The diagnosis of GDM is made when any of the following is met or exceeded:

- *Fasting:* 92 mg/dL (5.1 mmoL/L)
- *1 hour:* 180 mg/dL (10.0 mmoL/L)
- *2 hours:* 153 mg/dL (8.5 mmoL/L).

The two-step approach is a 1-hour (nonfasting) plasma glucose measurement after a 50-g oral glucose load in women at 24-48 weeks' gestation who were not previously diagnosed with diabetes. If the plasma glucose level after 1 hour is ≥130 mg/dL, 135 mg/dL, or 140 mg/dL (7.2 mmoL/L, 7.5 mmoL/L, or 7.8 mmoL/L, respectively), perform a fasting 100-g OGTT. The diagnosis of GDM is made if at least two of the following four plasma glucose levels (measured during OGTT) are met or exceeded:

1. *Fasting:* 95 mg/dL (5.3 mmoL/L)
2. *1 hour:* 180 mg/dL (10.0 mmoL/L)
3. *2 hours:* 155 mg/dL (8.6 mmoL/L)
4. *3 hours:* 140 mg/dL (7.8 mmoL/L).

■ MANAGEMENT

Gestational diabetes mellitus encompasses a wide range of glucose intolerance but most women can be managed without insulin. *Lifestyle change* is an essential component of management of GDM, including diet and exercise. Advice a healthy diet, and to switch from high to low glycemic index food. ADA recommends individualized nutrition plan developed by a registered dietitian familiar with the management of GDM. Advise to exercise regularly (walking for 30 minutes after a meal). There is no international consensus when to start pharmacological treatment. Almost 50% of newly diagnosed patients should meet the control criteria within 2 weeks of institution of dietary regulation and exercise. If BG targets are not met with diet and exercise changes within 2 weeks, offer metformin. If metformin is contraindicated or unacceptable, or if BG targets are not met with diet and exercise changes plus metformin, *offer insulin* (5th International Workshop conference on GDM in 2007 recommendation, NICE 2015).

Insulin treatment is globally considered the safest option for GDM treatment with an immediate effect on maternal glycemia. Human insulins do not cross the placenta and are not related to fetal complications. *Canadian diabetic association, ADA, and ACOG-*(2018) recommends: *Insulin as first-line therapy* if glycemic control is not achieved after 1-2 weeks of diet and lifestyle interventions. The International Federation of Gynecology and Obstetrics *(FIGO)* considers insulin and oral antidiabetics as safe and efficient options in the management of GDM after 20 weeks of pregnancy, but recommend insulin as first-line treatment in the management of hyperglycemia during first trimester due to the high risk of failing therapy on oral agents.

Total Daily Calorie Intake

Medical nutrition therapy (MNT) is the cornerstone of GDM treatment. Individualization of MNT depending on maternal weight and height is recommended. MNT should include the provision of adequate calories and nutrients to meet the needs of pregnancy and should be consistent with the maternal BG goals that have been established. MNT alone can assure glycemic targets in 80-90% of GDM patients. The first step in meal plan is to calculate optimum total daily calorie. Calorie intake with a normal BMI of 18.5-24.9 kg/m^2 is about 30 kcal/kg; 35-40 kcal for underweight women (<80%); 25 kcal for overweight (121-150%) and 12 kcal for morbid obese women. For majority GDM patients, total daily calorie will be between 2,000 and 2,500 kcal/day. In the third trimester when the calorie need is increased it is necessary to add extra 300 kcal. Total daily calorie should be distributed in such way that carbohydrate intake should be reduced to 33-45% of the total calories, while the rest of the calories should be equally divided between protein and lipids distributed over 3 meals and 2-4 snacks/day, thus reducing postprandial glucose peak. Simple carbohydrates release glucose rapidly from maternal gut, therefore, be avoided. The diet should emphasize monounsaturated and polyunsaturated fats while limiting saturated fats and avoiding trans fats.

Gestational weight gain: Should be based on the early pregnancy weight, as per the Institute of Medicine (IOM) guidelines, 12.5-18 kg weight gain for underweight (BMI <18.5 kg/m^2), 11.5-16 kg for normal weight (BMI 18.5-24.9 kg/m^2); 7-11.5 kg for overweight (BMI 25-29.9 kg/m^2), and 5-9 kg for obese (BMI ≥30.0 kg/m^2) women. The target should be set 10% lower from the recommended weight gain in normal pregnancy, although it is probably safe to restrict the overall weight gain to <5 kg in extremely obese women. Physical activity improves glycemic control in GDM women. The generally accepted recommendation is daily moderate-intensity regular exercise (walking 30 minutes/day or more if no contraindications, improves BG control).

Oral Medications

The goal of medical therapy is to reduce fetal macrosomia. Currently, there are two oral agents licensed in the treatment of GDM. Glibenclamide, a second-generation sulfonylurea that increases insulin release from the pancreatic β-cells. It differs from the other sulfonylureas in the high protein binding (99.8%) and short elimination half-life, resulting in very low transplacental transport. All published data up to date agree that glibenclamide is not inferior to insulin treatment in achieving desired glycemic control. Controversy remains regarding the safety profile for the fetus.

Metformin belongs to the biguanide class. It inhibits hepatic gluconeogenesis and increases insulin sensitivity in peripheral tissues. It is well-described that metformin crosses the placental barrier exposing the fetus to levels similar to maternal circulation.

The National Institute for Health and Care Excellence (NICE) guideline recommends use of metformin in GDM if glycemic target is not reached with lifestyle intervention.

Two recent randomized controlled trials (RCTs) showed glyburide and metformin failed to provide adequate glycemic control in 23% and 25-28% cases, respectively. Glyburide was associated with a higher rate of neonatal hypoglycemia and macrosomia than insulin or metformin. Metformin was associated with reduced risk of neonatal hypoglycemia and less weight gain than insulin, however, may slightly increase the risk of prematurity. The metformin in gestational diabetes: the offspring follow-up (MiG TOFU) study showed 9-year-old offspring exposed to metformin was heavier and had a higher waist-to-height ratio and waist circumference than those exposed to insulin (ADA, Diabetes Care, 2021).

INSULIN TREATMENT

Insulin treatment is globally considered the safest option for GDM treatment with an immediate effect on maternal glycemia. Human insulins do not cross the placenta and are not related to fetal complications and can lead to tight glycemic control. The goal is to maintain self-monitored glucose at the following levels: Fasting whole BG ≤95 mg/dL (5.3 mmoL/L), FPG ≤105 mg/dL (5.8 mmoL/L) or 1-hour postprandial whole BG ≤140 mg/dL (7.8 mmoL/L), 1-hour postprandial plasma glucose ≤155 mg/dL (8.6 mmoL/L) or 2-hour postprandial whole BG ≤120 mg/dL (6.7 mmoL/L), and 2-hour postprandial plasma glucose ≤130 mg/dL (7.2 mmoL/L). The target of HbA1c is <6-6.5% (42-48 mmoL/moL); lower HbA1c—6% (42 mmoL/moL) is optimal if it can be achieved without significant hypoglycemia; the target may be relaxed to 7% (53 mmoL/moL) to prevent hypoglycemia.

Treatment of GDM with lifestyle and insulin has demonstrated to improve perinatal outcomes in two large randomized studies as summarized in a United States (US) Preventive Services Task Force review. Insulin remains the gold standard treatment for GDM women that do not reach glycemic targets with lifestyle intervention as recommended by several guidelines. *FIGO* recommends insulin therapy under the following conditions:
- Oral therapy failure or
- One of the following risk factors:
  - Diagnosing diabetes before 20 weeks of gestation
  - Oral therapy for >30 weeks
  - Fasting plasma BG above 110 mg/dL
  - 1-hour postprandial glycemia above 140 mg/dL
  - Weight gain over 12 kg during pregnancy.

Types of Insulin

Regular insulin (U-100, U-500) is identical to human insulin, and is used as mealtime insulin to cover postprandial hyperglycemia. Rapid-acting insulin analogs include lispro, aspart, and glulisine. These can be used as mealtime insulin in multiple daily insulin injection (MDII) therapy, or in an insulin pump. Time to onset of regular insulin is about 30 minutes (10-75 minutes), the peak effect is in 3 hours (2.5-5 hours), and the effect ends at about 8 hours (up to 24 hours for U500). Aspart should be taken 5-10 minutes before a meal. Its peak action time is 40-50 minutes, and its duration of action is 3-5 hours. Insulin aspart produce less hypoglycemia than regular insulin. Insulin lispro (U-100 and U-200) is another rapid-acting insulin. Its onset of action is 10-15 minutes, the peak is at 30-90 minutes, and its duration of action is 3-4 hours. It can be used in insulin pumps or pens.

Insulin isophane [neutral protamine Hagedorn (NPH)] is an intermediate-acting insulin. It is similar to human insulin and is presented in a liquid suspension. Its onset of action is maximum 2 hours, with an average peak of 4 hours, full duration of action is 10-20 hours. There is no restriction on use in gestational diabetes or DM in pregnancy; it does not cross the placental barrier and it is Food and Drug Administration (FDA) pregnancy category B.

Long-acting insulin analogs include detemir and glargine. They are "peakless" and have a longer duration of action compared to NPH insulin. The time to onset of detemir insulin action can be 1-2 hours and action lasts for up to 24 hours; can be considered during pregnancy. The efficacy and safety of detemir has been established in a multinational RCT involving pregnant women with T1DM. Detemir has demonstrated lower fasting glucose levels, similar hypoglycemia rates and perinatal outcomes, and noninferior glycemic control compared to NPH. Detemir has been approved by the European Medicines Agency for use in pregnancy, and is FDA category B.

Glargine has a higher receptor affinity for the type 1 insulin-like growth factor receptor. Limited data on the glargine use in women with pregestational DM suggests comparable maternal, fetal, and neonatal outcomes compared with other basal insulins. Insulin glargine does not carry a FDA classification consistent with current labeling **(Fig. 2)**.

Insulin Regimens (FIGO)

There are many insulin regimens proposed for treating hyperglycemia, but the MDI is by far the most efficient and the most flexible. The insulin regimen should be chosen based on the BG profile. If fasting glycemia is higher than 90-95 mg/dL, basal insulin should be initiated. It can be a long-acting insulin analog or NPH. The basal insulin dose can be calculated according to the weight: *0.2 units/kg/day*. If hyperglycemia *follows a meal, rapid-acting insulin* or regular insulin should be initiated before that meal (begin with *1 unit of insulin for 10-15 g of carbohydrates*). Sometimes both fasting and postprandial glycemia are elevated, thereby needing MDI: 3 mealtime insulin and basal insulin. The total daily insulin requirement during the first trimester, is 0.7 units/kg/day, while in the second trimester it is 0.8 units/kg/day, and in the third trimester, it is 0.9–1.0 units/kg/day. This does not necessarily fit all pregnancies. Usually, in pregestational diabetes, the total insulin dose is up to twice higher than in GDM. In the case of morbid obesity, the initial doses of insulin can be increased to 1.5–2.0 units/kg to overcome the combined IR of pregnancy and obesity.

Usually, the calculated total daily dose of insulin should be divided in two as for type 1 and type 2 diabetes: 50% as basal insulin at bedtime, and 50% divided between 3 meals and given as rapid-acting, or regular insulin before meals. Rapid-acting insulin analogs are preferred over regular insulin in pregnancy because there is a lower risk of hypoglycemia, and because they provide a better postprandial BG control.

The doses of insulin have to be continuously optimized, so the self-monitoring blood glucose (SMBG) is essential. Fasting and postprandial SMBG are recommended in both gestational DM and preexisting diabetes in pregnancy to achieve optimal glucose levels.

Target capillary blood glucose (CBG)—to keep preprandial value under 95 mg/dL (5.3 mmoL/L), postprandial <140 mg/dL (7.8 mmoL/L) at 1 hour or <120 mg/dL (6.7 mmoL/L) at 2 hours (NICE, 2015; 5th International Workshop Conference Gestational Diabetes and International Association of Diabetes and Pregnancy Study Group, 2007; FIGO, 2015; CDA, 2018; and ADA, 2018).

Frequency of monitoring: As much as necessary (fasting, 1 or 2 hours postprandial) without customizing for treatment. Based on a randomized control trial (RCT) the initial recommendation *for SMBG is four tests per day*, with the possibility to lessen the number of determinations if the patient has good control and the fetal morphology is normal. In basal-bolus insulin-treated GDM, seven tests per day are recommended. A randomized clinical trial demonstrated that patients who adjusted insulin doses based on 1-hour postprandial glycemia had a lower risk of giving birth to a macrosomia, or to have a cesarean procedure; also, the risk for neonatal hypoglycemia was smaller **(Table 2)**.

Summary of target glucose and HbA1c levels for gestational diabetes from international guidelines has been given in **Table 3**.

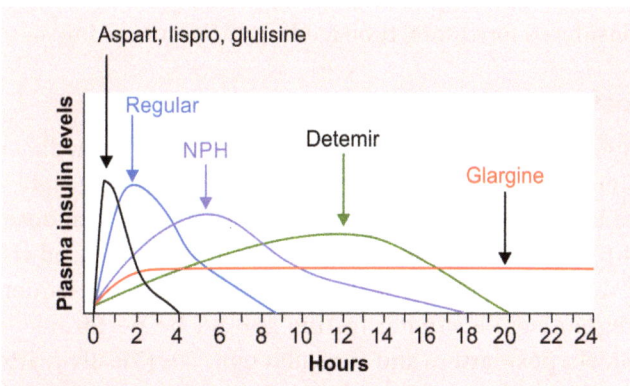

"Regular" insulin = Humalog, Novolog

Fig. 2: Subtypes and approximate durations of action of different insulin formulations. The duration of action of regular and NPH insulin increases at higher doses. Adapted from Kennedy and Masharani (2015) (NPH: neutral protamine Hagedorn)

TABLE 2: Monitoring blood glucose (American Association of Clinical Endocrinologist and American College of Endocrinology).

Regimen	SMBG
GDM with diet or oral antidiabetics	Fasting, 1 hour postprandial
GDM with basal insulin	Fasting, 1 hour postprandial, bedtime
GDM with premixed insulin	Fasting, 1 hour postprandial, Dinner preprandial, 1 hour postprandial
GDM with basal bolus	Fasting, preprandial (lunch, dinner), 1 hour postprandial

(GDM: gestational diabetes mellitus; SMBG: self-monitoring blood glucose)

TABLE 3: Summary of target glucose and HbA1c levels for gestational diabetes from international guidelines.

Guideline	Fasting/Preprandial (mmol/L)	1-hour postprandial (mmol/L)	2-hour postprandial (mmol/L)	HbA1c (mmol/mL, %)
The American College of Obstetricians and Gynecologists (ACOG), 2018	<5.3	<7.8	<6.7	NA
American Diabetes Association (ADA), 2020	<5.3	<7.8	<6.7	NA
The National Institute for Health and Care Excellence (NICE), 2015	<5.3	<7.8	<6.4	<48, 6.5
Australasian Diabetes in Pregnancy Society (ADIPS), (2014)	≤5.0	≤7.4	≤6.7	NA

■ FETAL SURVEILLANCE

Low-risk GDM patients with adequate control by diet and exercise and who have not developed macrosomia, polyhydramnios or preeclampsia do not require antepartum fetal surveillance tests. *High-risk* GDM patients or GDM diagnosed before 20 weeks of pregnancy, who are on glyburide or insulin, a detailed fetal anatomy scan including cardiac assessment, should be performed between 18 and 20 weeks. Women should attend antenatal clinics every 2 weeks or at least once monthly. Each visit should address lifestyle interventions, glycemic control, maternal blood pressure, proteinuria, and other obstetric complications. Growth scan should be performed at 28 weeks of pregnancy and repeated every 4 weeks. If fetal macrosomia or polyhydramnios is present, growth scan intervals should be reduced to 2 weeks.

Pregnancies complicated by GDM are at higher risk of stillbirth between 36 and 39 weeks, with a relative risk ranging from 1.45 to 1.84; therefore, nonstress test (NST) is recommended three times per week for medically treated pregnancies. Modified biophysical profile (MBPP) weekly or twice weekly is another option. Daily fetal activity assessment (fetus should kick at least 10 times within 2 hours after a meal) is an alternative when medical resources and access to assessment units are not available.

Timing of Delivery

Low-risk GDM: Do not need delivery before term. Waiting will increase the chance for spontaneous onset of labor. Offer tests of fetal well-being at 39 weeks. Advice women with uncomplicated gestational diabetes to deliver no later than 40 weeks plus 6 days. For cervical ripening misoprostol or prostaglandin E can be used. High-risk GDM, poorly controlled maternal diabetes or fetal macrosomia, is an indication for earlier induction of labor at 38 weeks. If fetus is macrosomic (>4.5 kg) deliver by elective CS. All women at risk of vaginal delivery between 24 and 36 weeks of gestation or elective CS before 39 weeks of gestation should have steroids to ensure fetal lung maturity. Two doses of betamethasone 12 mg, given intramuscularly, 24 hours apart is the steroid regimen of choice. Glucose levels are expected to rise up to 5 days after the second steroid dose and insulin requirements to increase by 40% within the first 2 days.

Labor and Delivery

The National Institute for Health and Clinical Excellence suggests continuous electronic fetal monitoring in pregnancies with diabetes. Neonatal hypoglycemia (glucose <2.5 mmoL/L) results from excessive fetal insulin production as a result of maternal hyperglycemia, during labor glucose levels should be controlled in order to minimize this risk. Patients with GDM controlled by dietary regulations alone avoidance of dextrose containing intravenous (IV) fluid during labor usually maintains excellent glucose control. Most insulin-dependent GDM patients do not need insulin during labor or after vaginal or CS delivery. CBG should be monitored hourly once patient is in established labor, if CBG found high, corrected with small dose of short-acting insulin or low dose IV insulin to keep BG between 4 and 7 mmoL/L. If woman has general anesthesia for CS, monitor glucose every 30 minutes from induction until baby is born and patient is fully conscious (NICE, 2015).

Neonatal Care

Tight glycemic control during labor may not be enough to prevent neonatal hypoglycemia, defined as capillary glucose level <45 mg/dL (2.5 mmoL/L). Poorly controlled diabetes during pregnancy may lead to hyperplasia of the fetal pancreas, resulting in persistent hyperinsulinemia during the immediate neonatal period. Current guidelines emphasize the need of early feeding and tight glucose monitoring in order to prevent hypoglycemia. Infants should be fed within the first 30 minutes after birth and at 2–3 hourly intervals thereafter, aiming to maintain a prefeed capillary glucose level >35 mg/dL (2 mmoL/L) at four consecutive glucose readings. Infants who remain hypoglycemic despite maximal feeding support should be considered for enteral tube feeding or IV glucose infusion.

Postpartum

Patients should stop glucose-lowering therapy immediately after birth. Breastfeeding should be encouraged given the beneficial effect of breast milk. All women diagnosed with GDM should be informed about the increased risk of developing type 2 diabetes and GDM in subsequent pregnancies. Postnatal testing should be performed at 6 weeks postpartum and at regular intervals (ideally yearly) thereafter. The method of postnatal testing varies between different guidelines and can be a fasting glucose sample, a HbA1c, or a 75-g OGTT. After the pregnancy ends, the woman should be reclassified as having either diabetes mellitus, or IGT, or normal glucose tolerance based on the results of a 75 g OGTT, 6 weeks or more after delivery.

Gestational diabetes mellitus recurs in 40–50% cases in subsequent pregnancies, particularly in obese or with prior macrosomic baby, women who required treatment with glyburide or insulin, had elevated fasting BG or had the diagnosis before 24 weeks. Ongoing evaluation includes annual A1c, annual FPG, or triennial 75-g OGTT using nonpregnant thresholds who have a negative postnatal test for diabetes. In addition, women should continue to follow lifestyle advice (weight reduction, diet, and exercise) (ADA, 2021 and NICE, 2015).

Lifestyle Recommendations for Women who have had Gestational Diabetes Mellitus

"Healthy lifestyle" diabetic diet recommendations—low saturated fat, lower glycemic index carbohydrate choices, eat regularly, and care with meal sizes. Encourage regular exercise (3-4 hours' brisk walking per week)—to reduce overall risk of type 2 diabetes by one-third and slow progression of IGT to diabetes. Obesity and weight gain following a GDM pregnancy are associated with two times increased risk of developing abnormal glucose tolerance; weight loss approximately halves this risk—aim for "healthy weight" range.

Obstetric Complications

Poor glycemic control increases the risk of maternal urinary tract, wound, and endometrial infections. The incidence of hypertension and preeclampsia is higher in women with GDM. The exact mechanism is not well described but IR seems to be one of the main contributing factors. Preeclampsia affects 10–25% compared to nondiabetics. Based upon the results of clinical trials, the US Preventive Services Task Force recommends the use of low-dose aspirin (81 mg/day) as a preventive medication after 12 weeks of gestation in women who are at high risk for preeclampsia. (ADA, 2018).

Polyhydramnios is increased in women with poorly controlled diabetes probably due to fetal osmotic diuresis induced by maternofetal hyperglycemia. Preterm labor occurs in approximately 20% of diabetic pregnancies, associated with polyhydramnios. β-mimetics and glucocorticoids used in such cases have its own side effects. β-mimetics cause hepatic glycogenolysis and both cause IR and high dose insulin is required to prevent hyperglycemia.

The association of GDM with increased risk of stillbirth and excessive fetal growth during the later-part of pregnancy has led clinical practice to earlier induction of labor. These may lead to increased operative delivery, the CS rate varies between 32% to more than 50% in different studies. Women who need insulin treatment at an early gestational age have a higher chance of delivering by CS. Furthermore, approximately 20% patients who deliver vaginally suffer from second to fourth degree perineal tear as well as increased risk of postpartum hemorrhage (PPH) due to uterine overdistension and high incidence of chorioamnionitis and postpartum endometritis.

Fetal and Neonatal Risks

Gestational diabetes mellitus poses both short- and long-term consequences for the infant. Large for gestational age (LGA) (commonly defined as fetal or neonatal weight at or above the 90th centile for gestational age) and macrosomia (usually defined as birth weight ≥4,500 g) are the most common adverse neonatal outcomes associated with GDM. In one report, the prevalence of LGA among women with GDM was almost twofold higher than those without GDM. The increase in placental transport of glucose, amino acids, and fatty acids stimulate fetal endogenous production of insulin and insulin-like growth factor 1 (IGF-1). Together, these can cause fetal overgrowth, often resulting in macrosomia at birth. Excess fetal insulin production can stress the developing pancreatic β-cells, contributing to β-cell dysfunction and IR even prenatally.

Maternal hyperglycemia induces fetal hyperinsulinism which in turn accelerates fetal asymmetric growth (normal head size but broader shoulders and increased thoracic and abdominal diameters). Macrosomia and fetal truncal asymmetry are associated with an increased risk of operative delivery (cesarean or instrumental vaginal) and adverse neonatal outcomes, such as shoulder dystocia and its associated complications—brachial plexus injury, humerus or clavicle fracture, and birth asphyxia. The level of glycemic control is strongly associated with the risk of shoulder dystocia. Athukorala and associates found a positive relationship between the severity of maternal fasting hyperglycemia and the incidence of shoulder dystocia, with a doubling risk with each 1 mmol increase in the FPG value on the OGTT.

Gestational diabetes mellitus is related not only to adverse neonatal size but also to altered body composition. Studies showed that neonates of GDM mothers have higher percentage of fat mass at birth, increased anterior abdominal wall thickness at 20 weeks of gestation (even before GDM was diagnosed), with findings persisting to 32 weeks, irrespective of GDM treatment. These observations imply that genetics, epigenetics, and intrauterine exposure to fuels other than glucose (e.g., lipids) may adversely program offspring's metabolic trajectories during the early stages of pregnancy resulting in long-lasting effects on the offspring.

Neonates born to GDM mothers are at increased risk of multiple, often transient morbidities, including hypoglycemia, hyperbilirubinemia, hypocalcemia, hypomagnesemia, polycythemia, respiratory distress, and/or cardiomyopathy. Maternal hyperglycemia resulting in fetal hyperinsulinemia inhibits cortisol and surfactant production, has detrimental effects on fetal lung maturation, leading to neonatal respiratory distress syndrome; in addition, fetal hyperinsulinemia causes neonatal hypoglycemia immediately after birth because of rapid drop of BG after cord clamping. Even in well-controlled diabetics the incidence of hypoglycemia is still high. Neonatal transient hypoglycemia could have implications in the neurocognitive development as was shown by magnetic resonance imaging.

Chronic maternal hyperglycemia leads to glycosylation of hemoglobin, reducing its oxygen carrying capacity. If the fetal adoptive mechanisms are not enough to counterbalance the hypoxemia, anaerobic metabolism promotes lactate production and acidemia, resulting in intrauterine fetal death.

In HAPO study, 0.56% of the 23,316 deliveries experienced a perinatal death. About 5–10% infants of diabetic mother develop hyperviscosity syndrome (hematocrit ≥65%), which may cause necrotizing enterocolitis, renal vein thrombosis or cerebral infarcts. Approximately 30% macrosomic plethoric fetuses of mothers with poorly controlled diabetes develop hypertrophy of the myocardium particularly of the ventricular septum, extremes of hypertrophic cardiomyopathy may lead to intrauterine fetal demise.

Long-term Outcome

Approximately 60% of women with a past history of GDM develop T2DM later in life. Each additional pregnancy confers a threefold increase in the risk of T2DM. Further, women with a previous case of GDM have a yearly risk of conversion to T2DM of ~2–3%. Emerging evidence also suggests that the vasculature of women with a prior case of GDM is permanently altered, predisposing them to CVD. A recent study reported a 63% increased risk of CVD among women with a history of GDM, which was partly, but not fully, explained by BMI.

In the long term, babies born of GDM pregnancies are at increased risk of obesity, T2DM, CVD, and associated metabolic diseases. Children born to mothers with GDM have almost double the risk of developing childhood obesity when compared with nondiabetic mothers, even after adjusting for confounders such as maternal BMI, IGT can be detected as young as 5 years old. Female babies are more likely to experience GDM in their own pregnancies, contributing to a vicious intergenerational cycle of GDM.

TYPE 1 DIABETES MELLITUS AND TYPE 2 DIABETES MELLITUS

Type 1 DM accounts for 5–10% of all diabetics and almost 1% of diabetes in pregnancy (ADA, 2008). Most are compliant and know self-administration of insulin and follow dietary regulations. Type 2 DM has a strong hereditary component and is rare before 25 years. Obesity especially abdominal obesity (waist hip ratio >0.9), hypertension, dyslipidemia, and low socioeconomic conditions are other risk factors.

Preconceptional Counseling

All women of childbearing age with diabetes should be informed about the importance of achieving and maintaining euglycemia as close to normal as is safely possible prior to conception and throughout pregnancy. Ideally, A1c <6.5% (48 mmoL/moL) to reduce the risk of congenital anomalies, preeclampsia, macrosomia, preterm birth, and other complications. Observational studies showed an increased risk of diabetic embryopathy, especially anencephaly, microcephaly, congenital heart disease, renal anomalies, and caudal regression, directly proportional to elevations in A1c during the first 10 weeks of pregnancy. Optimizing glycemia prior to conception, given that organogenesis occurs primarily at 5–8 weeks of gestation, with an A1c <6.5% (48 mmoL/moL) being associated with the lowest risk of congenital anomalies, preeclampsia, and preterm birth.

Pregnancy is a ketogenic state, women with type 1 diabetes, and to a lesser extent those with type 2 diabetes are at risk for DKA at lower BG levels than in the nonpregnant state. Women with type 1 diabetes, need ketone strips at home and education on DKA prevention and detection (ADA, Diabetes Care, 2019). Women with diabetes who are planning pregnancy should take folic acid (5 mg/day) until 12 weeks of gestation to reduce the risk of neural tube defects. Explain the role of diet, body weight control, exercise, and the risks of developing hypoglycemia. Stop oral hypoglycemic agents before pregnancy, and use insulin, isophane insulin (NPH insulin) as the first choice. Stop angiotensin-converting enzyme (ACE) inhibitors, angiotensin receptor blockers (ARBs), and statins before conception, or as soon as pregnancy is confirmed.

Management (Type 1 and Type 2)

Team approach: Women with preexisting type 1 and type 2 diabetes who are planning pregnancy should ideally be managed beginning in preconception in a multidisciplinary clinic involving an endocrinologist, maternal-fetal medicine specialist, registered dietitian nutritionist, and diabetes care and education specialist, when available.

Offer self-monitoring of BG, *glucose target* (ADA, 2019):
- Fasting <95 mg/dL (5.3 mmoL/L) and either
- 1-hour postprandial <140 mg/dL (7.8 mmoL/L) or
- 2-hour postprandial <120 mg/dL (6.7 mmoL/L)

In type 1 DM, retinal assessment should be done at first appointment. Tight glycemic control in the setting of retinopathy is associated with worsening of retinopathy, defer rapid optimization of BG. Offer renal assessment (including albuminuria), refer to a nephrologist before stopping contraception if serum creatinine is 120 µmoL/L (1.3 mg/dL) or more or the urinary albumin: creatinine ratio >30 mg/mmoL or estimated glomerular filtration rate (eGFR) <45 mL/minute/1.73 m^2. Monthly HbA1c in women who are planning pregnancy, risk of diabetic embryopathy is directly proportional to elevations in A1c during first 10 weeks of pregnancy. Good control (A1c <6–6.5%) before conception and during organogenesis is associated with lowest risk (ADA, 2021 and NICE, 2020). Women with type 2 DM, A1c <6% in second and third trimesters have the lowest risk of LGA infants, preterm delivery, and preeclampsia. Uncontrolled DM increases the risk of having LGA baby, increased likelihood of birth trauma, induction of labor, and instrumental and CS delivery (ADA, 2021 and NICE, 2020).

Insulin in Type 1 and Type 2 Diabetes Mellitus

Insulin has long been considered the standard of care to attain optimal glucose control in pregnancy. Insulin is the preferred agent for management of both type 1 and type 2 diabetes in pregnancy as it does not cross the placenta and because oral agents are generally insufficient to overcome the IR in type 2 diabetes and ineffective in type 1 diabetes. The physiology of pregnancy requires frequent titration to match changing requirements. In first trimester, women with type 1 diabetes will have lower insulin requirements and increased risk for hypoglycemia. Around 16 weeks, IR begins to increase, and total daily insulin doses increase linearly ~5% per week through week 36. A small proportion (<50%) of total daily dose is given as basal insulin and >50% as prandial insulin. Insulin requirement levels off toward the end of the third trimester with placental aging, usually results in a doubling of daily insulin dose compared with the prepregnancy requirement.

Choice of Insulin

Rapid-acting insulin (aspart and lispro) and intermediate-acting insulin are safe in pregnancy. Peak serum concentration of lispro three times higher and time to peak 4.2 times shorter, absorption rate double, and duration of action half as long over regular insulin. The total daily insulin requirement during the first trimester, is 0.7 units/kg/day, while in the second trimester it is 0.8 units/kg/day, and in the third trimester, it is 0.9-1.0 units/kg/day. Usually in pregestational diabetes, the total insulin dose is up to twice higher than in GDM. In case of morbid obesity, the initial doses of insulin can be increased to 1.5-2.0 units/kg to overcome the combined IR of pregnancy and obesity (FIGO).

Target CBG: Fasting 3.9-5.3 mmoL/L and either 1-hour postprandial glucose 6.1-7.8 mmoL/L or 2-hour postprandial glucose 5.6-6.7 mmoL/L. (NICE guideline, 2020 recommendation—to maintain capillary PG above 4 mmoL/L).

Dose: Although multiple methods are available to initiate insulin—weight-based dosing, weight plus gestational age-based dosing, and even a "one-dose-for-all" type of dosing have been used. The following guidelines can help in managing and adjusting insulin (Diabetes Spectrum, 2016):
- A combination of short- and intermediate-acting insulin is given.
- Typical regimen involves intermediate-acting insulin (NPH) before breakfast and at 10 pm; short-acting insulin before breakfast and dinner.
- Two-thirds of total insulin should be given in the morning and one-third in the afternoon and at bedtime.
- In the morning dose two-thirds NPH insulin and one-third insulin aspart or lispro.
- In the evening half lispro or aspart with dinner and half NPH insulin before bed.
- To avoid nocturnal hypoglycemia, NPH insulin should be given between 10 and 11 pm.
- Insulin adjusted no more frequently than weekly or biweekly.
- Pregestational diabetic patients should count the grams of carbohydrate in their meal and adjust short-acting insulin dosage accordingly.
- A typical meal of 60 g carbohydrate may require 4-6 U of lispro in nonpregnant state; during first trimester the typical ratio is 1:12, second trimester ratio is 1:10-1:6, and in the third trimester this may be 1:6-1:2.

Blood Glucose Monitoring

Type 1 diabetic and type 2 diabetic women who are on a MDI regimen test their fasting, premeal, 1-hour postmeal, and bedtime BG *daily*, which may later be reduced to three times. Those with *type 2* diabetes—to test their fasting and 1-hour postmeal BG daily if they are managing their diabetes with diet and exercise alone or taking oral therapy (with or without diet and exercise changes) or single-dose intermediate-acting or long-acting insulin.

Antenatal Care

Confirm gestational age by crown–rump length (CRL) measurement as there may be significant growth problem in diabetic pregnancies. Efforts to detect embryopathy should start soon after conception by measuring HbA1c. Value >8.5% is associated with 20-25% risk of congenital abnormality. All patients with type 1 and type 2 diabetes should have transvaginal scan (TVS) between 10 and 14 weeks to exclude aneuploidy [nuchal translucency (NT)]. Serum markers (triple test) should be done at 16 weeks to exclude neural tube defect and Down's syndrome. Values are lower in DM, should be taken into account during risk calculation. Comprehensive USG should be done at 18-20 weeks and fetal echo at 22-24 weeks to exclude cardiac anomaly. Serial measurement of head and abdominal circumference (A/C) every 2-4 weeks provides best means to identify fetal macrosomia.

Pregestational type 2 diabetes often associated with obesity. Recommended weight gain during pregnancy for overweight women is 15-25 lbs and for obese women is 10-20 lbs. Glycemic control is often easier to achieve in type 2 diabetes than in type 1 diabetes, but hypertension and other comorbidities often render pregestational type 2 diabetes as high or higher risk than pregestational type 1 diabetes. Women with type 1 or type 2 diabetes should be prescribed low-dose aspirin 100-150 mg/day from the end of the first trimester until the baby is born in order to lower the risk of preeclampsia.

Type 1 diabetic women have an increased risk of hypoglycemia in the first trimester. Frequent hypoglycemia can be associated with growth restriction. Antenatal visit should be every 2 weeks till 32–34 weeks and weekly thereafter. Because of increased risk of fetal growth restriction (FGR) and or preeclampsia, increased surveillance during last 6–10 weeks.

Cardiotocography (CTG) and biophysical profile (BPP)—little evidence to guide the frequency of monitoring. Twice weekly NST and weekly BPP in the third trimester have been shown to be associated with low perinatal mortality rate. Umbilical artery *(UA) Doppler* velocity assessment to exclude placental insufficiency and fetal compromise. Abnormal Doppler indicates need for more intense surveillance.

Labor and Delivery

Timing and mode of delivery must be balanced between risk of prematurity and risk of late intrauterine death (IUD) and birth trauma due to fetal macrosomia. Gestation-specific risk of stillbirths continue to fall up to around 38 weeks and rises thereafter. Most obstetricians are comfortable in delivering their patients between 38 and 39 weeks. Coexisting maternal hypertension, suboptimal glucose control, or suspicious fetal BPP are important cofactor influencing decision regarding early delivery. Because of delay in lung maturity, maturity should be verified in all patients delivered before 38 weeks by presence of >3% phosphatidylglycerol. It is not necessary to deliver all insulin-dependent diabetic patients by CS, though almost 50% will need delivery by CS for various reasons.

Management in Labor

Labor is a time of unpredictable glucose and insulin demand. Hyperglycemia during labor leads to perinatal asphyxia and neonatal hypoglycemia. Euglycemia throughout labor and before elective CS is vital. Maintaining glucose level in a range of 80–110 mg/dL (4.5–6.1 mmoL/L) by use of combined insulin and glucose infusion reduces incidence of neonatal hypoglycemia.

For delivery of well-controlled DM patients, usual dose of bedtime insulin is given, morning insulin is withheld. Following admission to labor ward determine capillary glucose (CG). Insulin infusion: begin continuous glucose infusion (5% D/A) @ 100 mL/hour throughout labor and insulin lispro or aspart @ 0.5 U/hour. Monitor maternal CBG hourly using capillary reflectance meter, and adjust insulin infusion as given in **Table 4**.

Intermittent subcutaneous (SC) injection: Give 0.5 (half) of regular insulin in the morning. Begin glucose infusion (5% D/A) @100 mL/h, monitor capillary glucose hourly. Give regular insulin in small dose (2–5 U) to maintain BG between 80 and 120 mg/dL (4.5–6.7 mmoL/L). Increase insulin when CBG increases.

TABLE 4: Monitoring of maternal CBG hourly using capillary reflectance meter.

Plasma/capillary glucose (mg/dL)	Infusion rate U/hour
<80 (4.5 mmoL/L)	0.5 U
80–100 (4.5–5.6 mmoL/L)	1.0 U
101–140 (5.6–7.8 mmoL/L)	1.5 U
141–180 (7.8–10 mmoL/L)	2.0 U
181–200 (10–11.1 mmoL/L)	2.5 U

(CBG: capillary blood glucose)

Labor analgesia: Adequate analgesia during labor is important. Pain stimulates catecholamine release and cause hyperglycemia. Epidural analgesia should be considered.

Cardiotocography: Continuous monitoring of fetal heart rate (FHR) and uterine contractions, because of increased risk of fetal distress (FD) in labor.

Partograph: For detailed records of progress of labor, prolonged labor should be avoided.

Cesarean Section

Cesarean section should be done in early morning to avoid prolonged fasting. On the previous night patient is instructed to take full dose of NPH insulin or glyburide; no morning insulin or glyburide. A glucose containing IV channel opened, if CBG is high, start hartsol or normal saline (NS). Short-acting insulin is given as IV bolus on sliding scale as needed every 1–4 hours to keep maternal BG between 80 and 160 mg/dL (4.5–8.9 mmoL/L).

Postpartum

Insulin resistance drops rapidly with delivery of the placenta, and women become very insulin sensitive, requiring much less insulin than antepartum period. Study showed insulin requirements in the immediate postpartum period roughly 34% lower than prepregnancy requirements, then returns to prepregnancy levels over the following 1–2 weeks. In T1DM, particular attention should be directed to hypoglycemia prevention in the immediate postpartum period. IV glucose insulin infusion should be continued specially in CS patients, until diet normalized, in T2DM after delivery short-acting insulin can be given on a sliding scale until regular diet is established. Weight loss is recommended in T2DM in the postpartum period (ADA, 2021).

Breastfeeding and Contraception

Breastfeeding reduces insulin requirement by 25% and may also confer longer-term metabolic benefits to both mother and neonates, therefore encouraged. In the light of immediate nutritional and immunological benefits of breastfeeding for the baby, all women including those with diabetes should be supported in attempts to breastfeed. Women taking insulin, particular attention should be directed to hypoglycemia prevention in the setting of breastfeeding and erratic sleep and eating schedules, and insulin dosing may need to be adjusted.

Contraception: Progesterone only pill *(mini pill)* virtually has no effect on carbohydrate or fat metabolism, suitable for patients who wants to breastfeed. Newer *low-dose oral contraceptive pill (OCP)* which has little effect on low or high-density lipoproteins can be given to younger insulin-dependent diabetics. *Injectable progesterone* produces IR and insulin dose needs to be increased but are not contraindicated. *Copper intrauterine contraceptive device (IUCD)* and newer progesterone containing IUCDs may also be used. Diabetic patients who have completed their families are encouraged to have permanent sterilization.

■ MATERNAL COMPLICATIONS

Maternal mortality: Pregnancy has negative effect on diabetes and cause worsening of diabetic associated complications. Prior to the availability of insulin, maternal mortality in diabetic women approached 50%. This rate fell immediately after insulin was discovered, and in the early 21st century occurred in 0.04% or less of diabetic pregnancies. Maternal death rate is still approximately four times higher than in the general obstetric population.

Diabetic ketoacidosis: Pregnancy increases the tendency toward starvation ketosis and DKA due to enhanced lypolytic activity. DKA is a life-threatening condition for the mother as well as for the fetus, ketoacidosis is more commonly seen in cases of type 1 diabetes, and can precipitate in conditions of extreme stress, diarrhea, infection, preterm labor, and others. The incidence of DKA is 0.5–3%. Maternal mortality due to DKA < 1% and fetal mortality rates of 9–36%. Perinatal mortality and morbidity appear to be directly related to the degree to which ambient maternal glucose levels during pregnancy exceed nondiabetic limits.

Diagnosis of DKA: Blood glucose >250 mg/dL, may occur at lower level in pregnancy, ketone bodies in blood and urine, arterial pH <7.3, serum bicarbonate level <15 mEq/L, and elevated anion gap >12 mEq/L.

Therapeutic management of DKA: Fluid replacement as severe dehydration may result in a large fluid deficit of as much as 6–7 L. Estimated fluid deficit must be replaced in around 12–24 hours. In the first hour, 1 L of NS is infused, followed by 300–500 mL/hour till pulse and blood pressure are back to normal. Insulin therapy is started as soon as possible:
- An intravenous bolus of 2.0 units/kg
- Then 0.1 unit/kg/hour in NS
- If the BG does not fall by 30% in the first 3 hours, the drip rate should be doubled

Once glucose level is between 200 and 250 mg/dL, NS is changed to 5% dextrose. Hypokalemia generally occurs with DKA. If <4 mEq/L, 30 mEq/hour KCI must be given; when the level rises >4 mEq/L the amount of KCI can be reduced to 10–15 mEq/hour. Bicarbonate administration is required if pH falls <6.8. Antibiotics are given. Treatment of the cause is important, as prompt management can prevent maternal and fetal mortality.

Retinopathy: Complicates both type 1 and type 2 diabetes. In women with early retinopathy 10% chance of progression and those with progressive retinopathy there is 50% chance of progression. The earliest manifestation includes microaneurysms, small vessel obstruction, cotton wool spots, intraretinal microvascular abnormalities (venous abnormalities and small retinal hemorrhages), and hard exudates. Vision is generally not threatened by background retinopathy unless macular edema or ischemia supervene. Hypertension and preeclampsia further increases the risk of retinopathy. Control of diabetes over the long term has been shown to slow the progression of retinopathy in both type 1 and type 2 diabetes.

Diabetic nephropathy: Overt diabetic nephropathy, generally detected by the presence of albuminuria ≥300 mg/day, complicates both type 1 and type 2 diabetes. Pregnant women with type 1 diabetes are considerably more likely to have nephropathy than are those with type 2 diabetes. Women with markedly decreased GFR prior to pregnancy, are at significant risk of permanent decline in renal function during pregnancy.

Urinary tract infections—appear to be generally more common among individuals with diabetes than nondiabetic patients. In Cousins' literature review pyelonephritis complicated approximately 3% of pregnancies in women with preexisting diabetes. Urinary tract infections are of particular significance in women with diabetes because metabolic control may be adversely impacted by such problems. DKA as well as more subtle derangements of control are commonly brought about by infections.

Hypertension: Hypertension is commonly present in diabetic gravidas with nephropathy. However, even in the absence of nephropathy women with diabetes are more likely than nondiabetic individuals to have hypertensive complications during pregnancy.

Endocrine disease: Type 1 diabetes is an autoimmune condition, so these women are at risk of other autoimmune disease particularly thyroid disease.

■ FETAL COMPLICATIONS

Perinatal mortality: Fetal deaths continue to be significantly higher among diabetic than nondiabetic pregnancies. The most recent available data indicate that the relative risk of stillbirth in pregnancies complicated by type 1 diabetes (compared to the general population) is 2.9–4.3 fold, and for type 2 diabetes 2.5–4.5 fold. Perinatal mortality rates are higher in poorly controlled diabetic pregnancies, as evidenced by the study of Karlsson and Kjellmer, in which perinatal deaths ranged from 4% when mean third trimester BG was <100 mg/dL, to 16% when glucose was maintained between 100 and 150 mg/dL, and 24% for diabetic patients whose mean glucose levels exceeded 150 mg/dL.

Congenital malformations: Infants of diabetic mothers are two to three times more likely than infants in general to manifest all types of birth defects. Cardiac, neural tube, and skeletal defects are most common, but a particular set of anomalies the "caudal regression syndrome," is highly specific for diabetic pregnancy. Tight metabolic control at the time of organogenesis is associated with congenital malformation rate similar to the general population.

Macrosomia: Macrosomia is considerably more prevalent in offspring of type 2 diabetic, as compared to nondiabetic, pregnancies. The cause of macrosomia in infants of diabetic mothers appears to be fetal hyperinsulinemia.

Neonatal hypoglycemia: Usually defined as a plasma glucose concentration <35 mg/dL in a term infant, or <25 mg/dL in a preterm infant. Its likelihood in an infant of a diabetic mother has been positively associated with maternal hyperglycemia at delivery and the rapid infusion of glucose-containing IV fluids during labor. Hypoglycemia is most likely to occur during the first 60–90 minutes of life, and is often asymptomatic. Infants who manifest symptoms usually are irritable, jittery, may have apneic spells, tachypnea, hypotonia, and at the extreme, convulsions. Early institution of oral feeding may be helpful in preventing hypoglycemia.

Neonatal respiratory problems: Respiratory distress syndrome (RDS), as well as other forms of neonatal respiratory difficulty, occurs with increased frequency in infants of diabetic mothers. Because maturation of the surfactant system may be delayed, it is advisable to test stable lung maturity, such as the presence of phosphatidylglycerol (PG) in amniotic fluid, prior to elective delivery of a diabetic pregnancy.

Other neonatal problems: A number of other problems are reported to occur with increased frequency in infants of diabetic mothers. These include polycythemia and hyperviscosity syndrome, hyperbilirubinemia, and hypocalcemia, and all are likely explainable on the basis of hyperinsulinemia. Transient cardiac dysfunction, presumably due to increased thickness of the intraventricular septum, has been reported in neonates of diabetic mothers even when metabolic control has been reportedly good during pregnancy.

SUGGESTED READING

1. American Diabetes Association. Gestational Diabetes Mellitus. Diabetes Care. 2003;26(Suppl 1):s103-5.
2. American Diabetes Association. Management of Diabetes in Pregnancy: Standards of Medical Care in Diabetes—2021. Diabetes Care. 2021;44(Suppl 1):S200-10.
3. American Diabetes Association. Management of diabetes in pregnancy. Diabetes Care. 2017;40(Suppl 1):S114-9.
4. Bagias C, Xiarchou A, Saravanan P. Screening, diagnosis, and management of GDM: An update. J Diabetol. 2021;12(5):43-51.
5. Broughton C, Douek I. An overview of the management of diabetes from pre-conception, during pregnancy and in the postnatal period. Clin Med. 2019;19(5):399-402.
6. Caughey AB, Werner EF, Barss VA. Gestational diabetes mellitus: Obstetric issues and management. UpToDate, 2021. [online] Available from https://www.uptodate.com/contents/gestational-diabetes-mellitus-obstetric-issues-and-management [Last accessed April, 2022].
7. CDC. Diabetes During Pregnancy. [online] Available from www.cdc.gov/reproductivehealth/maternalinfanthealth/ [Last accessed April, 2022].
8. Coustan DR. (2016). Diagnosis and Management of Diabetes Mellitus in Pregnancy. Glob Libr Women's Med. Available from 10.3843/GLOWM.10162 [Last accessed April, 2022].
9. Dabelea D, Hanson RL, Lindsay RS, Pettitt DJ, Imperatore G, Gabir MM, et al. Intrauterine exposure to diabetes conveys risks for type 2 diabetes and obesity: a study of discordant sibships. Diabetes. 2000;49(12):2208-11.
10. Detailed information on pathophysiology of diabetes mellitus. [online] Available from https://healthhearty.com/pathophysiology-of-diabetes-mellitus [Last accessed April, 2022].
11. Feig DS, Hwee J, Shah BR, Booth GL, Bierman AS, Lipscombe LL. Trends in incidence of diabetes in pregnancy and serious perinatal outcomes: a large, population-based study in Ontario, Canada, 1996-2010. Diabetes care. 2014;37(6):1590-6.
12. Galicia-Garcia U, Benito-Vicente A, Jebari S, Larrea-Sebal A, Siddiqi H, Uribe KB, et al. Pathophysiology of Type 2 Diabetes Mellitus. Int J Mol Sci. 2020;21(17):6275.
13. Guerin A, Nisenbaum R, Ray JG. Use of maternal GHb concentration to estimate the risk of congenital anomalies in the offspring of women with pre-pregnancy diabetes. Diabetes Care. 2007;30(7):1920-5.
14. Hameed AB, Combs CA. Society for Maternal Fetal Medicine Special Statement, Updated checklist for antepartum care for pregestational DM. Am J Obstet Gynecol. 2020;223(5):B2-B5.
15. Holmes VA, Young IS, Patterson CC, Pearson DW, Walker JD, Maresh MJ, et al. Optimal glycemic control, pre-eclampsia, and gestational hypertension in women with type 1 diabetes in the diabetes and pre-eclampsia intervention trial. Diabetes Care. 2011;34:1683-8.
16. Lam AYR, Lim W. (2021). Glob Libr Women's Med. Clinical Management of Diabetes in Pregnancy. [online] Available from DOI 10.3843/GLOWM.416423 [Last accessed April, 2022].
17. Liu J, Ren ZH, Qiang H, Wu J, Shen M, Zhang L, et al. Trends in the incidence of diabetes mellitus: results from the Global Burden of Disease Study 2017 and implications for diabetes mellitus prevention. BMC Public Health. 2020;20(1):1415.

18. Ludvigsson JF, Neovius M, Söderling J, Gudbjörnsdottir S, Svensson AM, Franzén S, et al. Maternal glycemic control in type 1 diabetes and the risk for preterm birth: a population-based cohort study. Ann Intern Med. 2019;170(10):691-701.
19. Moore TR, Mouzon SH, Catalano P, Resnik R, Creasey RK, Iams JD, et al. Diabetes in pregnancy. In: Creasy and Resniks Maternal Fetal Medicine, 7th edition. Philadelphia, PA: Elsevier; 2013. pp. 998-1021.
20. NICE. (2020). Diabetes in pregnancy: management from preconception to the postnatal period NICE guidelineNG18, december2020. [online] Available from https://www.guidelines.co.uk/diabetes/nice-diabetes-in-pregnancy-guideline/252595.article [Last accessed April, 2022].
21. Olatunbosun ST. What are the ADA diagnostic criteria for gestational diabetes mellitus (GDM)? Updated: Jul 08, 2020, Medscape. [online] Available from https://www.medscape.com/answers/119020-189164/what-are-the-ada-diagnostic-criteria-for-gestational-diabetes-mellitus-gdm [Last accessed April, 2022].
22. Pantea-Stoian A, Stoica RA, Stefan SD. Insulin therapy in gestational diabetes mellitus. Gestational Diabetes Mellitus—an overview with some recent advances. [online] Available from http://dx.doi.org/10.5772/intechopen.84569. FIGO 2019 [Last accessed April, 2022].
23. Plows JF, Stanley JL, Baker PN, Reynolds CM, Vickers MH. The Pathophysiology of Gestational Diabetes Mellitus. Int J Mol Sci. 2018;19(11):3342.
24. Suhonen L, Hiilesmaa V, Teramo K. Glycaemic control during early pregnancy and fetal malformations in women with type I diabetes mellitus. Diabetologia. 2000;43(1):79-82.
25. World Health Organization. (2013). Diagnostic criteria and classification of hyperglycaemia first detected in pregnancy. [online] Available from https://apps.who.int/iris/handle/10665/85975. WHO/NMH/MND/13.2 [Last accessed April, 2022].

CHAPTER 8

Cardiac Diseases in Pregnancy

INTRODUCTION

Cardiovascular disease (CVD) complicates 1–4% of pregnancies and is a leading cause of maternal death. Pregnant women with heart disease are at higher risk for cardiovascular complications during pregnancy and also have a higher incidence of neonatal complications. While in the Western world, congenital heart disease (CHD) is the most frequent (70–80%) CVD present during pregnancy, in non-Western countries, rheumatic valvular disease dominates (50–90%). As the number of adults with CHD is increasing over the last decades, there has been an increase in the number of pregnancies in women with CHD. Cardiomyopathy is rare but severe. Coronary heart disease is relatively uncommon in women of childbearing age.

In the United States, along with an increase in cardiac disease in pregnancy, "cardiovascular disease" related deaths have gradually increased over time from 7.2 to 17.2 deaths per 100,000 live births from 1987 to 2015 (Circulation, 2020) and are now the leading cause of death in pregnant women and women in the postpartum period. Most recent data indicates that CVD constitute 26.5% of US pregnancy-related deaths (ACOG Practice Bulletin 212; 2019). In the UK, the Confidential Enquiries into Maternal Deaths (CEMACH) have shown that the overall rate of mortality from cardiac disease has risen from 7.3/million births in the 1982–1984 triennium to 22.7/million births in the 2003–2005 triennium. The major part of this increase is attributable to acquired heart disease, deaths from which have risen from 4.7/million births to 20.8/million births. One-third of these deaths are a result of myocardial infarction/ischemic heart disease and a similar number of late deaths are associated with peripartum cardiomyopathy. Other significant contributors (5–10% each) are rheumatic heart disease, CHD, and pulmonary hypertension (HTN).

Cardiovascular disease has become a cause of increasing concern for Bangladesh with patients suffering from it topping the list of people with noncommunicable diseases. A National Institute of Cardiovascular Disease (NICVD), 2018 study found that the prevalence of the CVD among the Bangladeshi population is 4.5% regardless of the type. It is estimated that 1–4% of women entering pregnancy either have cardiac disease or are diagnosed with the cardiac disease while they are pregnant. In India, cardiac disease complicates 2% of pregnancies and contributes to one-fifth of all maternal deaths.

TYPES OF CARDIAC DISEASE IN PREGNANCY

Cardiac disease in pregnancy covers a wide range of conditions:
- Congenital heart disease
- Acquired disease, e.g., rheumatic valvular disease
- Cardiomyopathy
- Coronary artery disease.

Congenital Heart Disease

Acyanotic heart disease, e.g., atrial septal defect (ASD), ventricular septal defect (VSD), atrioventricular septal defect, patent ductus arteriosus (PDA), pulmonary stenosis, coarctation of the aorta.

Cyanotic heart disease, e.g., tetralogy of Fallot, Eisenmenger syndrome, transposition of the great arteries (TGA), Ebstein anomaly, double outlet right ventricle, single ventricle, tricuspid atresia.

Rheumatic Heart Disease

Mitral stenosis (MS), aortic stenosis, mitral regurgitation, aortic regurgitation.

Other Cardiac Diseases in Pregnancy

Ischemic heart disease, hypertensive disorder, thyrotoxicosis, conduction defects, infective endocarditis, and peripartum cardiomyopathy.

PHYSIOLOGICAL CHANGES IN CARDIOVASCULAR SYSTEM DURING PREGNANCY

Pregnancy induces changes in the cardiovascular system to meet the increased metabolic demands of the mother and fetus and to ensure adequate uteroplacental circulation for fetal growth and development **(Fig. 1)**. Most of these hemodynamic changes start in the first trimester, peak during the second trimester, and plateau during the third trimester. The total blood volume rises steadily during the first trimester and is increased by almost 50% by the 30th week. Several mechanisms are responsible for increasing blood volume in pregnancy including increasing steroid hormones; elevated plasma renin activity, elevated plasma aldosterone level, human placental lactogen, atrial natriuretic factors and other peptides may also play a significant role in governing changes in blood volume. The hematocrit level decreases due to a disproportionate increase in plasma volume that exceeds the rise in red cell mass leading to physiological anemia.

The cardiac output (CO) increases by 30–50% and half of this increase occurs by 8 weeks of gestation. The increase in CO is achieved by an increase in stroke volume in the first-half of pregnancy and a gradual increase in heart rate thereafter, which increases by 10–20 beats/min. The increase in stroke volume leads to a rise in the ventricular outflow tract velocity, and it mimics a hyperkinetic state, many women have audible systolic murmurs due to changes in blood flow. Despite an increase in intravascular volume, blood pressure decreases by 5–10 mm Hg (the majority of the decrease occurs early in pregnancy) owing to a decrease in systemic vascular resistance (SVR). SVR is progressively reduced (by 35–40%) until the middle of the second trimester when it plateaus before beginning to increase late in the third trimester.

During the third trimester, CO is further influenced by body position, where the turning from left lateral recumbent to supine position can cause a decrease in CO by 25–30%. Stroke volume normally increases in the first and second trimester and decreases in the third trimesters, due to partial vena cava obstruction. During labor and delivery CO, heart rate, blood pressure, and SVR increase with each uterine contraction. Significant fluid shifts at delivery lead to labile peripartum blood pressure, often rising before delivery and then falling within a week. Maternal cardiac and circulatory adaptations to pregnancy begin early in the first trimester and do not return to baseline until at least 6 weeks postpartum. Physiological changes in the cardiovascular system during pregnancy may bear a risk for those with CHD who are not able to sufficiently adapt. Heart failure, arrhythmia, and worsening of the cardiac condition may complicate pregnancy and expose mother and child to an increased risk of morbidity and mortality.

As well as the circulatory changes described above, there are also adaptive changes that occur in the great vessels and blood that are important to women with heart disease. Hormonal changes in pregnancy influence the integrity of the vessel wall. The structure of the aortic wall may have a subtle weaker composition, which is not of significant importance to healthy women, but may enhance the risk of aortic dissection in women with aortic disease. Pregnancy is a hypercoagulable state designed to reduce the risk of postpartum hemorrhage (PPH). This results in an increased risk of clotting, most commonly venous thromboembolism, and women who require anticoagulation for heart disease, e.g., mechanical prosthetic heart valve or Fontan circulation are at increased risk.

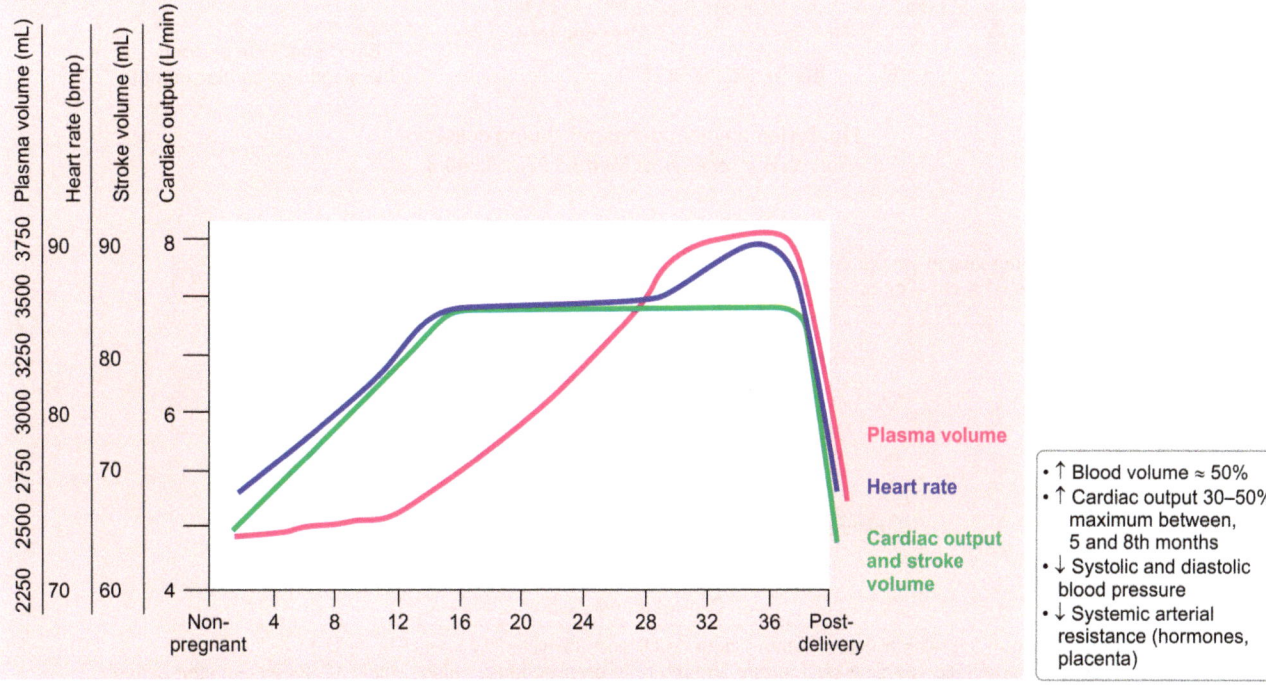

Fig. 1: Cardiovascular changes in pregnancy.
Source: Basic medical key (Modified from Thorn SA. Pregnancy in heart disease. Heart. 2004;90:450-56)

EFFECTS OF PREGNANCY ON DISEASED HEART

The risk of complications in pregnancy depends on the underlying cardiac diagnosis, ventricular and valvular function, functional class, presence of cyanosis, pulmonary artery pressures, and other factors. Heart failure usually occurs around the 28–32th weeks of pregnancy, during labor, or soon after delivery. Patients may develop cardiac arrhythmia, stroke, subacute bacterial endocarditis, and postpartum thromboembolic complication.

There are *five danger periods* in pregnancy. The *first danger period* is between 12 and 16 weeks when hemodynamic changes of pregnancy begin. Second critical period is between 28 and 32 weeks when hemodynamic changes are at peak and cardiac demands are at maximum. Another dangerous time is during labor and delivery. Each uterine contraction injects 300–500 mL of blood from uteroplacental circulation to maternal stream, which increases the CO to 15–20%. During *second stage,* maternal pushing decreases the venous return to heart causing a decrease in CO. This sudden and frequent variation in CO during the second stage of labor may be critical for some cardiac patients. Another danger time is immediately after delivery when there is sudden transfusion of blood from the lower extremity and uteroplacental vascular bed to the systemic circulation, which further challenges to maternal cardiac reserve that results from increased preload via vena caval decompression and extrusion of blood from the contracted uterus into the inferior vena cava. Augmented venous return increases maternal CO by 60–80% after vaginal delivery. The final danger time is 4–5 days after delivery, decreased peripheral resistance with the right to left shunting and pulmonary embolization from silent iliofemoral thrombus are two problems that may occur at this time **(Figs. 2 and 3)**.

Patients with primary pulmonary HTN, Eisenmenger syndrome, aortic stenosis, and cyanotic heart disease may go through labor and delivery without complications but sudden death may occur in early puerperium because of these physiological changes.

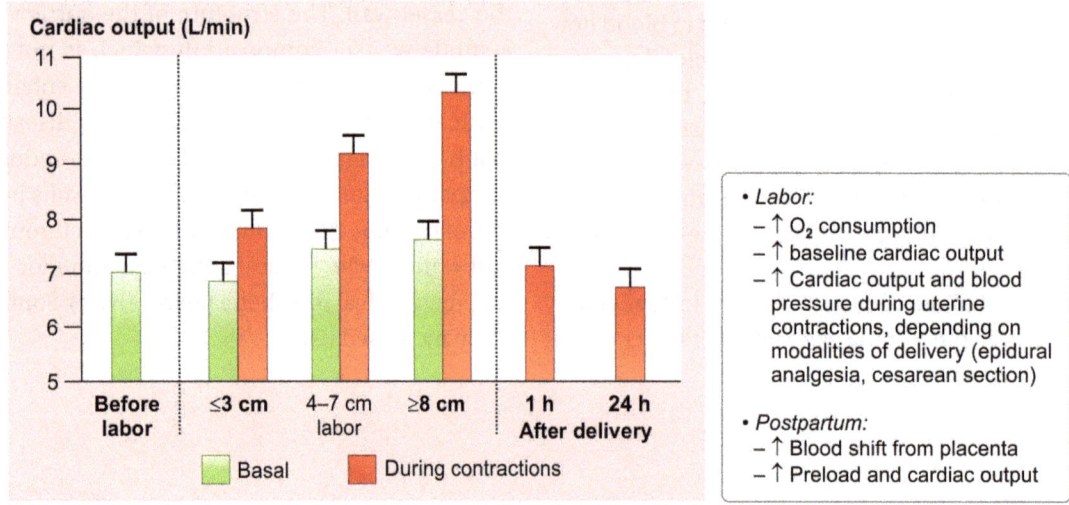

Fig. 2: Hemodynamic changes during delivery.
Source: Hunter et al. Br Med J. 1992;68:540-3.

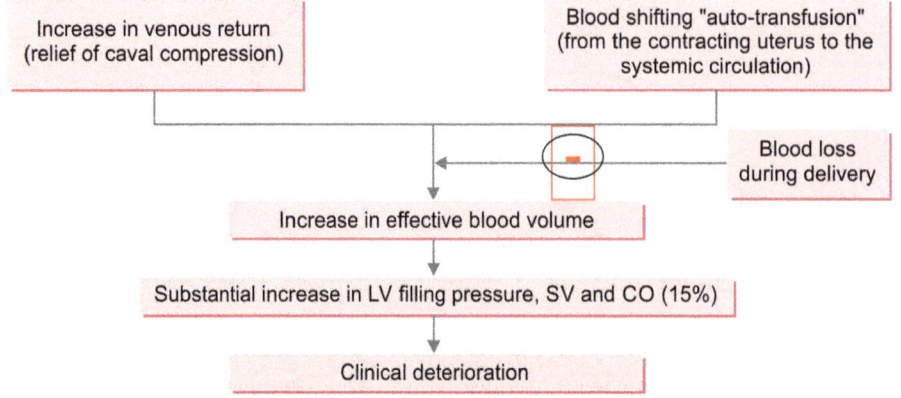

- HR and CO return to prelabor values within 1 hour. MAP and SV within 24 hours.
- Hemodynamic adaptation persists postpartum and return to prepregnancy values within 12–24 weeks after delivery

Fig. 3: Hemodynamic changes postpartum.
(CO: cardiac output; HR: heart rate; LV: left ventricle; MAP: mean arterial pressure; SV: stroke volume)

DIAGNOSIS OF HEART DISEASE IN PREGNANCY

Diagnosis of heart disease during pregnancy is difficult, because the physiological changes that occur during pregnancy may mimic CVD. However, many disorders can be identified by taking a careful history and a thorough physical examination.

SIGNS AND SYMPTOMS THAT SIMULATE OR OBSCURE HEART DISEASE

Table 1 shows signs and symptoms that simulate or obscure heart disease.

FINDINGS SUGGESTING SIGNIFICANT CARDIOVASCULAR ABNORMALITY

Table 2 enlists the findings suggesting significant cardiovascular abnormality.

FEATURES OF HEART FAILURE

Easy fatigue, shortness of breath, orthopnea, and pulmonary congestion are suggestive of left heart failure, while jugular venous pressure is increased in right heart failure. Some patients may develop paroxysmal nocturnal dyspnea or "cardiac asthma" but the most important sign of failure is bibasilar basal creps (secondary to left-sided congestive cardiac failure). Patients with MS predominantly have features of left-sided heart failure and those with peripartum cardiomyopathy have signs/symptoms of biventricular failure.

CARDIAC CONDITIONS NEED CORRECTION BEFORE PREGNANCY

There are some cardiac conditions that need correction before pregnancy, these include:

- Large intracardiac shunt, i.e., atrial or ventricular septal defect with mild-to-moderate pulmonary HTN, PDA with mild-moderate pulmonary HTN.
- Severe coarctation of the aorta
- Severe MS or regurgitation—valve area <1.0 cm^2 (normal mitral valve area—4-5 cm^2. Mild MS—valve area >1.5 cm^2, moderate MS—valve area 1–1.5 cm^2, severe MS—valve area <1 cm^2).
- Severe aortic stenosis or regurgitation—valve area <1.0 cm^2
- Tetralogy of Fallot (VSD, pulmonary stenosis, overriding of aorta and right ventricular hypertrophy)
- Various congenital malformation and acquired heart disease.

Note: After any palliative surgery 1 year or more time should be elapsed before pregnancy is contemplated.

MANAGEMENT

Principle of management include:
- Preconceptional counseling
- Assessment and stratification of maternal and fetal risk

TABLE 1: Signs and symptoms that simulate or obscure heart disease.

Symptoms	Signs	Investigation
• Dyspnea • Orthopnea • Easy fatigability • Dizziness • Syncope • Palpitation • Reduced exercise tolerance	• Pedal edema • Distended jugular veins • Increased heart rate (tachycardia) with wide pulse pressure • Systolic ejection murmur at left sternal border • Continuous murmur at second and fourth intercostals space (mammary souffle) • Shifting of apex beat • Loud first heart sound with splitting • Pulmonary bibasilar rales	• Electrocardiography nonspecific ST segment and T-wave abnormality • Echo—increased cardiac chamber diameter • Slight regurgitation through valves • Small pericardial effusion

TABLE 2: Findings suggesting significant cardiovascular abnormality.

Symptoms	Signs	Investigations
• Severe dyspnea • Syncope with exertion • Paroxysmal nocturnal dyspnea • Chest pain related to exertion • Nocturnal cough and hemoptysis	• Cyanosis • Clubbing • Diastolic murmur with thrill • Loud, harsh systolic murmur • Arrhythmia-rapid and irregular pulse • Decreased oxygen saturation in cyanotic heart disease	*ECG:* T wave inversion, bilateral enlargement, dysrhythmia • *Echocardiography:* It is indicated when disproportionate or unexplained dyspnea occurs during pregnancy and/or when a new pathological murmur (all audible diastolic murmurs are abnormal) is heard • Detects structural abnormalities (ASD, VSD), valve anatomy, valve area, function, left ventricular ejection fraction, pulmonary artery systolic pressure *Chest radiography:* Cardiomegaly, increased pulmonary vascular markings, enlargement of pulmonary veins *Cardiac MRI:* It can delineate complex anatomy (when it is not well evaluated by echocardiography) *Exercise testing:* Physiological exercise testing is an integral part of follow-up in adult congenital heart disease and valve disease and should be performed in patients with known heart disease who plan pregnancy *Cardiac enzymes:* Troponin I for diagnosing acute myocardial injury

(ASD: atrial septal defect; ECG: electrocardiography; MRI: magnetic resonance imaging; VSD: ventricular septal defect)

- Management of pregnancy and complications
- Determining timing, mode, and place of delivery.

Preconceptional Counseling

Team Approach (Fig. 4)

The prepregnancy counseling and management during pregnancy and around delivery should be conducted in an expert center by a multidisciplinary team (the pregnancy heart team). The minimum team requirements are a cardiologist, obstetrician, and anesthetist, all with expertise in the management of high-risk pregnancies in women with heart disease. Additional experts that may be involved, depending on the individual situation, are a geneticist, cardiothoracic surgeon, pediatric cardiologist, fetal medicine specialist, neonatologist, hematologist, nurse specialist, pulmonary specialist, and others where appropriate.

Counseling

The first step in a preconception counseling session is to obtain a thorough history, perform a physical examination, and to have an available information from the recent electrocardiogram and echocardiogram. This information will help to make a functional classification and place the patient in risk category. The cardio-obstetrics team will comprehensively review maternal cardiovascular risk, obstetric risk, and fetal risk, and discuss with the husband and family regarding necessity of careful planning of pregnancy. Several other aspects include long-term prognosis, fertility, and miscarriage rates, risk of genetic transmission to fetus, effect of pregnancy on heart, effect of cardiac disorder on fetal development, effect of maternal drugs on fetus, need for compliance, need for termination, are all that should be discussed.

Recurrence of CHD in the fetus varies widely from 3 to 5%, depending on the type of maternal heart disease. Maternal risk varies with specific form and severity of cardiac disease, from negligible to prohibitive. The cardio-obstetrics team will jointly develop a comprehensive strategy for the management of CVD during pregnancy, delivery, and postpartum. Women should be advised against pregnancy if she is in an extremely high-risk category [World Health Organization (WHO) risk class IV].

Counseling includes: Contemplated pregnancy may be—safe/will necessitate treatment/carries significant risk/would be extremely dangerous and should not be undertaken.

Coexisting conditions that may aggravate pre-existing CVD, such as anemia, arrhythmia, infection, and HTN, should be appropriately treated and controlled. Discuss safe and effective contraception, optimal medical/surgical treatment prepregnancy should be discussed, intervention is recommended before pregnancy with MS, valve area <1.0 cm^2.

Assessment and Stratification of Maternal and Fetal Risk

The functional classification universally used is that proposed by the New York Heart Association **(Table 3)**. The risk

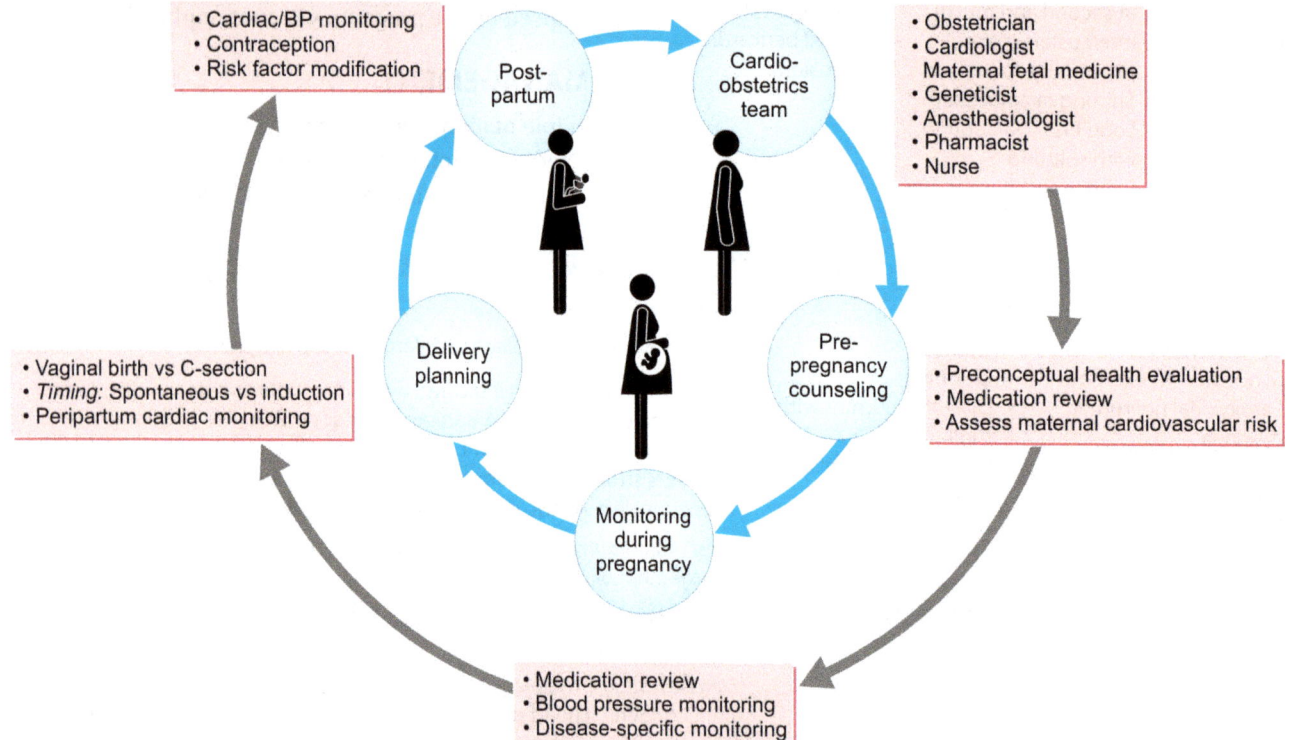

Fig. 4: The cardiac team.
Source: Mehta LS. Cardiovascular Considerations in Caring for Pregnant Patients: A Scientific Statement from the American Heart Association. Circulation. 2020;141:e884-e903.

TABLE 3: New York Heart Association (NYHA) Functional Classification of Cardiac Disease.

Class	Clinical impairments
Grade I	No limitation of physical activity; ordinary activity does not cause undue fatigue, palpitations, dyspnea, or angina
Grade II	Slight limitation of physical activity; ordinary activity causes undue fatigue, palpitations, dyspnea, or angina
Grade III	Marked limitation of physical activity; less than ordinary activity causes symptoms
Grade IV	Severely compromised cardiac function; inability to perform any physical activity without symptoms

categories are defined as low or minimal risk, intermediate or moderate risk, and high or major risk. The evaluation of risk provides a basis to explain to patient the need for extensive testing during pregnancy, increased frequency of visits, the need for prolonged hospitalization, and in some cases the need for medical or surgical correction before pregnancy. Risk assessment is also useful to determine the type of fatality and where the patient should go for delivery.

The risk of complications in pregnancy depends on the underlying cardiac diagnosis, ventricular and valvular function, functional class, presence of cyanosis, pulmonary artery pressures, and other factors. To assess the maternal risk of cardiac complications, the condition of the woman should be assessed, taking into account medical history, functional class, oxygen saturation, natriuretic peptide levels, echocardiographic assessment of ventricular and valvular function, intrapulmonary pressures, and aortic diameters, exercise capacity, and arrhythmias.

Several risk scores have been proposed to estimate the risk of maternal complications during and after pregnancy. The modified WHO (mWHO) risk classification provides an important step in the recognition of risks. The stratification is based on the underlying diagnoses and may also give directions as to who should be referred immediately and who may be evaluated in non-tertiary centers. Risk estimation should be further refined by taking into account predictors that have been identified in studies that included large populations with various diseases, such as the Cardiac Disease in Pregnancy (CARPREG), Zwangerschap bij Aangeboren Hartafwijking (ZAHARA), and Registry Of Pregnancy And Cardiac disease (ROPAC) study, of which CARPREG risk score is most widely known and used. Prediction of maternal cardiac complications in women with heart disease is enhanced by integration of general, lesion-specific, and delivery of care variables. Careful cardiovascular clinical assessment remains the foundation of risk stratification of pregnant women with heart disease.

Table 4 shows the disease-specific risk of maternal cardiovascular complication assessed by modified WHO (mWHO) classification and/or CARPREG study.

Predictors of Maternal Cardiovascular Events and Risk Score According to CARPREG (Canadian Cardiac Disease in Pregnancy Score) Study

The CARPREG risk score consists of four predictors and several cardiac conditions in pregnancy, increasing number of predictors corresponds to an increasing risk of maternal cardiac complications during pregnancy **(Table 5)**. The CARPREG risk index has a high sensitivity and negative predictive value with regard to cardiac complications in pregnant women with heart disease.

FETAL RISK

Maternal CHD is a major determinant of risk to the fetus and the neonate. Fetal complications occur in 18-30% of patients with a neonatal mortality rate of approximately 27.8%. There is a higher frequency of spontaneous abortions (15-25%), a higher frequency of recurrence of CHD (risk of fetal CHD 0-18% depending on the specific lesion (ASD, VSD—4-10%, aortic stenosis—4-18%). Preterm birth rate varies between 17 and 21%, higher especially in those with complex CHD (22-65%). In addition, a higher frequency of neonatal events, e.g., small for gestational age, respiratory distress syndrome, interventricular hemorrhage, and neonatal death may occur. The frequency of these problems is related to the severity of functional impairment of heart and the severity of chronic tissue hypoxia. Fetal death is usually secondary to chronic severe or acute maternal deterioration. Specific maternal risk factors such as subaortic ventricular outflow obstruction, maternal cyanosis, and reduced CO have been reported as predictors of adverse perinatal events. Perinatal mortality may be >fourfold higher than in the general population (<1%) and is common with premature delivery or recurrence of CHD. Perinatal mortality is highest in patients with Eisenmenger syndrome (27.7%).

PRENATAL MANAGEMENT

Existing adult CHD and pregnancy guidelines recommend that patients with complex CHD should be managed and delivered at a regional or tertiary center where a multidisciplinary team with knowledge and experience in adult CHD is available. Management in pregnancy depends on the New York Heart Association (NYHA) class of the patient and modified WHO classification of maternal cardiovascular risk.

- mWHO class I and II—advised for routine ANC at local hospitals.
- mWHO class II-III—care and delivery at referral hospitals.

TABLE 4: Modified World Health Organization classification of maternal cardiovascular risk.

	mWHO I	mWHO II	mWHO II–III	mWHO III	mWHO IV

Diagnosis (if otherwise well and uncomplicated)	• Small or mild:
	  – Pulmonary stenosis
	  – Patent ductus arteriosus
	  – Mitral valve prolapses
	• Successfully repaired simple lesions (atrial or ventricular septal defect, patent ductus arteriosus, anomalous pulmonary venous drainage)
	• Atrial or ventricular ectopic beats, isolated
		• Unoperated atrial or ventricular septal defect
		• Repaired Tetralogy of Fallot
		• Most arrhythmias (supraventricular arrhythmias)
		• Turner syndrome without aortic dilatation
			• Mild left ventricular impairment (EF >45%)
			• Hypertrophic cardiomyopathy
			• Native or tissue valve disease not considered WHO I or IV (mild MS, moderate aortic stenosis)
			• Marfan or other HTAD syndrome without aortic dilatation
			• Aorta <45 mm in bicuspid aortic valve pathology
			• Repaired coarctation
			• Atrioventricular septal defect
				• Moderate left ventricular impairment (EF 30–45%)
				• Previous peripartum cardiomyopathy without any residual left ventricular impairment
				• Mechanical valve
				• Systemic right ventricle with good or mildly decreased ventricular function
				• Fontan circulation. If otherwise the patient is well and the cardiac condition is uncomplicated
				• Unrepaired cyanotic heart disease
				• Other complex heart diseases
				• Moderate MS
				• Severe asymptomatic aortic stenosis
				• Moderate aortic dilatation (40–45 mm in Marfan syndrome or other HTAD; 45–50 mm in bicuspid aortic valve, Turner syndrome ASI 20–25 mm/m^2, tetralogy of Fallot <50 mm)
				• Ventricular tachycardia
					• Pulmonary arterial hypertension
					• Severe systemic ventricular dysfunction (EF <30% or NYHA class III–IV)
					• Previous peripartum cardiomyopathy with any residual left ventricular impairment
					• Severe MS
					• Severe symptomatic aortic stenosis, systemic right ventricle with moderate or severely decreased ventricular function
					• Severe aortic dilatation (>45 mm in Marfan syndrome or other HTAD, >50 mm in bicuspid aortic valve, Turner syndrome ASI >25 mm/m^2, tetralogy of Fallot >50 mm)
					• Vascular Ehlers–Danlos
					• Severe coarctation
					• Fontan with any complication

Risk	No detectable increased risk of maternal mortality and no/mild increased morbidity	Small increased risk of maternal mortality or moderate increase in morbidity	Intermediate increased risk of maternal mortality or moderate to severe increase in morbidity	Significantly increased risk of maternal mortality or severe morbidity	Extremely high risk of maternal mortality or severe morbidity
Maternal cardiac event rate	2.5–5%	5.7–10.5%	10–19%	19–27%	40–100%
Counseling	Yes	Yes	Yes	Yes: Expert counseling required	Yes: Pregnancy-contraindicated—if pregnancy occurs, termination should be discussed
Care during pregnancy	Local hospital	Local hospital	Referral hospital	Expert center for pregnancy and cardiac disease	Expert center for pregnancy and cardiac disease
Minimal follow-up visits during pregnancy	Once or twice	Once per trimester	Bimonthly	Monthly or bimonthly	Monthly
Location of delivery	Local hospital	Local hospital	Referral hospital	Expert center for pregnancy and cardiac disease	Expert center for pregnancy and cardiac disease

Source: Modified World Health Organization classification of maternal cardiovascular risk.
(ASI: Arterial stiffness index; CARPREG: Cardiac Disease in Pregnancy; HTAD: heritable thoracic aortic diseases; MS: mitral stenosis; NYHA: New York Heart Association; WHO: World Health Organization)

TABLE 5: Four predictors of CARPREG risk score.	
Prior cardiac event	Heart failure, transient ischemic attack (TIA), stroke before pregnancy, or arrhythmia
Baseline NYHA class	>2 or cyanosis (SO_2 <90%)
Left heart obstruction	Mitral valve area <2 cm^2, aortic valve area <1.5 cm^2, peak ventricular outflow gradient >30 mm Hg by echo
Reduced systemic ventricular systolic function	Ejection fraction <40%
CARPREG risk scores	For each above-mentioned CARPREG predictor that is present a point is assigned: • 0 points 5% • 1 point 27% • >1 point 75%

(CARPREG: Cardiac Disease in Pregnancy; NYHA: New York Heart Association)
Source: https://researchgate.net/figure/CARPREG-risk-score-predictive-factors-1.

- mWHO class III, IV—care and delivery at tertiary hospitals with coronary care unit (CCU) facilities.

Principle of Management

It includes—activity restriction, diet modification, infection control, immunization, prophylaxis against bacterial endocarditis, cardiovascular surgery, cardiovascular drugs, interruption of pregnancy, contraception, or sterilization.

Bed Rest

It is the most important measure for attenuating effect of pregnancy. Rest increases venous return, improves renal perfusion, induces diuresis, promotes elimination of water, and reduces the metabolic needs of various organs, as blood flow to these organs reduces it markedly ameliorates the workload on heart. Patients with significant MS and cardiomyopathy may require strict bed rest during pregnancy, particularly in the last trimester. Advice against undue strain.

Diet Modification

Salt restriction (4–6 g/day) prevents excessive retention of salt and water.

Diuretics

Are advised if a moderate salt restriction is insufficient to limit normal IV volume expansion. Most commonly used diuretic is *chlorothiazide*. Risks of using diuretics are—severe neonatal electrolyte imbalance, jaundice, occasional occurrence of neonatal thrombocytopenia, and decreased plasma volume with compromised placental and fetal growth. Serial hematocrit should be done to see the effects on plasma volume and dose adjusted accordingly.

Prophylactic Digitalization

Its objective is to improve contractility of the heart and to relieve symptoms, e.g., fatigue, orthopnea, and weakness. Digitalization avoids ventricular tachycardia and rapid atrial rhythms.

Early Prevention of Heart Failure

Prevention of heart failure through adequate rest, activity restriction, depending upon severity of disease, and treatment of stimulating factors of heart failure, e.g., infection, anemia, pregnancy-induced hypertension (PIH), multiple pregnancies.

Treatment of Heart Failure

Strategy for treatment of heart failure includes reducing workload with bed rest, reducing preload with diuretics, improving cardiac contractility with digitalis, reducing afterload with vasodilators. For women with *NYHA class III or IV* symptoms, hospital admission by the mid-second trimester may be advisable.

Cardiovascular Drugs

Beta-adrenergic blocking agents are commonly used for HTN, maternal tachyarrhythmia, myocardial ischemia, MS, hypertrophic cardiomyopathy, hyperthyroidism, and Marfan syndrome. Used late in pregnancy has been associated with neonatal RDS, sustained bradycardia, and hypoglycemia. Judicious use is well tolerated in case of cardiomyopathy and heart failure. Atenolol has been associated with low birth weight and therefore is not the β-blocker of choice during pregnancy. *Angiotensin-converting enzyme (ACE) inhibitors* and *angiotensin receptor blockers (ARBs)* used for HTN have a deleterious effect on fetal renal function, absolutely contraindicated in pregnancy. These are pregnancy category D drugs because of the risk of reduced fetal renal function and increased fetal and neonatal morbidity and death, especially with use during the second and third trimesters. Women taking an ACE inhibitor or angiotensin receptor blocker who desire to become pregnant should be advised to stop taking these drugs before conception to minimize the risk of fetal abnormality. Amlodipine with hydralazine can be used if needed.

Treatment of Arrhythmias

Premature atrial or ventricular beats are common in pregnancy. Sustained tachyarrhythmia such as atrial flutter or atrial fibrillation should be treated promptly. Digoxin and β-blockers are antiarrhythmic drugs of choice in view of their known safety profiles. *Quinidine, adenosine,* and *lidocaine* are also "safe". Amiodarone has been associated with a 9% incidence of fetal hypothyroidism and a 21% incidence of intrauterine growth retardation and should be reserved for cases of refractory ventricular arrhythmias. Electrical cardioversion is safe in pregnancy.

Maternal Monitoring

Women with cardiac disease have an increased risk of obstetric complications, including premature labor, preeclampsia, and PPH, in addition to increased maternal mortality and morbidity.

Antenatal Care

Should be given every 2-4 weeks until 20 weeks of gestation, then every 2 weeks until 24 weeks, then weekly thereafter (RCOG: good practice guideline, 2011). At each visit—look for signs and symptoms of heart failure and factors which aggravate heart failure. At each visit note—palpitation, cough, dyspnea, weight, anemia, pulse rate, blood pressure (BP), pedal edema, auscultation of lung bases. Re-evaluate functional grade and ensure treatment compliance.

Infection Control

Search for any evidence of urinary tract, dental, respiratory tract infection, infective endocarditis; dental care, and dental hygiene to prevent any infection.

Patients with structural heart disease, complex cyanotic heart disease, prosthetic heart valves, and h/o infective endocarditis need endocarditis prophylaxis before any dental and surgical procedure.

Thromboprophylaxis

The risk of thrombosis is increased during pregnancy. Anticoagulation reduces the risk of thrombosis by 75%. Indications include:
- Mechanical valve replacement
- Congenital heart disease with pulmonary HTN
- Atrial fibrillation.

Cardiac Surgery

Although not contraindicated, is usually not required during pregnancy, best delayed until postpartum. If needed surgery should be done between 13 and 28th weeks. Types of surgery are—balloon catheterization or even closed heart operation, valve replacement, and cardiopulmonary bypass in life-threatening cases. Cardiac surgery with cardiopulmonary bypass increases fetal mortality risk (10-15%).

Place of Therapeutic Termination

Eisenmenger syndrome, Marfan syndrome with aortic involvement (aortic root dilatation >4 cm), primary pulmonary HTN/severe pulmonary HTN from any cause (pulmonary pressure >75% of systemic pressure), coarctation of aorta with aortic valvular involvement, dilated cardiomyopathy or left ventricular dysfunction (EF < 40%), are few examples where medical termination is advised though medical termination of pregnancy (MTP) also carries risk for life.

Both medical and surgical methods (surgical dilation and suction curettage represent the most common method of pregnancy termination through 12 weeks gestation) are effective with similar rates of major complications, and suction evacuation is preferred. Medical terminations can be considered up to 9 weeks of gestation using a reduced misoprostol dose of 100 µg.

High/Prohibitive Risk where Pregnancy Needs to be Avoided

It includes pulmonary arterial HTN, severe ventricular dysfunction, severe left-sided heart obstruction, and significant aortic dilatation with underlying connective tissue disease.

Hospital Admission

Elective Admission

- NYHA I—2 weeks before estimated date of delivery (EDD)
- NYHA II—28-30 weeks
- NYHA III/IV—irrespective of period of gestation as soon as patient comes.

Emergency Admission

If deterioration of functional grade or if patient develops symptoms and signs of complications—fever/persistent cough/basal crepitations/tachyarrhythmia (P/R > 100 min)/JVP > 2 cm/anemia/infections/PE/abnormal weight gain/other medical disorders.

Fetal Monitoring

Screening for Congenital Heart Disease

Genetic ultrasonography test [USG $(11-13^{+6})$] with NT > 3.5 mm is an indication for detailed follow-up USG between 18 and 22 weeks. For major CHD, a 12 weeks ultrasound has a sensitivity and specificity of 85% [95% confidence interval (CI) 78-90%] and 99% (95% CI 98-100%), respectively. The incidence of CHD with normal nuchal translucency (NT) is about 1/1,000.

Fetal Echocardiography

All women with CHD should be offered fetal echocardiography in the 19th to 22nd weeks of pregnancy. Women with pregestational diabetes mellitus (DM), increased NT, abnormal anomaly scan, previously affected siblings, and family history of congenital cardiac disease should have fetal echocardiography done. Maternal medical history, e.g., medical disorders, viral illness, or teratogenic medication are other indications for fetal echocardiography.

Genetic Evaluation

It should be made available to all women with CHD to determine recurrence, particularly in those patients with a family history of CHD and those with possible autosomal dominant lesions (e.g., 22 q11 deletion) and appropriate referral to a fetal medicine specialist, pediatric cardiologist, geneticist, and neonatologist. Delivery in an institution that can provide neonatal cardiac care.

Assessing Fetal Well-being

Fetal growth and surveillance should be assessed between 32 and 34 weeks by USG, biophysical profile (BPP), and Doppler USG. When there is an increased risk of fetal growth restriction, serial USG every 2–4 weeks in the third trimester should be done.

Predictors of Neonatal Events

Pregnancy outcome is compromised by the presence of cardiac disease. Fetal morbidity is usually secondary to preterm birth and fetal growth restriction. Fetal death is mostly seen in mothers with cyanotic heart disease. Though predictors of offspring outcomes have been identified, there is no validated prediction model. The poor fetal outcome associated with maternal cardiac disease has been drastically modified with adequate ANC, prolonged hospitalization, and intensive care.

Thromboprophylaxis during Pregnancy (Table 6)

The optimal strategy for maintenance of anticoagulation during pregnancy in women with prosthetic heart valves remains controversial. Given the known dose-dependent teratogenicity, the 2014 AHA/American College of Cardiology Guideline for the Management of Patients with Valvular Heart Disease and the 2018 European Society of Cardiology Guideline for the Management of CVD during Pregnancy recommend continuing warfarin if therapeutic anticoagulation can be maintained at a dose ≤5 mg/day. Suggested alternatives include low molecular weight heparin (LMWH) or unfractionated heparin (UFH) and aspirin. Warfarin is contraindicated in the first trimester, can be resumed safely in the second trimester, and then transitioned to heparin after 36 weeks in patients on an anticoagulant.

With regard to labor and delivery, the use of epidural anesthesia is contraindicated in the anticoagulated patient. The American Society of Regional Anesthesia and the Society for Obstetric Anesthesia and Perinatology recommend holding UFH for 4–6 hours and LMWH for 24 hours before the administration of epidural anesthesia. The 2018 European Society of Cardiology guidelines for the management of CVD during pregnancy recommend planned delivery in women with mechanical valves. These women should be hospitalized and placed on intravenous UFH or LMWH with close monitoring at 36 weeks, and at approximately 36 hours before planned delivery, they should be on intravenous UFH, which is recommended to be discontinued 4–6 hours before delivery. Intravenous UFH can be restarted as early as 4–6 hours after delivery, depending on the type of delivery and whether there were bleeding complications or not. Warfarin should be started following delivery and continue along with heparin. After 3–5 days when therapeutic International Normalized Ratio (INR) has reached, UFH can be stopped.

Emergency Delivery

For women on UFH or LMWH in case of emergency delivery protamine should be considered. Patients on warfarin—fresh frozen plasma (FFP) prior to C-section to achieve INR ≤2 along with oral vitamin K (0.5–1 mg). It takes 4–6 hours to influence INR. For newborns—FFP and vitamin K.

Anticoagulant Regimen with Dose

Table 7 shows the anticoagulant regimen with dose.

Anticoagulation Regimens for Mechanical Prosthetic Heart Valve (Flowchart 1)

Low Dose Aspirin

Additional use of low-dose aspirin should be considered, particularly in women with high-risk valves, patients with

TABLE 6: ACC/AHA/European Society of Cardiology Anticoagulation Guidelines.	
NYHA class III/IV or cyanosis during baseline prenatal visit	Cardiac medication before pregnancy "At birth" cyanotic heart disease
Maternal left heart obstruction	Mechanical valve prosthesis
Smoking during pregnancy	Maternal cardiac event during pregnancy
Low maternal oxygen saturation (<90%)	Maternal decline in cardiac output during pregnancy
• Multiple gestations • Use of anticoagulants throughout pregnancy	• Abnormal uteroplacental • Doppler flow
(NYHA: New York Heart Association) *Source:* Modified from Siu et al. (Carpreg investigators), Reper et al. (Zahara investigators).	

cyanosis, with intracardiac shunts, with previous transient ischemic attacks (TIAs) and/or strokes, and women with atrial fibrillation.

MANAGEMENT DURING LABOR AND DELIVERY

Spontaneous vaginal delivery is preferred. Most patients with cardiac disease go into spontaneous labor and deliver without difficulty. Vaginal delivery is associated with less blood loss and lower risk of infection, venous thrombosis and embolism, and a lower risk of an acute shift of blood volume that happens during C/S, therefore, should be advised for most women.

Induction of Labor

The ACOG recommends elective induction of labor for pregnant women with cardiac disease between 39 and 40 weeks of gestation in patients who do not have spontaneous onset of labor or clinical indications for preterm delivery. This reduces the risk of emergency cesarean section by 12% and the risk of stillbirth by 50% in women without heart disease, and the benefit is likely to be greater for women with heart disease who have higher rates of obstetric complications. The ACOG literature does not provide specific information about delivery timing in WHO class IV maternal cardiac conditions; thus, these decisions are frequently made on a case-by-case basis by the high-risk cardio-obstetric team. Timing of induction will depend on cardiac status, obstetric evaluation including cervical assessment and fetal well-being.

Artificial rupture of membranes and infusion of oxytocin can be used safely in women with heart disease. Intracervical foley instillation might be preferable in patients with CHD where a drop in SVR would be detrimental. Both misoprostol [25 µg, prostaglandin E1 (PGE_1)] or dinoprostone [1–3 mg or slow-release formulation of 10 mg (PGE_2) or gel (0.5 mg)] can be used safely to induce labor. Induction of labor to be avoided in decompensated heart disease.

TABLE 7: Anticoagulant regimen with dose.				
Regimen	Dosing	Monitoring	Therapeutic goal	Risks

LMWH throughout pregnancy category C	Begin with Enoxaparin 1 mg/kg SC q12 hours	• Antifactor Xa level 4 hours after dose in-hospital daily, anti-Xa levels until target, then weekly	• Manufacturers' upper therapeutic range
			• *Target anti-Xa levels:* 1.0–1.2 U/mL (mitral and right-sided valves) or 0.8–1.2 U/mL (aortic valves) 46 hours postdose (I); -predose anti-Xa levels >0.6 U/mL
				• Risk of thrombosis 4.4–8.7%
				• Use in mechanical heart valve is controversial
				• *Advantage over UFH:*
				  – More predictable therapeutic effect
				  – Lower risk of maternal bleeding, osteoporosis, thrombocytopenia

UFH throughout pregnancy category C	Begin at 17,500–20,000 U q12 hour IV or dose adjusted SC	• aPTT or anti-factor Xa level 4–6 hours after dose • In-hospital daily after a stable aPTT has been achieved, UFH should be monitored weekly	>2x control 0.35–0.70 U/mL	• Risk of thrombosis 9–33% • Osteoporosis, thrombocytopenia
• LMWH or UFH through 13 weeks and after 36 weeks and • Warfarin (category D) from 14 to 36 weeks	Heparin q 12 hours Warfarin (>5 mg) daily	As above for heparin INR	As above for heparin INR—2.5–3.5	*Less fetal consequences of warfarin* Warfarin risk: • ↑ risk of miscarriage • Embryopathy (4–10%, dose dependent, ↑ if >5 mg) • Risk of fetal bleeding and neurological abnormalities • ↑ risk of maternal bleeding
Warfarin throughout the pregnancy (up to 36 weeks)	Warfarin <5 mg/day	After target INR, monitor INR at least 2 weekly	INR—2.5–3.5	• Risk of thrombosis is low (0–4%) • Warfarin risk as above
Aspirin added to all above regimen	75–100 mg/day	None		

(aPTT: activated partial thromboplastin time; INR: international normalized ratio; LMWH: low-molecular-weight heparin; UFH: unfractionated heparin)
Source: Edited from Researchgate. ACC/AHA/European Society of Cardiology Anticoagulation Guidelines.

Flowchart 1: Anticoagulation in mechanical valves.

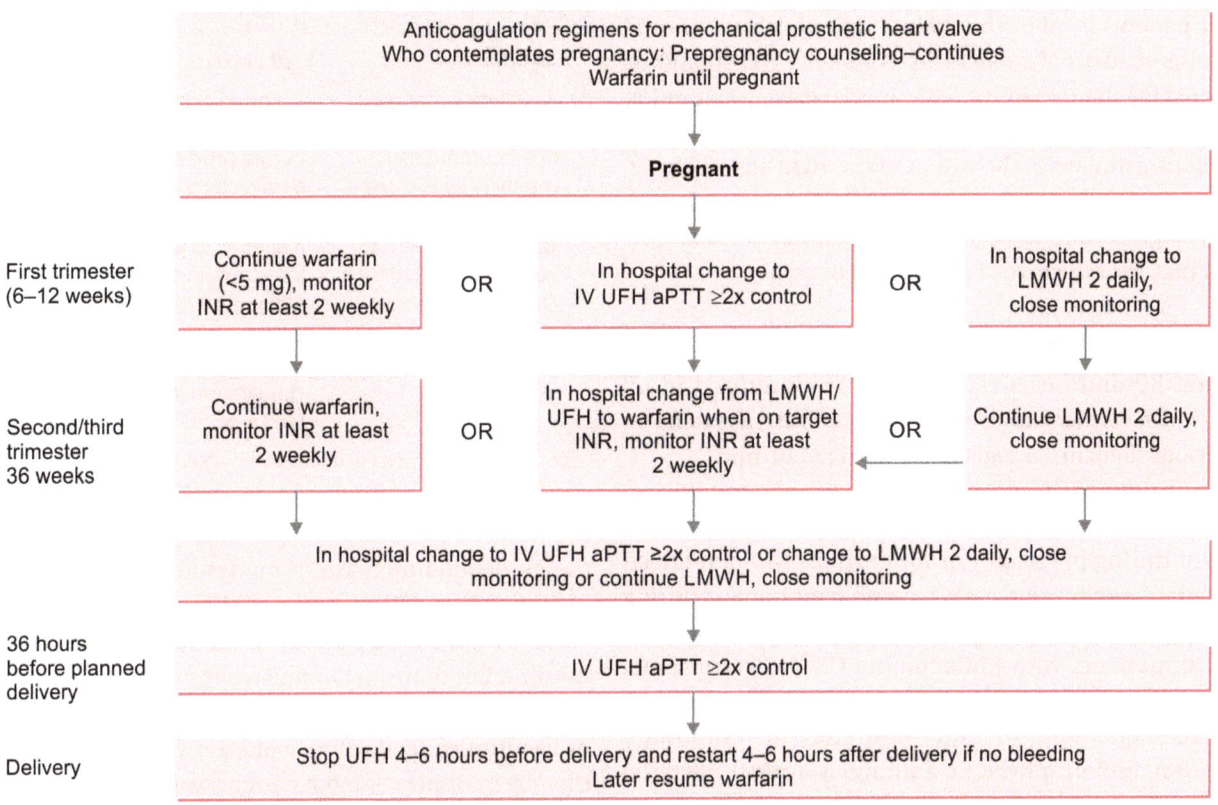

(aPTT: activated partial thromboplastin time; INR: international normalized ratio; IV: intravenous; LMWH: low molecular weight heparin; UFH: unfractionated heparin)
Source: Researchgate

Cesarean Section

It should be considered for obstetric indications and for patients presenting in labor on oral anticoagulants (OACs), with aggressive aortic pathology, acute intractable HF, and in severe forms of PH (including Eisenmenger syndrome).

INTRAPARTUM MANAGEMENT

First Stage of Labor

Labor results in important hemodynamic changes, including an increase in heart rate, central venous pressure, and CO. In the supine position, uterine contractions are associated with an approximately 15% rise in CO; in the lateral position, cardiac output rises only approximately 8–11%. Cardiac patients should be in the lateral recumbent position throughout labor and during delivery. Uterine contractions augment maternal CO as a result of enhanced sympathetic activity (via anxiety, pain) and expulsion of uterine blood into the central venous circulation. During a contraction, the uterus expels up to 400 mL of blood into the central venous circulation, leading to a rise in central venous pressure, right atrial pressure, CO, and arterial pressure. The labor-induced augmentation of CO is attenuated by effective epidural anesthesia.

Adequate Pain Relief

Pain increases CO 50% above that in second stage. The labor-associated rise in arterial pressure can be attenuated by effective pain control (e.g., epidural blockade) and lateral tilting of the patient. Pain relief—reduces tachycardia, myocardial work, and CO. Epidural narcotics (e.g., fentanyl) can be used in epidural anesthesia where regional anesthesia is relatively contraindicated such as severe aortic stenosis (AS), severe MS, and aortic coarctation, Marfan syndrome with dilated root or hypertrophic obstructive cardiomyopathy. Because epidural anesthesia via venodilatation can reduce return of blood to the heart, cautious incremental dosing is advised, especially in gravidas whose CO is sensitive to falls in preload.

Fluid Management

In spontaneous labor, allow oral fluid. Intravenous crystalloid administered when necessary for hydration with close monitoring of fluid balance. All patients with right-to-left shunts should have filtered vascular lines to prevent paradoxical air embolization. In induced/augmented labor—use fluids cautiously not >75 mL/hour (15–18 drops/min) (150 mL/hour—AS).

Oxygen Saturation

Cardiac patients in labor should be continuously monitored with pulse oximetry. Patients with complex CHD should be monitored for changes in systemic arterial oxygen saturation (SaO_2). In those with right-to-left shunts, SaO_2 provides a continuous estimate of the extent of the right-to-left shunt. Intermittent/continuous oxygen inhalation of 5-6 L/min should be given if required. Desaturation not corrected by oxygen may be indicative of pulmonary edema.

Hemodynamic Monitoring

Maternal BP and heart rate should be monitored in all patients with cardiac disease. Rapid digitalization is done by intravenous digoxin 0.5 mg if pulse rate is >110/min.

Continuous ECG monitoring (e.g., via telemetry) is indicated for patients with a history of arrhythmias before or during pregnancy or for gravidas with a reduced ventricular function who have become symptomatic during gestation to detect early signs of decompensation. In some high-risk patients with Philadelphia (PH) chromosome, central venous pressure monitoring may be considered. Other managements include—diuretics in pulmonary congestion, and prophylactic antibiotics against bacterial endocarditis.

Prevention of Infection

Repeated vaginal examination should be avoided if needed to be done under the strict aseptic precautions. Artificial rupture of membranes (ARM)—should be avoided unless indicated because of risk of infection.

Subacute bacterial endocarditis prophylaxis: Patients with complex CHD and those with artificial valve prosthesis may be given antibiotic prophylaxis at the time of delivery to avoid subacute bacterial endocarditis. The European Society of Cardiology, American College of Cardiology/American Heart Association Guidelines do not recommend antibiotic prophylaxis for heart disease in pregnancy but it is a common practice in developing countries to give intravenous antibiotics routinely during labor and if any procedure is contemplated **(Table 8)**.

Fetal Monitoring

In all patients with CVD continuous fetal heart rate (FHR) monitoring by cardiotocography (CTG) during labor is indicated.

TABLE 8: SABE (Subacute bacterial endocarditis) prophylaxis during delivery.

Indications	Prophylaxis
• Antibiotic prophylaxis is controversial. It is not recommended routinely by ESC and American college of cardiology/American heart association) • Only given to those who are at risk of infection and severe lesion	• A single IV dose of ampicillin 2 g + Gentamicin 1.5 mg/kg 30–60 minutes before procedure • 6 hours later: Ampicillin—1 g IV/IM or 1 g PO • If allergic to penicillin • Vancomycin 1G IV or clindamycin—600 mg IV+ Gentamicin—1.5 mg/kg • Others—penicillin, amoxicillin (2 g), erythromycin, cephalosporin, clindamycin (600 mg), teicoplanin (400 mg)

Source: European Society of Cardiology guideline, 2015.

Second Stage of Labor

The uterine contractions of the second stage of labor are normally augmented by maternal Valsalva maneuvers. Historically, Valsalva maneuvers have been discouraged for patients with significant cardiac disease because of the associated increase in maternal O_2 consumption and reduction in cardiac return and CO.

Delivery should be considered in propped up position, minimizing maternal expulsive effort by passive delivery and facilitating the second stage by assisted delivery (forceps or vacuum extraction) to avoid the Valsalva maneuver and thereby minimize hemodynamic perturbations in those with critical obstructive lesions (e.g., aortic stenosis [AS]), fragile aortas (bicuspid aortic valve with aortopathy, coarctation), and pulmonary HTN. Strict cardiovascular monitoring and delayed cord clamping is preferred.

Third Stage of Labor

Maternal blood loss in the first postpartum hour averages 600 mL for vaginal and 1,000 mL for cesarean delivery. Excessive blood loss is associated with maternal tachycardia and decreased stroke volume. For active management of the third stage of labor (AMTSL)—give 10 U oxytocin IM, and avoid bolus oxytocin. A slow intravenous infusion of oxytocin (2 U of oxytocin given over 10 minutes immediately after birth, followed by 12 mU/min for 4 hours) reduces the risk of PPH. Slight blood loss is not detrimental, avoid bolus syntocinon®/ergometrine.

Immediately after delivery management includes—propped up position, oxygen inhalation, diuretics to avoid fluid overload (furosemide 40 mg IV), watch for signs of congestive heart failure (CHF) and pulmonary edema. Treat PPH energetically—misoprostol (200–1,000 µg) can be used to treat PPH.

Postpartum Hemodynamic Changes

Immediately after delivery, the intravascular volume is augmented by an "autotransfusion" of about 500 mL of blood from the involuting uterus. This increases the stroke volume and CO immediately by 71% and 60–80%, respectively.

This physiologic phenomenon may exceed the pumping ability of the heart resulting in acute pulmonary edema. To decrease this risk patient should be placed in a sitting position following delivery as it allows more gradual hemodynamic adaptation by increasing venous pooling in the lower extremity and thereby reducing venous return to heart.

The hemodynamic changes begin to reverse shortly after delivery and continue to decrease over the next 24 hours, resolving over the next 6–8 weeks but may persist for up to 6 months. Mean arterial pressure can be elevated for 1–2 days postpartum before declining over the ensuing 2 weeks. Pulmonary vascular resistance (PVR) rises to preconception values within 6 months postpartum.

Postpartum Monitoring

The recommendations for postpartum monitoring are largely dependent on the patient's underlying congenital cardiac abnormality, predisposition to arrhythmias, presence or absence of signs or symptoms of heart failure, and clinical course during pregnancy and delivery. Telemetry cardiac monitoring should continue for at least 24 hours for those patients with symptoms or signs of significant antepartum or intrapartum arrhythmias. For the patient considered at highest risk or who has demonstrated signs of decompensation during the pregnancy or delivery period, management in an intensive care unit/critical care unit setting for the first 24–48 hours after delivery for hemodynamic monitoring should be considered. Meticulous leg care, elastic support stockings, and early ambulation are important to reduce the risk of thromboembolism.

Breastfeeding

It is not contraindicated. In cases of intrauterine fetal death (IUD), peripartum cardiomyopathy (PPCM) inhibition of lactation can be obtained with standard doses of cabergoline (0.25 mg every 12 hours for 2 days), or bromocriptine (2.5 mg on the day of delivery, followed by 2.5 mg twice daily for 14 days) if cabergoline is not available.

With preceding beta-blockade, monitoring of the baby for 48 hours is recommended. Newborn should be screened for ASD, VSD, and coarctation of aorta.

■ ADVICE DURING DISCHARGE

Continue medical treatment, iron and calcium supplementation. Avoid infection.

Contraception (Fig. 5)

Oral desogestrel, progestin-only pills, progestin implants, and emergency contraception can be used in all cardiac

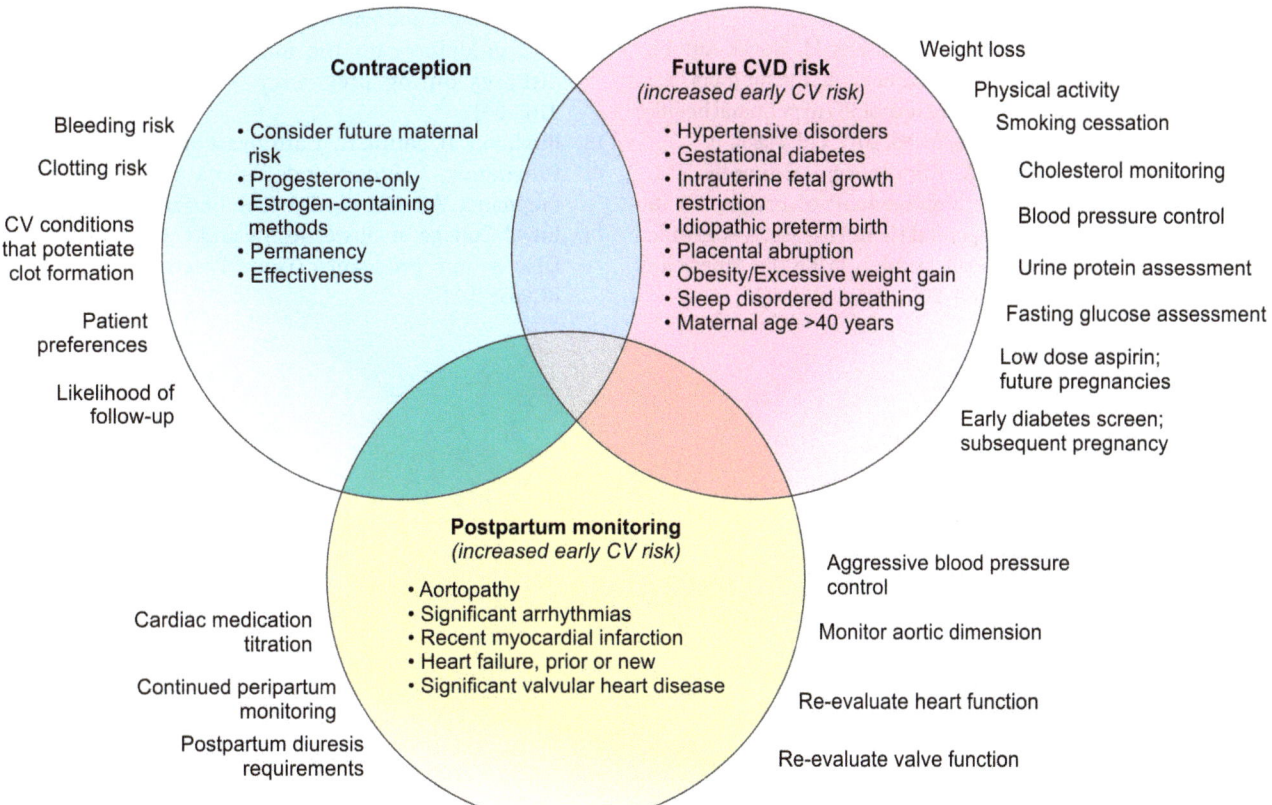

Fig. 5: Postpartum monitoring, contraception, and future risk.
(CVD: cardiovascular disease)
Source: Mehta LS. Cardiovascular Considerations in Caring for Pregnant Patients: A Scientific Statement from the American Heart Association. Circulation. 2020;141:e884-e903.

patients. Depo-Provera—avoided in patients on warfarin, copper intrauterine device (CU-T IUD) avoided, but levonorgestrel-releasing IUD (Mirena®) can be used. Ethinyloestradiol-containing oral contraceptive pills (OCP) have the greatest risk of thrombosis, avoid in patients with a mechanical heart valve, those with history of myocardial infarction (MI). Barrier methods are unreliable but reduce the risk of pelvic inflammatory disease. A good approach is the combination of barrier methods and long-acting reversible contraception (levonorgestrel-based long-acting reversible contraception, progestin-releasing implant, or progestin-releasing intrauterine devices). *Sterilization*—tubal ligation, hysteroscopic insertion of Essure device, vasectomy in selected cases.

FOLLOW-UP

Reassess after 6 weeks or earlier if complications occur, by a multidisciplinary team. Subsequent pregnancy needs to be avoided if patient develops heart failure, cardiomyopathy, or is in a high-risk group.

SUGGESTED READING

1. American College of Obstetricians and Gynecologists' Presidential Task Force on Pregnancy and Heart Disease and Committee on Practice Bulletins—Obstetrics. ACOG Practice Bulletin No. 212: Pregnancy and Heart Disease. Obstet Gynecol. 2019;133(5):e320-56.
2. Bouvier-Colle MH, Mohangoo AD, Gissler M, Novak-Antolic Z, Vutuc C, Szamotulska K, et al. What about the mothers? An analysis of maternal mortality and morbidity in perinatal health surveillance systems in europe. BJOG. 2012;119(7):880-9.
3. Canobbio MM, Warnes CA, Aboulhosn J, Connolly HM, Khanna A, Koos BJ, et al. Management of Pregnancy in Patients With Complex Congenital Heart Disease: A Scientific Statement for Healthcare Professionals From the American Heart Association. Circulation. 2017;135(8):e50-87.
4. Cantwell R, Clutton-Brock T, Cooper G, Dawson A, Drife J, Garrod D, et al. Saving mothers' lives: Reviewing maternal deaths to make motherhood safer: 2006-2008. The eighth report of the confidential enquiries into maternal deaths in the United Kingdom. BJOG. 2011;118(Suppl 1):1-203.
5. Chowdhury MZI, Haque MA, Farhana Z, Anik AM, Chowdhury AH, Haque SM, et al. Prevalence of cardiovascular disease among Bangladeshi adult population: a systematic review and meta-analysis of the studies. Vasc Health Risk Manag. 2018;14:165-81.
6. Drenthen W, Boersma E, Balci A, Moons P, Roos-Hesselink JW, Mulder BJ, et al. Predictors of pregnancy complications in women with congenital heart disease. Eur Heart J. 2010;31(17):2124-32.
7. Elkayam U, Goland S, Pieper PG, Silverside CK. High-risk cardiac disease in pregnancy: Part I. J Am Coll Cardiol. 2016,68(4):396-410.
8. James DK, Steer PJ, Weiner CP, Gonik B, Robson SC. High Risk Pregnancy, 5th edition. New Delhi: Cambridge University Press; 2018.
9. Krishna L. Obstetrics Protocols, 2nd edition. New Delhi: Jaypee Brothers Medical Publishers; 2016.
10. Lockwood CJ, Moore TR, Copel J, Silver RM, Resnik R. Maternal-Fetal Medicine: Principles and Practice, 8th edition. Philadelphia: Saunders; 2019.
11. Mehta LS, Warnes CA, Bradley E, Burton T, Economy K, Mehran R, et al. Cardiovascular Considerations in Caring for Pregnant Patients: A Scientific Statement from the American Heart Association. Circulation. 2020;141(23):e884-903.
12. Regitz-Zagrosek V, Roos-Hesselink JW, Bauersachs J, Blomström-Lundqvist C, Cífková R, De Bonis M, et al. 2018 ESC guidelines for the management of cardiovascular diseases during pregnancy. Eur Heart J. 2018;39(34):3165-241.
13. Rovinsky JJ, Jaffin H. Cardiovascular Hemodynamics in Pregnancy. I. Blood and Plasma Volumes in Multiple Pregnancy. Am J Obstet Gynecol. 1965;93:1-15.
14. Royal College of Obstetricians and Gynaecologist. Cardiac Disease and Pregnancy (Good Practice No. 13). London: RCOG; 2011.

CHAPTER 9

Liver Diseases in Pregnancy

INTRODUCTION

Liver disease is a serious complication of pregnancy and poses a challenge for the obstetricians and hepatologists. Among the causes are the preexisting liver disease, liver disease acquired during pregnancy, especially viral hepatitis, pregnancy-related liver diseases including hyperemesis gravidarum (HG), intrahepatic cholestasis of pregnancy (ICP), preeclampsia, hemolysis, elevated liver enzymes, low platelet count (HELLP) syndrome and fatty liver of pregnancy. Pregnancy-associated liver diseases affect up to 3% of pregnant women in developed countries and are the most frequent cause of liver dysfunction in pregnancy.

Pregnancy-associated liver disorders exhibit trimester-specific occurrence, while nonpregnancy-related liver diseases can occur at any time. The timing of the occurrence of clinical manifestations and abnormal liver function tests (LFTs) are critical for determining diagnosis and treatment strategies. Therapeutic decisions must be made considering the implications for both mother and the baby. A rapid evaluation to distinguish between these dysfunctions are essential, in order to facilitate appropriate management. The main factors determining maternal prognosis are the type of liver disease, the degree of impaired synthetic, metabolic, and excretory functions of the liver, and timing of delivery. Severe liver diseases are associated with significant morbidity and mortality for both the mother and the infant and urgent delivery needed if at the severe end of the spectrum. These cases require rapid management by a multidisciplinary team including maternal-fetal medicine specialists, hepatologists, gastroenterologists, and interventional radiologists. Availability of liver transplantation is also important for obtaining good outcomes.

CLASSIFICATION

Liver disease during pregnancy is classified into two main categories—(1) those related to pregnancy, and (2) those unrelated to pregnancy or coincidental to pregnancy. Those unrelated to pregnancy can present *de novo* in pregnancy, or pregnancy can occur in women with preexisting liver pathology.

Classification of Liver Diseases in Pregnancy

Table 1 shows the classification of liver diseases in pregnancy.

NORMAL PHYSIOLOGICAL CHANGES IN PREGNANCY

In normal pregnancy, many physiological and hormonal changes occur within the human body, some of which can mimic those seen in women with liver disease. There is a rise in maternal heart rate, cardiac output increases by 40%, the circulating plasma volume increases by 30% and there is a reduction in peripheral vascular resistance. These physiological changes result in hyperdynamic circulation, a physiological state that is common in patients with decompensated chronic liver disease. Physical examination of a pregnant woman may show *palmar erythema* and the presence of multiple spider nevi in up to 70% of cases. Blood flow to the liver remains constant during pregnancy and liver becomes impalpable in advanced gestation as it is displaced little upwards in the thoracic cavity by the enlarged uterus. Gallbladder motility decreases resulting in an increased risk of developing gallstones in the women.

TABLE 1: Classification of liver diseases in pregnancy.

Pregnancy-related liver diseases	Pregnancy-unrelated liver diseases preexisting	Pregnancy-unrelated liver diseases Coincidental with pregnancy
• Hyperemesis gravidarum • Cholestasis of pregnancy • Acute fatty liver of pregnancy • Preeclampsia and eclampsia • HELLP syndrome	• Hepatitis B, C, and E • Cirrhosis and portal hypertension, autoimmune liver disease • Wilson disease • Postliver transplantation state • Nonalcoholic fatty liver disease	• Acute viral hepatitis • Biliary diseases (e.g., cholelithiasis, primary sclerosing cholangitis) • Vascular alterations (Budd–Chiari syndrome) • Liver tumors • Drug-induced hepatotoxicity

(HELLP: hemolysis, elevated liver enzymes, low platelet count)

Biochemical and *hematological indices* need to be interpreted in light of altered normal ranges in pregnancy. Albumin, total protein, and antithrombin III concentrations decrease. Total serum protein concentration decreases 20-40%, because of reduction of albumin concentration as well as because of hemodilution. Maternal alkaline phosphatase (ALP) increases in the third trimester, as ALP is produced both from the placenta and as a result of fetal bone development. The alpha-fetoprotein (AFP) level is increased as AFP is produced by the fetal liver. Other common biochemical and hematological tests including urea, hemoglobin levels and the prothrombin time, remain unchanged or slightly reduced due to hemodilution. Elevations in transaminases, bilirubin or the prothrombin time are abnormal and indicate a pathological state which requires further assessment. Pregnancy is a procoagulant state, and clotting factors (I, II, V, VII, X, and XII) and fibrinogen are increased.

Small clinically insignificant esophageal varices can occur in up to 50% of pregnant women in the late second and third trimester due to compression of the inferior vena cava (IVC) by the enlarging uterus and a reduction in venous return. Liver biopsy is rarely indicated in pregnancy, but if performed does not carry additional risks.

■ HYPEREMESIS GRAVIDARUM

Introduction

Characterized by severe persistent nausea and vomiting with subsequent dehydration, weight loss, electrolyte imbalance, and nutritional deficiency. Hyperemesis gravidarum occurs in about 0.3-2% of pregnancies, usually begins very early in gestation and resolves by 20 weeks.

Etiology

Exact etiology is unclear, but has been proposed to involve liver cell injury due to multiple factors, including dehydration, starvation, and placental-derived cytokines, including tumor necrosis factor alpha (TNF-α). Numerous theories based on genetic, psychiatric, psychological, cultural, and hormonal factors have been put forward. Others include gastric motility alterations, changes in the autonomic nervous system and *Helicobacter pylori* infection. It is noted that liver enzymes return to normal levels after resolution of HG, no long-term sequelae of HG on liver-related health.

The first trimester peak human chorionic gonadotropin (hCG) is correlated with the severity of HG, hyperthyroidism occurs in 60% of patients with HG. hCG activates thyroid stimulating hormone (TSH) receptors leading to thyroid suppression and increased thyroxine levels. Clearly identified risk factors in HG include molar and twin pregnancies, previous history of HG, and previous history of fetal abnormalities, increased body mass index, psychiatric diseases, and diabetes.

Biochemical Changes in Hyperemesis Gravidarum

Biochemical changes in HG include elevations in aspartate transaminase (AST) and alkaline transaminase (ALT) levels, which are typically mildly elevated but have been observed to rise as high as 1,000 in some patients. Fifty percent of affected patients have LFTs 2-3X normal, seen 1-3 weeks after onset of the condition. Jaundice is rare, occurring more commonly in severe cases.

Patients may present with renal dysfunction and electrolyte disorders such as hyponatremia, hypokalemia, and hypochloremic alkalosis. In severe cases, dehydration can lead to orthostatic hypotension, tachycardia, and lethargy. Vomiting can lead to bleeding from esophageal lacerations and vitamin deficiency produce neurological disorders in very rare cases.

Treatment

Treatment is supportive, involves administration of intravenous fluid, nutritional support, hydration, and control of emesis. Less than 1% of patients require admission to the hospital, symptoms usually resolve with progression of gestational age. Intravenous rehydration, correction of electrolyte disorders, and thiamine replacement are indicated for prevention of Wernicke's encephalopathy, especially in patients who receive dextrose solutions. Vitamin B_6 for control of nausea and vomiting is considered the first-line therapy while *antiemetics* are considered as the *second line*. Second line therapies including dopamine antagonists (metoclopramide), phenothiazines (chlorpromazine, prochlorperazine), and anticholinergics (dicycloverine) have a reasonable safety data.

Systemic steroids and ondansetron can be considered for refractory patients, but their safety profiles must be taken into account. Patients who cannot maintain weight and do not respond to antiemetics require advanced enteral nutrition and may even require total parenteral nutrition. Dietary modification should focus on consumption of small, frequent, low-fat meals with high carbohydrate content.

Biochemical abnormalities usually improve with resolution of vomiting and do not leave permanent liver sequelae. Hyperemesis gravidarum is a reversible condition, often recurs in subsequent pregnancies. If liver tests are not normalized with resolution of vomiting, other causes should be suspected.

■ INTRAHEPATIC CHOLESTASIS OF PREGNANCY

Introduction

Intrahepatic cholestasis of pregnancy also known as *obstetric cholestasis* is the most common pregnancy-specific liver disease characterized by cholestasis and pruritus, with onset in the late second and third trimester of pregnancy. Obstetric cholestasis is diagnosed when otherwise unexplained pruritus involving the palms and soles occurs in pregnancy along with abnormal LFTs and/or raised bile acid, both resolve after delivery.

Risk Factors

Intrahepatic cholestasis of pregnancy is more common in multiple gestations (twins 20.9 vs. singletons 4.7% in one study from Chile; triplets 43% versus 14% in twins in a study from Finland). Other epidemiologic factors include chronic hepatitis C, prior history or family history of intrahepatic cholestasis, and advanced maternal age. Some studies suggest a higher prevalence in patients with cholelithiasis and nonalcoholic fatty liver disease (NAFLD).

Incidence

The reported incidence of ICP varies widely worldwide, ranging from <1 to 27.6%, for reasons that are incompletely understood. Incidence varies with geographical location and ethnicity, across Europe the incidence ranges from 0.5 to 1.5%, with the highest rates in Scandinavia. The incidence is 1.2-1.5% in the Indian Asian and Pakistani Asian populations, 3-5% among pregnant women in Chile, 1% in Europe, 0.7% in the UK, 0.3-1.0% in USA, and rarely reported in African countries. Geographic variations may reflect differences in susceptibility between ethnic groups and differences in environmental factors. Seasonal variations indicate a higher incidence in the winter months in some countries. The araucanian Indians in Chile have the highest incidence worldwide at 27.6%.

Pathogenesis

The pathogenesis of ICP is unknown. Approximately 15% cases have genetic variation in one of the hepatocanalicular transport proteins. Multidrug resistance protein 3 (MDR3) is the major phospholipid transporter, and mutation of the gene which express it leads to a loss in function and increased levels of serum bile acids. The *MDR3* mutation is located on chromosome 7q21. Other mutations include the *ABCB11* gene mutation, which is a mutation in the bile salt export pump (BSEP).ABnormal placental transport of bile acids from fetal to the maternal circulation increases maternal bile acids while the immature fetal transport system can contribute to increased bile acid levels in the fetus itself.

Symptoms

A typical symptom of ICP is intense pruritus, predominantly nocturnal and usually affecting palms and soles, characteristically improves within 48 hours of delivery. Some patients may complain of other symptoms, e.g., choluria, acholia, anorexia, fatigue, epigastric pain, and steatorrhea due to fat malabsorption. Right upper quadrant pain, nausea, poor appetite, sleep deprivation, or steatorrhea may occur. Pruritus and other symptoms usually develop during the late second or third trimester.

Biochemical Changes

An increase in serum total bile acid concentration is the key laboratory finding (present in >90% of affected pregnancies) and may be the first and only laboratory abnormality. Typical laboratory findings include elevated serum bile acid levels >10 µmol/L and increased activity of liver aminotransferases. Serum aminotransferases (elevated in 60% of cases), which are usually <2X the upper limit of normal, but may reach values >1,000 unit/L, making a distinction from viral hepatitis important. ALT has been found to be a more sensitive marker than AST, ALT levels increase between 2 and 10 times more than AST. ALP, which may be elevated fourfolds but is not specific for cholestasis during pregnancy due to expression of the placental isoenzyme.

The serum concentration of gamma-glutamyl transpeptidase (GGT) is normal or modestly elevated (30% of cases), which is unusual in most other forms of cholestatic liver disease in which GGT levels parallel other cholestatic markers. The prothrombin time is usually normal. When prolonged, it is typically secondary to vitamin K deficiency from fat malabsorption due to severe steatorrhea or secondary to the use of bile acid sequestrants (such as cholestyramine), rather than liver dysfunction.

Adverse outcomes are rarely reported in pregnancies where the maternal bile acid level is below 40 µmol/L. Once obstetric cholestasis is diagnosed, it is reasonable to measure LFTs weekly until delivery. Clinical jaundice occurs in 10-15% of pregnant women with bilirubin levels not exceeding 100 µmol/L or 5.85 mg/dL, which appears after the onset of pruritus. If jaundice is the initial symptom, further evaluation is necessary.

Diagnosis

Serum bile acids are the most sensitive and specific test for diagnosis and monitoring of this condition. When a diagnosis of ICP is ruled out, other causes of cholestasis should be sought. Serum autotaxin, a lysophospholipase D, essential for angiogenesis and neuronal development during embryogenesis, was found to be a highly sensitive and specific diagnostic marker that distinguishes ICP from other pruritic disorders of pregnancy and pregnancy-related liver diseases. Ultrasonography should be performed to exclude cholelithiasis.

Liver biopsy shows bile plugs in hepatocytes and canaliculi predominately in zone 3. The portal tracts are unaffected, with no features of inflammation. However, histopathology is rarely available as liver biopsy is not necessary for diagnosis.

Treatment

The first line of treatment is ursodeoxycholic acid (UDCA), which results in improved maternal symptoms and liver biochemistry in approximately 75% of cases, and have possible beneficial effects on perinatal outcomes. UDCA enhances the biliary transport of bile—acids, it is antiapoptotic and increases the excretion of pruritogens such as progesterone sulfate. Both in-vitro and in-vivo experiments demonstrate that UDCA enhances the transplacental transport of bile acids from the fetus to the mother and reduces placental damage.

Dose

Usually started at a dose of 500 mg twice daily. It may be increased maximum up to 2 g/day for symptomatic and biochemical improvement till delivery. If prothrombin time is prolonged, the use of vitamin K in doses of 5-10 mg daily is indicated. Aqueous cream with menthol improves symptoms but not the disease process.

Treatment in Refractory Cases

S-Adenosyl Methionine

The glutathione precursor S-adenosyl methionine (SAMe) influences the composition and fluidity of hepatocyte plasma membranes and increases the methylation and biliary excretion of hormone metabolites, usually administered intravenously, but it is inconvenient as prolonged therapy is required.

Cholestyramine

It decreases ileal absorption of bile salts, thereby increasing fecal excretion. Cholestyramine is given orally in divided doses starting at 2-4 g/day and gradually increased to a maximum dose of 16 g/day if needed, for symptom control. However, its effect on pruritus in ICP is limited and cholestyramine may cause constipation, abdominal discomfort, and malabsorption of fat including fat-soluble vitamins (e.g., vitamin K) at higher doses (>4 g/day).

Rifampicin

It is a potent pregnane X receptor agonist which mediates many detoxification and hepatobiliary processes. It relieves pruritus associated with cholestasis in nonpregnant patients. Potential adverse effects include nausea, decreased appetite, hemolytic anemia, renal failure, and hepatitis.

Combined use of UDCA and rifampicin has been postulated to have synergistic beneficial effects in nonobstructive cholestasis. Given the favorable safety data for rifampicin in the third trimester of pregnancy, it is used as a second-line agent in patients whose symptoms or biochemistry don't respond to UDCA. Nevertheless, it should only be used if transaminases are not too high.

Fetal Risk

Maternal bile acids cross the placenta and accumulate in the fetus and amniotic fluid, which carries significant risks for the fetus including increased risks for intrauterine demise, meconium-stained amniotic fluid, preterm delivery (spontaneous and iatrogenic), neonatal respiratory distress syndrome and unexplained intracerebral hemorrhage (due to vitamin K deficiency). Fetal/perinatal mortality is 0.4-1.4%. Fetal risk is high when serum bile acid is >40 µmol/L and risks of stillbirth is high when serum bile acid levels are 100 µmol/L or higher. A large Swedish cohort demonstrated that the likelihood of the development of meconium-stained fluid, spontaneous preterm birth, and fetal asphyxia increased by 1-2% for every µmol/L increase of bile acid.

Preterm births in ICP result from bile acid-induced release of prostaglandins; in addition, bile acid stimulates gut motility or toxic effect on the gut causing meconium passage. The likelihood of meconium passage is more in preterm than in term obstetric cholestasis (25% compared with 12%). The pathophysiology of fetal death in ICP is poorly understood but may be related to the sudden development of a fetal arrhythmia or vasospasm of the placental chorionic surface vessels induced by high levels of bile acids.

Timing of Delivery

At present, there is no recommended specific method of antenatal fetal monitoring for the prediction of fetal death. Ultrasound and cardiotocography are not reliable methods for preventing fetal death in obstetric cholestasis.

Because of possible impact on perinatal outcome, delivery may be undertaken at term (37-38 weeks) or as soon as fetal lung maturity has been documented because of inability to predict stillbirth if the pregnancy continues. Poor fetal outcomes cannot currently be predicted by biochemical results and delivery decisions should not be based on it alone. Obstetricians should advise women regarding premature delivery, especially iatrogenic prematurity (4-12%). Continuous fetal monitoring in labor should be offered.

Maternal Risk

Cesarean section rates are high, ranging from 10 to 36% and there is an increased risk of postpartum hemorrhage (PPH).

Postnatal Management

Symptoms and liver profile changes usually disappear after delivery, but sometimes they continue. Bile acid and liver enzyme levels should be tested 6-8 weeks after delivery. If enzyme levels have not improved, other causes of cholestasis should be sought. Chronic pancreatitis (CP) has a high recurrence rate (40-90%) in subsequent pregnancies.

Drugs that cause cholestasis in susceptible individuals should be avoided, e.g., erythromycin, flucloxacillin, amoxicillin with clavulanic acid.

Intrahepatic cholestasis of pregnancy-affected women also have an increased risk of hepatobiliary disease later in life, most commonly gallstones, hepatobiliary malignancies and immune-mediated or metabolic syndrome at some point in their lifetime.

ACUTE FATTY LIVER OF PREGNANCY

Introduction

Acute fatty liver of pregnancy (AFLP) is a life-threatening obstetric emergency typically occurring during the last trimester of pregnancy, between 30 and 38 weeks although it can appear at early postpartum. It is characterized by microvesicular steatosis in the hepatocytes of zone 3 (centrilobular), rapid loss of liver function, jaundice, and coagulopathy requiring maternal supportive care. Delivery is necessary to assure maternal survival.

Acute fatty liver of pregnancy can be fatal for both mother and baby as without early recognition and appropriate management, can lead to acute liver failure and if diagnosis is delayed, to death of the fetus and the mother. Maternal mortality is 10–15%, and fetal mortality is up to 20%.

Risk Factors

Risk factors include the history of previous episodes of AFLP, multiple gestation, male fetal sex, the coexistence of other liver diseases during gestation (HELLP, preeclampsia), and a body mass index under 20 kg/m^2.

Incidence

Acute fatty liver of pregnancy is a rare disorder that occurs in about 1:7,000–1:15,000 pregnancies. A prospective population study conducted in the UK with a cohort of 1.1 million pregnancies estimated an incidence of 1:20,000 births. Acute fatty liver typically occurs in the third trimester between week 30 and 38, but sometimes it is not recognized until after delivery.

Pathophysiology

It is thought that AFLP is caused by inherited deficiencies of enzymes that are involved in the mitochondrial metabolism of fetal fatty acids. Impairment in fatty acid oxidation in the fetus and placenta can lead to an increase in the levels of intermediate products of metabolism that accumulate in the placenta and maternal blood, leading to maternal hepatotoxicity. The most investigated fatty acid oxidation defect that is thought to contribute to AFLP is deficiency in long-chain 3-hydroxyacyl-coenzymeA-dehydrogenase (LCHAD), which is a part of the mitochondrial trifunctional protein (MTP). G1528C and E474Q mutations of MTP are thought to be the cause of LCHAD deficiency and development of AFLP.

Approximately 20% of neonates born to mothers with AFLP have been shown to have defects in β-oxidation and deficient in LCHAD due to mutation on one or both alleles of the α-subunit of the trifunctional protein. Due to the genetic defect, affected fetuses do not metabolize long-chain fatty acids completely resulting in the accumulation of abnormal and highly toxic intermediates in the heterozygote mother's liver.

Fetal fatty acid oxidation disorders are inherited in an autosomal recessive way with both parents being heterozygotes. AFLP develops in mothers who are heterozygous for fetal fatty acid oxidation defects and pregnant with homozygous fetuses. A heterozygous mother has a reduced hepatic capacity to metabolize long-chain fatty acids. Although there is sufficient capacity in the nonpregnant state but during pregnancy liver has to metabolize fatty acids from the fetoplacental unit, in addition to its own, resulting in hepatotoxicity.

Mothers of neonates with LCHAD deficiency have been shown to have a 79% chance of developing AFLP or HELLP syndrome, both of which are multifactorial disorders that have a requirement to excrete pathologically high concentrations of β-fatty acid oxidation metabolites which is likely to unmask susceptibility to both disorders.

Symptoms

Initial symptoms of AFPL are generally nonspecific starting in the third trimester with 1-2 weeks of nausea, vomiting, abdominal pain, malaise, and anorexia; along with higher levels of transaminases and bilirubin in a short period of time, polyuria and polydipsia may also occur. It is often difficult to differentiate AFL from HELLP syndrome. Those with severe disease may develop disseminated intravascular coagulation (DIC).

Signs and *symptoms* of acute liver failure such as encephalopathy, jaundice, and coagulopathy may appear with rapid development of moderate to severe hypoglycemia. Approximately 50% of these patients present with preeclampsia, although hypertension is generally not severe.

Diagnosis

Biochemical abnormalities include aminotransferase elevations up to 20 times the upper limit of normal and hyperbilirubinemia. Proteinuria, a diagnostic feature of preeclampsia/eclampsia, can also occur. Coagulopathy with prolongation in prothrombin times can also present. Thus, the presentation of AFLP is often suggestive of liver dysfunction whereas the presentations of preeclampsia/eclampsia and HELLP syndrome are typically more suggestive of significant liver injury with less impact on hepatic synthetic function.

The definitive diagnostic method for AFLP is a liver biopsy. The characteristic histological finding is microvesicular fat infiltration, which affects the pericentral zone and respects the periportal zone **(Fig. 1)**. When a biopsy is performed at an early stage of the disease, the hepatocytes appear ballooned in the absence of large amounts of fat and giant mitochondria. At later stages, hepatocyte destruction can cause loss of the liver parenchyma and cellular atrophy. There is no adequate correlation between the degree of alterations found in laboratory tests and the severity of histological compromise.

Imaging modalities that help in diagnosis includes ultrasonography test (USG), magnetic resonance imaging (MRI) and computed tomography (CT) scan. Ultrasound and CT scan findings are inconsistent for detection of fatty infiltration, so diagnosis is usually based on clinical and laboratory findings. Liver biopsy is not typically required for diagnosis, and the associated coagulopathy of AFLP may preclude performance of liver biopsy. The Swansea criteria for diagnosis of AFLP are a proposal that includes symptoms, laboratory findings, and imaging. When at least six of 15 criteria are present, AFLP is likely. These criteria have demonstrated a sensitivity of 100% [95% class interval (CI): 77-100%], a specificity of 57% (95% CI: 20-88%), a positive predictive value of 85%, and a negative predictive value of 100%.

Swansea Criteria

- *Signs and symptoms:*
  - Vomiting, abdominal pain
  - Polydipsia/polyuria
  - Encephalopathy, ascites
- *Laboratory findings:*
  - Bilirubin >0.8 mg/dL
  - Hypoglycemia <72 mg/dL
  - Urea elevated >950 mg/dL
  - Leukocytosis >11 × 10^9/L
  - ALT >42 U/L
  - Ammonium >66 μmoL
  - Creatinine >1.7 mg/dL
  - PT coagulopathy >14s or PTT >34 seconds
- *Others:*
  - Ascites or "bright liver" found by ultrasound
  - *Biopsy:* Microvesicular steatosis

Liver enzymes should not be used as marker of severity as hepatocytes cannot release transaminase if they have been destroyed by severe injury. Disseminated intravascular coagulation with increased lactic dehydrogenase (LDH) is frequently observed. Potential complications include ascites, pleural effusion, acute pancreatitis, respiratory, and renal failure. Infections are common as in vaginal bleeding or bleeding from cesarean section wounds.

Management

As soon as the diagnosis of AFLP is confirmed, maternal stabilization should be followed by delivery regardless of the gestational age. Mother should be cared in an intensive care setting. Blood should be taken every 6 hours to ensure that biochemical and hematological abnormalities are diagnosed and corrected.

Monitor prothrombin time and other markers of coagulopathy, plasma glucose, platelets, creatinine, LFT and arterial blood gas.

- Glucose assessment every 2 hourly
- Tests for liver function (LF) and prothrombin time (PT)—6 hourly
- Renal function test, serum electrolytes, complete blood count (CBC)—6 hourly
- Level of consciousness hourly, all vital signs should be recorded.

Supportive Therapy

Hypoglycemia corrected with IV glucose, coagulopathy—fresh frozen plasma (FFP) should be given as required. Patients should be assessed for encephalopathy. Mild encephalopathy may manifest as confusion, unpleasant breath, and liver flap. In case of persistent deterioration and development of liver failure, liver transplantation should be considered. Encephalopathy with elevated blood lactate is associated with poor prognosis.

Plan Delivery

Once maternal condition is stable. There is no contraindication against vaginal delivery, although a small study published in 2010 showed a lower maternal mortality rate in the cesarean group than in the vaginal delivery group (16.2% vs. 48.1%). Initial recovery is observed in most patients after terminating pregnancy.

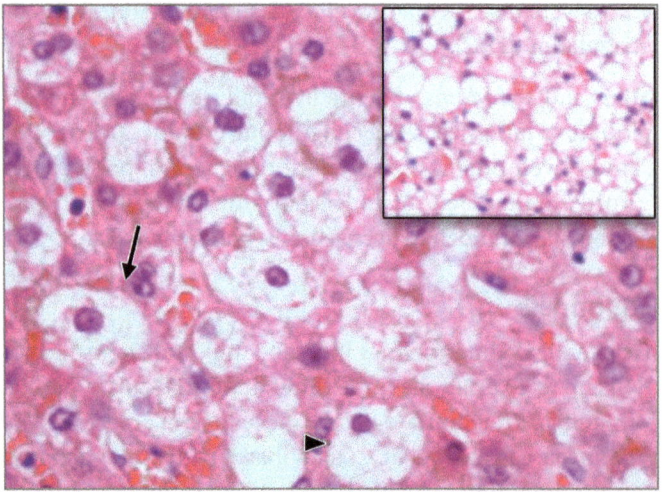

Fig. 1: Micro- and macrovesicular fat droplets with ballooned hepatocytes containing dense central nuclei. The periportal areas are often spared.
Source: Westbrook RH, Dusheiko G. Pregnancy and liver disease. Journal of Hepatology. 2016;64(4):933-45.

Postnatal Management

Acute fatty liver of pregnancy is usually reversible with complete liver function recovery and no sequelae. Monitoring in subsequent pregnancies is recommended since recurrence risk of 25% exists particularly in cases with defects of fatty acid-β-oxidation. The offspring of mothers affected by AFLP should be monitored carefully for manifestations of deficiency of LCHAD, including hypoketotic hypoglycemia and fatty liver. International recommendation suggests that all women with AFLP and their children should have molecular testing for LCHAD/TFP. Fetuses born to mothers with AFLP should be monitored for manifestations of deficiency of LCHAD as they are at risk of developing liver failure, cardiomyopathy, nonketotic hypoglycemia, myopathy, and neuropathy (American College of Gastroenterology, 2016).

LIVER DISEASE COINCIDENTALLY ARISING WITH PREGNANCY

Viral Hepatitis (Table 2)

Acute viral infections caused by hepatitides A, B, C, D, or E; herpes simplex, *Cytomegalovirus (CMV)* and Epstein–Barr virus—accounts for 40% of jaundice in pregnant women in the United States. Hepatitides A, B, and C have the same frequency in the pregnant and nonpregnant populations and during each of the three trimesters of pregnancy.

Most cases of acute viral hepatitis are subclinical and anicteric. Clinical presentation is similar in all with nausea, vomiting, headache, malaise, and subsequent development of jaundice. Viruses may not be hepatotoxic; however, the immunological response is the cause of hepatocellular necrosis. All cases of hepatitis A will recover completely, and so will most cases of hepatitis B. However, complete clinical and biochemical recovery will be seen only in a small proportion of cases of hepatitis C.

Viral hepatitis does not appear to affect the pregnant state adversely; an exception to this is hepatitis E, which in the third trimester of pregnancy may lead to fulminant liver failure and may carry a high mortality (up to 31.1%). Women with hepatitis E virus (HEV) infection during pregnancy have a higher risk of obstetric complications including antepartum hemorrhage, intrauterine fetal death and worse fetal outcomes including prematurity and stillbirth.

In general, the management of the pregnant patient with acute viral hepatitis is supportive, and viral hepatitis is not an indication for termination of pregnancy, performance of a cesarean section, or discouragement for breastfeeding. Early treatment with antiviral therapy such as acyclovir or vidarabine is life-saving; ribavirin use is precluded because of the teratogenic effects.

Hepatitis A

Introduction: Hepatitis A virus (HAV) is a small (27 nm) RNA virus that causes either symptomatic or asymptomatic infection in humans. Incidence during pregnancy is 1:1,000. Hepatitis A in pregnancy has a clinical course similar to the nonpregnant population and fulminant hepatitis is rare with hepatitis A virus.

Incubation period: The incubation period is 28 days (range, 15–50 days). Hepatitis A virus replicates within the liver and is excreted in the bile, with the highest viral concentrations in the stool late in the incubation period. This represents the window of greatest infectivity.

Transmission: The virus is transmitted from person to person through feco-oral contamination, facilitated by poor hygiene and poor sanitation through contaminated food and water. Intrauterine transmission of hepatitis A virus is rare; however, perinatal transmission could occur. The management of acute HAV in pregnancy does not differ from that used in nonpregnant patients.

Symptoms: Include malaise, headache, fatigue, anorexia, nausea, vomiting, and diarrhea. Cholestasis follows jaundice, acholic stool, and dark urine. LFTs—ALT higher than AST, level peaks prior to appearance of jaundice, may remain elevated over a month.

TABLE 2: Viral hepatitis with their mode of transmission, effect on pregnancy and management.

Type of virus	Mode of transmission	Effect on pregnancy	Management
Hepatitis A	Fecal oral	Perinatal transmission rare, acute infection associated with preterm labor and maternal complications	• Supportive care • Postexposure immunoglobulin safe, breastfeeding not contraindicated
Hepatitis B	Perinatal, sexual, parenteral	Acute infection can cause fetal neonatal hepatitis	• Supportive care • Active and passive immunization recommended, lamivudine can be given during second and third trimester, breastfeeding not contraindicated
Hepatitis C	Perinatal, sexual, parenteral	No effects on pregnancy and fetal outcome	Supportive care, breastfeeding appears to be safe
Hepatitis E	Fecal oral	Preterm labor and increased maternal mortality in third trimester	Supportive care, breastfeeding appears to be safe, no therapy to prevent transmission

Diagnosis: The detection of presence of hepatitis A IgM Antibody (anti-HAV IgM) in serum. Immunoglobulin M (IgM) antibody appears 1 month after exposure and may persist up to 6 months. Immunoglobulin G (IgG) appears 35–40 days after exposure and provides lifelong immunity. Presence of IgG antibody indicates post infection status and immunity, hepatitis A immunoglobulin G (Anti-HAV) IgG remain positive for years.

Management: Acute infection rarely requires more than general supportive care. Hepatitis A is a self-limiting disease without chronic process; recovery follows within 4–6 weeks. Although hepatitis A virus infection in pregnancy is not a major cause of maternal or neonatal morbidity, in utero infection has been associated with fetal meconium peritonitis, neonatal cholestasis, and preterm labor. It is, therefore, appropriate that women at increased risk of hepatitis A are vaccinated.

Vaccination: The safety of hepatitis A vaccination during pregnancy has not been determined; however, because hepatitis A vaccine is produced from an inactivated hepatitis A virus, the theoretical risk to the developing fetus is expected to be low. It is proposed that all pregnant women should be screened at delivery for anti-HAV antibodies and children born to anti-HAV–negative mothers should be vaccinated early during the first year of life, whereas vaccination may be postponed in children born to anti-HAV–positive mothers if necessary.

Hepatitis B

Introduction: Hepatitis B virus (HBV) infection is a significant public health problem worldwide and a major cause of chronic liver disease, cirrhosis, and hepatocellular carcinoma (HCC). HBV infection occurs worldwide; the areas of highest prevalence are China, Southeast Asia, sub-Saharan Africa, and Alaska. Prevalence of hepatitis B surface antigen (HBsAg) can exceed 8% in some areas. In the areas with intermediate prevalence such as Japan and India the seroprevalence is 3–5%. In low-prevalence areas, such as the United States, Western Europe, and Australia, the rate of HBsAg positivity is 0.1–2%. With this background, women at childbearing age and pregnant women living in the areas of high or intermediate prevalence would be at risk of getting the infection. Fortunately, since the implementation of universal vaccination in 1980s, together with public health measures to educate the general public on transmission risks, the number of cases of acute HBV infection has declined substantially in recent years. The incidence of acute HBV infection in the United States has declined from 11.5 cases per 100,000 population in 1985 to 1.5 per 100,000 population in 2007.

Clinical course: The *incubation period* is 6 weeks to 6 months. There is no difference with regard to mortality and incidence of fulminant hepatitis between pregnant women and nongravid women. Although many such patients may be asymptomatic, nausea, vomiting, jaundice, and abdominal pain can be seen, particularly in acute HBV infection. Ninety-five percent of acute infections in pregnant women spontaneously resolve, and the risk of liver failure is about 1%. If an infection occurs early in pregnancy, it can cause a miscarriage, but it usually resolves without consequences for the mother or the fetus.

Diagnosis: Hepatitis B virus (HBV) is a double-stranded deoxyribonucleic acid (DNA) virus having three structural antigen—(1) outer surface coat antigen [hepatitis B surface Ag (HBsAg)], (2) inner core protein [hepatitis B core antigen (HBc Ag)], and (3) hepatitis B e antigen (HBeAg). The core antigen is present only in the hepatocyte and does not circulate in the serum.

Hepatitis B surface Ag appearance is the first evidence of infection, appears 2–8 weeks before symptoms or biochemical evidence of liver disease. Detection of HBsAg implies infectivity and remains detectable until convalescent phase. Hepatitis B e antigen becomes detectable after HBsAg, indicates viral replication and infectivity, persistence beyond 6 m indicates likelihood of chronicity. The diagnosis of acute HBV infection requires detection of HBsAg and IgM Ab to HBcAg (IgM anti-HBc). Clinical recovery is accompanied by clearance of HBV DNA followed by HBeAg and HBsAg antigenemia within 1–3 months along with presence of IgG antibody to HBcAg and antibody to HBeAg. The presence of HBsAb may indicate recovery and immunity from HBV infection, or successful immunization against HBV.

Pregnancy with hepatitis B virus: Acute infection with HBV occurs in 1–2/1,000 pregnancies. In addition, 0.5–1.5% of pregnant women are carriers. In Bangladesh about 4–7% of populations are HBV infected and 3.5% of pregnant women have this virus. Pregnancy does not have a major effect on the liver disease in mothers with chronic hepatitis B, except in the context of cirrhosis; which is relatively uncommon in young childbearing women with HBV infection. Development of an acute HBV infection during pregnancy has been associated with gestational diabetes, increased postpartum hemorrhage, preterm delivery, and low birth weights.

Pregnant women should be tested for hepatitis B surface antigen (HBsAg) early in pregnancy regardless of previous testing or vaccination. All HBsAg-positive women should be tested for HBeAg, anti-HBe, and HBV DNA level, to identify pregnancies at increased risk. Blood clotting profile should be checked for once at least during acute HBV infection, and to be repeated if there is coagulopathy or hepatitis is getting worse. Vitamin K should be given if international normalized ratio (INR) >1.5, while FFP is reserved for patients who have clinical bleeding or before invasive procedures (including delivery). Short-term use (7 days or shorter) of corticosteroid in case of preterm labor/delivery, is generally very safe; yet if prolonged corticosteroid is anticipated, tenofovir disoproxil fumarate (TDF) would prevent HBV reactivation in the pregnant women.

Mother-to-child transmission: Mother-to-child transmission (MTCT) and early childhood acquisition of HBV infection are modes of transmission in 50% of persons worldwide who develop chronic HBV infection. The presence of HBeAg positivity and levels of hepatitis B viremia are the two most significant maternal risk factors for MTCT. High viral load being associated to 80–90% risk of transmission compared to 10–30% transmission rates in patients with undetectable viral load. Transmission can occur directly via the placenta, during breastfeeding, or during delivery through infected maternal secretions and blood. Vertical transmission occurs in 70–90% cases if mother is positive for both HBsAg and HBeAg, which becomes 10% if mother is HBsAg positive but HBeAg negative. The risk of MTCT is also dependent on the timing of the exposure and highest in the third trimester of pregnancy. Although there is a 10% likelihood of transmission to the newborn if maternal infection occurs in the first trimester, the risk of HBV transmission is as high as 60% if exposure occurs in the third trimester. Maternal transmission leads to more severe morbidity and mortality than horizontal transmission because chronic infection, which lasts for decades, develops in approximately 95% of those who acquire HBV in neonatal period.

Timely immune-prophylaxis with hepatitis B immuno-globulin (HBIG) and vaccine after birth prevents approximately 90% of mother-to-infant transmission. However, despite immune-prophylaxis, a small proportion of infants are still infected. The causes of immunoprophylactic failure include—(1) intrauterine infection, which cannot be prevented by immune prophylaxis after birth, (2) breakthrough infection occurring at perinatal period (because of high maternal viral load), and (3) rarely postnatal infection, occurring in a small number of children who have inadequate antibody response to neonatal immune prophylaxis.

Management: The goals of treatment in pregnancy are to maintain stable liver function in the mother and to prevent neonatal infection. Levels of aminotransferases should be regularly evaluated during pregnancy.

To reduce transmission, many professional organization guidelines recommend highly viremic pregnant women with stable HBV disease activity to receive short-term antiviral therapy starting between 28th and 32nd week of pregnancy since organogenesis is complete but there is still enough time to reduce HBV DNA levels significantly. Medications should be continued up to 12 weeks after delivery due to the possibility of exacerbation of HBV, particularly in patients who are HBeAg positive, whose risk is 2.56 times higher than patients who are negative. American Association for the Study of Liver Diseases (AASLD) guidance on hepatitis B recommends antiviral therapy for mothers with HBV DNA levels of greater than 200,000 IU/mL. Immunoprophylaxis has been shown to significantly reduce the rate of MTCT of HBV infection. In patients with chronic hepatitis B carrier status but HBeAg negative and with viral loads of 200,000 IU/mL or less, antiviral prophylaxis is not indicated. If an adequate immune prophylaxis is offered, the perinatal transmission rate falls to 2%.

Three available antiviral drugs whose fetal safety profile is adequate are: (1) lamivudine, (2) telbivudine, and (3) tenofovir. Lamivudine use has been falling due to resistance rates which can be as high as 70% over 5 years. This limits future maternal treatment options since use for even a short period promotes resistant viral variants in 20% of cases. Tenofovir has been suggested as the first line nucleoside analogue in pregnancy by the Society for Maternal-Fetal Medicine. It should be administered orally in doses of 300 mg/day. It is the most potent nucleoside analog, has the lowest resistance rates and extensive safety data are available for use during pregnancy. Most studies of antiviral therapy during pregnancy to prevent mother-to-infant HBV transmission reported short-term outcomes no longer than 1 year after delivery. A systematic review and meta-analysis of antiviral therapy in pregnant HBV-infected women concluded that the use of lamivudine, telbivudine, and TDF is safe in pregnancy with no increased adverse maternal complications such as postpartum hemorrhage, cesarean section, and elevated creatinine kinase rates, and with no increased adverse fetal outcomes such as congenital malformation and prematurity rates.

Delivery: Mode of delivery should be decided by obstetric indications and cesarean section is not recommended for the sole indication for reduction of vertical transmission. Elective cesarean delivery may have a potential role to reduce transmission in highly viremic mothers. However, elective cesarean delivery is not recommended solely for HBV prevention, according to the practice guidelines from leading professional organizations. All hepatitis B positive women should be monitored closely during pregnancy and in the postpartum period for exacerbations of disease. The risk of flares in serum aminotransferases is somewhat raised during pregnancy and postpartum but deaths fortunately are rare.

Prevention of neonatal infection (Fig. 2): Infection of infants born to HBsAg positive mothers, or of children early in life confers a high risk of chronic infection. World Health Organization (WHO) published the first global health sector strategy on viral hepatitis in June 2016; a

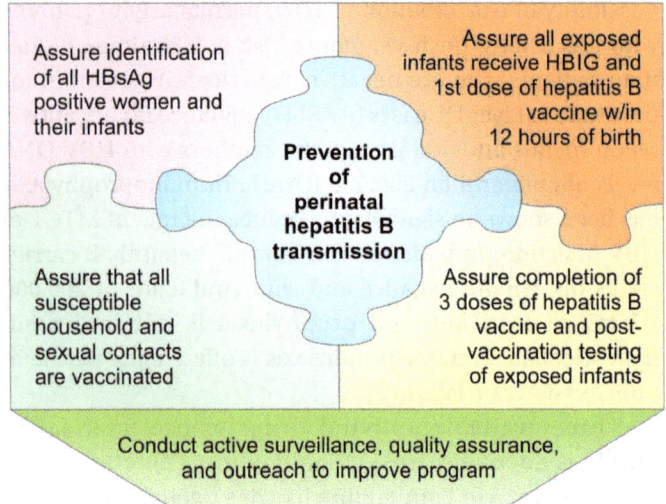

Fig. 2: Six responsibilities of perinatal hepatitis B prevention program. (HBIG: hepatitis B immunoglobulin)
Source: Slide serve. Pat Fineis: "Perinatal hepatitis B prevention Programme".

strategy that contributes to the proposed targets for the reduction of chronic viral hepatitis incidence and mortality by 2030. WHO recommends universal vaccination of all infants against HBV. All infants born to HBsAg positive mothers should receive hepatitis B vaccine and HBIG as soon as possible after birth. Hepatitis B immune globulin is recommended immediately after birth and hepatitis B vaccine within 12 hours of birth. Three doses of HBV vaccine series should be completed according to recommended schedules. Infants who received HBIG and the first dose of hepatitis B vaccine at birth can be breastfed. Completion of HBV vaccine is important for the newborn to gain maximal protection and consists of the birth dose followed by two subsequent doses. Neonatal immune prophylaxis is effective in preventing 85–95% HBV infection. Centers for Disease Control and Prevention (CDC) recommends testing of infants HBsAg and HBsAb at 12 months to ensure presence of antibody. Approximately 25% of infected infants will become chronic carriers.

Hepatitis C

Introduction: Hepatitis C virus (HCV) infection constitutes one of the leading causes of chronic liver disease worldwide. The natural history of this entity varies greatly from minimal histological changes to cirrhosis, with or without hepatocellular carcinoma. Worldwide, there are approximately 71 million people who have chronic HCV infections. Estimated 1–8% of pregnant women have HCV.

Screening: There is no universal consensus on screening for HCV during pregnancy. Society for Maternal-Fetal Medicine (SMFM) recommends HCV screening in the first visit for mothers who are at an increased risk. The American College of Obstetricians and Gynecologists and the Centers for Disease Control and Prevention also recommends screening for women with risk factors.

Recommendations for prenatal HCV screening:
- Illegal drug injections (current or past, even those who injected only once)
- Intranasal illicit drug use
- Hemodialysis use
- History of piercing or tattoos in an unregulated environment
- HIV or HBV infection
- Recipients of transfusions or transplants before 1992 or clotting factors before 1987
- Background of incarceration
- In-vitro fertilization with anonymous donors
- Sexual partners of people with HIV, HBV, or HCV
- Women with unexplained chronic liver disease (including persistently elevated ALT)

Diagnosis of maternal infection:
- HCV Ab +ve, by third generation enzyme immunoassays (EIAs).
- *Chronic HCV:* HCV Ab +ve and HCV RNA positive (lower limit of detection of 50 units/mL or less)
- *Chronic active HCV:* HCV Ab +ve and HCV RNA positive with abnormal LFT.

Perinatal transmission: A 2014 meta-analysis reported vertical transmission rates of 5.8% in viremic women and 10.8% for those who were coinfected with HIV. Transmission occurs almost exclusively from mothers who are HCV ribonucleic acid (RNA)-positive, and risk correlates with the mother's viral load titers. Transmission is four times higher for patients with 6 log copies/mL than for those who have lower viral loads (14.3% vs. 3.9%).

Transmission of infection from mother to child can occur during three different periods. *Intrauterine transmission* is defined by HCV RNA in the serum of the newborn within the first 3 days of life. It accounts for 30–40% of cases. Among the proposed mechanisms are the passage of viral particles from mother to fetus, maternal-fetal flow of infected mononuclear cells, and infection of trophoblasts. *Peripartum transmission* is defined by a finding of HCV RNA in the serum of a newborn within the first 28 days after birth. This is the most important period in vertical transmission (60% of cases). It correlates with exposure to maternal blood. The main risk factors are invasive obstetric procedures as well as lacerations of the vaginal or perineal mucosa during vaginal delivery and prolonged rupture of the membranes. *Postpartum transmission* is rare and is attributed to breast feeding. However, despite the fact that HCV RNA is detectable in human colostrum, breastfeeding is not considered a risk factor for MTCT.

Treatment: There are no adequate human data for the use of second-generation direct acting antivirals during pregnancy, but data obtained from animal studies demonstrate that they do not confer risk to the fetus. Due to the lack of human studies, no direct acting antiviral therapy has yet been approved for treating HCV infections during pregnancy. The use of interferon and ribavirin is contraindicated in pregnancy due to teratogenic effects.

Obstetric outcomes: Most HCV infected pregnant women are carriers of chronic asymptomatic infection and maternal outcomes are similar to patients who are not pregnant. However, there are conflicting data about obstetrical outcomes. Although some data have suggested that HCV infection does not affect obstetrical outcomes, other data have indicated associations of HCV infection with gestational diabetes, preterm delivery, low birth weight, requirements for neonatal intensive care, and the presence of ICP.

No evidence that cesarean section decreases transmission of HCV and recommended that fetal scalp monitoring is avoided due to reports of an increased risk of HCV transmission with this mode of monitoring. Breastfeeding is not contraindicated except in cases of cracked or bleeding nipples.

Hepatitis E

Background: Hepatitis E is an inflammation of the liver caused by infection with the HEV. Every year there are an estimated 20 million HEV infections worldwide, leading to an estimated 3.3 million symptomatic cases of hepatitis E and 60,000 deaths worldwide. WHO estimates that hepatitis E caused approximately 44,000 deaths in 2015 (accounting for 3.3% of the mortality due to viral hepatitis). Hepatitis E is found worldwide, most common in East and South Asia. The disease is common in low- and middle-income countries with limited access to essential water, sanitation, hygiene and health services. In these areas, the disease occurs both as outbreaks and as sporadic cases.

The epidemiologic features of HEV are similar to those of hepatitis A. Hepatitis E virus is a single-stranded RNA virus with 4 genotypes, genotype 1 and 2 infect human. Transmission is through fecal-oral route, principally via contaminated water. The virus is shed in the stools of infected persons, occasionally leading to fulminant hepatitis (acute liver failure) which can be fatal.

Hepatitis E in pregnancy

Clinical course: Acute viral hepatitis with hepatitis E is the most common cause of jaundice in pregnancy worldwide. *Incubation period* ranges from 2 to 10 weeks, with an average of 5 to 6 weeks. The infection is usually self-limiting and resolves within 2–6 weeks.

The clinical manifestations of HEV infection are varying from asymptomatic to fulminant hepatic failure. HEV usually causes an acute self-limiting hepatitis. The prodromal phase lasts up to 1 week, and the symptoms may be nonspecific, such as malaise, fever, joint pain, nausea, and vomiting. Subsequently, a series of typical symptoms related to acute icteric hepatitis, including jaundice, darkened urine, and pale stools may occur, similar to those seen in HAV infection. The jaundice of acute HEV infection is likely much less in severity. Serum alanine aminotransferase (ALT) and aspartate aminotransferase (AST) levels are markedly elevated. In immunocompetent individuals, the infection and symptoms typically resolve spontaneously within 4–6 weeks. Compared to nonpregnant women, clinical features do not differ in pregnant women initially; however, acute liver failure can develop rapidly in patients with HEV infection during pregnancy.

Pregnant women with hepatitis E infection in the second or third trimester, particularly with genotype 1 is associated with more severe infection and might lead to fulminant hepatic failure and maternal death. Although the mechanism of liver injury is not yet clear, it is possible that interplay of hormonal and immunologic changes during pregnancy, along with a high viral load of HEV, renders the woman more vulnerable.

Several clinical studies and case reports from developing countries have shown there is a well described but unexplained increased mortality as high as 50%, ranging from 20 to 25% from acute hepatitis E in pregnant women. Hepatic encephalopathy is the most common cause of death among these patients. Several complications of fulminant hepatic failure, including cerebral edema, DIC, and encephalopathy are seen in 70% of HEV infected pregnant women. Additionally, HEV infection in pregnancy is also associated with high rates of preterm labor, vertical transmission of infection, low birth weight, stillbirth and neonatal death.

Although the mechanism of liver injury is not yet clear, possible explanations for the severe course in pregnant women with HEV infection are hormonal, genetic and immunological changes that render the woman more vulnerable **(Fig. 3)**. It has been suggested that a reduced expression of the progesterone receptor or a mutation of the human methylenetetrahydrofolate reductase (*MTHFR*) gene might be associated with development of fulminant hepatitis E in pregnant women.

Diagnosis: Definitive diagnosis of hepatitis E infection is usually based on the detection of specific anti-HEV immunoglobulin M (IgM) antibodies to the virus in a person's blood; this is usually adequate in areas where the disease is common. IgM anti-HEV antibodies develop nearly 4 weeks after the infection and can be detected in

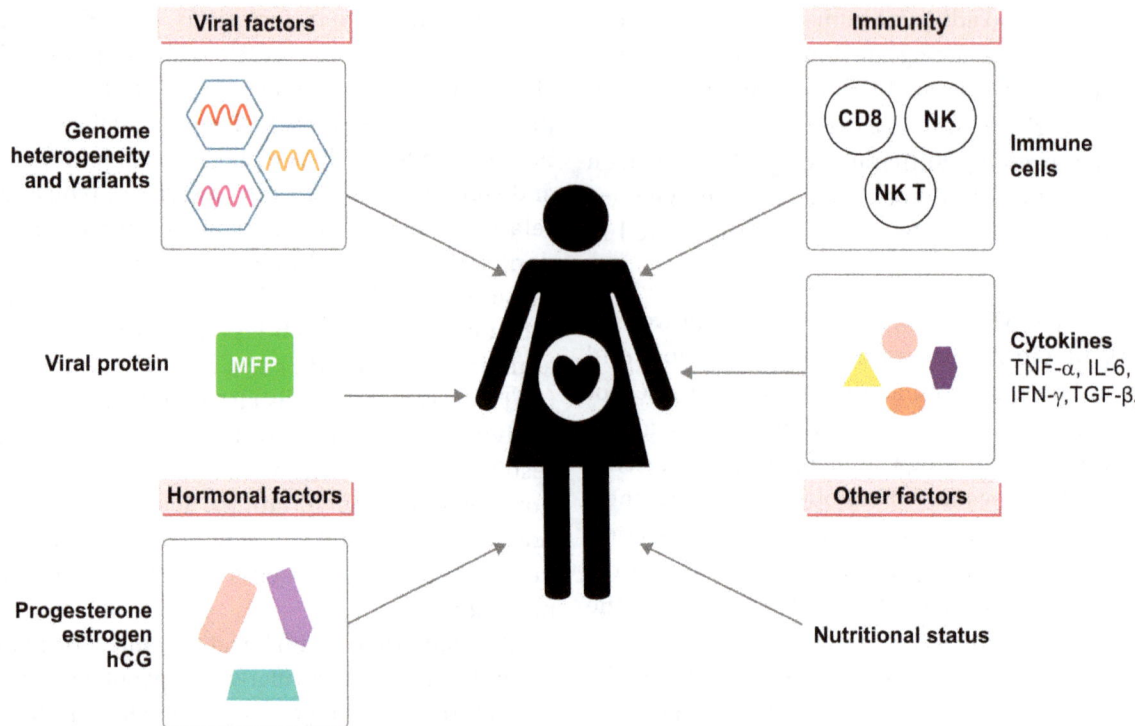

Fig. 3: Mechanisms underlying severe liver injury due to hepatitis E virus (HEV) infection in pregnancy.
(The altered status of immunity, hormone levels and viral factors may be related to the severity of the disease. Viral factors include HEV genome heterogeneity and variants, as well as viral proteins, such as multifunctional protein (MFP), encoded by HEV ORF3, may be associated with the severity of the disease. Host immune factors, such as CD8+ T-cells, NK and NKT cells, may be involved in the pathogenicity of HEV during pregnancy. In addition, some cytokines, such as TNF-α, IL-6, IFN-γ, and TGF-β1, may also be involved in this process. The dramatically elevated levels of hormonal factors, including progesterone, estrogen and human chorionic gonadotropin (hCG) play a considerable role in altering immune regulation in pregnancy may also contribute to liver injury. Other host factors, such as nutritional status, may also influence the severity of HEV infection in pregnant wo men)
Source: Chunchen Wu, Xiaoxue Wu. Hepatitis E virus infection during pregnancy. Virology. 2020;17:73.

the sera for nearly 6 months, hence indicating an acute or recent infection from HEV. IgG antibodies usually also develop simultaneously with IgM antibodies early after the infection and last for years, indicating either a recent or a past infection. HEV RNA in blood or stool is the gold standard for the detection of HEV infection. It becomes detectable even before the patient becomes clinically symptomatic and may persist for nearly 4 weeks in the blood and 6 weeks in the feces.

Fetal and neonatal outcomes: There is a very high risk of vertical transmission of HEV from the mother to the fetus. Maternal–fetal transmission of hepatitis E virus ranges between 33.3 and 50%. HEV infection in animal experimental model has demonstrated vertical transmission with replication of HEV in the placenta, perhaps explaining the adverse pregnancy outcomes. During an epidemic in Delhi, a hospital-based study revealed that HEV infection during pregnancy was associated with miscarriage, stillbirth, or neonatal death in 56% of infants. One recent study highlights that HEV infection might be responsible for 2,400–3,000 stillbirths each year in developing countries, with many additional fetal deaths linked to antenatal maternal deaths. There is a very high risk of preterm delivery in pregnant women with HEV infection, with poor neonatal survival rates. In two separate studies from India, 15–50% of live-born infants of mothers with HEV infection died within 1 week of birth.

Management: Management is supportive, there is no specific treatment capable of altering the course of acute hepatitis E as the disease is usually self-limiting, and no vaccine is available. Immunosuppressed people with chronic hepatitis E benefit from specific treatment using ribavirin, an antiviral drug. In some specific situations, interferon has also been used successfully. Use of ribavirin and IFNα is precluded in pregnancy because of the high risks of teratogenicity.

Currently, there is no evidence of any therapeutic benefit of termination of pregnancy in HEV induced ALF. European Association for the Study of Liver (EASL) recommends treatment of HEV genotypes 1 and 2 infections during pregnancy in high-dependency units and prompt transfer to Liver Transplant Unit if liver failure develops.

Breastfeeding is considered safe in asymptomatic women infected with HEV despite the presence of anti-HEV antibodies and HEV RNA in the colostrum. However, it is considered unsafe if the mother has acute hepatic disease or an increased viral load. In these cases, feeding formula is advised, as there is a possibility of transmission from infected breast milk or lesions on the nipple through suckling. At the present time, it is important to continue breastfeeding during epidemics of HEV in underdeveloped and endemic areas to prevent a greater risk of infant mortality from other infectious diseases.

Prevention: Currently, there is no commercially available HEV vaccine. Hepatitis E vaccine using recombinant capsid protein has been shown in phase 2 and 3 clinical trials to be safe and effective in the general adult population. The recombinant hepatitis E vaccine, the first prophylactic vaccine against HEV infection, was approved in China in December 2011. Since HEV infection is water and foodborne, women traveling to HEV-endemic countries should strictly follow food and water precautions, such as drinking only bottled water, not adding ice cubes to beverages, avoiding unpeeled fruits and vegetables, and washing hands, fruits, and vegetables thoroughly with safe water before eating. Immunosuppressed and chronic liver disease patients are advised to refrain from eating raw, undercooked meat and shellfish. It has been recommended to cook meat thoroughly at temperatures of 70°C and above before consumption.

Management guidelines for severe hepatitis:
- Protect the liver
- Prevention of encephalopathy
- Prevention of DIC
- Prevention of hepatorenal syndrome.

Hepatic Encephalopathy

Hepatic encephalopathy is the occurrence of *confusion, altered level of consciousness, and coma as a result of* liver failure. It is caused by accumulation in the bloodstream of toxic substances such as ammonia that are normally removed by the liver. Toxins build up in the bloodstream and potentially get into the brain. The diagnosis is typically based on the symptoms after ruling out other potential causes. It may be supported by blood ammonia levels, an electroencephalogram, or a CT scan of the brain.

Hepatic encephalopathy may be triggered by infections such as pneumonia, constipation, use of medications (such as barbiturates or benzodiazepine tranquilizers) that suppress the central nervous system, electrolyte imbalance, especially a decrease in potassium after vomiting or taking diuretics.

Pathogenesis: Hepatic encephalopathy or portosystemic encephalopathy (PSE) is a reversible syndrome of impaired brain function occurring in patients with advanced liver failure. In healthy subjects, nitrogen-containing compounds from the intestine, generated by gut bacteria from food, are transported by the portal vein to the liver, where 80–90% are *metabolized* through the urea cycle and/or excreted immediately. This process is impaired in all subtypes of hepatic encephalopathy, either because the hepatocytes are incapable of *metabolizing* the waste products or because portal venous blood bypasses the liver through collateral circulation; Nitrogenous waste products accumulate in the systemic circulation. The most important waste product is ammonia (NH_3). This small molecule crosses the blood–brain barrier and is absorbed and *metabolized* by the astrocytes, a population of cells in the brain that constitutes 30% of the cerebral cortex. Astrocytes use ammonia when synthesizing glutamine from glutamate. The increased levels of glutamine lead to an increase in osmotic pressure in the astrocytes, which become swollen. There is increased activity of the inhibitory γ-aminobutyric acid (GABA) system, and the energy supply to other brain cells is decreased. This can be thought of as an example of brain edema of the "cytotoxic" type.

Treatment: Hepatic encephalopathy is possibly reversible with treatment. This typically involves supportive care and addressing the triggers of the event. Lactulose is frequently used to decrease ammonia levels. Certain antibiotics (such as rifaximin) and probiotics are other potential options. A liver transplant may improve outcomes in those with severe disease.

SUGGESTED READING

1. Brady CW. Liver Disease in Pregnancy: What's New. AASLD. 2020;4(2):137-324.
2. Chaudhry SA, Verma N, Koren G. Hepatitis E infection during pregnancy. Can Fam Physician. 2015;61(7):607-8.
3. García-Romero CS, Guzman C, Cervantes A, Cerbón M. Liver disease in pregnancy: Medical aspects and their implications for mother and child. Ann Hepatol. 2019;18(4):553-62.
4. Joueidi Y, Peoc'h K, Le Lous M, Bouzille G, Rousseau C, Bardou-Jacquet E, et al. Maternal and neonatal outcomes and prognostic factors in acute fatty liver of pregnancy. Eur J Obstet Gynecol Reprod Biol. 2020;252:198-205.
5. Kar P, Karna R. A Review of the Diagnosis and Management of Hepatitis E. Curr Treat Options Infect Dis. 2020;12:310-20.
6. Lee RH, Chung RT, Pringle P. In: Resnik R, Creasy RK, Iams JD, Moore T, Greene MFLockwood CL (Eds). Diseases of the Liver, Biliary System and Pancreas. Creasy & Resnik's Maternal Fetal Medicine, 8th edition. Philadelphia: Elsevier; 2019.
7. Nelson DB, Yost NP, Cunningham FG. Acute fatty liver of pregnancy: clinical outcomes and expected duration of recovery. Am J Obstet Gynecol. 2013;209(5):456.e1-7.

8. Rector RS, Ibdah JA. Fatty acid oxidation disorders: maternal health and neonatal outcomes. Semin Fetal Neonatal Med. 2010;15(3):122-8.
9. Royal College of Obstetricians and Gynaecologists. (2011). Obstetric Cholestasis (Green-top Guideline No. 43). [online] Available from https://www.rcog.org.uk/guidance/browse-all-guidance/green-top-guidelines/obstetric-cholestasis-green-top-guideline-no-43/. [Last accessed April, 2022].
10. Toro LG, Correa EM, Calle LF, Ocampo A, Vélez SM. Liver diseases and pregnancy. Rev Col Gastroenterol. 2019;34(4).
11. Tran TT, Ahn J, Reau NS. ACG Clinical Guideline: Liver Disease and Pregnancy. Am J Gastroenterol. 2016;111(2):176-94.
12. UpToDate. (2021). Acute fatty liver of pregnancy (Lee RH, Reau N). [online] Available from https://www.uptodate.com/contents/acute-fatty-liver-of-pregnancy#:~:text=Acute%20fatty%20liver%20of%20pregnancy%20(AFLP)%20is%20an%20obstetric%20emergency,full%20recovery%20for%20the%20mother [Last accessed April, 2022].
13. UpToDate. (2021). Intrahepatic cholestasis of pregnancy (Lindor KD, Lee RH). [online] Available from https://www.uptodate.com/contents/intrahepatic-cholestasis-of-pregnancy. [Last accessed April, 2022].
14. Westbrook RH, Dusheiko G, Williamson C. Pregnancy and liver disease. J Hepatol. 2016;64(4):933-45.
15. Wong GL, Wen WH, Pan CQ. Hepatitis B-management of acute infection and active inflammation in pregnancy-a hepatologist's perspective. Best Pract Res Clin Obstet Gynaecol. 2020;68:54-65.
16. World Health Organization. (2021). Hepatitis E. [online] Available from https://www.who.int/news-room/fact-sheets/detail/hepatitis-e. [Last accessed April, 2022].
17. Wu C, Wu X, Xia J. Hepatitis E virus infection during pregnancy. Virol J. 2020;17(1):73.

CHAPTER 10

Coagulation Disorders in Pregnancy

INTRODUCTION

The process of hemostasis is a dynamic and delicate equilibrium between coagulation and fibrinolysis **(Figs. 1A and B)**. Coagulation results from an interaction among vessel walls, platelets, and coagulation factors. Following endothelial damage, platelets adhere to the subendothelium forming a platelet plug which then becomes permanent with fibrin deposition. Clot formation is limited by antithrombin (AT) and proteins C and S. The fibrinolytic system functions to maintain the fluid state of blood through the breakdown of fibrin by plasmin. Plasmin is generated from plasminogen by the action of tissue plasminogen activator (t-PA). The mechanism of hemostasis is complex and is further complicated by the physiological changes of pregnancy, such as physiological anemia and fluctuating coagulation factor concentrations, which alter the balance between bleeding and clot formation in preparation for peripartum blood loss.

Coagulopathies in pregnancy can present with or lead to obstetric emergencies and vary from prothrombotic/microangiopathic events such as HELLP syndrome (Hemolysis Elevated Liver Enzymes Low Platelets), thrombotic thrombocytopenia purpura (TTP), and other microangiopathies, especially disseminated intravascular coagulopathy (DIC), to deep venous thrombosis (DVT) and recurrent pregnancy losses. Coagulopathy can result from massive stored blood transfusion following bleeding events such as antepartum and postpartum hemorrhage (PPH). Patients who present with bleeding disorders should be treated by a multidisciplinary team consisting

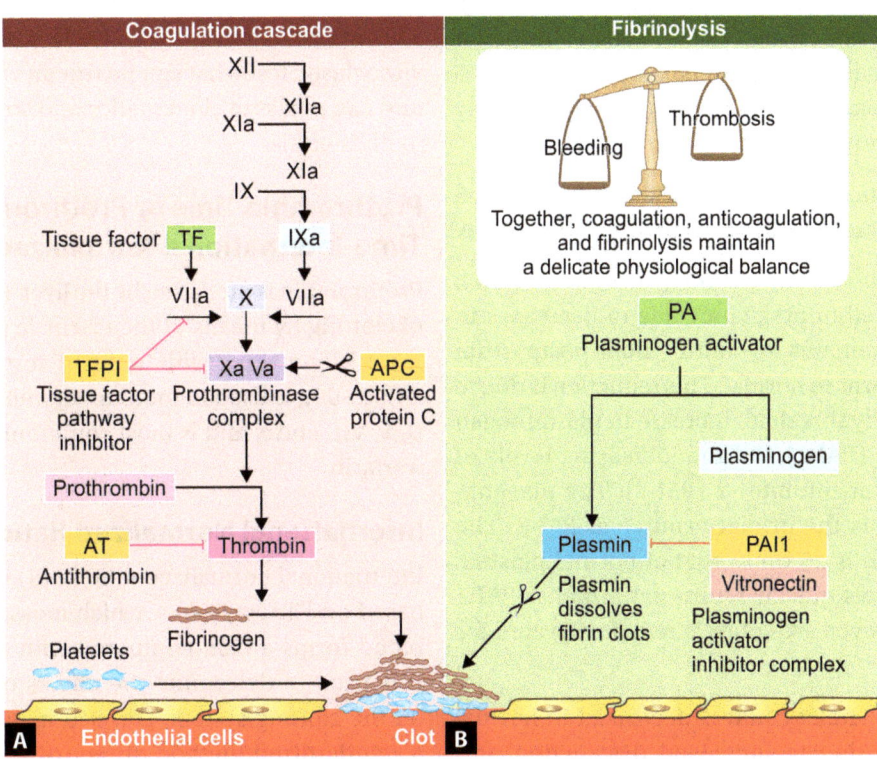

Figs. 1A and B: (A) Coagulation cascade; (B) Fibrinolysis.

of an obstetrician, anesthetist, hematologist, and support personnel (such as a hemophilia nurse to aid in dispensing of medication and neonatologists to care for the potentially affected neonate) when indicated. With proper planning and care delivered by an experienced knowledgeable team, the majority of women can carry a pregnancy to term and safely deliver a healthy neonate.

PHYSIOLOGICAL CHANGES TO COAGULATION DURING PREGNANCY

The coagulation system undergoes significant changes during pregnancy; physiological changes in pregnancy affect the coagulation and fibrinolytic systems, including an increase in the majority of clotting factors, a decrease in the quantity of natural anticoagulants, and a reduction in fibrinolytic activity. These changes result in a state of hypercoagulability, are likely due to hormonal change, and thus increase the risk of thromboembolism. Preexisting coagulopathies may affect the course of pregnancy and the nature of coagulopathy may also be modified by pregnancy. The increase in clotting activity is greatest at the time of delivery with placental expulsion, releasing thromboplastic substances. This substance stimulates clot formation to stop maternal blood loss. Coagulation and fibrinolysis generally return to prepregnant levels 3–4 weeks postpartum.

EFFECTS OF PREGNANCY ON THE CLOTTING SYSTEM

Increase of clotting factors: There is an increase of factors VIII, VII, X, XII, fibrinogen, and von Willebrand factor (vWF), while factors II, V, IX, and XI are stable. Levels of factor VII (FVII) increase gradually during pregnancy (up to 1,000% increase), and fibrinogen also increases during pregnancy with levels reaching very high levels (up to 100%) by term.

Reduction of coagulation inhibitors: Reduction in protein S (up to 50% decrease) and AT while protein C remains stable.

Reduction of fibrinolysis inhibition (hypofibrinolysis): Fibrinolysis is reduced in pregnancy due to decreases in t-PA activity, which remains low until 1-hour postpartum when the activity returns to normal. This reduction is due to the gradual, eventually threefold, increase in plasminogen activator inhibitor-1 (PAI-1) and the increasing levels of plasminogen activator inhibitor-2 (PAI-2). The placenta produces PAI-1 and is the primary source of PAI-2. The level of PAI-2 at term is 25 times that of normal plasma. Postpartum, t-PA levels quickly return to normal as PAI-1 levels decrease; however, PAI-2 levels remain elevated for a few days.

Effects on platelets: Platelet count is decreased in normal pregnancy possibly due to increased destruction and hemodilution with a maximal decrease in the third trimester.

ASSESSMENT OF COAGULATION DISORDERS

A coagulation test measures blood's capability to clot and if it clots how long it takes to clot. Although a thorough bleeding history is likely to be the best screening tool for global coagulation function, laboratory assessment is often sought to confirm or diagnose potential disorders. Currently, routine screening for coagulation deficits is not recommended in the face of a negative bleeding history owing to the low prevalence of inherited coagulation disorders.

Parturients who present with known disorders or bleeding history (mucocutaneous bleeding or menorrhagia) are at an increased risk of bleeding complications during pregnancy and childbirth. Investigation for coagulation disorders is also warranted in patients with a history of PPH without other known causes. Simple laboratory tests such as a global coagulation panel including a complete blood count (CBC), prothrombin time (PT), partial thromboplastin time/partial thromboplastin time with kaolin (PTT/PTTK), and plasma fibrinogen could predict a coagulopathy. A prolonged PT could suggest an underlying liver disease or FVII deficiency, a prolonged activated partial thromboplastin time (aPTT)/PTTK could suggest deficiency of the intrinsic pathway (factors XII, XI, IX, VIII), and a prolongation of both could suggest a defect in the global coagulation system, especially DIC or coagulopathy of PPH or of massive transfusion. A short (less than the control) value of the coagulation tests (PT, aPTT/ PTTK) may actually warn us of a prothrombotic state such as preeclampsia (PE) or early DIC in a given clinical situation. Thromboelastography (TEG®) and ROTEM® are two viscoelastic tests that can be run on whole or citrated blood and can measure clot kinetics and strength from formation to fibrinolysis.

Prothrombin Time or Prothrombin Time-International Normalized Ratio

Prothrombin is produced by the liver. PT measures the speed of clotting by means of the extrinsic pathway. Usually, this test is done along with an aPTT test. Specifically, PT and INR testing is used to monitor vitamin K–dependent factors II, V, VII, and X and is most commonly used for patients on warfarin.

International Normalized Ratio

International normalized ratio (INR) is a type of calculation based on PT test results, which measures how quickly your blood forms a clot, compared with normal clotting time. It is used to determine the effects of oral anticoagulants on the clotting system. Devised in 1983, the INR provides a standardized method of reporting the effects of an oral anticoagulant such as warfarin on blood clotting. A normal

INR is 1.0. Each increase of 0.1 means the blood is slightly thinner (it takes longer to clot).

Partial Thromboplastin Time

Partial thromboplastin time measures the overall speed at which blood clots by means of two consecutive series of biochemical reactions known as the intrinsic pathway and common pathway of coagulation. Testing of aPTT was designed to assess factors VIII, IX, and XI for patients either with factor deficiency or on heparin therapy. As such, they are poor tests to assess clinical coagulopathy, especially in the bleeding patient.

Thrombin Time

Thrombin time, also known as the thrombin clotting time (TCT), measures the time it takes for a clot to form in the plasma of a blood sample containing anticoagulant, after an excess of thrombin has been added. If the time it takes for the plasma to clot is prolonged, a quantitative (fibrinogen deficiency) or qualitative (dysfunctional fibrinogen) defect is present. The test may be used to help diagnose problems such as inherited conditions that lead to low fibrinogen or fibrinogen disorders; liver diseases such as cirrhosis, hepatitis, and liver cancer; and other conditions, e.g., lupus and DIC. Use of heparin and warfarin can also lead to a longer thrombin time.

Bleeding Time

Bleeding time analyzes how soon small blood vessels in the skin close and stop bleeding.

Thromboelastogram

Thromboelastogram (TEG) is a simple bedside test with a fast turnaround time that may identify and guide appropriate component therapy in case of bleeding, especially in a patient with PPH or postoperative state where the physician/obstetrician would like to differentiate between a coagulopathy and a local surgical cause for bleeding. TEG provides information about the various stages of coagulation and fibrinolysis. The maximum amplitude (MA) is thought to represent platelet function. TEG is used by some centers to predict the risk of bleeding from coagulation abnormalities; however, the sensitivity and specificity of TEG in pregnancy remain unproven. An abnormal test has not been shown to be predictive for the development of a neuraxial hematoma, but most anesthetists will not provide regional anesthesia if the MA is abnormal.

Platelet Function Analyzer

Platelet function analyzer (PFA) measures the speed of formation of a platelet plug in vitro, expressed as closure time in seconds. Studies in parturients suggest that it is an effective bedside test of platelet function; however, evidence is lacking to support its routine use.

More common tests of blood coagulation include PT (INR) and PTT (aPTT) which measure coagulation factor function; TEG can assess platelet function, clot strength, and fibrinolysis which these other tests cannot do.

TABLE 1: Tests to check coagulation.

Test	Normal Value	Measures
Bleeding time	3–10 minutes	Platelet count, vascular integrity
Platelet count	150,000–400,000 cells mm^{-3}	
Prothrombin time	12–14 seconds	Factors I, II, V, VII, X
Partial thromboplastin time	25–35 seconds	Factors I, II, V, VIII, IX, X, XI, XII
Thrombin time	12–20 seconds	Factors I, II
Fibrinogen	200–400 mg/dL	
Fibrin degradation products	<4 µg/mL	

Preoperative coagulation screening should be done if:
- History or physical examination suggests a possibility of coagulation disorder
- A patient is on anticoagulant or antiplatelet drugs
- A medical disease is present that could alter coagulation. Tests to check coagulation are given in **Table 1**.

CLASSIFICATION

Disorders of coagulation in pregnancy can be classified as follows:

Bleeding Disorders

- *Congenital bleeding disorders:*
  - von Willebrand disease (VWD)
  - Hemophilia A and B
  - Others, e.g., factor V, VII, X, XIII, prothrombin deficiency
- *Acquired bleeding disorders:*
  - DIC (e.g., placental abruption, retained dead fetus, amniotic fluid embolism, molar pregnancy)
  - Microangiopathic hemolytic anemia (MAHA; PE, eclampsia, HELLP syndrome, TTP)
  - Liver disease
  - Anticoagulants: Aspirin and heparin.

Disorders Promoting Thrombosis in Pregnancy

- *Genetic hypercoagulable states:*
  - AT deficiency
  - Protein C deficiency
  - Protein S deficiency
  - Factor V Leiden (FVL)

- Hyperhomocysteinemia
- Prothrombin G20210A variation
■ *Acquired thrombophilia:* The most common cause is antiphospholipid syndrome (APS).

Platelet Disorders

■ *Quantitative abnormalities (not enough platelets):*
- Gestational thrombocytopenia
- Idiopathic thrombocytopenic purpura
- Increased consumption (HELLP syndrome, DIC)
- Systemic lupus erythematosus/antiphospholipid antibody syndrome (SLE/APS)
- Thrombotic thrombocytopenic purpura (TTP)
- Drug-induced thrombocytopenia
- Decreased platelet production (marrow suppression), e.g., sepsis, HIV

■ *Qualitative disorders (poor platelet function).*

Inherited Disorders of Coagulation

von Willebrand Disease

von Willebrand disease is an autosomal dominant inherited coagulopathy. It affects the vWF, which is a part of the factor VIII complex. The vWF helps in coagulation in two ways:
1. It combines with factor VIII to produce a procoagulant factor VIIIc.
2. It helps platelets to bind to the damaged endothelium.

Additionally, it stabilizes factor VIII, which degrades rapidly when not attached to vWF.

von Willebrand disease is the most common bleeding disorder encountered in the general population, with an estimated prevalence of ~1% of the US population. There are three types of this disease:
1. *Type 1:* It is a mild-to-moderate bleeding disorder and there is a partial deficiency of vWF.
2. *Type 2a:* There is a qualitative defect in vWF.
   Type 2b: There is a qualitative defect in vWF with increased binding to platelets causing mild thrombocytopenia.
3. *Type 3:* This is a severe bleeding disorder in which there is a complete absence of vWF and reduced levels of factor VIII.

Diagnosis: A good history of past episodes of bleeding and history of mucosal bleeding from childhood, especially menorrhagia, along with a family history of bleeding can warn of a congenital bleeding disorder such as VWD. Patients with VWD have a prolonged bleeding time, raised aPTT, and normal platelet count except in type 2b disease.

Management in pregnancy and labor: During pregnancy, there is a three- to four-fold increase in vWF (increases 200–375%). Patients suffering with type 1 disorder improve during pregnancy as the vWF levels increase up to the normal range. Women suffering with type 2 and 3 disorders do not improve during pregnancy. Pregnancy outcome is generally good, but PPH is encountered in up to 50% of cases. PPH can occur as the levels of vWF fall to the prepregnancy level after delivery. Vaginal delivery is considered safe if vWF is >40 IU/dL; if operative delivery is necessary, the level has to be >50 IU/dL. The type of disease, platelet count, and levels of factor VIII and vWF should be known before considering regional anesthesia in these patients. Regional anesthesia is safe in patients with type 1 disease; central neuraxial block is not recommended for women with type 2 and 3 diseases.

Treatment: Prophylaxis and treatment in selected patients can be achieved with tranexamic acid (TXA), DDAVP (desmopressin), antihemophilic factor (FVIII), plasma, cryoprecipitate, or a combination of these. The use of DDAVP in antepartum is controversial because of a theoretical risk of vasoconstriction and placental insufficiency. TXA blocks the binding of plasminogen to fibrin, thus stabilizing a formed clot. Dosing is oral or IV.

Hemophilia

Hemophilia is an X-linked condition associated with reduction or absence of clotting factor VIII (hemophilia A) or IX (hemophilia B), causing bleeding. Females are usually carriers of this disease as they have only one affected chromosome. The clotting factor level activity is expected to be around 50% of the normal. But a wide range of values have been reported as a result of random inactivation of one of the two X chromosomes.

A detailed history of bleeding problems and full coagulation profile with factor VIII and IX levels should be sought. Women with low factor levels have the same risk of bleeding, as do affected males. Pregnancy issue usually focuses on the fetus because 50% of male offspring born to female carrier are affected. Carrier state and the risk of her fetus should be determined early in pregnancy by genetic testing.

Pregnancy should be managed in close collaboration with a hematologist. The factor levels should be checked at booking and at 28 and 34 weeks and before invasive procedures. The levels of factor VIII and vWF increase during pregnancy. The levels of factor VIII may double pre-pregnant values, but there is no increase in factor IX levels. The maternal factor levels do not rise significantly until the second trimester. An invasive procedure such as first-trimester abortions can be complicated by serious hemorrhage. A plasma level ≥40 IU/dL is generally regarded as safe for normal vaginal delivery and a level ≥50 IU/dL is sufficient for caesarean section. If the factor level is <50 IU/dL, then prophylactic factor supplementation is needed to maintain levels ≥50 IU/dL throughout labor and up to 7 days postdelivery.

Patients with hemophilia, because of prior treatment with factor VIII or IX, may develop antibodies directed against these factors which may lead to life-threatening hemorrhage. Rarely in puerperium, women may develop severe, protracted, repetitive PPH starting a week or so after an apparently uncomplicated delivery. The aPTT is markedly prolonged. Treatment of hemophilia A is factor VIII concentrates, cryoprecipitate, and intranasal or intravenous DDAVP. The increase in coagulation factor remains for 6 hours. There is a theoretical risk of uterine contractions and possible harm to the fetus with the use of DDAVP. This is not a contraindication to use DDAVP during labor, which is the usual time when it is administered. Treatment of hemophilia B includes factor IX concentrates and fresh frozen plasma (FFP).

The use of regional block is controversial. Unless factor levels are ≥50 IU/dL, and APTT and PT are normal, regional anesthesia should not be considered. The epidural catheter should be removed soon after delivery as factor levels fall quickly in the postpartum period.

Hypoprothrombinemia

This disorder is a deficiency in prothrombin, or factor II, a glycoprotein formed and stored in the liver. Some patients may show no symptoms, and others will suffer severe hemorrhage. Patients may experience easy bruising, profuse nose bleeds, PPH, excessively prolonged or heavy menstrual bleeding, and postsurgical hemorrhage. Hypoprothrombinemia may also be acquired rather than inherited and usually results from a vitamin K deficiency caused by liver diseases.

Acquired Coagulopathy

Acquired coagulopathies are due to uncontrolled activation of the coagulation system causing DIC. Once triggered, the uncontrolled activation of procoagulants leads to widespread intravascular coagulation. This leads to a fall in the levels of clotting factors to such a low level that they are insufficient to stop further bleeding.

Causes of consumption coagulopathy in pregnancy:
- Injury to vascular endothelium—PE, hypovolemic shock, septicemic shock
- Release of tissue factor (TF)—placental abruption, amniotic fluid embolism, retained dead fetus, placenta accreta, acute fatty liver
- Production of procoagulants—fetomaternal hemorrhage, incompatible blood transfusion, septicemia, intravascular hemolysis.

Placental Abruption

Placental abruption is the most common cause of obstetric consumptive coagulopathy (60% of cases; 5% of all abruptions). The syndrome is uncommon unless the abruption is severe enough to cause fetal death. Initially, increased intrauterine pressure forces TF-rich decidual fragments into the maternal circulation; in severe abruption, hypovolemic shock, large volume transfusion and high levels of fibrin degradation products (FDPs) that act as anticoagulants themselves exacerbate the situation.

Retained Dead Fetus

Retained dead fetus may cause chronic consumptive coagulopathy by release of TF from the dead fetus into the maternal circulation, but generally only if the fetus is at least of 20 weeks' size and the period of death is more than 4 weeks.

Amniotic Fluid Embolism

Amniotic fluid embolism can occur during labor, cesarean section or within a short time of delivery. Amniotic fluid is rich in TF that may enter uterine veins when there has been a tear in the uterine wall. The condition may lead to maternal death due to severe pulmonary hypertension (HTN) following embolization of the fetal squames in the pulmonary vessels. If the mother survives this acute event, there may be an anaphylactoid reaction to the presence of the fetal tissues in the maternal circulation associated with cardiovascular collapse, pulmonary edema, and the development of consumptive coagulopathy.

Sepsis

Sepsis causes consumptive coagulopathy via the release of proinflammatory cytokines such as tumor necrosis factor-α (TNF-α), interleukin 1 (IL-1), and IL-6, which may trigger TF expression by monocytes and endothelial cells.

Preeclampsia

Preeclampsia affects approximately 6% of all pregnancies; thrombocytopenia develops in approximately 50% of patients, with the severity usually proportional to the severity of PE. The current understanding of the pathogenesis of thrombocytopenia in PE is that it is due to excessive platelet activation, adhesion of platelets to damaged or activated endothelium, and/or clearance of IgG-coated platelets by the reticuloendothelial system.

Activation of the coagulation cascade occurs in most patients with PE although coagulation tests are usually normal initially. In severe PE, the activation of coagulation results in consumption of clotting factors; coagulation screening shows prolonged bleeding time and PTT with increased levels of fibrin-split products and a fall in plasma fibrinogen.

HELLP Syndrome

The HELLP (hemolysis, elevated liver enzymes and low platelets) syndrome is often considered to be a variant of

PE and is the most common cause of severe liver disease in pregnant women. Incidence—0.2 to 0.6% of all pregnancies.

The HELLP syndrome is characterized by hepatic endothelial disruption followed by platelet activation, aggregation, and consumption, ultimately resulting in ischemia and hepatocyte death. Criteria for the diagnosis include MAHA (low Hb%), low serum haptoglobin, raised aspartate aminotransferase (AST; >70 U/L) and thrombocytopenia, with a platelet count <100 × 10^9/L. Serum lactate dehydrogenase (LDH) >600 IU/L, high serum bilirubin (>1.2 mg/dL), abnormal peripheral blood film (PBF), smear positive burr cells, schistocytes, spherocytosis, triangular cells, helmet cells, reticulocytosis, anisocytosis, and polychromasia.

Management of the PE/HELLP syndrome is supportive and should be focused on stabilizing the patient medically prior to early delivery of the fetus. Platelet transfusion may be needed, particularly if the count is <50,000/mm³, if bleeding occurs, or if thrombocytopenia is severe and cesarean delivery is planned, although the survival time of transfused platelets in PE is diminished. The consumptive coagulopathy resulting from PE should be treated with FFP, but if severe hypofibrinogenemia is present, plasma fibrinogen levels can be raised with cryoprecipitate or fibrinogen concentrate.

Acute Fatty Liver in Pregnancy

Acute fatty liver in pregnancy (AFLP) is most aptly viewed as part of the pregnancy-associated microangiopathies; up to 50% of patients with AFLP may also meet the criteria for PE. The extent of microangiopathic hemolysis and thrombocytopenia is generally mild compared with that observed in HELLP, TTP, or hemolytic–uremic syndrome (HUS).

Delivery is the most important aspect of management, as it starts the reversal of the pathological process. Coagulation defects are managed supportively with FFP, cryoprecipitate or fibrinogen concentrate and platelet concentrates. In these patients, normalization of hemostatic abnormalities may not occur for up to 10 days after delivery.

Disseminated Intravascular Coagulation

Disseminated intravascular coagulation is an acquired clinicopathologic syndrome, characterized by a concomitant overactivation of the coagulation and fibrinolytic systems, leading to widespread microvascular thrombosis, disruption of blood supply to different organs, ischemia, and multiorgan failure. This extensive activation of the coagulation cascade leads to consumption and depletion of platelets and coagulation proteins, which can provoke concurrent severe bleeding. This condition may occur in the setting of sepsis, major trauma, and obstetric calamities including placental abruption, amniotic fluid embolism, retained dead fetus, and acute fatty liver of pregnancy.

Disseminated intravascular coagulation can present as an acute, life-threatening emergency or a chronic, subclinical process, depending on the degree and tempo of the process and the contribution of morbidities from the underlying cause (**Fig. 2**). Acute DIC results from an acute trigger of coagulation (e.g., sepsis or trauma). This leads to abrupt and exuberant depletion of coagulation factors, leading to hemostatic imbalances. Chronic DIC, sometimes termed "chronic compensated DIC" observed in cases of retained dead fetus, chronic abruption, and retained placenta accreta, causes gradual consumption of coagulation factors, which can be compensated by the production of additional clotting factors. The "hyperfibrinolytic" form of DIC as often observed in postpartum DIC and abruption results from an extremely rapid burst of thrombin generation, whereas a "procoagulant" form of DIC (e.g., PE-related DIC) may result from an excessive but slower and more gradual form of thrombin generation. Although both procoagulant and hyperfibrinolytic processes may proceed simultaneously in DIC, the clinical presentation of thrombosis or bleeding is determined by the predominant mechanism at a particular time. Obstetric DIC more typically presents with bleeding complications, rather than thrombotic complications, and is usually acute in onset (except in retained dead fetus). Placental abruption is the most common cause; up to 30% of patients may develop coagulopathy.

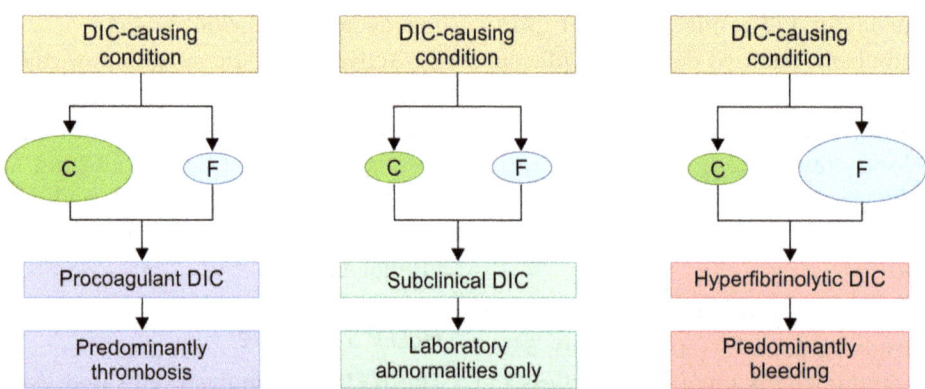

Fig. 2: Different types of disseminated intravascular coagulation (DIC).

Incidence: The incidence of DIC during pregnancy is not well defined and varies from 0.03% in North America to 0.35% in developing countries.

Pathophysiology: DIC is triggered by several mechanisms including release of TF into the circulation, endothelial damage to small vessels, and production of procoagulant phospholipids in response to intravascular hemolysis. Blood loss itself with massive transfusion and volume replacement may also trigger consumptive coagulopathy. These triggers may lead to the generation of thrombin, cause defects in inhibitors of coagulation, and suppress fibrinolysis. Thrombin promotes platelet activation and aggregates formation, which occlude the microvasculature and result in thrombocytopenia. The DIC in obstetric hemorrhage activates coagulation and triggers fibrinolysis. Activation of fibrinolysis leads to the production of D-dimers and fibrin-degradation products. These will interfere with platelet function and can impair myometrial contractility **(Flowchart 1)**.

Diagnosis and Management: The hallmark of successful management of this dire complication depends on prompt and accurate recognition of DIC. Unfortunately, often the diagnosis is based mainly on clinical presentation of the patient and often made relatively late in the course of the disease. During pregnancy, there is a physiologic change in the plasma concentrations of many of the coagulation parameters leading to a false perception that the status of the coagulation system is normal in cases when the patient is already developing coagulopathy. Moreover, often there is underestimation of the amount of bleeding and the relevant laboratory tests are performed too late when the patient is already compromised.

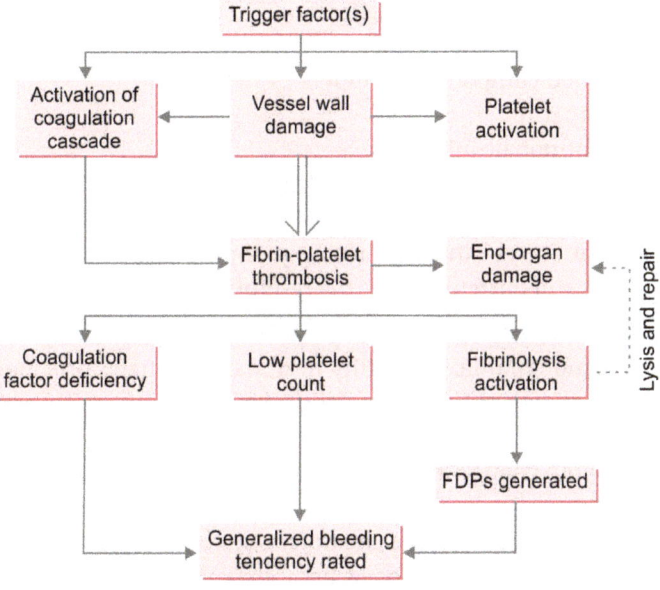

Flowchart 1: Pathogenesis of disseminated intravascular coagulation (DIC).

(FDPs: fibrin degradation products)

Symptoms: Symptoms are those of the underlying cause and those due to complications of DIC. Consumption of clotting factors usually leads to a bleeding diathesis. A small percentage of affected individuals may go on to develop widespread thrombosis with peripheral organ ischemia. Hemorrhagic manifestations include ecchymosis, petechiae, bleeding from the gum, hematuria, venipuncture oozing, intracranial or intracerebral hemorrhage, and gastrointestinal (GI) bleeding. Although some degree of consumptive coagulopathy accompanies most forms of obstetric hemorrhage, the highest risk usually arises from consumption of clotting factors and platelets as a result of massive obstetric hemorrhage.

Laboratory tests: There is no single laboratory or clinical test that is sensitive and specific enough to diagnose DIC and the risk to develop DIC is not evident in all cases. DIC screening laboratory test includes:
- CBC
- INR or PT, PTT
- Fibrinogen
- D-dimer.

PT/INR—increased, APTT—increased, thrombin time—prolonged, fibrinogen level—decreased (normal 200–400 mg/dL), platelet count markedly decreased, markedly increased FDPs, D-dimer—raised. PBF will show features of MAHA including schistocytes (fragmented RBCs) and microspherocytes.

In order to facilitate the diagnosis and management of DIC, a scoring system was developed by the International Society on Thrombosis and Hemostasis (ISTH); later, a pregnancy-modified DIC score was constructed by Erez et al. for patients who have obstetrical complications that put them at risk for DIC, which includes the PT difference (the differences between the PT values of patients and the laboratory controls in seconds), fibrinogen concentration, and platelet count, adjusted to the reference ranges of pregnancy. At a cutoff of ≥26 points, the pregnancy-specific DIC score has 88% sensitivity, 96% specificity, a positive likelihood ratio (LR) of 22, and a negative LR of 0.125.

Bedside tests that may can give useful information and help in tackling the crisis are: (1) bleeding time, (2) coagulation time, (3) clot observation test, (4) peripheral smear, and (5) circulatory fibrinolysis test.

Clot observation test (Weiner): Clot observation test is a useful bedside test. It can be repeated at 2–4-hour intervals. 5 mL of venous blood is placed in a 15-mL dry test tube and kept at 37°C. Usually, blood clot forms within 6–12 minutes. This test provides a rough idea of the blood fibrinogen level. If the clotting time is less than 6 minutes, the fibrinogen level is >150 mg%. If a clot does not form within 30 minutes, the fibrinogen level is probably <100 mg%.

TABLE 2: Components of the pregnancy specific DIC score with assigned weight.

	Effect of Individual Analytes		Effect of individual analytes adjusted to other tests		Assigned weight*
	Relative risk	p value	Relative risk	p value	
PT difference (seconds)					
<0.5	1.0		1.0		0
0.5–1	12.7	0.031	29.3	<0.001	5
1.0–1.5	27.7	0.005	68.8	<0.001	12
>1.5	60.3	<0.001	558.1	<0.001	25
Platelets (10^9/L)					
<50	3.1	0.06	89.2	<0.001	
50–100	5.2	<0.001	56.2	<0.001	2
100–185	2.9	0.001	12.8	<0.001	1
>185	1.0		1.0		0
Fibrinogen (g/L)					
<3.0	59.0	<0.001	662.9	<0.001	25
3.0–4.0	13.4	<0.001	59.1	<0.001	6
4.0–4.5	2.4	0.320	6.8	0.03	1
>4.5	1.00		1.0		0

*Weight was calculated as relative risk of each of the adjusted factors to the relative risk of a factor with minimal effect.
Source: Adapted from Erez O, Novack L, Beer-Weisel R, Dukler D, Press F, Zlotnik A, et al. DIC score in pregnant women—a population based modification of the International Society on Thrombosis and Hemostasis score. PLoS One. 2014;9:e93240.

Peripheral blood smear: Peripheral blood smear when stained with Wright's stain may be of help. (1) If less than four platelets per high-power field are seen, thrombocytopenia is diagnosed. Thrombocytopenia is a feature of DIC but not of the fibrinolytic process. (2) RBC morphology—the cell shape will be "helmet shaped" or fragmented, schistocytes, and microspherocytes whereas in the fibrinolytic process, the cell morphology will be normal.

Circulatory fibrinolysis test: The measurement of FDP is indirect evidence of fibrinolysis. Determination of a low platelet count is of far more diagnostic significance than the finding of a raised FDP level in the fibrinolytic process. The most valuable and rapid clotting screen is thrombin time. Thrombin time of normal plasma is 12–20 seconds. Thrombin time is prolonged when fibrinogen is depleted.

Standard laboratory tests have limitations, including absence of real-time data and incapacity to determine the functionality of the hemostatic system of whole blood (i.e., the strength of blood clot and platelet function). Point-of-care viscoelastic tests—TEG and ROTEM—are the most widely studied viscoelastic tests which provide a rapid assessment of in vivo coagulation. ROTEM/TEG allows early detection and dynamic monitoring of clotting abnormalities, and fibrinogen transfusion needed; hence, they could potentially be used as guidance for administration of blood components. FIBTEM is a kind of ROTEM which specifically studies fibrinogen function by using cytochalasin D to inhibit the platelet function, so clot formation is only contributed by the fibrinogen. FIBTEM helps a physician to make a proper decision for blood component transfusion. FIBTEM amplitude at 10 minutes (A10) has been widely used to identify hypofibrinogenemia, a threshold of <11-mm-guided fibrinogen replacement in bleeding trauma patients **(Flowchart 2)**.

Management: The principles of management include the following:
- Remove underlying cause
- Replenish depleted factors
- Volume replacement
- Blood component therapy
- Heparin
- Fibrinolytic inhibitors.

Most obstetric DIC are intrapartum and women have severe uterine bleeding. The goal of management is to identify and to correct the underlying pathology. In most cases, delivery of the fetus brings the resolution of coagulopathy.

Assess hemodynamic stability: Make a provisional diagnosis of hemodynamic instability in nonanesthetized pregnant patients with one or more of the following:
- Systolic blood pressure <100 mm Hg
- Acute change in heart rate or systolic blood pressure by >15%
- Shock index (SI) (i.e., heart rate/systolic blood pressure), which is a predictor of hemodynamic compromise in obstetric patients. It performed better than conventional

Flowchart 2: Algorithm for the treatment of obstetrical hemorrhage based on FIBTEM and fibrinogen concentrations.

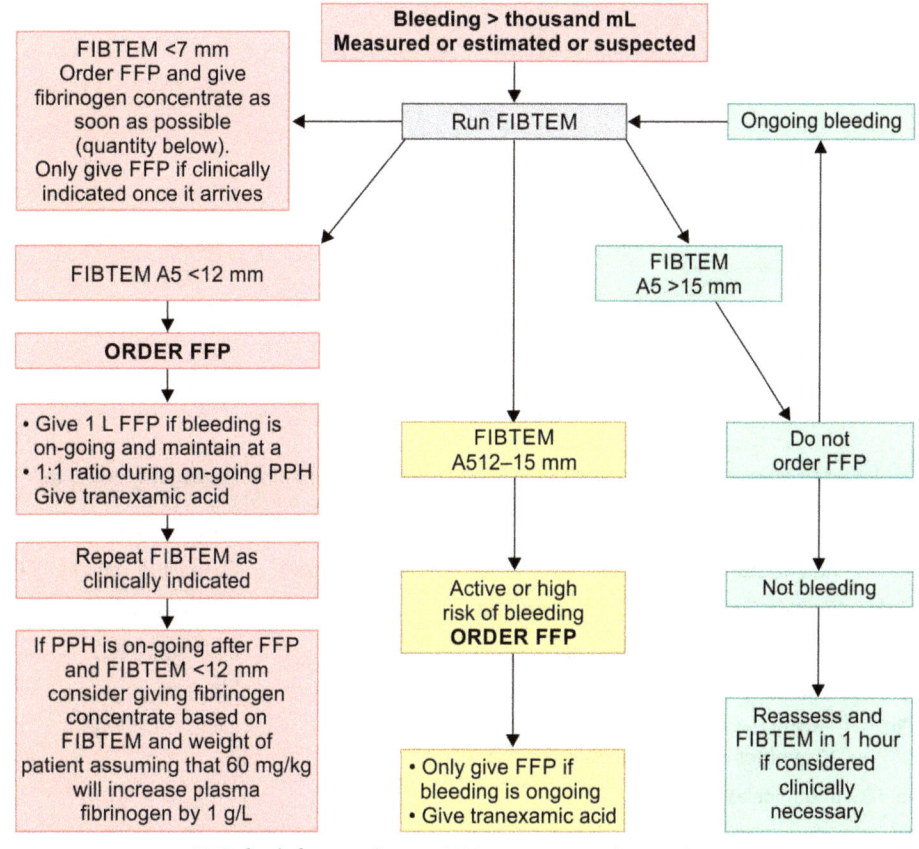

(FFP: fresh frozen plasma; PPH: postpartum hemorrhage)

vital signs alone in one study in which SI ≥1.7 was predictive of blood transfusion ≥4 units. Patients with PE/eclampsia and PPH tend to have lower mean SI values as compared to nonpreeclamptic/eclamptic patients, suggesting that SI may not be a reliable indicator in patients with PE/eclampsia.

- Urine output <30 mL/hr
- Heart rate >100 beats per minute (although the 97th percentile in normal pregnant people is approximately 115 beats per minute in the third trimester).

Other signs and symptoms of hemodynamic instability may be present, such as altered level of consciousness, shortness of breath, cold, clammy skin, and pallor.

Resuscitation: Resuscitation aims to treat the condition that caused the DIC, achieve euvolemia, normalize tissue oxygen delivery, and resolve acidosis and coagulopathy. This is achieved by appropriate fluid therapy and transfusion [using a 1:1:1 ratio of packed red blood cells (PRBCs), plasma, and platelets], warming the patient, and providing appropriate airway and ventilatory management. The other part of the management is to achieve a platelet count >50,000/μL and a fibrinogen level >100 mg/dL.

Volume replacement: Volume replacement is initially done by crystalloids (Ringer's solution) or by colloid solution (hemaccel or gelofusine or human albumin 5%), which will reduce the amount of whole blood needed to restore the blood volume. The crystalloids remain in the vascular compartment for less time compared to colloids. As colloid, dextran should be avoided as it adversely affects platelet function and blood crossmatching tests.

Blood products: Blood is rapidly administered to actively bleeding patients. In massive hemorrhage, rapid transfusion of blood components and avoiding associated hyperkalemia and hypocalcemia are essential for ensuring adequate tissue perfusion and for preventing the combination of acidosis, coagulopathy, hypothermia, and electrolyte abnormalities, which is often lethal ("lethal quad").

Whole blood transfusion: Whole blood transfusion is the sheet anchor to replenish not only the fibrinogen but also the other procoagulants. 500 mL of fresh blood will increase the blood volume, the fibrinogen level approximately by 12.5 mg/100 mL, and add 10,000–15.000 platelets/mm^3. However, whole blood is rarely used in modern obstetrics due to its disadvantages.

Packed red blood cells: Packed red blood cells are most effective to improve oxygen-carrying capacity in a euvolemic patient. Oxygen-carrying capacity is reduced when the hemoglobin level is <8 g/dL and transfusion reactions are less compared to whole blood transfusion. Each unit

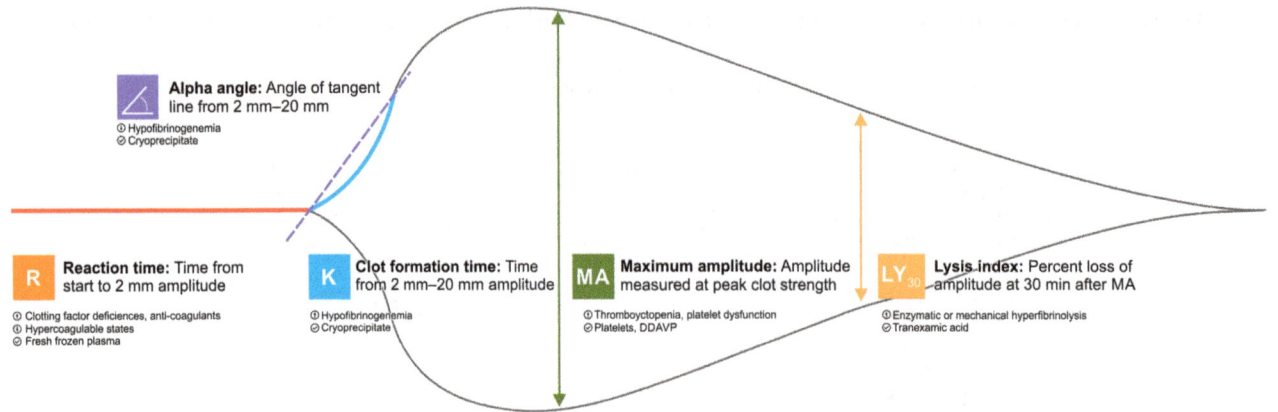

Fig. 3: Thromboelastogram (TEG).
Source: Researchgate

TABLE 3: Thromboelastogram-based component use.				
Components	**Definition**	**Normal values**	**Problem with...**	**Treatment**
R time	Time to start forming clot	5–10 minutes	Coagulation factors	FFP
K time	Time until clot reaches a fixed strength	1–3 minutes	Fibrinogen	Cryoprecipitate
Alpha angle	Speed of fibrin accumulation	53–72°	Fibrinogen	Cryoprecipitate
Maximum amplitude	Highest vertical amplitude of the TEG	50–70 mm	Platelets	Platelets and/or DDAVP
Lysis at 30 minutes (LY30)	Percentage of amplitude reduction 30 minutes after maximum amplitude	0–8%	Excess fibrinolysis	Tranexamic acid and/or aminocaproic acid

(FFP: fresh frozen plasma; TEG: thromboelastography)
Source: Researchgate

contains about 300 mL (250 mL RBC and 50 mL of plasma). One unit of PRBC will raise the hemoglobin by 1 g/dL and hematocrit by 3%. Massive transfusion protocols should be followed in the presence of severe bleeding. The commonly used protocol includes 6 units of PRBCs, 4 units of FFP, and 1 unit of platelet concentrate (6:4:1).

Replenish depleted factors: Fresh frozen plasma contains fibrinogen and provides the source of most factors (factors II, V, VIII, IX, X, and XI and AT III); cryoprecipitate is rich in fibrinogen, factor VIII, von Willebrand's factor, and XIII (each unit contains 300 mg of fibrinogen which raises plasma concentration 6 mg/dL). Cryoprecipitate provides less volume (40 mL) compared to FFP (250 mL) and should not be used for volume replacement. Cryoprecipitates may be necessary if fibrinogen levels are low, when large amounts of fibrinogen must be administered in a low-volume product. One unit of cryoprecipitate increases the fibrinogen level by 5–10 mg/dL.

A fibrinogen level <200 mg/dL should trigger fibrinogen replacement in a patient with ongoing bleeding. In general, transfusion of 15 units of FFP or 3 g of fibrinogen concentrate is necessary to increase the blood fibrinogen level by >100 mg/dL. As a working rule, give 1 unit of FFP after the initial 4–6 units of whole blood, and thereafter 1 unit for every 2 units of whole blood is required. Many massive transfusion protocols recommend transfusion of FFP, platelets, and RBCs in a ratio of 1:1:1.

Platelet target: The risk of severe bleeding due to thrombocytopenia only increases substantially with platelet counts below 50,000/mm^3. One unit of platelets can raise the number of platelets to about 5,000–10,000/mm^3. For women with platelet counts <50,000 and severe bleeding (bleeding into a closed space, bleeding requiring transfusion, bleeding that will not stop) or bleeding that is expected to become severe, platelet transfusion should be given immediately, regardless of the underlying cause of thrombocytopenia.

In most women, swift treatment of the initiating cause and maintenance of organ perfusion are all that is required for successful treatment. Once the cause of DIC has been removed, the liver will replenish adequate levels of most coagulation factors within 24 hours. The platelet count may take 5–6 days to return to normal, but will probably reach adequate levels for hemostasis within 24 hours.

Desmopressin-1-deamino-8-D-arginine vasopressin (DDAVP): The synthetic antidiuretic hormone analog increases factor VIII concentrations and VWF release from endothelial cells, promoting platelet aggregation and adhesion. DDAVP can reduce bleeding resulting from obstetrical hemorrhage with a good safety profile. The current evidence although limited suggests that DDAVP may be beneficial in DIC resulting from abnormal platelet activity.

Heparin: Heparin can be used when the vascular compartment remains intact. In an acute condition such as amniotic fluid embolism, intravenous heparin 5,000 units repeated 4–6-hour intervals is useful to stop DIC and may be lifesaving. In a retained dead fetus, there is progressive but slow defibrination due to DIC. In such cases, the process can be arrested by intravenous heparin. In acute DIC, heparin may aggravate bleeding.

Fibrinolytic inhibitors: The place of fibrinolytic inhibitors is very limited. Fibrinolysis may be a protective phenomenon. Commonly available antifibrinolytic agents are: (1) Epsilon amino caproic acid (EACA)—inhibits plasminogen and plasmin, (2) trasylol—inhibits plasmin, and (3) aprotinin—nonspecific enzyme inhibitor. Fibrinolytic inhibitors are mainly indicated in PPH following abruptio placentae in spite of a firm and contracted uterus and when the blood fibrinogen level is 200 mg% or more. However, these drugs can increase the risk of thrombosis.

HYPERCOAGULABLE STATES IN PREGNANCY

Pregnancy is a hypercoagulable state and certain disorders increase the risk of thrombosis. Patients with inherited thrombophilia have an increased tendency to venous thromboembolism.

Inherited Thrombophilia

Thrombophilia is defined as a predisposition to thrombosis, secondary to any persistent or identifiable hypercoagulable state. Although these disorders are collectively present in about 15% of population, they are responsible for more than 50% of all thromboembolic events during pregnancy and should be considered in patients with RPL, unexplained intrauterine fetal demise (IUFD) and early onset severe FGR. Thrombophilia associated with a high risk of venous thromboembolism (VTE) includes AT deficiency, protein C or S deficiency, compound heterozygosity for FVL and prothrombin gene mutation (PGM; G20210A) or other combinations of thrombophilia, and homozygosity for these conditions. Low-risk thrombophilia includes heterozygosity for FVL or the PGM. In women with an inherited deficiency of antithrombin, factor C or S the incidence of thromboembolism is increased eightfold during pregnancy and puerperium. The incidence of thrombotic risk in females with FVL is 1 in 400–500.

Antithrombin Deficiency

Antithrombin III is a naturally occurring anticoagulant. It inactivates thrombin and factors IXa, Xa, XIa, and XIIa. The clinical manifestation of deficiency is thrombosis. This is an autosomal-dominant condition. The risk of thrombosis during pregnancy among AT-deficient women without a personal or family history is 3–7%, and 11–40% with such a history.

More than 250 mutations in AT gene have been identified, producing a highly variable phenotype. Acquired deficiency may be due to liver impairment, increased consumption of AT with sepsis or DIC, and increased renal excretion with nephrotic syndrome. Inherited or acquired deficiency is associated with VTE. Deficiency is also associated with significantly increased risk of stillbirth after 28 weeks, modest association before 28 weeks, and associated with increased risk of FGR.

Protein C Deficiency

Protein C is a vitamin K-dependent anticoagulant. Protein C downregulates coagulation cascade, inhibits activated clotting factors V and VIII, and stimulates fibrinolysis; deficiencies lead to unregulated fibrin formation. There is a positive family and personal history of thromboembolic phenomenon at a young age in patients with protein C deficiency. These patients are on prophylactic anticoagulants.

Protein C deficiency results from more than 160 mutations, producing highly variable phenotype. The reported risk of VTE with protein C deficiency is 2–8%. Because of its rarity, few reports link protein C deficiency and adverse pregnancy outcome. A rare homozygous deficiency variety may cause neonatal purpura fulminans and need for lifelong anticoagulation.

Protein S Deficiency

More than 130 mutations have been linked to deficiency of protein S. Because protein S drops substantially during pregnancy, screening during pregnancy should not be done. Value <55% in nonpregnant women is consistent with diagnosis. A meta-analysis reported deficiency with recurrent late pregnancy loss (after 22 weeks). Another meta-analysis found strong association with stillbirth, intrauterine growth restriction (IUGR), PE, and eclampsia.

Factor V Leiden

Factor V Leiden is the most common inherited hypercoagulable disorder. Prevalence is 3–5% in the White population and rare in Blacks, Asians, and Native Americans.

Factor V is normally cleaved and inactivated by activated protein C (APC). Patients with a single point mutation in the gene coding for factor V produce a mutated factor V (called FVL) that is resistant to inactivation by APC, resulting in increased thrombin production and increased risk of thromboembolism. This mutated gene is inherited as an autosomal dominant trait and is the most common cause of thrombosis and familial thrombophilia.

Majority of patients resistant to activated protein C are heterozygous for FVL. Heterozygotes have seven times increased lifetime risk of thrombosis and 15 times increased risk during pregnancy or oral contraceptive pill (OCP) use. Homozygotes have 50–100 times increased lifetime risk of thrombosis. There appears to be modest association between FVL mutation and pregnancy loss; no clear association exists with PE and stillbirth.

Prothrombin Gene Mutation

The gene involved in the synthesis of prothrombin is located on chromosome 11. The prothrombin gene polymorphism is a point mutation causing a guanine to adenine switch at nucleotide position 20210 in the 3′ unsaturated region of the gene. This nucleotide switch results in increased translation of messenger RNA. There is increased prothrombin concentration, which augments thrombin generation. About 1 in every 50 white people in Europe and North America has the heterozygous PGM, making it the second most common inherited clotting disorder, while 1 of every 250 Black people in America has PGM.

Prothrombin gene mutation has been associated with an increased risk of pregnancy loss and small for gestational age (SGA) below the 5th centile. A recent review suggests a strong association between PGM and RPL before 25 weeks.

Hyperhomocysteinemia

Homocysteine is a nonessential amino acid that derives from the biosynthesis and metabolism of methionine (Met). Within the Met metabolic pathway, HCys can be either irreversibly degraded to cysteine (Cys) via the trans-sulfuration pathway or re-methylated back to methionine. About 50% of homocysteine is converted back to methionine by remethylation via the methionine synthase pathway. This requires active folate [known as 5-methyltetrahydrofolate (5-MTHF)] and vitamin B_{12}, in order to donate a methyl group. Another pathway for the conversion of homocysteine back to methionine involves methylation with trimethylglycine as a methyl donor. The remaining homocysteine is converted to cysteine via trans-sulfuration pathway, with vitamin B6 as the co-factor. Hyperhomocysteinemia is inherited as an autosomal recessive form; the most common acquired form is due to folate deficiency. There is increased homocysteine in combination with B_{12} deficiency.

The normal fasting homocysteine level is <12 nmol/mL. Moderate hyperhomocysteinemia: homocysteine value 15–30 nmol/mL (or µmol/L), intermediate hyperhomocysteinemia: homocysteine level between 30 and 100 nmol/mL, severe hyperhomocysteinemia: homocysteine level >100 nmol/mL. Hyperhomocysteinemia can result from a number of mutations in the methionine metabolic pathway. Homozygosity for mutation C677T polymorphism in methylene tetrahydrofolate reductase gene (*MTHFR*) is the most common cause of hyperhomocysteinemia and occurs in 10–16% of all Europeans; most heterozygotes have *A1298C* mutations. Hyperhomocysteinemia is associated with VTE and has adverse pregnancy outcomes (PE, thrombosis, and premature vascular disease).

■ ACQUIRED THROMBOPHILIA

Antiphospholipid Antibodies

Antiphospholipid antibodies (aPL) are a heterogenous group of antibodies and interfere with the normal function of phospholipids or phospholipid-binding proteins such as β2-glycoprotein. Women with moderate to high level of these antibodies may have aPL syndrome characterized by thromboembolism or recurrent early pregnancy fetal loss. It is postulated that they interfere with the normal function of phospholipids or phospholipid-binding protein involved in coagulation regulation, including prothrombin, protein C, annexin V, and tissue factor. Many of these glycoproteins are directed against β2-glycoprotein, which may itself function as a natural anticoagulant. aPLs are associated with 3.4% of early pregnancy loss.

Mechanisms by which APLA cause pregnancy morbidity include induction of syncytiotrophoblast apoptosis, inhibition of villous cytotrophoblast differentiation and extravillous cytotrophoblast invasion into the decidua, activation of complement pathways at the maternal–fetal interface resulting in a local inflammatory response and in later pregnancy, and thrombosis of the uteroplacental vasculature.

Anticoagulation for VTE Prophylaxis (ACOG)

Assess the risk of the women, whether she falls in the high- or low-risk group.
- *High-risk thrombophilia:*
  - AT deficiency
  - APS
  - FVL or PGM—homozygosity or compound heterozygotes
- *Low-risk thrombophilia:*
  - FVL or prothrombin gene variant (heterozygote state)
  - Protein C or protein S deficiency.

Management
- *Low-risk thrombophilia without personal history of (H/O) VTE:*
  - Antepartum—surveillance without anticoagulant
  - Postpartum—surveillance without anticoagulant or prophylactic anticoagulant therapy in those with risk factors, e.g., obesity, immobilization, and caesarean section
- *Low-risk thrombophilia with first-degree relative with VTE:*

- Antepartum—surveillance without anticoagulant or prophylactic low-molecular-weight heparin (LMWH)/unfractionated heparin (UFH)
- Postpartum—prophylactic anticoagulant or intermediate dose LMWH/UFH
- *Low-risk thrombophilia with personal H/O single episode of VTE (not on anticoagulant):*
  - Antepartum—prophylactic dose or intermediate-dose LMWH/UFH
  - Postpartum—prophylactic dose or intermediate-dose LMWH/UFH
- *High-risk thrombophilia without H/O VTE:*
  - Antepartum—prophylactic dose or intermediate-dose LMWH/UFH
  - Postpartum—prophylactic anticoagulant or intermediate-dose LMWH/UFH
- *High-risk thrombophilia with previous one episode of VTE or affected first-degree relative (not on long-term anticoagulant):*
  - Antepartum—prophylactic dose or intermediate-dose LMWH/UFH or adjusted dose LMWH/UFH
  - Postpartum—prophylactic dose or intermediate-dose LMWH/UFH or adjusted dose LMWH/UFH for 6 weeks (therapy equal to selected antepartum treatment)

NB: Counseled against oral anticoagulant. Full-dose LMWH initiated immediately if VTE occurred in the past month, three-fourth of treatment dose if it occurred within 12 months earlier and prophylactic dose if it VTE happened >12 months back.

- *High-risk thrombophilia with previous ≥2 episodes of VTE (not receiving long-term anticoagulant):*
  - Antepartum—intermediate-dose/adjusted dose LMWH/UFH
  - Postpartum—intermediate-dose LMWH/UFH or adjusted dose LMWH/UFH for 6 weeks (therapy equal to selected antepartum treatment)
- *Thrombophilia with previous ≥2 episodes of VTE:*
  - Antepartum—adjusted dose LMWH/UFH
  - Postpartum—resumption of long-term anticoagulant therapy. Oral route may be considered depending on breast feeding/patient preference.

Dose of LMWH/UFH:
- Antepartum *prophylactic dose*—5,000 IU of UFH subcutaneously once daily or every 12 hours after 20 weeks plus low-dose aspirin (81 mg/d) OR 0.5 mg/kg/d of LMWH (enoxaparin).
- *Therapeutic dose*—full anticoagulant doses, e.g., 1 mg/kg every 12 hours of enoxaparin, or 10–12,000 units UFH every 12 hours in those who have had prior thrombosis.
- *Intermediate dose*—one-half to three-fourth of therapeutic dose. Treatment begins at conception and continues for 6–12 weeks postpartum if there is no history of thrombosis and indefinitely if there is.

Treatment dose must be monitored by anti-factor Xa activity, since PTT is usually abnormal in patients with LAC. The goal of UFH is to keep APTT 1.5–2.5 of control value. The last dose of LMWH given 24 hours before induction and a split dose every 12 hours should be started 12–24 hours postpartum. UFH to stop 12 hours before surgery and restart after 12 hours of delivery. When postpartum thromboprophylaxis is needed, warfarin may be used. To avoid paradoxical thrombosis, UFH or LMWH should be continued with warfarin for 5 days until INR is 2.0–3.0 for 2 consecutive days before being withdrawn.

PLATELET ABNORMALITIES

Platelet abnormalities can be qualitative (poor platelet function) or quantitative and are the most common hematological disorders during pregnancy after anemia. Thrombocytopenia is a reduction in platelet number below 1,50,000/μL. It complicates 7–10% of all pregnancies.

Thrombocytopenia in Pregnancy
- *Gestational* thrombocytopenia
- Autoimmune thrombocytopenia (ITP)
- Activated clotting mechanism—PE, HELLP syndrome, DIC
- SLE/APS
- TTP
- Decreased platelet production (marrow suppression), e.g., sepsis, HIV
- Malignant marrow infiltration.

Gestational Thrombocytopenia
Gestational thrombocytopenia affects 5–8% of healthy pregnant women and is the most common (75%) cause of thrombocytopenia during pregnancy. The platelet counts are in the lower range of normal and can be as low as 1,00,000/μL. The quantitative decrease in platelets is balanced by enhanced platelet activity. Women with this disorder are not at risk of bleeding. It is a diagnosis of exclusion.

Cause: Accelerated platelet consumption plus increased plasma volume generally occurs in the third trimester. Platelets are normal before pregnancy and return to normal within 2–12 weeks postpartum. As the quantitative decrease is normally balanced by enhanced platelet activity, women with this disorder are not at risk of bleeding or fetal thrombocytopenia.

Once low platelet count is diagnosed, other causes of low count should be excluded, e.g., PE, SLE, APS, HIV or hepatitis C virus, drug-induced thrombocytopenia, liver disorder, bone marrow disorder, thrombotic thrombocytopenia, hereditary thrombocytopenia, and DIC. Assessment is required to exclude severe complications and evaluate bleeding risk for the mother and the fetus, especially when platelets <1,00,000/μL.

Idiopathic Thrombocytopenia

Idiopathic thrombocytopenia, commonly called immune thrombocytopenia, is an autoimmune disorder characterized by isolated thrombocytopenia in the absence of conditions known to cause thrombocytopenia, such as infections, other autoimmune disorders, and drugs. Patients develop autoantibodies against platelet-specific antigens and antibodies (IgG) against platelet glycoproteins (GPIIb/IIIa and GPIb/IX). The antibody (Ab)-coated platelets get destroyed in the reticuloendothelial system (spleen).

Idiopathic thrombocytopenia comprises 3% of thrombocytopenia in pregnancy. Moderate thrombopenia (platelet count 50-100,000/μL) may be present before conception or early in pregnancy. Major bleeding is rarely seen unless the platelet count is <10,000/μL, when there is risk of maternal bleeding as well as fetal thrombopenia (IgG crosses the placenta causing neonatal thrombocytopenia). 4-10% of neonates are at risk of having severe thrombocytopenia at birth or during the first week of life **(Fig. 4)**.

Diagnosis: Most women with ITP have H/O petechiae, ecchymoses, easy bruising, gingival bleeding, menorrhagia, or other bleeding manifestations. Diagnosis is by exclusion based on history, physical examination, CBC, and PBF.

Features suggestive of thrombocytopenia:
- CBC—count normal except platelet count <100,000/μL
- Smear—increased platelet volume
- Bone marrow—increased numbers of immature megakaryocytes.

Treatment: The goal of treatment in pregnancy is to minimize the risk of hemorrhage and to restore a normal platelet count. Asymptomatic women with ITP—platelet count >50,000/μL—do not require treatment. For nonpregnant women, most authorities recommend to start treatment when the platelet count is <10,000/μL or in the presence of bleeding. During pregnancy, the aim is to keep platelet count >30,000/μL during pregnancy and >50,000/μL near term. The American Society of Hematology ITP recommends treating pregnant women between platelet count 10-30,000/μL. Count >50,000/μL is sufficient for vaginal delivery and count 70-80,000/μL for spinal/epidural anesthesia for caesarean section in otherwise normal women.

Glucocorticoids: Glucocorticoids are the cornerstone of treatment of thrombocytopenia in pregnancy. A dose of 0.5-2.0 mg/kg/day is the initial treatment. Improvement in platelet count occurs in 3-7 days and reaches maximum

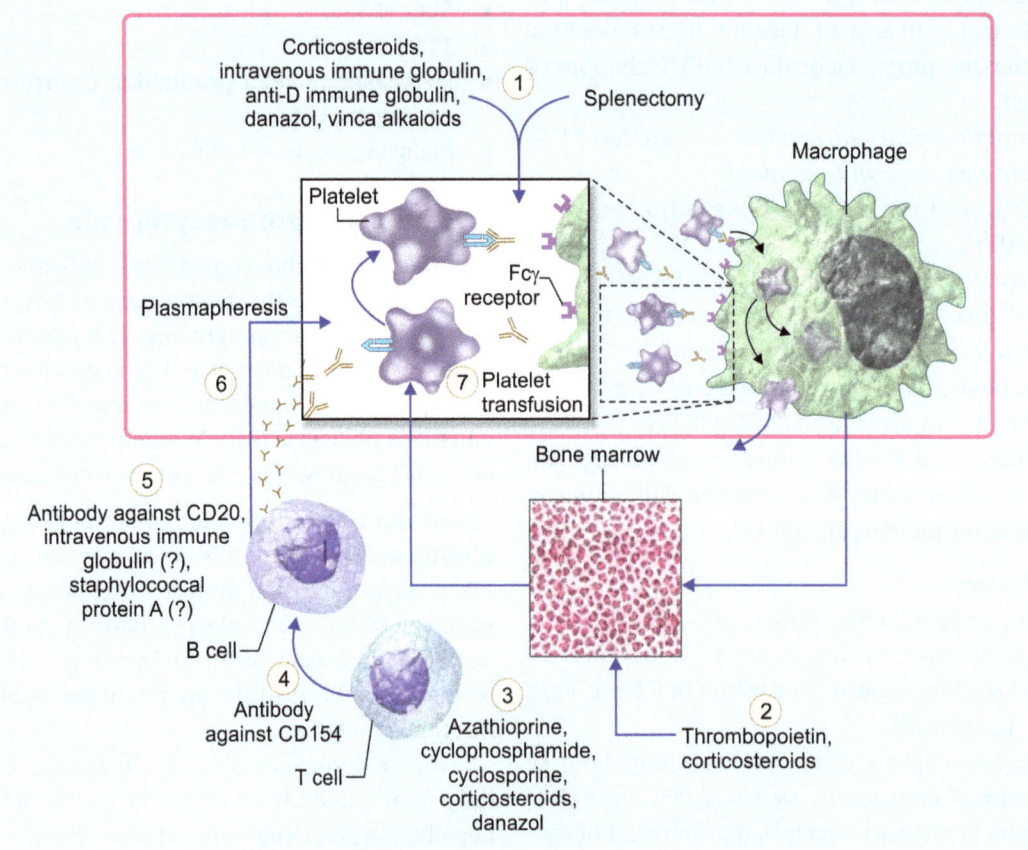

Fig. 4: Pathophysiology of idiopathic thrombocytopenia (ITP).
Source: Liberaldictionary.com

in 2–3 weeks. After improvement of count, the dose can be tapered by 10–20% per week until the lowest dose required to maintain platelet count at an acceptable level is reached. The mechanism of action of glucocorticoids is uncertain and may include increased platelet production, decreased production of platelet Ab and platelet-associated IgG, decreased clearance of Ab-coated platelet by the reticuloendothelial (RE) system, and decreased capillary fragility. Side effects of glucocorticoid include glucose intolerance, osteoporosis, HTN, psychosis, moon face, risk of preterm premature rupture of membranes (PPROM).

Intravenous immunoglobulin: Intravenous immunoglobulin (IVIG) is the treatment of choice for patients who have ITP refractory to corticosteroids and in an urgent situation, e.g., preoperatively, peripartum period, or when the count is below 10,000/μL (30,000/μL in a bleeding patient). IVIG is prepared from pooled concentrate of immunoglobulin collected from many donors.

Dose: A high dose of 1,000 mg/kg/day for 2–5 days induces platelet peak in 7–9 days. In 80% of the patients, platelet peaks to >50,000 with this treatment and lasts for more than 30 days. Untoward effects include flushing, headache, chills, nausea, transient neutropenia, autoimmune hemolytic anemia, and anaphylactic reaction.

Rhesus immunoglobulin: Anti-RhD immunoglobulin has been successfully used to treat ITP in RhD positive individuals. A dose of 75 μg/kg of maternal weight works as well as corticosteroids. It is more costly than steroids and has fewer side effects.

Platelet transfusion: Platelet transfusion is generally contraindicated but can be used in the setting of acute hemorrhage, used as a temporary measure to control life-threatening bleeding. Survival of platelets is decreased as antiplatelet Ab binds to transfused platelets also. The usual elevation of approximately 10,000/μL per unit of platelet concentrate in case of single donor; most cases need 8–10 packs.

Splenectomy: Occasionally, splenectomy is required during pregnancy. This may be safely accomplished in the second trimester or with caesarean section at term. It is indicated in women whose count is <10,000/μL who are bleeding and not responding to corticosteroids or IVIG; complete remission is obtained in 80% cases.

Refractory Patients: Immunosuppressive agents such as Vinca alkaloids, colchicine, cyclophosphamide, rituximab, and thrombopoietin receptor antagonists have been used; these are best avoided in pregnancy. Azathioprine and rarely cyclosporine may be considered in pregnancy.

Neonatal Thrombocytopenia

Antiplatelet Ab can cross the placenta and may cause fetal thrombopenia (5% of neonates have platelets <20,000/μL) and 10–15% have below 50,000, but intracranial hemorrhage is uncommon. Evaluation of the fetal platelet count by cordocentesis or fetal scalp sampling is not recommended as there are more risks. Avoid using forceps or ventouse during delivery. Measure cord platelets count and monitor platelets until nadir (2–5 days after delivery). In life-threatening hemorrhage, treatment with IVIG and platelet transfusion is recommended. If a neonate's platelet count is <30–50,000/μL, give IVIG 1 g/kg; no treatment is given if platelet >50,000/μL.

Drug-induced Thrombocytopenia

This is caused by drug-dependent binding of Fab part of the pathological IgG with the platelets, causing their destruction. In drug-induced thrombocytopenia, recovery of platelets occurs in 5–7 days after withdrawal of the offending drug **(Table 4)**.

TABLE 4: Drugs causing thrombocytopenia.

Drug category	Drugs implicated in five or more reports	Other drugs
Heparins	Unfractionated heparin, low-molecular-weight heparin	
Cinchona alkaloids	Quinine, quinidine	
Platelet inhibitors	Abciximab, eptifibatide, tirofiban	
Antirheumatic agents	Gold salts	D-penicillamine
Antimicrobial agents	Linezolid, rifampin, sulfonamides, vancomycin	
Sedatives and anticonvulsant agents	Carbamazepine, phenytoin, valproic acid	Diazepam
Histamine-receptor antagonists	Cimetidine	Ranitidine
Analgesic agents	Acetaminophen, diclofenac, naproxen	Ibuprofen
Diuretic agents	Chlorothiazide	Hydrochlorothiazide
Chemotherapeutic and immuno suppressant agents	Fludarabine, oxaliplatin	Cyclosporine, rituximab

Thrombotic Thrombocytopenic Purpura

Thrombotic thrombocytopenic purpura and HUS share the central features of MAHA and thrombocytopenia. Though neither disease occurs exclusively during pregnancy, up to 10% of all cases of TTP occur in pregnant patients. TTP is defined by a pentad of symptoms that include MAHA, thrombocytopenia, neurological abnormalities, fever, and renal dysfunction. Complete pentad is present at the time of diagnosis in <40% of patients.

Blood picture shows thrombocytopenia (platelet count <20,000/μL), anemia (HB <10 g/dL), hemolysis (elevated reticulocytosis, LDH, indirect bilirubin, haptoglobin), and schistocytes in peripheral smear. The clinical manifestations of HUS are similar but neurological abnormalities are a particular feature with TTP; renal dysfunction (increased creatinine) is more severe in patients with HUS.

Pathogenesis

Congenital or acquired deficiency of vWF cleaving protease, ADAMTS 13, and the consequent increased level of high-molecular-weight multimers of vWF play a central role in the pathogenesis of TTP.

TTP and HUS may be difficult to discern from one another and from other pregnancy-associated microangiopathies such as PE or the HELLP syndrome. The extent of microangiopathic hemolysis is more severe in TTP or HUS than in PE or HELLP, and the former disorders are not associated with HTN. The time of onset of these disorders is also helpful in differentiating between them. TTP usually presents in the second trimester, HUS in the postpartum period, and PE and the HELLP syndrome almost exclusively in the third trimester. Plasma AT levels are normal in TTP and HUS and reduced in PE and HELLP. Another distinguishing feature of these disorders is their response to delivery. Whereas PE and the HELLP syndrome usually improve following delivery, the course of TTP and HUS does not.

Thrombotic thrombocytopenic purpura responds equally well to plasma exchange with more than 75% of patients achieving remission. Plasma exchange should be instituted as soon as possible after the diagnosis and repeated plasma exchange cycles are usually maintained until delivery. There is a rationale for use of immunosuppressive therapy in those patients with inhibitors of ADAMTS 13. The use of low-dose aspirin has been advocated when the platelet count increases to >50×10^9/L. Platelet transfusion is contraindicated and may lead to rapid worsening of the condition. Management of HUS is supportive and includes renal dialysis and red cell transfusion. Plasma exchange has no proven benefit in the treatment of HUS.

■ SUGGESTED READING

1. ACOG guidance on thrombophilia in pregnancy. ACOG Practice Bulletin 197: Inherited thrombophilias in pregnancy. [online] Available from https://www.obgproject.com/2018/07/18/acog-guidance-on-thrombophilia-in-pregnancy [Last accessed July, 2022].
2. Alarm International. Coagulation and hematological disorders in pregnancy. Alarm International Program, 4th edition. Chapter 10. [online] Available from https://www.glowm.com/pdf/AIP%20Chap10%20Coagulation.pdf [Last accessed July, 2022].
3. Belfort MA. Disseminated intravascular coagulation (DIC) during pregnancy: Clinical findings, etiology, and diagnosis. UpToDate. [online] Available from https://www.uptodate.com/contents/disseminated-intravascular-coagulation-dic-during-pregnancy-clinical-findings-etiology-and-diagnosis [Last accessed July, 2022].
4. Bhave AB. Coagulopathies in pregnancy: What an obstetrician ought to know! J Obstet Gynecol India. 2019;69(6):479-82.
5. Erez O, Othman M, Rabinovich A, Leron E. DIC in Pregnancy – Pathophysiology, Clinical Characteristics, Diagnostic Scores, and Treatments. Macclesfield: Dovepress; 2022. pp. 21-44.
6. Ganchev RV, Ludlam CA. Acquired and congenital hemostatic disorders in pregnancy and the puerperium. In: Arulkumaran S, Karoshi M, Keith KG, Lalonde AB, Lynch CB, A Textbook of Postpartum Hemorrhage. [online] Available from https://www.glowm.com/resource-type/resource/textbook/title/a-comprehensive-textbook-of-postpartum-hemorrhage-2supnd-sup-edition/resource-doc/1275 [Last accessed July, 2022].
7. Katz D, Beilin Y. Disorders of coagulation in pregnancy. British J Anaesth. 2015;115(S2):ii75-ii88.
8. Management of Inherited Bleeding Disorders in Pregnancy. RCOG Green-top Guideline No. 71 (joint with UKHCDO). BJOG: An International Journal of Obstetrics & Gynaecology. 2017;124(8):e193-e263.
9. Rabinovich R, Abdul-Kadir R, Thachil J, Iba T, Othman M, Eerez O. DIC in obstetrics: Diagnostic score, highlights in management, and international registry-communication from the DIC and Women's Health SSCs of the International Society of Thrombosis and Haemostasis. J Thromb Hameost. 2019;17(9):1562-6.
10. Rodger M, Silver RM. Coagulation disorders in pregnancy In: Lockwood C, Moore T, Copel J, Silver R, Resnik R (Eds), Creasy & Resnik's Maternal Fetal Medicine, 8th edition. Philadelphia: Elsevier; 2019.
11. Royal College of Obstetricians and Gynaecologists. (2015). Thromboembolic disease in pregnancy and the puerperium: acute management. RCOG Green-top Guideline No. 37b. [online] Available from https://www.rcog.org.uk/media/wj2lpco5/gtg-37b-1.pdf [Last accessed July, 2022].
12. Sharma R, Bewlay A. (2005). Coagulation disorders in pregnancy. World Federation of Society of Anesthesiologist. [online] Available from https://resources.wfsahq.org/atotw/coagulation-disorders-in-pregnancy/ [Last accessed July, 2022].
13. Strong J. Bleeding disorders in pregnancy. Current Obstet Gynaecol. 2003;13:1–6.
14. Thornton P, Douglas J. Coagulation in pregnancy. Best Pract Res Clin Obstet Gynaecol. 2010;24:339-52.

Placenta Previa

INTRODUCTION

Placenta previa is a condition in which placenta gets implanted in the lower uterine segment or cervix, presenting ahead of the leading pole of the fetus. It occurs in 2.8/1,000 *singleton pregnancies* and 3.9/1,000 *twin pregnancies* and represents a significant clinical problem. This situation prevents a safe vaginal delivery and requires cesarean delivery. Placenta previa increases a woman's risk for placenta accreta spectrum (PAS), which substantially increases the delivery complications. It is a major risk factor for antepartum, intrapartum, and postpartum hemorrhage. Uncontrolled hemorrhage from placenta previa or PAS may necessitate massive transfusion, hysterectomy (0.2%), admission to an intensive care unit (ICU), or even death. The incidence of hysterectomy after cesarean section (CS) for placenta previa is 5.3% [risk ratio (RR) 33, as compared with those undergoing CS without placenta previa]. Perinatal mortality rates in women with placenta praevia are three to four times higher than in normal pregnancies. A multidisciplinary team approach and delivery at a center with adequate resources, including those for massive transfusion are both essential to reduce neonatal and maternal morbidity and mortality.

CLASSIFICATION

Placenta previa was originally defined using transabdominal sonography (TAS) as a placenta developing within the lower uterine segment and graded according to the relationship and/or the distance between lower edge of the placenta and the internal os of cervix as follows **(Fig. 1)**:

- *Grade I or minor previa*—defined as lower edge inside the lower uterine segment
- *Grade II or marginal previa*—as a lower edge reaching the internal os
- *Grade III or partial previa*—placenta partially covering the os
- *Grade IV or complete previa*—when the placenta completely covers the os.

Grades I and II are also often defined as "minor" placenta previa whereas grades III and IV are referred to as "major" placenta previa.

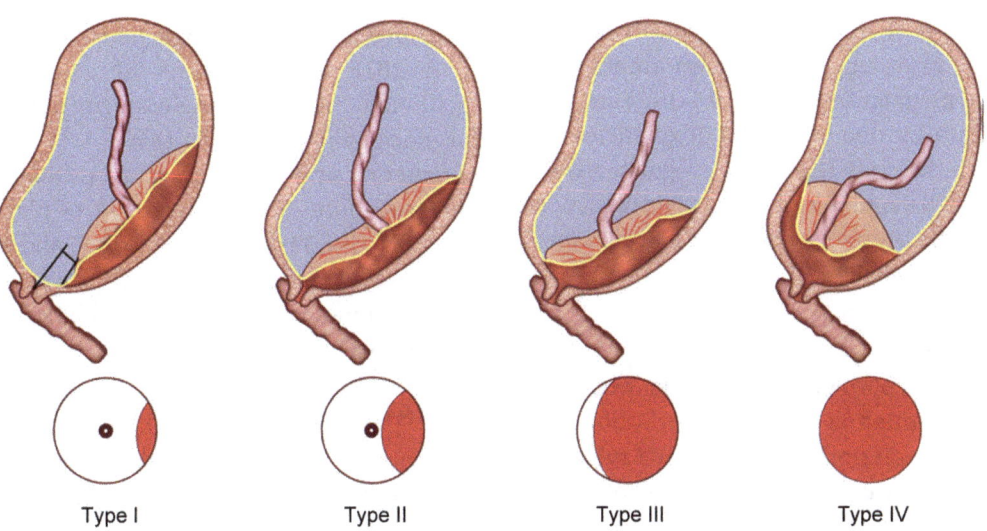

Fig. 1: Types of placenta previa.

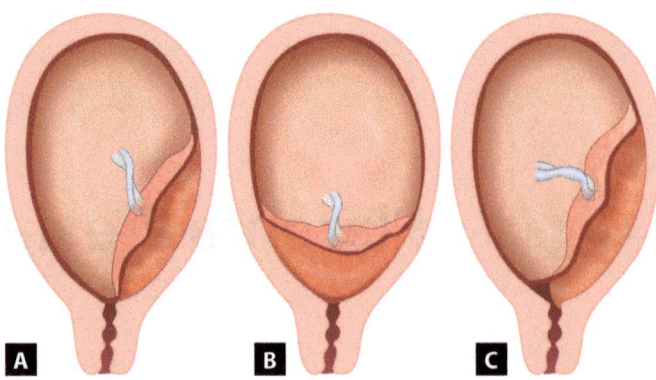

Figs. 2A to C: (A) Low lying placenta; (B and C) Placenta previa.

The introduction of transvaginal scanning (TVS) in obstetrics in the 1980s has allowed a more precise evaluation of the distance between the placental edge and the internal os. A recent multidisciplinary workshop of American Institute of Ultrasound in Medicine (AIUM) and The National Institute of Child health and Human Development panel on fetal imaging recommended replacement of all prior definitions with two terms: (1) placenta previa and (2) low-lying placenta **(Figs. 2A to C)**. The term "placenta previa" should be used when the placenta lies directly over the internal os/placental edge covers the internal os. For pregnancies >16 weeks of gestation, the placenta be reported as "low-lying" when the placental edge is <20 mm from the internal os and as normal when the placental edge is 20 mm or more from the internal os on TAS or TVS. This new classification could better define the risks of perinatal complications, such as antepartum hemorrhage and major postpartum hemorrhaged (PPH), and has the potential of improving the obstetric management of placenta previa.

■ PREVALENCE

A systematic review of the literature found the estimated global prevalence of placenta previa as 5.2/1,000 pregnancies [95% class interval (CI): 4.5–5.9]. However, there was a regional variation; prevalence was highest among Asian studies (12.2/1,000 pregnancies; 95% CI: 9.5–15.2) and lower among studies from Europe (3.6/1,000 pregnancies; 95% CI: 2.8–4.6), North America (2.9/1,000 pregnancies; 95% CI: 2.3–3.5) and Sub-Saharan Africa (2.7/1,000 pregnancies; 95% CI: 0.3–11.0). The prevalence of major placenta previa was 4.3/1,000 pregnancies (95% CI: 3.3–5.4).

■ PATHOGENESIS

The underlying cause of placenta previa is unknown. Nearly 90% of placenta identified as "low-lying" will ultimately resolve by the third trimester due to placental migration. The placenta itself does not move but grows toward the increased blood supply at the fundus, leaving the distal portion of the placenta at the lower uterine segment with relatively poor blood supply to *regress* and *atrophy*. Migration can also take place by the growing lower uterine segment thus increasing the distance from the lower margin of the placenta to the internal os of the cervix.

The development of placenta previa is hypothesized to be related to abnormal vascularization of the endometrium caused by scarring or atrophy from previous trauma, surgery, or infection. These factors may reduce differential growth of lower segment, resulting in less upward shift in placental position as pregnancy advances. The trophoblast adheres to uterine scar leading to placenta covering the cervical os or the placenta invading the walls of the myometrium.

■ RISK FACTORS

The exact etiology is unknown, major risk factors for placenta previa are previous placenta previa (4–8%), previous CS, and uterine surgery, previous or recurrent abortions. Other risk factors include increased maternal age >35 years, multiparity (5% in grand multiparous patients), large placenta as in multiple pregnancy, erythroblastosis, diabetes mellitus, maternal history of smoking, cocaine, previous manual removal of placenta, and pregnancy following assisted conception.

The risks of placenta previa increase 1.5–5-fold with a history of cesarean delivery. A meta-analysis showed that the rate of placenta previa increases with increasing numbers of cesarean deliveries, with a rate of 1% after one cesarean delivery, 2.8% after three cesarean deliveries, and as high as 3.7% after five cesarean deliveries. Advanced maternal age has been also associated with a slight increase in the risk of placenta previa [odds ratios (OR) 1.08, 95% CI 1.07–1.09]. The relationship between advanced maternal age and placenta previa may be confounded by higher parity and a higher probability of previous uterine procedures or fertility treatment. The incidence of placenta previa after the age of 35 years reported to be 2%. A further increase to 5% is seen after age 40 years, which is a ninefold increase when compared to females younger than 20 years.

A 2016 meta-analysis of assisted reproduction technology (ART) on singleton pregnancy reported a RR for placenta previa of 3.71 (95% CI 2.67–5.16). The impact of maternal smoking on placental position, in a 2017 meta-analysis, found an increased risk of placenta previa (OR 1.42, 95% CI 1.30–1.50). The nicotine and carbon monoxide in cigarettes act as potent vasoconstrictors of placental vessels; compromise the placental blood flow thus leading to abnormal placentation.

■ DIAGNOSIS

Placenta previa was originally defined using TAS. Most cases are diagnosed early in pregnancy via ultrasonography and others may present to the emergency room with painless vaginal bleeding in the second or third trimester of pregnancy. Diagnosis, nowadays, is usually made from midpregnancy routine fetal anomaly scan for placental localization, thereby identifying women at risk of persisting placenta previa or a low-lying placenta. If there is a concern for placenta previa, then a transvaginal sonogram should be performed to confirm the location of the placenta.

Transvaginal sonography is now well established as the preferred method for the accurate localization of a low-lying placenta. TAS is associated with a false positive rate for the diagnosis of placenta previa of up to 25%. Sixty percent of women who undergo TAS may have a reclassification of placental position when they undergo TVS. With TAS, there is a poor visualization of the posterior placenta, the fetal head can interfere with the visualization of the lower segment, and obesity and underfilling or overfilling of the bladder also interferes the accuracy. Accuracy rates for TVS are high (sensitivity 87.5%, specificity 98.8%, positive predictive value 93.3%, negative predictive value 97.6%), establishing TVS as the gold standard for the diagnosis of placenta previa (RCOG, 2018). TVS for the diagnosis of placenta previa or a low-lying placenta is superior to transabdominal approach, and is safe even when there is established vaginal bleeding (ACOG).

In women with low lying placenta (<20 mm from the internal os), or previa (covering the os), a follow-up ultrasound including a TVS is recommended at 32 weeks to diagnose persistent low-lying placenta and/or placenta previa, particularly with previous history of cesarean delivery or in the presence of other associated risk factors to clarify the diagnosis and allow planning for third-trimester management. Nearly 90% of placenta identified as "low-lying" will ultimately resolve by the third trimester. At the time of sonography, evaluation for PAS is also necessary. In women with a persistent low-lying placenta or placenta previa at 32 weeks of gestation who remain asymptomatic, an additional TVS is recommended at around 36 weeks of gestation to discuss the mode of delivery. Transvaginal ultrasonography with color and pulsed Doppler is recommended to rule out placenta previa and vasa previa, as resolution of a low-lying placenta can be associated with vasa previa **(Figs. 3 and 4)**.

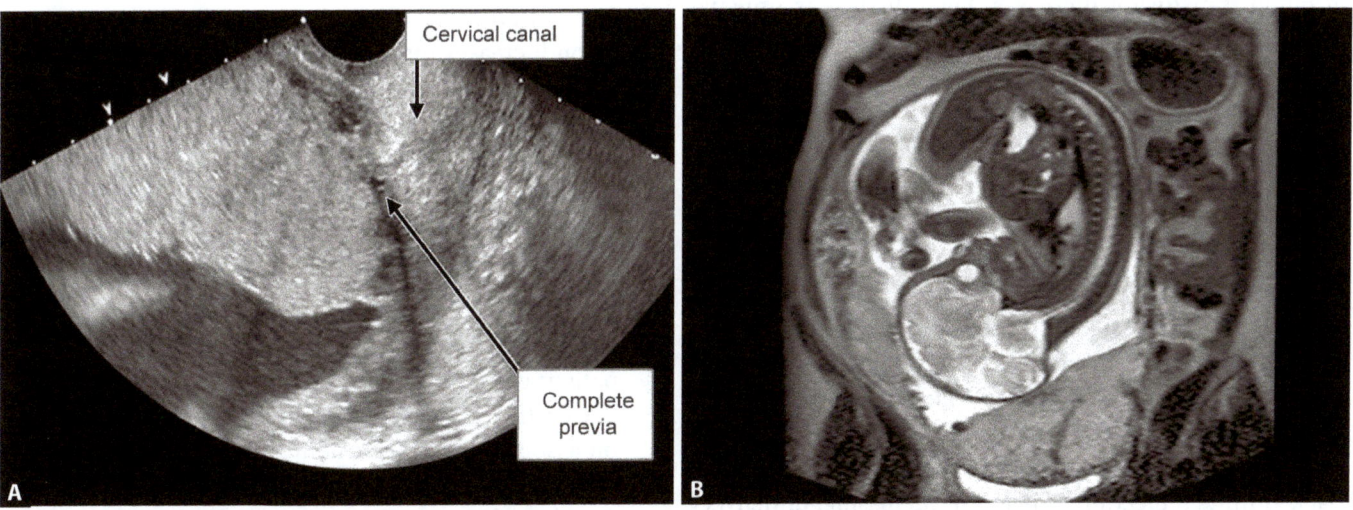

Figs. 3A and B: *Placenta previa:* (A) Transvaginal sonography (TVS); (B) Magnetic resonance imaging (MRI).

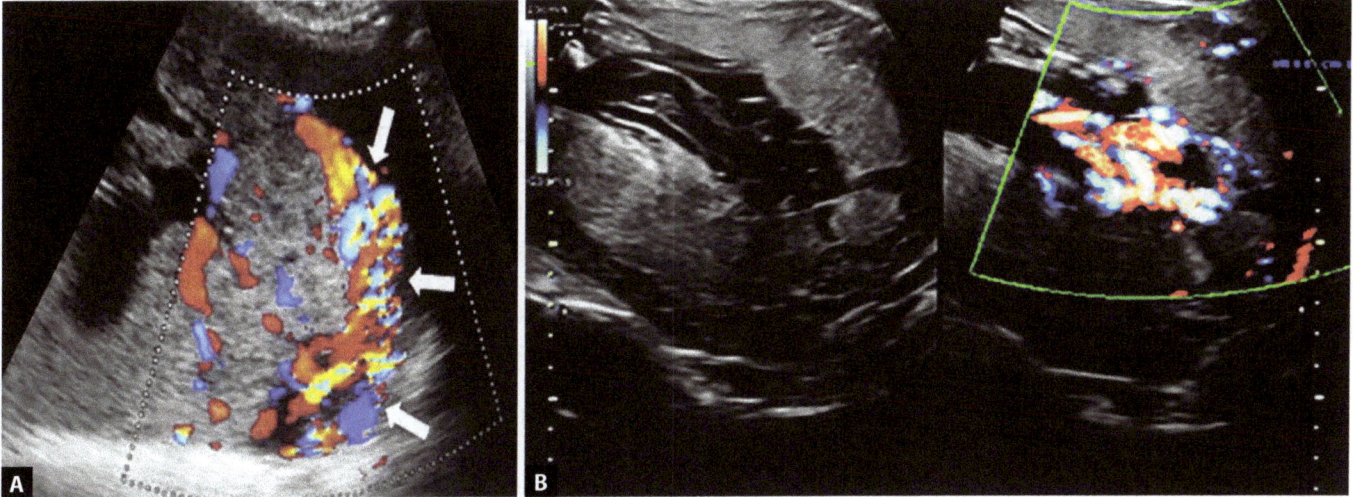

Figs. 4A and B: Color Doppler images of placenta previa.

Magnetic Resonance Imaging

It can accurately image the placenta and is superior to TAS. It is unlikely that it confers any benefit over TVS for placental localization, but can be complemented in equivocal cases to distinguish those women at the special risk of placenta accreta.

■ CLINICAL PRESENTATION

Painless vaginal bleeding during the second or third trimester of pregnancy is the usual presentation. The bleeding may be provoked from intercourse, vaginal examinations, labor, and at times there may be no identifiable cause. The first episode of bleeding typically occurs at 27–32 weeks—(in one-third cases before 30 weeks; one-third cases between 30–35 weeks and one-third cases after 36 weeks. The mean is 29.6 weeks).

Initial bleeding usually stops within few hours and usually not associated with adverse outcomes. The earlier the gestational age (GA) of first bleeding worse is the outcome, especially when it occurs before 28 weeks. With subsequent episodes of bleeding, the severity and need of blood transfusion increases. Fetal distress is unusual unless hemorrhage is severe enough to cause maternal hypovolemic shock. Abdomen is usually soft and nontender but uterine contraction commonly occurs in association with per vaginal (PV) bleeding and may provoke further bleeding (**Flowchart 1**). Avoid digital vaginal examination or speculum examination in suspected placenta previa.

■ LABORATORY INVESTIGATIONS

There is no consensus about the components of routine laboratory assessment of patients with bleeding placenta previa. At a minimum, blood should be sent for baseline CBC, type and antibody screen. The blood bank should be notified that patient may need transfusion. Cross-match 2–4 units of packed RBCs if bleeding is heavy or increasing, or delivery is likely.

Massive blood loss or suspicion of coexistent abruption should prompt evaluation for coagulopathy—fibrinogen level, activated partial thromboplastin time, prothrombin time including bed side clotting time. A Kleihauer–Betke test on a specimen of vaginal blood can diagnose fetal bleeding from disruption of fetal vessels in placental villi, vasa previa, or a velamentous cord; however, fetal bleeding typically results in fetal demise or a nonreassuring fetal heart rate tracing necessitating emergency delivery.

■ MANAGEMENT

The management of pregnancies complicated by placenta previa is best addressed in terms of the clinical setting:
- *Asymptomatic* women with low-lying placenta or placenta previa
- Women who are *actively bleeding*
- Women who are *stable after one or more episodes of active bleeding*.

Asymptomatic Women (Low-Lying Placenta or Placenta Previa)

Goal of Management
- Determine whether previa resolves with increasing GA.
- Determine whether associated with PAS or not.
- Reduce the risk of bleeding.
- Determine the optimal time for planned cesarean birth if previa persists.

Prediction of bleeding—it is not possible to accurately predict whether a bleed will occur, nor the volume, or frequency of bleeding. Sonographic features reported to be associated with a higher likelihood of bleeding include placenta completely covering the os, placenta with a thick edge (>1 cm), placenta with an echo-free space in the edge overlapping the os, and cervical length ≤3 cm.

Cervical length measurement—may help facilitate management decisions in asymptomatic women with placenta previa. A short cervical length on TVS before 34 weeks of gestation increases the risk of preterm emergency delivery and massive hemorrhage at CS. Women with a cervical length of <31 mm have 16 times (OR 16.4, 95% CI 3.4–75.9) higher risk of emergency CS due to massive hemorrhage. Consider hospitalization if CL is ≤15 mm or rapid cervical shortening (e.g., >10 mm over a one- to two-weeks period) on TVS.

Reduce the risk of bleeding:
- Avoid sexual activity after 20 weeks or earlier if the patient gives history of vaginal bleeding. The rationale is that this activity, especially if orgasm occurs, may be associated with transient uterine contractions that can provoke further bleeding.
- Avoid moderate and strenuous exercise, heavy lifting (>20 pounds), or standing for prolonged periods of time (e.g., >4 hours). This degree of activity has been linked to small but statistically significant increases in preterm birth in a meta-analysis.

Inpatient vs. Outpatient Management

Most cases can be cared as out-patients however; patient-specific risk factors need to be taken into account.
- Short cervical length on transvaginal ultrasound examination (<1.5 cm or rapid cervical shortening (e.g., >10 mm over 1–2 weeks of period)—consider hospitalization
- Inability to get to the hospital promptly (within 20 minutes)
- Lack of home support in case of an emergency.

If the woman is managed at home, it should be ensured that she has safety precautions in place, including having

Flowchart 1: Placenta previa: pathogenesis and clinical findings.

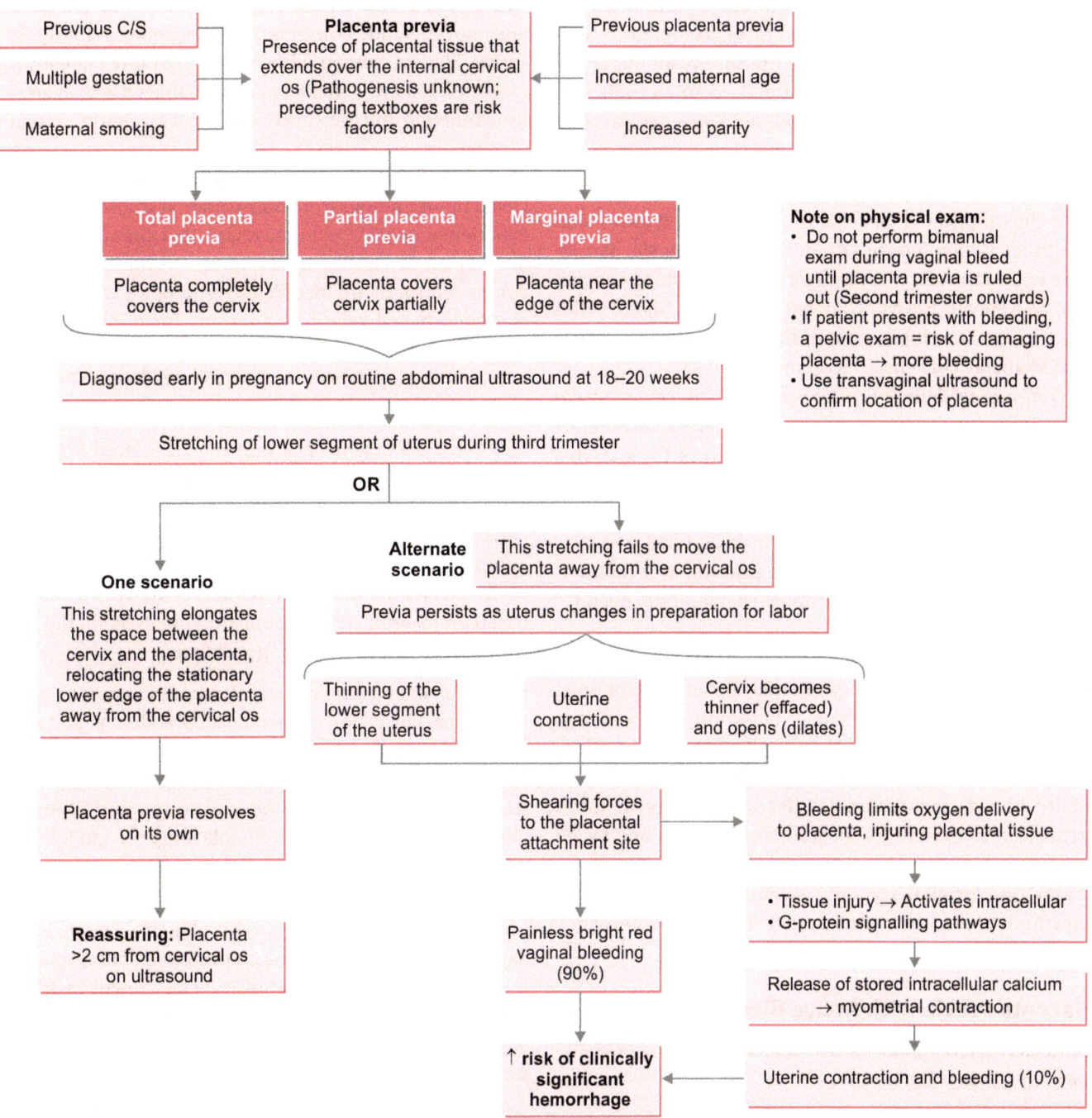

someone available to help her should need arise, and particularly, having ready access to the hospital. It should be made clear to any woman being managed at home that she should attend immediately if she experiences any bleeding, contractions or pain (including vague suprapubic period-like aches).

Antenatal corticosteroids (ACS): Administer a course of ACS 48 hours before a scheduled cesarean delivery if GA <37 weeks and if she did not already received ACS (UpToDate). A single course of antenatal corticosteroid therapy is recommended between 34+0 and 35+6 weeks of gestation for pregnant women with a low-lying placenta or placenta previa and is appropriate prior to 34+0 weeks of gestation in women at higher risk of preterm birth (RCOG, 2018).

Time and Mode of Delivery

Delivery timing should be tailored according to antenatal symptoms and, for women presenting with uncomplicated placenta previa should be accomplished at 36 weeks 0 days to 36 weeks 6 days, without documentation of fetal lung maturity by amniocentesis. The rationale behind this recommendation is that the risks associated with continuing the pregnancy (severe bleeding, emergency unscheduled delivery) are greater than the risks associated with prematurity at this GA (ACOG and the Society for Maternal-Fetal Medicine). RCOG recommends in uncomplicated placenta previa, delivery be considered between 36+0 and 37+0 weeks of gestation or before 36–37 weeks of gestation for suspected placenta accreta.

Note: Uncomplicated placenta previa is defined as no fetal growth restriction, no superimposed preeclampsia, and no other issues that take precedent for delivery decision-making (Eunice Kennedy Shriver National Institute of Child Health and Human Development and the Society for Maternal-Fetal Medicine consensus recommendations).

Optimizing delivery of women with placenta previa (RCOG): Placenta previa covering the internal os and anterior placentation are independent risk factors for massive hemorrhage during CS with risk of blood loss of >1000 mL and also have a higher risk of cesarean hysterectomy. Prior to delivery, all women with placenta previa and their partners should have a discussion regarding timing and mode of delivery, indications for blood transfusion and the need for hysterectomy.

Maternal hemorrhagic morbidity is more common when associated with predelivery anemia, thrombocytopenia, diabetes, and magnesium use. Screening, prevention, and treatment of anemia during the antenatal period, is important. Delivery should be arranged in place with onsite blood transfusion facility and access to adult critical care. Planned CS should be carried out by an appropriately experienced operator in presence of a senior obstetrician (usually a consultant) and senior anesthetist (usually a consultant) to handle emergency situation.

Placenta Previa with Active Bleeding

Management of Patients with Blood Loss 500–1,000 mL without Clinical Signs of Shock

Immediate measures:
- Hospitalization till free of P/V bleeding for at least 48 hours
- Intravenous access and blood sent immediately for grouping (if not done previously), complete blood count (CBC), coagulation screen
- Pulse, blood pressure (BP). Respiratory rate every 15 minutes
- Commence warmed crystalloid infusion.

Conservative management after an acute blood loss: Most women who initially present with symptomatic placenta previa respond to supportive therapy and do not require immediate delivery. Observational studies found, 50% of women with a symptomatic previa (any amount of bleeding) were not delivered for at least four weeks. Even a large bleed does not preclude conservative management. In one large series, 50% of women whose initial hemorrhagic episode exceeded 500 mL were successfully managed with aggressive use of antepartum transfusions and had a mean prolongation of pregnancy of 17 days.

Management of placenta previa after acute bleeding is based upon findings from observational studies and clinical experience. A 2003 Cochrane review that attempted to assess the impact of clinical interventions in these pregnancies concluded there are insufficient data upon which to make evidence-based recommendations for clinical practice. After the patient has been stabilized, the following *expectant management* approach may be followed with the goal of prolonging the pregnancy:

Expectant management: It may be considered for up to at least 36 weeks. Bed rest with limited bathroom facilities after patient has been asymptomatic. Tocolysis may be considered for 48 hours to facilitate administration of antenatal corticosteroids. As tocolytic nifedipine 10–20 mg orally every 4–6 hours is preferable. If delivery is indicated based on maternal or fetal concerns, tocolysis should not be used in an attempt to prolong gestation.

Correction of anemia: Iron supplementation may be needed for optimal correction of anemia. Stool softeners and a high-fiber diet help to minimize constipation and avoid excess straining that might precipitate bleeding.

Anti-D immune globulin: Administering anti-D-immune globulin to D-negative women following the guidelines for prevention of RhD alloimmunization.

Fetal assessment: There is no proven value of nonstress testing or performing a biophysical profile in pregnancies with asymptomatic placenta and no evidence of uteroplacental insufficiency (e.g., preeclampsia, fetal growth restriction, oligohydramnios) or other indications for antepartum fetal assessment; active vaginal bleeding is an indication for fetal monitoring.

Cervical cerclage: Cervical cerclage has been used in an attempt to minimize early development of the lower uterine segment, which is thought to promote placental separation. However, the efficacy of this approach is unproven. The use of cervical cerclage to reduce bleeding and prolong pregnancy is not supported by sufficient evidence to recommend its use outside of a clinical trial (RCOG). A meta-analysis of two, small randomized trials that evaluated cerclage for improving pregnancy outcome in placenta previa reported that cerclage reduced the risk of delivery before 34 weeks (RR 0.45, 95% CI 0.23–0.87) and the birth of a baby weighing <2,000 g (RR 0.34, 95% CI 0.14–0.83), the lack of consistency between trials and methodological issues prevent making a clear conclusion of benefit.

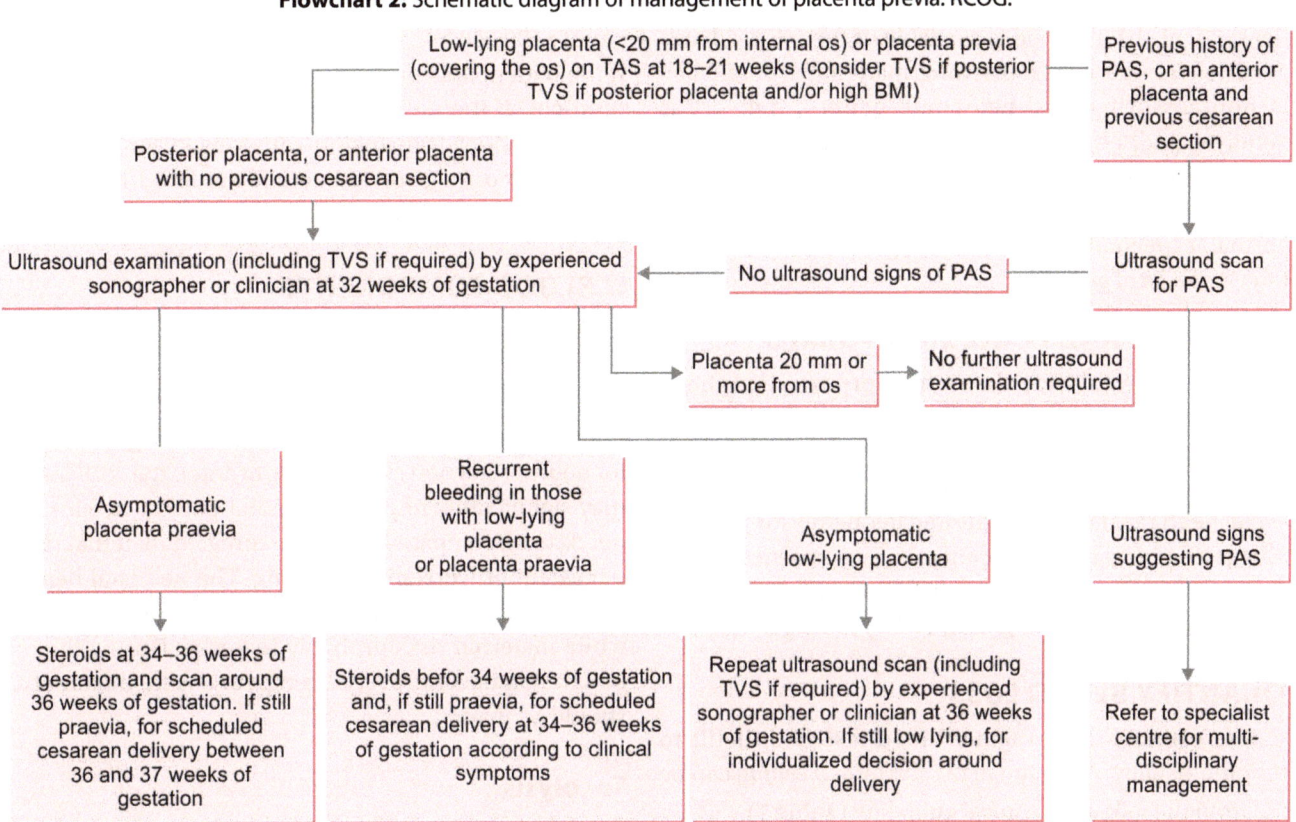

Flowchart 2: Schematic diagram of management of placenta previa: RCOG.

(PAS: placenta accreta spectrum)

Home management: Can be considered with proper counseling if fulfill the discharge criteria—

Discharge criteria:
- GA <36 weeks.
- Bleeding free for 72 hours in hospital and no abdominal pain.
- Understand the risks entailed by outpatient management.
- Be able to return to the hospital within 20 minutes.
- Have an adult companion available 24 hours/day who can immediately transport the woman to the hospital if there is light bleeding or call an ambulance for severe bleeding.
- Limited physical activity.
- Stable serial Hct ≥35%.
- Reactive nonstress test (NST) at the time of discharge.
- Weekly clinical follow-up until delivery.

Delivery: Timing of delivery depends on the patient's status. Delivery of stable patients with placenta previa (no bleeding or minimal bleeding) should be accomplished at 36–37 weeks, without documentation of fetal lung maturity by amniocentesis. For women with a low-lying placenta where the placental edge is 0–10 mm from the edge of the internal os, planned cesarean delivery as these pregnancies are at high (>50%) risk for intrapartum hemorrhage necessitating emergency cesarean delivery. Trial of labor—for those with placental edge to internal os distance 11–20 mm. These women have a >80% chance of successful vaginal delivery.

However, these are shared decisions between clinician and patient (UpToDate).

Acute Care of Bleeding Placenta Previa (Major Obstetric Hemorrhage with Blood Loss >1000 mL or Clinical Shock)

- A potential obstetric emergency
- Major goals of management are as follows:
  - Immediate admission in an equipped center with maternal and fetal monitoring and facilities for handling difficult CS
  - Achieve and/or maintain maternal hemodynamic stability
  - Determine if emergency cesarean delivery is indicated
  - The obstetric expert team, blood bank and anesthesia team should be notified.

■ MATERNAL STABILITY

Keep the patient warm. Airway: Start 10–15 L/minute of O_2 via face mask. Circulation: Establish IV channel with two wide bore IV cannula (at least 18 G) and a send a sample of blood for CBC, coagulation screen, serum creatinine, serum electrolyte, and cross-matching for at least 6 units of blood.

Intravenous access and crystalloid—crystalloid (ringer lactate or normal saline) is infused to achieve/maintain hemodynamic stability and adequate urine output (at least 30 mL/h) till blood is available. If there is evidence of persistent severe vaginal bleeding, maternal hypotension, or a nonreassuring fetal heart rate pattern, delivery is generally expedited via CS regardless of GA. If bleeding is not persistent and severe, the mother is hemodynamically stable or quickly stabilized, and the fetal heart rate pattern is normal, expectant management is preferable to delivery before 34 weeks of gestation.

■ MATERNAL AND FETAL MONITORING

- Monitor maternal BP, pulse, respiratory rate, peripheral oxygen saturation, and urine output. Tachypnea, tachycardia, hypotension, low oxygen saturation, and air hunger are signs of hypovolemia.
- Fetal heart rate is to be monitored frequently for patterns suggestive of hypoxemia or anemia. The presence of fetal hypoxia or anemia may result in category 2 or 3 fetal heart rate on cardiotocography (CTG) tracings.

■ QUANTIFY BLOOD LOSS

Accurate estimation of vaginal blood loss is difficult to determine visually. Assessment of *severity of bleeding* can be made from the following clinical guideline **(Table 1)**.

Transfusion

Transfusion of blood products in a woman with an actively bleeding placenta previa should be guided by the volume of blood loss over time and changes in hemodynamic parameters (e.g., BP, maternal and fetal heart rates, peripheral perfusion, and urine output), as well as the hemoglobin level. A reasonable approach is to begin red cell transfusions in hypotensive patients whose BP fails to improve after 2 L of crystalloid have been rapidly infused. It is important to not get behind in replacement of blood products.

Cross-match at least 6 units of blood when bleeding is heavy or increasing or delivery is likely for any reason. Initially, transfuse 2–4 units of typed and crossed-packed red blood cells (RBCs), without fresh frozen plasma or platelets as long as the fibrinogen level is >250 mg/dL and the platelet count >100,000/μL; goal is final hemoglobin value >10 g/dL. If the patient fails to stabilize, initiate a massive transfusion protocol. If the patient continues to bleed, use the same blood product transfusion ratios used for patients with severe hemorrhage of other etiologies (1:1:1 ratio of packed RBC: fresh frozen plasma: platelets).

■ BLOOD COMPONENTS

Indications and dosing in adults are given in **Table 2**.

Administration of Magnesium Sulfate

If gestational age is less than 32 weeks, magnesium sulfate for neuroprotection and a course of antenatal corticosteroids may significantly improve neonatal outcomes. This benefit needs to be compared with the estimated maternal risk from persistent or worsening bleeding. The neonatal benefits of avoiding expeditious delivery decrease with advancing GA, while maternal risks probably increase. During the period of decision making, every attempt to ensure maternal safety should be made.

Tocolysis

Do not administer tocolytic drugs to actively bleeding patients. Women presenting with symptomatic placenta previa or a low-lying placenta tocolysis may be considered for 48 hours to facilitate administration of antenatal corticosteroids (RCOG, 2018). If tocolytics are used, *indomethacin* has an inhibitory effect on platelet function and should be avoided in women with placenta previa due to the risk of increased blood loss.

Antishock Garments

Antishock garments have been used to restore adequate BP in pregnant/postpartum women who are hemodynamically unstable due to severe bleeding in low resource settings. However, these devices have not been used when the fetus was viable and there is no information on their effect on uteroplacental blood flow and the fetus.

TABLE 1: Assessment of severity of blood loss.

Parameters	I	II	III	IV
Blood loss in mL	<750 mL <15%	750–1500 mL 15–30%	1500–2000 mL 30–40%	>2000 mL >40%
Pulse rate (bpm)	<100	100–120	120–140	>140
Blood pressure	Normal	Decreased	Decreased	Decreased
Respiratory rate/min	14–20	20–30	30–40	>40
Urine output mL/h	>30	20–30	5–15	Negligible
CNS symptoms	Normal	Anxious	Confused	Lethargic

(CNS: central nervous system)

TABLE 2: Indications and dosing in adults.

Component (volume)	Contents	Indications and dose
Whole blood (1 unit = 500 mL)	RBCs, platelets, plasma	• Rarely required • May be appropriate when massive bleeding requires transfusion of >5–7 units of RBCs
RCC in additive solution (1 unit = 350 mL)	RBCs	• Anemia, bleeding • 1 unit will approximately raise Hb 1 g/dL; the increase in hematocrit will be 3%/unit
FFP or other plasma product* (1 unit = 200–300 mL)	All soluble plasma proteins and clotting factors	• Bleeding associated with DIC, liver disease, massive transfusion, warfarin overdose • In the rare event that FFP is used to replace a clotting factor, the dose is 10–20 mg/kg. This dose will raise the level of any factor, including fibrinogen, by close to 30%, which is typically sufficient for hemostasis
Platelets (1 unit of apheresis platelets or a 5 to 6 units of pooled platelets from whole blood = 200–300 mL)	Platelets	• The platelet count increase from 5 to 6 units of whole blood-derived platelets or 1 unit of apheresis platelets will be approximately 30,000/μL in an average-sized adult

Note: Frozen blood products* (FFP, cryoprecipitate) take 10–30 minutes to thaw. It may take the same amount of time to perform an uncomplicated cross match.
(DIC: disseminated intravascular coagulation; FPP: fresh frozen plasma; RBCs: red blood cells; RCC: red cell concentrates)

■ DELIVERY

Cesarean delivery is indicated if any of the following occurs:
- A nonreassuring fetal heart rate tracing unresponsive to resuscitative measures.
- Life-threatening maternal hemorrhage refractory to standard interventions (transfusion, tocolysis, rest)
- Significant vaginal bleeding after 34 weeks of gestation
- Active labor

Anesthesia

General anesthesia is typically administered for emergency cesarean delivery, especially in hemodynamically unstable women or if the fetal status is nonreassuring. However, regional anesthesia (epidural anesthetic) is an acceptable choice in hemodynamically stable women with reassuring fetal heart rate tracings. When prolonged surgery is anticipated in women with prenatally diagnosed placenta accreta, general anesthesia may be preferable, and regional analgesia could be converted to general anesthesia if undiagnosed accreta is encountered.

Cesarean Procedure

Two to four units of packed RBCs should be available for the delivery. Appropriate surgical instruments for performance of a cesarean hysterectomy should also be available since these patients are at increased risk of placenta accreta, even in the absence of a prior cesarean delivery. Evaluation for placenta previa-accreta should have been performed antenatally, with appropriate preparations for management. The surgeon should try to avoid disrupting the placenta when entering the uterus. If the placenta is incised, hemorrhage from fetal vessels can result in significant neonatal anemia.

A vertical skin incision is the recommended incision for optimal exposure. Preoperative or intraoperative sonographic localization is helpful in determining the position of the hysterotomy incision. A high vertical uterine incision may be required if the placenta is covering the lower uterine segment, or if the lower uterine segment is underdeveloped. If the placenta is transected during the uterine incision, immediately clamp the umbilical cord after delivery of the fetus to avoid excessive fetal blood loss.

After fetal delivery, sometimes, the placenta gets detached, and the uterine incision can be closed. However, severe bleeding may occur from the placental bed, secondary to the decreased contractability of the lower uterine segment, which can be managed with bimanual uterine massage, uterotonics, intrauterine tamponade using balloon or gauze, B-Lynch sutures, uterine artery or internal iliac artery ligation, and uterine artery or internal iliac artery embolization. At times the massive hemorrhage may not be controlled with conservative measures, and a hysterectomy is necessary.

Vasopressin

After removal of the placenta, subendometrial injection of vasopressin at the placental implantation site may be beneficial. The favorable effect has been attributed to binding to the vasopressin V1α receptor, which is highly expressed in smooth muscle cells in the lower segment of the uterus. Intravascular injection should be avoided, as it can cause severe adverse cardiovascular effects (bradycardia, cardiac arrhythmia, ischemia, right heart failure, shock, cardiac arrest, limb ischemia.

POSTPARTUM HEMORRHAGE

In a systematic review, 16–29% of patients with a placenta previa had a postpartum hemorrhage. The reason for the increased risk of postpartum hemorrhage is thought to be that the myometrium of the lower uterine segment does not contract as effectively as the upper uterine segment, and thus may impede physiologic hemostasis from a lower segment placental bed. In some cases, hemorrhage is due to focal placenta accrete. Postpartum hemorrhage is approached in the following ways:

Step one: Administer uterotonic drugs and tranexamic acid; consider temporizing maneuvers.

Oxytocin—the dose of oxytocin can be increased, as needed, to control heavy bleeding.

Tranexamic acid—if oxytocin alone does not control hemorrhage, administer tranexamic acid as soon as possible. *Dose:* 1 g IV over 10–20 minutes, Infusion of more than 1 mL/min can cause hypotension. If bleeding persists after 30 minutes, a second 1 g dose is administered. Tranexamic acid can be given concomitantly with other uterotonic drugs and procedures to reduce bleeding.

Tourniquets—tourniquets like a bladder catheter or soft drain tube can be tied tightly around the uterus as low as possible to occlude the uterine vessels in the broad ligaments and then secured with a clamp as a temporary measure while going for medical therapy or surgical interventions.

Step two: Ligation of myometrial vessels at the placental site will control focal bleeding in patients who have a focal placenta accreta and some patients who responded poorly to intravenous uterotonic therapy.

Treat focal bleeding by *the following options:*
- *Affronti endouterine hemostatic square*—ligation of myometrial vessels at the placental site, techniques involve making 4-6, 2 × 2 cm² in the area of placental bed bleeding by 1.0 Polyglactin sutures. The ends of the sutures are tied down tightly to compress the enclosed vessels, the suture should penetrate the decidua and extend into the myometrium but not beyond the uterine serosa **(Fig. 5B)**.
- Placement of *fibrin glue* or *patch over area* of oozing to promote clotting
- Application of ferric subsulfate (Monsel's solution) to the oozing area
- Placental site injection of vasopressin: Evidence based on two small studies. Local injection of 4 units of vasopressin in 20 mL of saline into the placental implantation site significantly reduced blood loss without increasing morbidity.
- *Excision*, if the area is small and easily accessible particularly in cases of focal placenta accreta with persistent bleeding.

Step three: Ligation of the uterine and utero-ovarian arteries (O'Leary stitch) **(Fig. 5A)**.

It can decrease diffuse uterine bleeding by reducing perfusion pressure in the myometrium.

Step four: If bleeding persists, the next step is either intrauterine balloon tamponed and/or uterine compression sutures. Uterine compression sutures may be more effective for atony and fundal bleeding, whereas the balloon may be more effective for lower segment bleeding.

TECHNIQUE OF INTRAUTERINE BALLOON TAMPONED DURING CS

The stem of a balloon/condom catheter can be passed through the uterine incision, through the cervical os, and

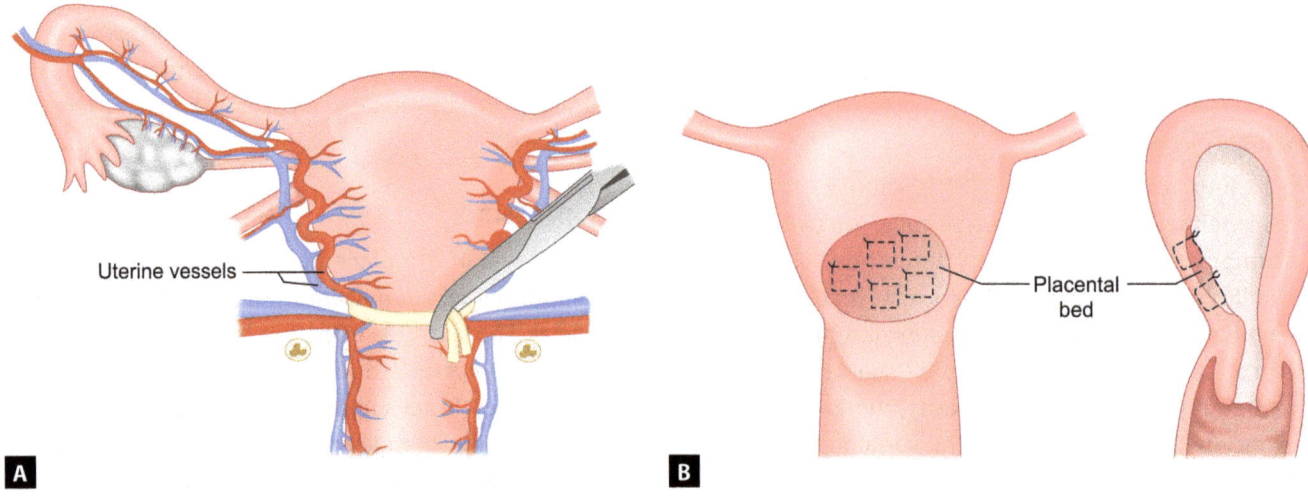

Figs. 5A and B: *Treatment of focal bleeding:* (A) By Tourniquets; (B) By hemostatic square sutures.

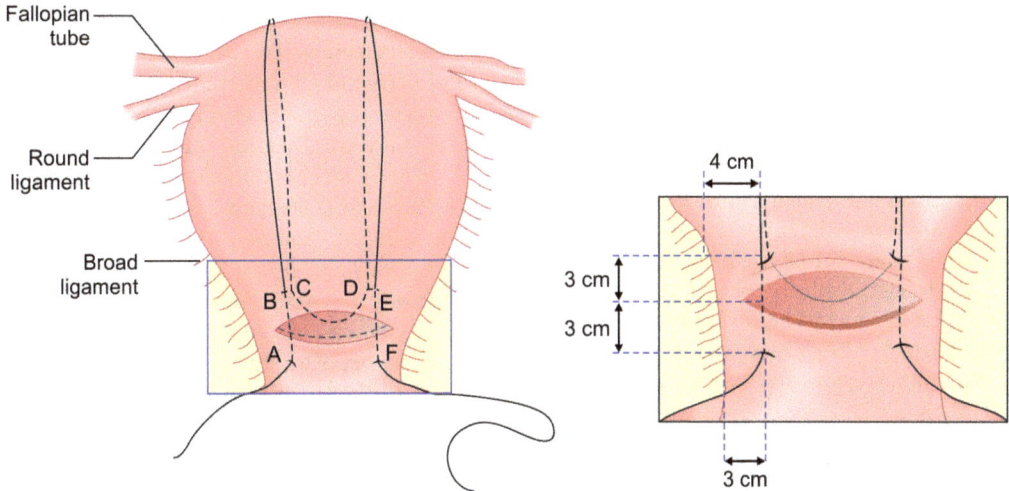

Fig. 6: Application of B-Lynch suture. A large needle with #2 chromic catgut is used to enter and exit the uterine cavity at A and B. The suture is looped over the fundus and then re-enters the uterine cavity posteriorly at C, which is directly below B. The suture should be pulled very tight at this point. It then enters the posterior wall of the uterine cavity at D. It is then looped back over the fundus, and anchored by entering the anterior lateral lower uterine segment at E and crossing through the uterine cavity to exit at F. The free ends at A and F are tied down securely to compress the uterus. The procedure was originally described by Christopher B-Lynch.

then into the vagina; an assistant then pulls the end of the catheter out of the introitus. The balloon can be left deflated or inflated with 50–100 mL sterile saline to reduce the risk of puncture when the hysterotomy incision is closed. After the uterine incision is closed, the assistant inflates the balloon to its maximum volume with sterile fluid while the surgeon inspects the uterus from above.

Uterine compression sutures: If a balloon tamponade is ineffective, the balloon can be deflated and a B-Lynch uterine compression suture is applied **(Fig. 6)**. The hysterotomy site is then closed, the uterus replaced in the pelvis (if previously exteriorized), and the balloon is reinflated, thereby applying pressure to both the outer and inner surfaces of the myometrium. It is important to observe the myometrium and stop instilling fluid before undue blanching occurs at the compression suture sites, which might lead to rupture or uterine necrosis.

REFRACTORY PATIENT

Consider arterial embolization: When the above measures have failed, uterine, or hypogastric artery embolization in an operating room with the full surgical team in attendance is an option if the facility has a hybrid operating room, or an operating room that allows simultaneous surgery and embolization, embolization is preferable to surgical internal iliac artery ligation.

Hysterectomy: As a last resort, ideally, it should be performed before severe hypovolemia, tissue hypoxia, hypothermia, electrolyte abnormalities, and acidosis have developed, which further compromise the patient's status.

CONCLUSION

Placenta previa can lead to serious consequences and requires immediate attention to the presentation of vaginal bleeding. An interprofessional team approach must be taken to provide the utmost care for the patient. Patients diagnosed with placenta previa prior to vaginal bleeding should have multiple discussions between clinician and patient with husband regarding management and expectations. Patients should consent for possible blood transfusions, uterine artery embolization, and possible cesarean hysterectomy. Various interprofessional team approach management can save life of the patient in emergencies.

SUGGESTED READING

1. American College of Obstetricians and Gynecologists' Committee on Obstetric Practice, Society for Maternal-Fetal Medicine. Medically Indicated Late-Preterm and Early-Term Deliveries: ACOG Committee Opinion, Number 831. Obstet Gynecol. 2021;138(1):e35-9.
2. Anderson-Bagga FM, Sze A. Placenta Previa. StatPearls [Internet]. Treasure Island (FL): StatPearls Publishing; 2022.
3. Arduini M, Epicoco G, Clerici G, Bottaccioli E, Arena S, Affronti G. B-Lynch suture, intrauterine balloon, and endo-uterine hemostatic suture for the management of postpartum hemorrhage due to placenta previa accreta. Int J Gynaecol Obstet. 2010;108(3):191-3.
4. Bakker R. (2018). Placenta Previa. [online] Available from https://emedicine.medscape.com/article/262063-overview. [Last Accessed April, 2022].
5. Bose P, Regan F, Paterson-Brown S. Improving the accuracy of estimated blood loss at obstetric haemorrhage using clinical reconstructions. BJOG. 2006;113(8):919-24.

6. Caric V, Bhide A. Antepartum Haemorrhage. Arias' Practical Guide to High-Risk Pregnancy and Delivery, 5th edition. Gurugram, India: Elsevier; 2015. pp. 137-41.
7. Cresswell JA, Ronsmans C, Calvert C, Filippi V. Prevalence of placenta praevia by world region: a systematic review and meta-analysis. Trop Med Int Health. 2013,18(6):712-24.
8. Hull AD, Resnik R, Silver RM. Placenta previa and Accreta, Vsa Previa, subchorionic Hemorrhage and Abruptio Placentae in Creasy & Resniks' Maternal-Fetal Medicine, 8th edition. Gurugram, India: Elsevier; 2018. pp. 786.
9. Jansen C, de Mooij YM, Blomaard CM, Derks JB, van Leeuwen E, Limpens J, et al. Vaginal delivery in women with a low-lying placenta: a systematic review and meta-analysis. BJOG. 2019(9);126:1118-26.
10. Jansen C, de Mooij YM, Blomaard CM, Derks JB, van Leeuwen E, Limpens J, et al. Vaginal delivery in women with a low-lying placenta: a systematic review and meta-analysis. BJOG. 2019(9);126:1118-26.
11. Jauniaux E, Alfirevic Z, Bhide AG, Belfort MA, Burton GJ, Collins SL, et al. Placenta praevia and placenta accreta: diagnosis and management: Green-top Guideline No. 27a. BJOG. 2019;126(1):e1-48.
12. Kavak SB, Atilgan R, Demirel I, Celik E, Ilhan R, Sapmaz E. Endouterine hemostatic square suture vs. Bakri balloon tamponade for intractable hemorrhage due to complete placenta previa. J Perinat Med. 2013;41(6):705-9.
13. Lam CM, Wong SF, Chow KM, Ho LC. Women with placenta praevia and antepartum haemorrhage have a worse outcome than those who do not bleed before delivery. J Obstet Gynaecol. 2000;20(1):27-31.
14. Lockwood CJ, Russo-Stieglitz K. (2022). Placenta previa: Management. [online] UpToDate website. Available from https://www.uptodate.com/contents/placenta-previa-management. [Last accessed April, 2022].
15. Lockwood CJ, Russo-Stieglitz K. Management of placenta previa. UpToDate. 2017.
16. Ottawa OL. Diagnosis and management of placenta previa. SOGC Clin Prac Guideline. 2007;189:261-6.
17. Pacheco LD, Hankins GDV, Saad AF, Costantine MM, Chiossi G, Saade GR. Tranexamic acid for the management of obstetric hemorrhage. Obstet Gynecol. 2017;130(4):765-9.
18. Reddy UM, Abuhamad AZ, Levine D, Saade GR; Fetal Imaging Workshop Invited Participants. Fetal imaging: executive summary of a joint Eunice Kennedy Shriver National Institute of Child Health and Human Development, Society for Maternal-Fetal Medicine, American Institute of Ultrasound in Medicine, American College of Obstetricians and Gynecologists, American College of Radiology, Society for Pediatric Radiology, and Society of Radiologists in Ultrasound Fetal Imaging Workshop. Obstet Gynecol. 2014;33(5):745-57.
19. Shin JE, Shin JC, Lee Y, Kim SJ. Serial change in cervical length for the prediction of emergency cesarean section in placenta previa. PLoS One. 2016;11(2):e0149036.
20. Society for Maternal-Fetal Medicine (SMFM). Electronic address: pubs@smfm.org, Gyamfi-Bannerman C. Society for Maternal-Fetal Medicine (SMFM) Consult Series #44: Management of bleeding in the late preterm period. Am J Obstet Gynecol. 2018(1);B2-8.
21. Suarez S, Conde-Agudelo A, Borovac-Pinheiro A, Suarez-Rebling D, Eckardt M, Theron G, et al. Uterine balloon tamponade for the treatment of postpartum hemorrhage: a systematic review and meta-analysis. Am J Obstet Gynecol. 2020;222(4):293.e1-52.

CHAPTER 12

Placenta Accreta Spectrum Disorders

■ INTRODUCTION

The term placenta accreta spectrum (PAS) is a spectrum of disorders ranging from abnormally adherent to deeply invasive placental tissue including which have invaded into the adjacent viscera (percreta). PAS describes a clinical situation where the placenta does not get detached spontaneously after delivery or cannot be forcibly removed without causing a massive and potentially life-threatening hemorrhage.

The clinical implication of this obstetric complication includes massive hemorrhage, which leads to secondary complications including coagulopathy, multisystem organ failure, and death. Other complications include damage to adjacent organs, cesarean hysterectomy, and significant maternal morbidity. Research suggests that up to 7% of women with this condition may die and up to 60% experience significant morbidities.

■ PREVALENCE

The prevalence of PAS disorders in the general population of pregnant women is around 1.7 per 10,000 pregnancies. The incidence is 4.1% in women with one prior cesarean delivery and 13.3% in women with two or more previous cesarean sections.

The recent increase in the prevalence of PAS disorders is a consequence of the change in risk factors, most notably the increased rate of cesarean delivery. Over the last 40 years, cesarean section rates have risen globally from <10% to over 30% and at the same time, a 10-fold increase in the incidence of PAS has been reported. Recent publications from all over the world reported a notable increase in the prevalence of this condition, with an incidence of one in 533 births to even one in 321 births in populations with higher rates of the cesarean section [The International Federation of Gynecology and Obstetrics (FIGO)]. A 2016 study conducted in the United States using the National Inpatient Sample found that the overall rate of placenta accreta was 1 in 272 for women who had a hospital birth, higher than any other published study.

■ RISK FACTORS

Direct Surgical Scar

The most common risk factor is a previous cesarean delivery, the incidence of PAS increases with the number of prior cesarean deliveries. In a systematic review, the rate of PAS increased from 0.3% in women with one previous cesarean delivery to 6.74% for women with five or more cesarean deliveries. The 2016 Nordic Obstetric Surveillance Study found that the risk of invasive placentation increases sevenfold after one prior cesarean section. A large multicenter US cohort study found that for women presenting with placenta previa and prior cesarean deliveries, the risk of accreta was 3%, 11%, 40%, 61%, and 67% for first, second, third, fourth, and fifth or more cesareans respectively. These risks were independent of other maternal characteristics, such as parity, body mass index, tobacco use, and coexisting hypertension or diabetes.

Surgical Techniques

Single-layer closure in cesarean operation could play a role in the etiology of PAS disorders, and may be associated with thinner residual *myometrial thickness* as evaluated by postoperative ultrasound.

Placenta Previa

The placenta previa is another significant risk factor. PAS occurs in 3% of women diagnosed with placenta previa with no prior cesarean deliveries.

Other Surgical Trauma

Placenta accreta spectrum is not exclusively a consequence of cesarean delivery. Other surgical trauma to the integrity of the uterine endometrium and/or superficial myometrium, such as those following uterine curettage, endometrial resection, manual removal of the placenta, myomectomy has been associated with accreta placentation in subsequent pregnancies. Overall, the adjusted odds ratio (aOR) for PAS after previous uterine surgery is 3.40 [95% confidence interval (CI) 1.30–8.91]. Nonsurgical scars such as uterine artery embolization, chemotherapy, and radiation, endometritis, and intrauterine devices are additional risk factors for PAS.

Uterine Pathology

Development of PAS disorders has also been reported in women with no prior uterine surgery, but with uterine pathology such as the bicornuate uterus, adenomyosis, submucous fibroids, and myotonic dystrophy.

Other Risk Factors

Other risk factors include advanced maternal age, grand multiparity, smoking, and conception by in vitro fertilization (IVF).

Placental Biomarkers as Predictors of Placenta Accreta Spectrum Disorders

Abnormal results of placental biomarkers increase the risk of PAS. Unexplained elevation in maternal serum α-*fetoprotein* is associated with an increased risk of PAS. However, maternal serum α-fetoprotein is not accurate enough to be clinically useful. Other placental analytes linked to PAS include pregnancy-associated plasma protein-A (PAPP-A), pro-B-type natriuretic peptide, troponin, and free human chorionic gonadotropin (β-hCG) [messenger ribonucleic acid (mRNA)], and human placental lactogen (cell-free mRNA). In addition, other proposed markers of aberrant trophoblast invasion, such as total placental cell-free mRNA, may be associated with PAS. As with α-fetoprotein, they are too nonspecific for clinical use.

PATHOPHYSIOLOGY

The most favored hypothesis regarding the etiology of PAS is that a defect of the endometrial-myometrial interface leads to a failure of normal *decidualization* in the area of a uterine scar, which allows abnormally deep placental anchoring villi and trophoblast infiltration.

Disruption of the decidua, for example by a previous cesarean delivery incision, may result in loss of the inherent regulation and uncontrolled invasion of extravillous trophoblast through the entire depth of the myometrium. The extent of penetration of the villous tissue within the myometrium is likely to be related to the degree of deciduous-myometrial damage. Conditions such as manual removal of the placenta, uterine curettage, and endometritis are more likely to result in abnormally adherent placentation (accreta). On the other hand, a full-thickness surgical scar is associated with both the absence of endometrial re-epithelialization and vascular remodeling around the scar area, and this may lead to abnormally invasive placentation (increta/percreta). However, this explanation fails to explain the rare occurrence of PAS in nulliparous women without any previous uterine surgery or instrumentation.

Conception by IVF is a risk factor for PAS. A characteristic hormonal milieu at the time of implantation and placentation resulting from IVF may enhance trophoblast invasion and cause PAS. Aberrant placentation may be the effect of elevated serum estrogens at the time of embryo implantation, which may lead to excessive trophoblastic invasion through the endometrium. Alternatively, lower serum estradiol levels together with the presence of a thinner decidualized endometrium may result in abnormal trophoblastic growth leading to PAS.

TYPES OF PLACENTA ACCRETA SPECTRUM DISORDERS

Placenta accreta spectrum encompasses three histopathological diagnoses depending on depth of villus tissue invasion—(1) placenta accreta, (2) placenta increta, and (3) placenta percreta.

1. *Placenta accreta (also called placenta creta, vera or adherenta)*, where the placental villi adhere superficially to the myometrium without invading it. The cases of placenta accrete are often subdivided into *total, partial,* or *focal* according to the amount of placental tissue involved and the different depths of accreta placentation found to coexist in the same case.
2. *Placenta increta:* Villi penetrating deep in the myometrium up to the serosa.
3. *Placenta percreta:* Villi invade full thickness of the myometrium including the uterine serosa and sometimes to adjacent pelvic organs (**Fig. 1**), e.g., the bladder.

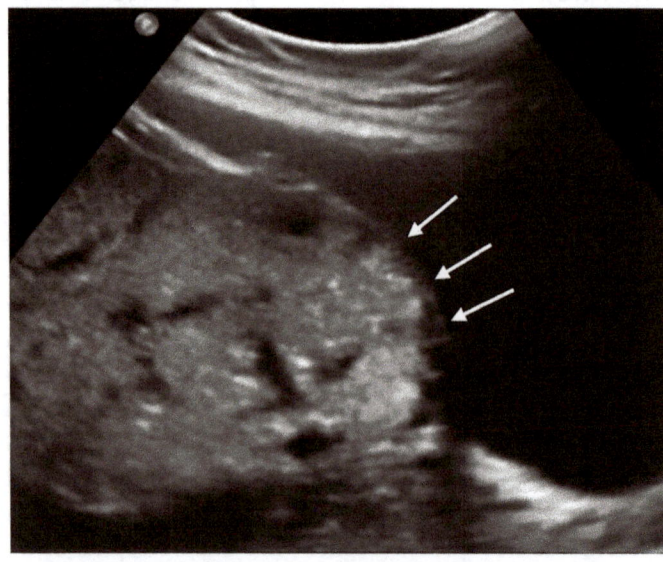

Fig. 1: Placenta percreta with invasion of bladder (arrows).

DIAGNOSIS

Clinical Features

- There may be no signs or symptoms antenatally.
- There might be possible hematuria if there is percreta in the bladder.

The presence of any risk factors needs prompt sonographic search for accreta especially when any part of the placenta lies under the previous C/S scar. Accurate antenatal diagnosis of PAS is highly crucial because outcomes are optimized when delivery occurs at a level III or IV maternal care facility before the onset of labor or bleeding and with avoidance of placental disruption. While antenatal diagnostic accuracy reaches 95% in a series from experienced centers, several population studies found that PAS remains undetected before delivery in half of the cases in the overall population. Therefore, women with relevant clinical risk factors for PAS (e.g., placenta previa and a cesarean scar) should undergo ultrasound evaluation in a center with expertise in this condition.

Ultrasonogram

Ultrasound imaging is highly accurate when performed by a skilled operator with experience in diagnosing *placenta accreta spectrum*. The International Society for PAS proposed a standardized definition of the PAS for ultrasound descriptors, in order to improve the comparability among studies, increase the diagnostic accuracy, and facilitate the international collaboration on the study of PAS.

Women with a history of previous cesarean section seen to have an anterior low-lying placenta or placenta previa at the routine fetal anomaly scan (18–22 weeks) should be specifically screened for PAS [Royal College of Obstetricians and Gynaecologists (RCOG)]. In cases with asymptomatic suspected major placenta previa or a question of placenta accrete; imaging should be performed again at around 32 weeks of gestation (ACOG). This will allow for the assessment of previa resolution, placental location to optimize the timing of delivery, and possible bladder invasion and allow planning for third-trimester management, further imaging, and delivery.

In 2016, the "European Working Group on Abnormally Invasive Placenta (AIP)" standardized the definitions of AIP by analysis of all 23 studies in a systematic review of the antenatal sonographic diagnosis.

Ultrasound criteria for diagnosis are as follows:
- *Grayscale (Figs. 2A and B):*
  - Loss of clear zone—loss or irregularity of the retroplacental sonolucent zone (hypoechoic plane in myometrium underneath placental bed known as *clear zone*).
  - Abnormal placental lacunae—the presence of numerous lacunae including some that are large

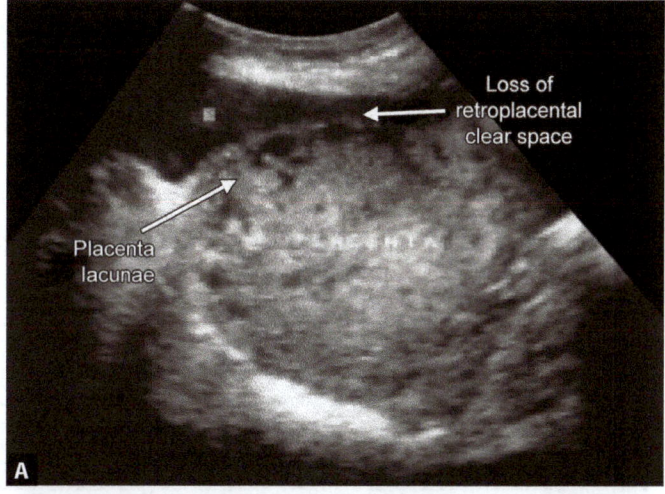
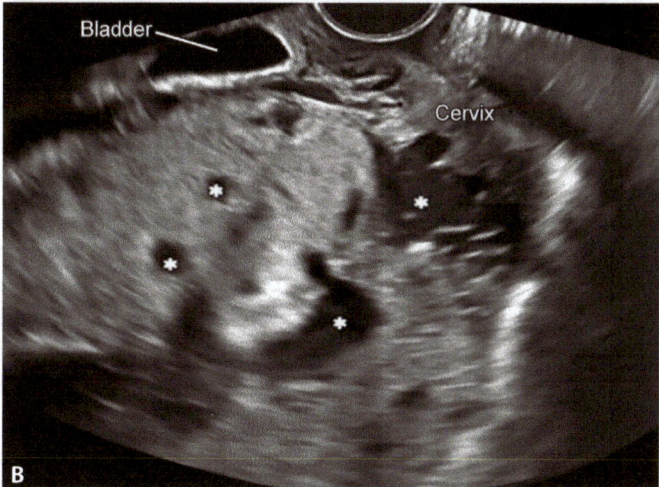

Figs. 2A and B: Gray scale of placenta previa.

and irregular (Finberg grade 3), often containing a *turbulent flow* visible on grayscale imaging.
- Bladder wall interruption—loss or interruption of bright bladder wall (hyperechoic band or "line" between uterine serosa and bladder lumen).
- Myometrial thinning—thinning of myometrium overlying placenta to <1 mm or undetectable.
- Placental bulge—deviation of uterine serosa away from the expected plane, caused by abnormal placental tissue into a neighboring organ, typically bladder; uterine serosa appears intact but outline shape is distorted.
- Focal exophytic mass—placental tissue seen breaking through uterine serosa and extending beyond it; most often seen inside the urinary bladder.

Color Doppler

The use of color flow Doppler imaging may facilitate the diagnosis:
- *Intraplacental hypervascularity*—complex, irregular arrangement of numerous placental vessels, exhibiting tortuous courses, and varying calibers.

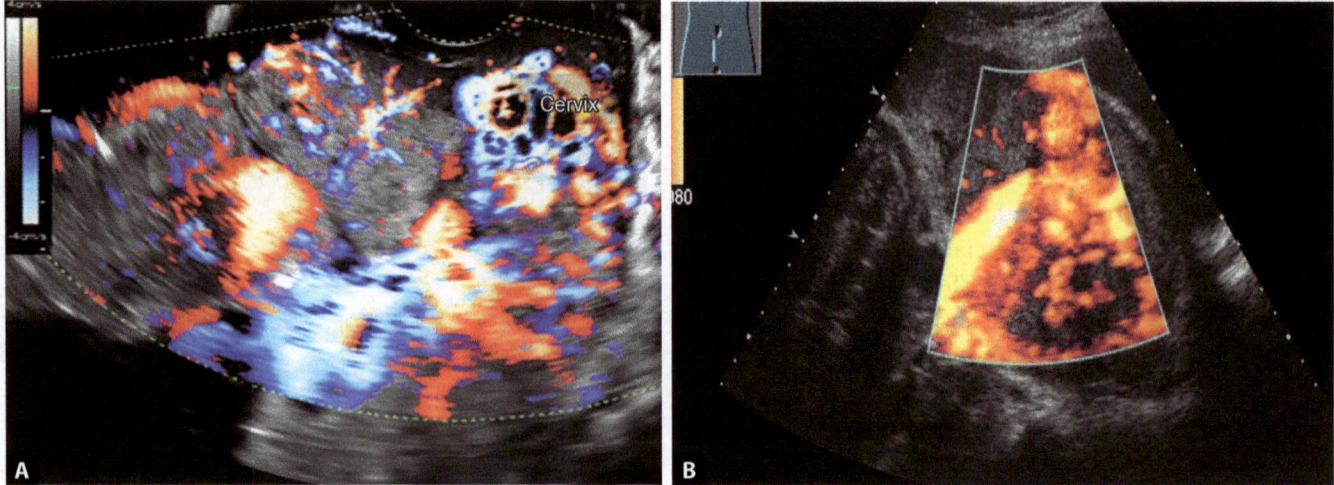

Figs. 3A and B: (A) Color Doppler of placenta percreta; (B) Extensive vascularity in the area of invasion.

- *Turbulent lacunar blood flow*—vessels with high-velocity blood flow leading from myometrium into placental lacunae, causing turbulence upon entry, is the most common finding of PAS on color flow Doppler imaging.
- *Hypervascularity of serosa bladder interface*—the striking amount of color Doppler signal seen between myometrium and posterior wall of the bladder; this sign probably indicates numerous, closely packed, tortuous vessels in that region (demonstrating multidirectional flow and aliasing artifact).
- *Bridging vessels*—vessels appearing to extend from placenta, across myometrium, and beyond serosa into bladder or other organs; often running perpendicular to myometrium.

Three-dimensional power Doppler shows the following (**Figs. 3A and B**):
- Numerous coherent vessels involving the whole uterine serosa—bladder junction (basal-view)
- Hypervascularity (lateral-view)
- Inseparable cotyledonal and intervillous circulations, chaotic branching, detour vessels (lateral-view).

Magnetic Resonance Imaging

The role of magnetic resonance imaging (MRI) in diagnosing placenta accreta is still debated. A recent systematic review found that most studies are of a small sample size, and thus sensitivity and specificity of MRI in diagnosing accreta placentation varies widely between 75 and 100%, and 65 and 100%, respectively. Currently, MRI may be used to complement ultrasound imaging to assess the depth of invasion and lateral extension of myometrial invasion, especially with posterior placentation and/or in women with ultrasound signs suggesting parametrial invasion. Two recent comparative studies have shown sonography and MRI to be comparable; (sensitivity 93% versus 80% and specificity 71% versus 65% for ultrasound versus MRI).

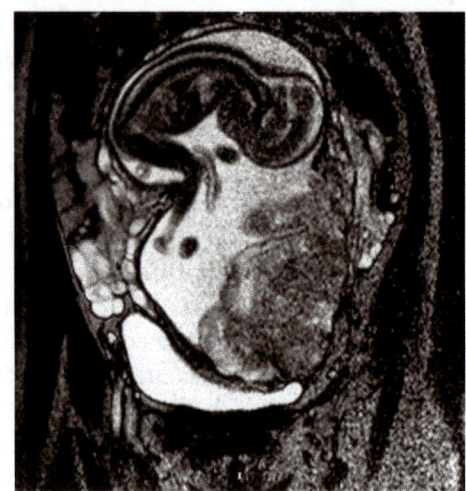

Fig. 4: MRI showing placenta previa with percreta.

Figure 4 shows MRI in placenta percreta. The main MRI features suggestive of placenta accreta include:
- Indistinctness or the absence of a myometrial wall at the placental site
- Loss of the thin T2 dark uteroplacental interface
- A nodular interface between the placenta and the uterus, a mass effect of the placenta on the uterus causing a uterine outer bulge
- Heterogeneous signal intensity within the placenta
- Dark intraplacental bands on *T2-weighted images*, and abnormal dilated venous lakes within the placenta.

MANAGEMENT

Key steps to management:
- Accurate prenatal diagnosis
- Thorough counseling
- Careful planning.

The depth of placental invasiveness is one of the main factors affecting the maternal outcomes. Therefore, accurate prenatal prediction, assessment of the degree of the invasion,

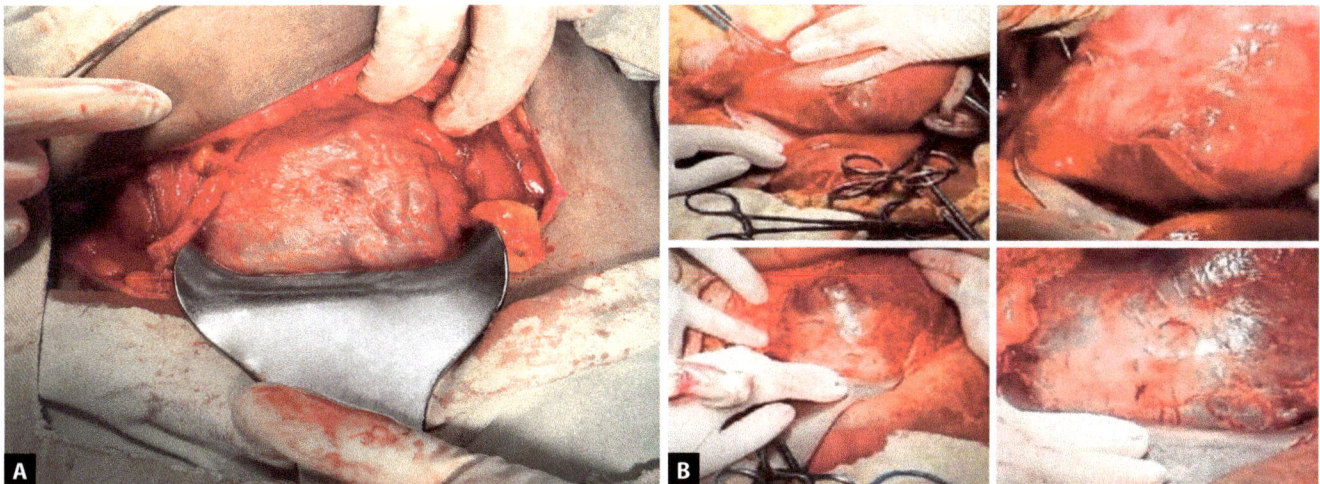

Figs. 5A and B: (A) Peroperative features of engorged vessels; (B) Peroperative image of placenta percreta.

and stratification of women, in order to identify the best strategies for the management helps to minimize clinical complications by enabling obstetricians to plan for resources that may be required during cesarean delivery, including obstetric anesthesia, appropriate surgical expertise, available blood products, and interventional radiology for uterine artery embolization.

American College of Obstetricians and Gynecologists (ACOG) and the Society for Maternal Fetal Medicine recommend these patients receive level III (subspecialty) or higher care. This level includes continuously available medical staff with appropriate training and experience in managing complex maternal and obstetric complications, including PAS, and consistent access to interdisciplinary staff with expertise in critical care (i.e., critical care subspecialists, hematologists, cardiologists, and neonatologists). The general resources needed to attain improved health outcomes in the setting of a known or suspected placenta accreta include planning for delivery with appropriate subspecialists and having access to a blood bank with protocols in place for massive transfusion.

Maternal morbidity has been proven to be significantly reduced when care is provided in a center of excellence (level III or IV) for the PAS conditions. A hallmark feature of a center of excellence is usually a tertiary referral hospital, which can provide a multidisciplinary team (MDT) with significant experience in managing the most invasive forms of PAS providing both antenatal diagnosis and preoperative planning. This team is likely to include experienced obstetricians and maternal-fetal medicine subspecialists, pelvic surgeons with advanced expertise or female pelvic medicine, and reconstructive surgeons, urologists, interventional radiologists, obstetric anesthesiologists, critical care experts, general surgeons, trauma surgeons, and neonatologists. Because of extensive vascular engorgement with challenging anatomy is the rule, having the most experienced pelvic surgeons involved from the outset is recommended. The MDT should be available 24 hours a day, 7 days a week, to ensure that expertise is available for emergency situations. Notification and collaboration with the blood bank are recommended in concert with delivery and surgical planning given the frequent need for large-volume blood transfusion. Cross-matched blood and blood products should be readily available in anticipation of massive hemorrhage.

The different risks and treatment options should have been discussed and the management plan agreed, which should be reflected clearly in the consent form. This should include the anticipated skin and uterine incisions and whether conservative management of the placenta or proceeding straight to hysterectomy is preferred in the situation where accreta is confirmed at surgery. Additional possible interventions in the case of massive hemorrhage should also be discussed, including cell salvage, and interventional radiology when available.

■ DELIVERY

Planned delivery at a center experienced with this condition involving a MDT with surgical expertise in managing the spectrum of accreta complexity.

Timing of delivery: Scheduled delivery—between 35^{+0} and 36^{+6} weeks to avoid emergency (RCOG, 2018)/between $34^{0/7}$ and $35^{6/7}$ weeks (ACOG).

■ PREOPERATIVE WORK-UP

Counseling

Prior to delivery, all women with placenta accrete spectrum and their partners should have a discussion regarding massive obstetric hemorrhage, increased risk of lower urinary tract damage, need for cesarean hysterectomy, and possible need of obstetric intensive care unit (ICU), interventional radiology where available. Any concerns, queries, or refusals of treatment should be dealt with effectively and documented clearly.

Maximizing Hemoglobin Level

Maximizing the hemoglobin level by oral or intravenous iron therapy (in iron deficiency anemia)/blood transfusion as the situation demands to achieve Hb level at least 11 g/dL. Where resource permits—erythropoietin therapy is combined with concomitant intravenous iron treatment.

Notification and Collaboration with the Blood Bank

Notification and collaboration with the blood bank is recommended in concert with delivery and surgical planning given the frequent need for large-volume blood transfusion. Arrangement of blood, at least 4 units blood and 4 donors prior to surgery.

Preoperative Ureteric Stents and Cystoscopy

When the urinary bladder is invaded by the placental tissue, preoperative cystoscopy, and placement of ureteral stents have been recommended. However, the evidence is not strong enough to recommend routine placement of ureteric stents for all suspected cases of PAS. Opening the bladder to identify percreta villus tissue and removal of the involved bladder area has been recommended by different authors.

Cell Salvage

It offers a way to minimize allogeneic red blood cell transfusion in selected patients, such as those with high-risk of massive obstetric hemorrhage, low preoperative hemoglobin concentrations, rare blood types (e.g., Bombay blood group), and/or those who refuse such products. Autologous cell salvage is now being adopted in many obstetric centers managing PAS disorders, with observational studies showing improved outcomes and reduced need for allogeneic blood transfusion.

Interventional Radiology

It may be life saving for the treatment of massive postpartum hemorrhage, and therefore, having this facility available locally is desirable. These devices are inserted by interventional radiologists into the aorta, common iliac, internal iliac or uterine arteries under fluoroscopic guidance and are inflated after delivery of the baby when hemorrhage is encountered.

SURGICAL MANAGEMENT: CESAREAN HYSTERECTOMY (FIG. 6)

Cesarean hysterectomy is considered as the gold standard for the treatment of invasive placentation. This radical approach, however, is associated with high rates (40–50%) of severe maternal morbidity, mostly related to hemorrhage and insult to surrounding organs during surgery, and mortality rates as high as 7% due to massive untreatable hemorrhage have been reported. A recent meta-analysis suggested that when prenatal diagnosis and multidisciplinary expert management are available, mortality rates reduced in the range of 0.05%.

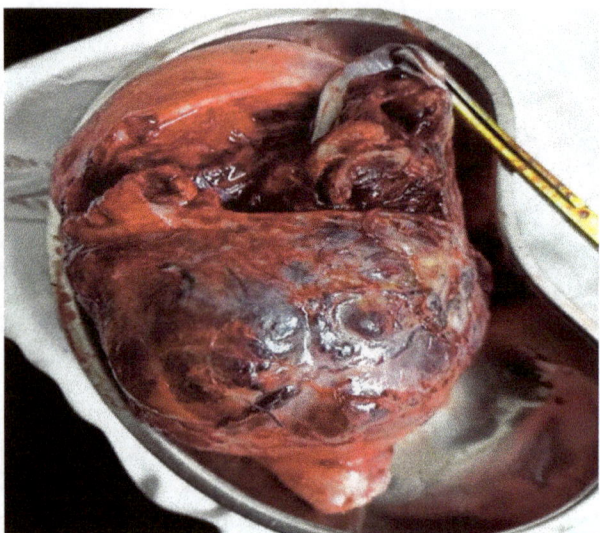

Fig. 6: Post-hysterectomy specimen of placenta percreta.

Intraoperative Considerations

Anesthesia: It involves senior anesthetic team. The choice of anesthetic technique must be made by the anesthetic team conducting the procedure. There is insufficient evidence to support one technique over another. Close monitoring of volume status, urine output, ongoing blood loss, and overall hemodynamics is critically important in managing such cases.

Abdominal incision: Abdominal incision can be midline or transverse but must allow sufficient access to the uterus to choose a location for uterine incision above the placental margin. A midline incision is recommended by most authors.

Uterine incision: Avoiding the placenta at planned cesarean hysterectomy reduces blood loss; consider using preoperative and/or intraoperative ultrasonography to precisely determine placental location and the optimal place for uterine incision (RCOG, 2018). A high *upper-segment transverse uterine incision* above the upper margin of the placenta without disturbing the placenta or a *fundal transverse hysterotomy* for delivery of the baby.

Placental removal: Any attempt to manually remove the placenta typically provokes heavy bleeding and is associated with high maternal morbidity and mortality and are strongly discouraged. If the placenta fails to separate with the usual measures, leaving it in place and closing, or leaving it in place, closing the uterus and proceeding to a hysterectomy are both associated with less blood loss than trying to separate it.

If the placenta partially separates, the separated portion(s) need to be delivered and any hemorrhage that occurs needs to be dealt within the normal way. Adherent portions can be left in place, but blood loss in such circumstances can be large and massive hemorrhage management needs to follow in a timely fashion.

Prophylactic Endovascular Balloon Catheters

Endovascular balloon occlusion of the pelvic vessels has been proposed as a method to reduce intraoperative blood loss, in order to improve maternal outcome related to hemorrhage and to allow the surgeon to operate in a cleaner field with improved visibility.

Uterotonic agents: These agents should not be administered unless placental removal is imminent or complete placental separation ruling out PAS disorders.

Tranexamic acid: It inhibits the enzymatic breakdown of *fibrinogen* and *fibrin* by *plasmin*. (1 g slow IV or 1,000–1,300 mg orally) immediately prior to or during cesarean delivery for PAS disorders appears beneficial in reducing blood loss. Prophylactic use in PAS has not been studied.

Fibrinogen therapy: Other clotting factors, e.g., fibrinogen therapy may help in cases of refractory bleeding. The goal is to achieve levels of 200 mg/dL or greater, cryoprecipitate is preferred to reduce the risk of transmitting viral pathogens. Recombinant activated factor *VIIa* has been used with success but there is a risk of thrombosis. Use in PAS should be limited to posthysterectomy bleeding with failed standard therapy.

Subtotal/total hysterectomy: Subtotal hysterectomy is associated with decreased blood loss, blood transfusions, perioperative complications, and shorter operating time but may not be effective in the management of placenta increta or percreta if cervical involvement is present and a total hysterectomy should be the preferred option in these cases.

Intraoperative Measures to Treat Life-threatening Hemorrhage

Several operators recommend different strategies for the management of massive intraoperative bleeding in case of PAS. The surgical treatments proposed include internal iliac artery ligation, uterine devascularization, uterine compression sutures, uterine balloon tamponade, and pelvic tamponade.

If massive bleeding occurs after placental removal, the first-line measure should be the intrauterine tamponade (e.g., balloon tamponade). If this measure is not effective, or the placenta remains in situ, an additional useful measure is uterine devascularization, with or without uterine compressive sutures.

Hypogastric artery ligation may decrease blood loss, but may be ineffective because of collateral circulation. The last measure to be tried is the ligation of the internal iliac artery; this procedure is associated with the highest risk of postoperative complications.

The use of interventional radiology to embolize the hypogastric arteries in cases of persistent or uncontrolled hemorrhage may be useful. Interventional radiology is especially helpful when there is no single source of bleeding that can be identified at surgery.

Other methods to address severe and intractable pelvic hemorrhage include pelvic pressure packing and aortic compression or clamping. Pelvic packing, although not standard management, can be highly-effective for patient stabilization and blood product replacement when experiencing acute uncontrolled hemorrhage. Packing may be left in situ for 24 hours (with an open abdomen and ventilatory support) to allow for optimization of clotting and hemostasis.

When the woman is unstable or life-threatening bleeding, in such cases an emergency hysterectomy should be performed rapidly.

■ CONSERVATIVE SURGERY

The cases where the extent of *placenta accreta is limited in depth* and surface area and the entire placental implantation area is accessible and visualized, the *uterine preserving surgery* may be appropriate including *partial myometrial resection*.
- Aim is to avoid peripartum hysterectomy and related morbidity and consequences.
- Indicated for women who desire future childbearing and agree to high continuous long-term monitoring in centers with an adequate expertise.

Techniques

Four different primary methods of conservative management have been described in the international literature:
1. The *extirpative technique* (manual removal of the adherent part of placenta).
2. Leaving the placenta in *situ* (or the expectant approach).
3. One-step conservative surgery (removal of the accreta area).
4. The Triple-P procedure (suturing around the accreta area after resection).

These methods have been used alone or in combination and in many cases with additional procedures such as those proposed by interventional radiology.

■ THE EXTIRPATIVE TECHNIQUE

This procedure consists of forcibly removing the placenta manually in an attempt to empty the uterus at delivery. The aim of this approach is to avoid leaving retained placental tissues in the uterine cavity and is recommended by established worldwide guidelines as one of the first steps. This procedure often results in massive obstetric hemorrhage, because it may leave placental tissues within the myometrium, connected to large feeding vessels, which are responsible for uncontrolled massive obstetric hemorrhage and the need for salvation hysterectomy. Uncontrolled bleeding may lead to coagulopathy and will also complicate the surgical procedure.

Successful conservative management strategies will preserve fertility and thus reduce the impact on a woman's societal status and self-esteem associated with the loss of her uterus.

"LEAVING THE PLACENTA IN SITU" APPROACH

Delivering the fetus avoiding the placenta and repair of the incision keeping the placenta in situ waiting for its complete spontaneous resorption.

In this conservative approach, the umbilical cord is ligated close to its placental insertion, and without any attempt of removal. By leaving the placenta accreta in situ after the delivery of the fetus, one can expect a progressive decrease in blood circulation within the uterus, parametrium, and the placenta. This will result in secondary necrosis of the villous tissue and theoretically the placenta should progressively detach itself from the uterus and the percreta villi from the adjacent pelvic organs and involution is postulated to facilitate delayed surgery. However, there is an associated risk of coagulopathy, hemorrhage, and sepsis during the interim period. Patients must be compliant with follow-up and resources to manage patients urgently if complications arise should be available 24 hours a day.

Complications including sepsis, septic shock, peritonitis, uterine necrosis, fistula, acute pulmonary edema, acute renal failure, deep vein thrombophlebitis or pulmonary embolism, even *maternal death* (in 6% cases) has been reported. Delayed hysterectomies are performed between 3 and 12 weeks postpartum. The residual villous tissue may require up to 6 months to be completely absorbed.

Follow-up schedule of the patients are as follows:
- In the first 2 months β-hCG and ultrasound by an expert on a weekly basis. If there is no complication, then monthly until complete resorption of placenta.
- Frequent clinical examination [per vaginal (P/V) bleeding, temperature, pelvic pain]
- Laboratory tests for infection (Hb% and leukocytes count, vaginal sample for bacteriological analysis).

Methotrexate should not be used as an expectant management. The low rate of trophoblastic cell turnover in later gestation compared with that in early pregnancy indicates a much lower efficacy of methotrexate in late compared with early pregnancy. In addition, it has significant adverse effect.

One-step Conservative Surgery

It consists of resecting the invasive accreta area (partial myometrial resection) followed by immediate uterine reconstruction and bladder reinforcement. This strategy aims to combine the advantages of both the "leaving in situ approach" of preserving the uterus and cesarean hysterectomy with minimal risk of secondary bleeding or infection. It is advantageous for low- and middle-income countries where expensive additional treatments such as interventional radiology may not be available.

Steps
- Vascular disconnection of newly-formed (feeder) vessels and the separation of invaded uterine tissues from invaded vesical tissues.
- Upper-segmental hysterotomy and delivery of the fetus.
- Resection of all invaded myometrial tissue and the entire placenta in one piece with *previous local vascular control*.
- Myometrial reconstruction in two planes.
- Bladder repair, if necessary.

In appropriately selected cases with no placental invasion into the uterine cervix and/or parametrium, local resection is a reasonable option and may reduce blood loss and improve maternal morbidity compared to hysterectomy. The International Society for Abnormally Invasive Placenta (IS-AIP) expert consensus defined an "appropriate case" for local resection, a case with *focal disease*, with an adherent/invasive area which is <50% of the anterior surface of the uterus.

Triple-P Procedure (Suturing Around the Accreta Area after Resection)

A novel uterine-sparing procedure for PAS disorders called the "Triple-P procedure" has been recently proposed. This procedure avoids incising through the vascular placental venous sinuses and excises the myometrium with PAS disorder tissue and reconstitutes the uterine defect.

The main steps of this procedure include:
- Perioperative placental ultrasound localization of the superior edge of the placenta and delivery of fetus by an incision above the placenta.
- Pelvic devascularization by inflating radiologically preplaced occlusion balloons in anterior division of internal iliac arteries.
- No attempt to remove the placenta, large myometrial excision and reconstruction of the uterine wall. If the posterior wall of the bladder is involved, the placental tissue invading the bladder is left in situ to avoid cystotomy.

Special point: Uterus preserving surgical techniques should only be attempted by surgeons working in teams

POSTOPERATIVE CONSIDERATIONS AND MANAGEMENT

Given the extensive surgery, PAS patients require intensive hemodynamic monitoring in the early postoperative period. This often is best provided in an intensive care unit setting to ensure hemodynamic and hemorrhagic stabilization. Close and frequent communication between the operative team and the immediate postoperative team is strongly encouraged. Postoperative PAS patients are at particular risk of ongoing abdominopelvic bleeding, fluid overload from resuscitation, and other postoperative complications given the nature of the surgery, degree of blood loss, potential for multiorgan damages, and the need for supportive efforts.

Continued vigilance for ongoing bleeding is particularly important. Obstetricians and other healthcare providers should have a low threshold for reoperation in cases of suspected ongoing bleeding. Pelvic vessel interventional radiologic strategies may be useful, but not all cases are amenable to these less invasive approaches and their use should be considered on a case-by-case basis. Clinical vigilance for complications such as renal failure, liver failure, infection, unrecognized ureteral, bladder, or bowel injury, pulmonary edema, and diverse intravascular coagulation is warranted.

CONCLUSION

Placenta accreta spectrum disorder is a potentially life-threatening condition. Given the increasing rates of cesarean section worldwide, the incidence of PAS will be likely to increase further over time. Therefore, clinicians should be aware of the difficulties related with the diagnosis and the challenges associated with the management of this condition.

SUGGESTED READING

1. Allen L, Jauniaux E, Hobson J, Papillon-Smith J, Belfort MA, FIGO Placenta Accreta Diagnosis and Management Expert Consensus Panel. FIGO consensus guidelines on placenta accreta spectrum disorders: nonconservative surgical management. Int J Gyanecol Obstet. 2018;140(3):281-90.
2. American College of Obstetricians and Gynecologists, Society for Maternal-Fetal Medicine. Obstetric Care Consensus No. 7: Placenta Accreta Spectrum. Obstet Gynecol. 2018;132(6):e259-75.
3. American College of Obstetricians and Gynecologists. Obstetric Care Consensus No. 2: Levels of maternal care. Obstet Gynecol. 2015;125(2):502-15.
4. Collins SL, Ashcroft A, Braun T, Calda P, Langhoff-Roos J, Morel O, et al. Proposal for standardized ultrasound descriptors of abnormally invasive placenta (AIP). Ultrasound Obstet Gynecol. 2016;47(3):271-5.
5. Comstock CH, Bronsteen RA. The antenatal diagnosis of placenta accreta. BJOG. 2014;121(2):171-81.
6. Eshkoli T, Weintraub AY, Sergienko R, Sheiner E. Placenta accreta: risk factors, perinatal outcomes, and consequences for subsequent births. Am J Obstet Gynecol. 2013;208(3):P219.E1-7.
7. Fitzpatrick KE, Sellers S, Spark P, Kurinczuk JJ, Brocklehurst P, Knight M. Incidence and risk factors for placenta accreta/increta/percreta in the UK: a national case-control study. PLoS One. 2012;7(12):e52893.
8. Garmi G, Salim R. Epidemiology, Etiology, Diagnosis, and Management of Placenta Accreta. Obstet Gynecol Int. 2012;2012:873929.
9. Hull AD, Resnik R, Robert M. Silver Placenta Previa and Accreta, Vasa Previa, subchorionic Hemorrhage, and Abruptio Placentae. Creasy and Resnik's Maternal-Fetal Medicine: Principles and Practice, 8th edition. Philadelphia: Elsevier, 2018. pp. 786-97.
10. Jauniaux E, Alfirevic Z, Bhide AG, Belfort MA, Burton GJ, Collins SL, et al. Placenta Praevia and Placenta Accreta: Diagnosis and Management: Green-top Guideline No. 27a. BJOG. 2019;126(1):e1-48.
11. Jauniaux E, Bhide A, Kennedy A, Woodward P, Hubinont C, Collins S, et al. FIGO consensus guidelines on placenta accreta spectrum disorders: Prenatal diagnosis and screening. Int J Gynaecol Obstet. 2018;140(3):274-80.
12. Jauniaux E, Chantraine F, Silver RM, Langhoff-Roos J, FIGO Placenta Accreta Diagnosis and Management Expert Consensus Panel. FIGO consensus guidelines on placenta accreta spectrum disorders: Epidemiology. Int J Gynaecol Obstet. 2018;140(3):265-73.
13. Marshall NE, Fu R, Guise JM. Impact of multiple cesarean deliveries on maternal morbidity: a systematic review. Am J Obstet Gynecol. 2011;205(3):262.e1-8.
14. Mogos MF, Salemi JL, Ashley M, Whiteman VE, Salihu HM. Recent trends in placenta accreta in the United States and its impact on maternal-fetal morbidity and healthcare-associated costs, 1998-2011. J Matern Fetal Neonatal Med. 2016;29(7):1077-82.
15. Morlando M, Collins S. Placenta Accreta Spectrum Disorders: Challenges, Risks, and Management Strategies. Int J Womens Health. 2020;12:1033-45.
16. RCOG. Placenta previa, Placenta previa accrete, Vasa previa: Diagnosis and management. RCOG Green top Guideline No. 27. London: RCOG; 2011.
17. Sentilhes L, Kayem G, Chandraharan E, Palacios-Jaraquemada J, FIGO Placenta Accreta Diagnosis and Management Expert Consensus Panel. FIGO consensus guidelines on placenta accreta spectrum disorders: Conservative management. Int J Gynaecol Obstet. 2018;140(3):291-8.
18. Tanimura K, Yamada H. Management of Placenta Accreta in Pregnancy with Placenta Previa. Placenta. United Kingdom: IntechOpen Limited; 2018.
19. Usta IM, Hobeika EM, Musa AA, Gabriel GE, Nassar AH. Placenta previa-accreta: risk factors and complications. Am J Obstet Gynecol. 2005;193(3Pt2):1045-9.

CHAPTER 13

Thyroid Disorders in Pregnancy

INTRODUCTION

Thyroid disorders are the most common endocrinopathies of women of childbearing age after diabetes. Thyroid hormone plays a crucial role for fetal development, especially in growth and neurodevelopment. The thyroid gland controls the rate of metabolic processes throughout the body via the production of two hormones triiodothyronine (T_3) and thyroxine (T_4). The hormonal and immunological perturbations of pregnancy and postpartum period and the dependence of fetus on maternal iodine and thyroid hormone have profound influence on maternal thyroid function and consequently of fetal well-being. Abnormalities in thyroid function, including hyperthyroidism and hypothyroidism, can have an adverse effect on reproductive health and result in reduced rates of conception, increased early pregnancy loss, and adverse pregnancy, and neonatal outcomes.

Evidence suggests that treating thyroid disorders and keeping thyroid-stimulating hormone (TSH) levels at the lower end of normal in euthyroid women may improve conception rates in subfertile women and reduce early pregnancy loss.

NORMAL THYROID PHYSIOLOGY

Regulation of Thyroid Hormone Production

Thyroid hormone production is controlled by the hypothalamic-pituitary-thyroid (HPT) axis and approximately 100 µg of thyroid hormone is released daily from the thyroid gland. Thyroid-releasing hormone (TRH) from the hypothalamus causes the release of a glycoprotein hormone TSH from the anterior pituitary gland.

Thyroid-stimulating hormone has many actions, e.g., increased release of T_4 and T_3 via increased iodide transport into follicular cells, organification and release of thyroglobulin (Tg) into the follicular lumen, and endocytosis of colloid. More T_4 than T_3 is produced by the thyroid gland, T_4 is converted in some peripheral tissues such as liver, kidney, and muscle to the more potent T_3. In the plasma, 99% of all T_3 and T_4 remain bound to the carrier proteins known as thyroid-binding globulin (TBG), transthyretin (previously known as thyroid-binding albumin), and albumin. Only the free hormones (FT_4 and FT_3) are biologically active (0.04% of total T_4 and 0.5% of total T_3). That is why ideally only free hormone measurements are done.

Formation and Secretion of Thyroid Hormone

Dietary iodine absorbed through the small intestine is transported in the plasma to the thyroid gland, where it is concentrated, oxidized, and then incorporated into Tg to form MIT (monoiodotyrosine) and DIT (diiodotyrosine) and later to T_4 (DIT + DIT) and T_3 (DIT + MIT), which are stored in colloid bound to Tg. Tg colloid is taken into the follicular cells by endocytosis. After a variable period of storage in thyroid follicles, Tg is subjected to proteolysis and the released hormones are secreted into the circulation, where specific binding proteins carry them to target tissues **(Fig. 1)**.

Physiological Alterations in Thyroid Status during Pregnancy

Physiologic thyroid changes during pregnancy are considerable and can be confused with maternal thyroid abnormalities. Maternal thyroid volume increases anywhere from 10 to 30% during the third trimester and is attributable to increases in extracellular fluid and blood volume during pregnancy. In addition, there are changes to thyroid hormone levels and thyroid function throughout pregnancy.

Normal pregnancy is associated with an increase in renal iodine excretion, an increase in T_4-binding proteins, an increase in thyroid hormone production, and thyroid stimulatory effects of human chorionic gonadotropin (hCG). All of these factors influence thyroid function tests (TFTs) in the pregnant patient. The healthy thyroid adapts to these alterations through changes in thyroid hormone metabolism, iodine uptake, and the regulation of the HPT axis. These hormonal changes of pregnancy result in profound alterations in the biochemical parameters of thyroid function.

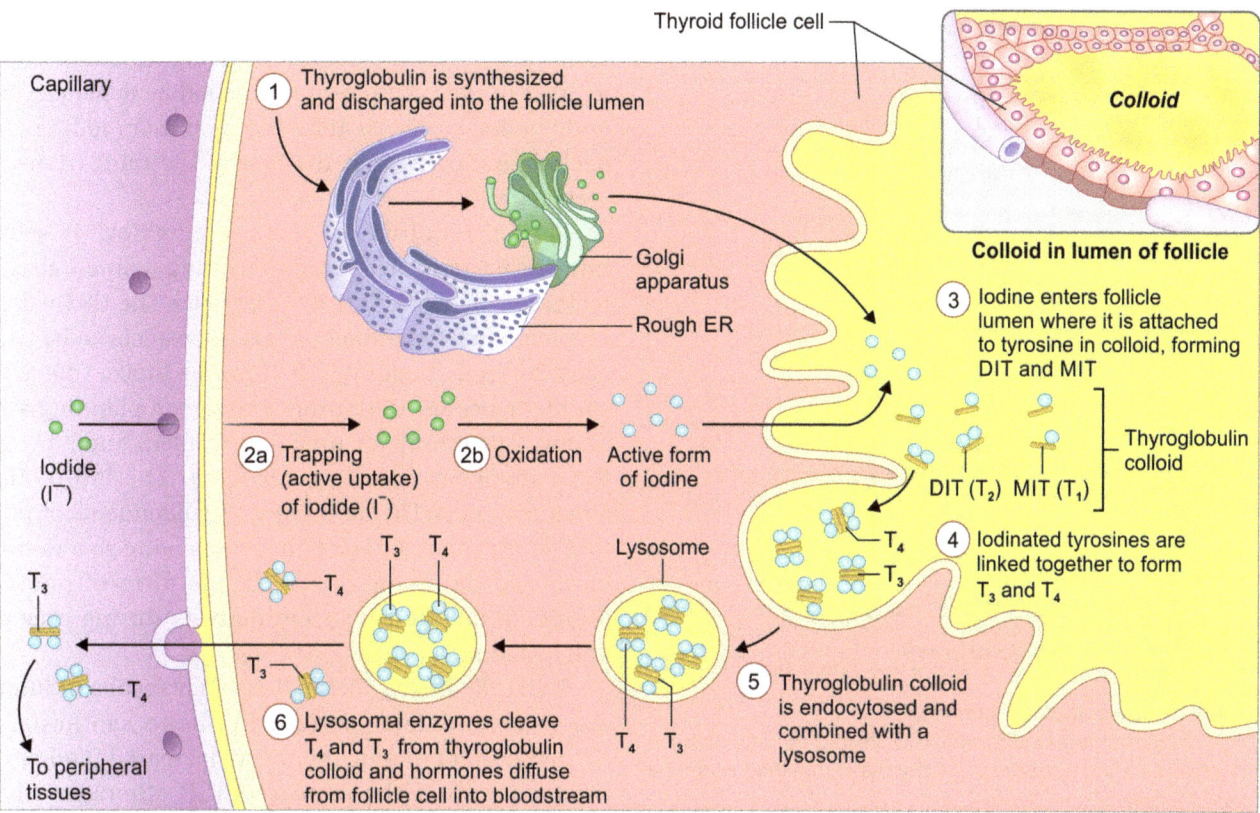

Fig. 1: Formation and secretion of thyroid hormone.
(DIT: diiodotyrosine; ER: endoplasmic reticulum; MIT: monoiodotyrosine; T_3: tri-iodothyronine; T_4: thyroxine)
Source: Bioscience notes. Synthesis of thyroid hormones, June, 2018.

Three series of events occur at different times of gestation. Increasing circulating estrogen concentration increases TBG by gestational age of 7 weeks and peaking at around 16 weeks and continuing till term. This increase is accompanied by a trend toward lower free T_4 and T_3 concentration. Under condition of iodine sufficiency, this decrease is marginal (10–15%) and a trend toward increase in TSH concentration from first trimester to term.

The second event takes place transiently in the first trimester, and is a consequence of thyroid stimulation due to increased serum β-hCG. There is partial inhibition of the pituitary and transient lowering of TSH between 8 and 14 weeks. TSH is a glycoprotein consisting of two subunit alfa (α) and beta (β). Alfa subunit is identical to hCG and beta subunit is unique to TSH. The thyrotropic activity of ∝-hCG causes a decrease in serum TSH in the first trimester so that pregnant women have lower serum TSH concentrations than the nonpregnant women. A TSH below the nonpregnant lower limit of 0.4 mU/L is observed in as many as 15% of healthy women during the first trimester of pregnancy. The TSH falls to about 10% in the second trimester, and 5% in the third trimester. A downward shift of the TSH reference range with a reduction in both the lower (decreased by about 0.1–0.2 mU/L) and the upper limit of maternal TSH (decreased by about 0.5–1.0 mU/L), relative to the typical nonpregnant TSH reference range.

The *American Thyroid Association (ATA)* recommends that when local reference ranges are not available, the lower reference range for TSH can be reduced by 0.4 mU/L and the upper reference range for TSH can be reduced by 0.5 mU/L in the late first trimester of pregnancy. Beyond the first trimester, TSH normalizes toward the nonpregnant reference ranges, and nonpregnant reference ranges can be used. Reference ranges for total T_4 and total T_3 also should be adjusted for pregnancy. The upper reference range limits for total T_4 and total T_3 can be increased by approximately 50% after 16 weeks of gestation. Before 16 weeks of gestation, there is a gradual increase in total T_4 and total T_3 compared with nonpregnant adults. These adjustments to total T_4 and total T_3 reference ranges are necessary to account for the increase in TBG in pregnancy.

In the third series of events, alteration in peripheral metabolism of thyroid hormones occurs throughout pregnancy, more prominent in the second half. Three enzymes deiodinate thyroid hormones, type 1 is not significant; type 2 converts T_4 to T_3, which is critical in the presence of low maternal T_4 level. Type 3 enzyme catalyzes the conversion of most fetal T_4 to reverse T_3 (inactivated) and T_3 to T_2. This explains low T_3 and high reverse T_3 concentration characteristic of fetal thyroid metabolism. Fetal brain tissue that depends on T_3 for development is supplied by local T_4-T_3 conversion by type 2 deiodinase **(Fig. 2)**.

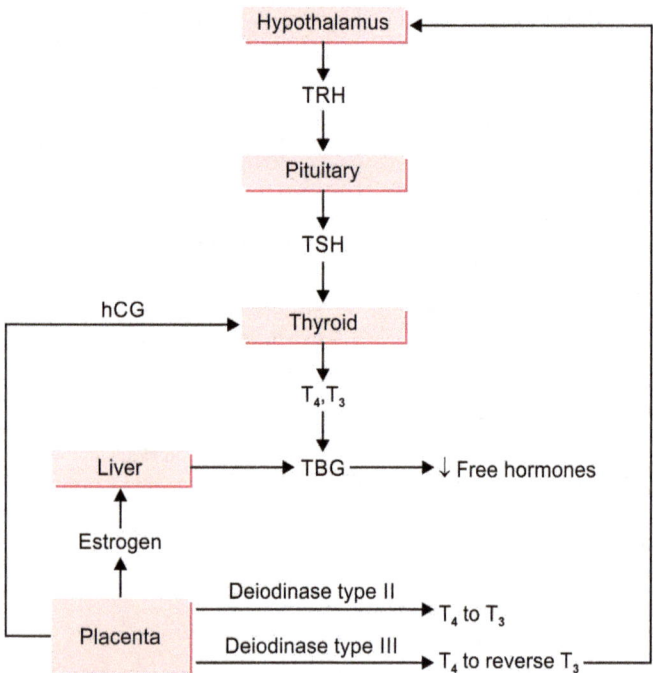

Fig. 2: Metabolism of thyroid hormone.
(hCG: human chorionic gonadotropin; TBG: thyroid-binding globulin; TRH: thyroid-releasing hormone; TSH: thyroid-stimulating hormone; T_3: triiodothyronine; T_4: thyroxine)

This physiological adaptation is attained without much difficulty by the normal thyroid gland in a state of iodine sufficiency, which does not apply in presence of iodine insufficiency or when thyroid function is abnormal.

Iodine Requirement in Pregnancy

Iodine, a key component of thyroid hormone, is crucial for fetal neurological development. Pregnancy is a state of relative iodine deficiency secondary to an increase in renal loss [increased glomerular filtration rate (GFR) in early first trimester] as well as due to transfer of iodine to the developing fetus. Pregnancy has a profound impact on the thyroid gland and its function. During pregnancy, the thyroid gland increases in size by 10% in iodine replete countries and by 20–40% in areas of iodine deficiency. Thyroid gland increases the iodine uptake from the blood, which may lead to the development of cellular hyperplasia and physiological thyroid goiter. Production of the thyroid hormones, T_4, and T_3, increases by nearly 50%, in conjunction with a separate 50% increase in the daily iodine requirement.

Because of increased thyroid hormone production, increased renal iodine excretion, and fetal iodine requirements, dietary iodine requirements are higher in pregnancy than they are for nonpregnant adults. Women with adequate iodine intake before and during pregnancy have adequate intrathyroidal iodine stores and have no difficulty adapting to the increased demand for thyroid hormone during gestation. In these women, total-body iodine levels remain stable throughout pregnancy. However, in areas of even mild-to-moderate iodine deficiency, total-body iodine stores, as reflected by urinary iodine values, decline gradually from the first to the third trimester of pregnancy.

Iodine, required for infant's nutrition, is secreted into breast milk. Therefore, lactating women also have increased dietary iodine requirements. The US Institute of Medicine recommended dietary allowances to be used as goals for individual total daily iodine intake (dietary and supplement) are 150 μg/day for women planning a pregnancy, 220 μg/day for pregnant women, and 290 μg/day for women who are breastfeeding. The World Health Organization (WHO) and The ATA guideline recommends that all pregnant and lactating women ingest a minimum of 250 μg/daily—optimally, in the form of potassium iodide, to ensure consistent delivery during pregnancy and lactation.

Maternal dietary iodine deficiency results in impaired maternal and fetal thyroid hormone synthesis. Low thyroid hormone values stimulate increased pituitary TSH production, and the increased TSH stimulates thyroid growth, resulting in maternal and fetal goiter. In areas of severe iodine deficiency, thyroid nodules can be present in as many as 30% of pregnant women. Low maternal urinary iodine concentration (UIC) in pregnancy has been associated with reduced placental weight and neonatal head circumference. In areas with adequate dietary iodine intake, maternal UICs have a limited influence on physical developmental outcomes. Mild-to-moderate maternal iodine deficiency has been associated with attention deficit and hyperactivity disorders in children as well as impaired cognitive outcomes. Severe iodine deficiency in pregnant women has been associated with increased rates of pregnancy loss, stillbirth, and increased perinatal and infant mortality.

Since 1990, the number of households worldwide using iodized salt has risen from <20 to >70%. Use of iodized salt has reduced the incidence of low UIC. Studies in rural Bangladesh found 6% of pregnant women had low UICs, whereas in Pakistan 80% had low urinary iodine concentration (UICs). Universal salt iodization is the most cost-effective way of delivering iodine and improving maternal and infant heath. In areas of severe iodine deficiency, iodine supplementation to mothers prior to conception or in early pregnancy results in children with improved cognitive performance relative to children of mothers given a placebo. The prevalence of cretinism and other severe neurological abnormalities is significantly reduced. Maternal iodine supplementation in severely iodine-deficient areas also decreases rates of stillbirth and neonatal and infant mortality. Oral administration of iodized oil can increase birth weight in addition to correcting iodine deficiency. In low-resource countries and regions where neither salt iodization nor daily iodine supplements are feasible, a single annual dose of ~400 mg of iodized oil for pregnant women and women of childbearing age can be used as a temporary measure to protect vulnerable populations.

Fetal Thyroid Development

Fetal thyroid gland begins to develop from about 4-5 weeks of gestation, having some function at 10 weeks. The fetal thyroid gland begins concentrating iodine and synthesizing thyroid hormone by approximately 12 weeks. Hypothalamic TRH is detectable at 8-9 weeks and pituitary portal circulation is functional by 10-12 weeks. Until midgestation, TSH and T_4 concentration remains low. By 18-20 weeks, iodine uptake by fetal thyroid and serum T_4 concentration begins to increase. Concentration of T_4 increases from 2 µg/dL at 20 weeks to 10 µg/dL at term, free T_4 concentration increases from 0.1 to 1.5 ng/mL, TSH rises from 4 to 8 mIU/L between 12 weeks and term. Maternal T_4 is transferred to the fetus throughout the entire pregnancy but placenta is impermeable to TSH and T_3. Increase in T_3 and FT_3 is small, because of inactivation by placental type 3 deiodinase. T_4 is important for normal fetal brain development, especially before the fetal thyroid gland begins functioning. Fetal brain tissue development, dependent on T_3, is supplied by catalyzation of local T_4 to T_3 by type 2 deiodinase enzyme.

Normal levels of thyroid hormone are essential for neuronal migration, myelination, and other structural changes of the fetal brain. First phase of growth velocity of developing brain structure occurring during the second trimester corresponds to a phase during which the supply of thyroid hormones to the fetus is almost exclusively of maternal origin. The second phase of maximum fetal brain growth velocity from the third trimester up to 2-3 years of life depends on thyroid hormone of fetal and neonatal origin. Approximately 30% of T_4 in umbilical cord serum at delivery is maternal in origin.

Maternal and fetal iodine deficiency in pregnancy have adverse effects on the cognitive function of offspring. Children whose mothers were severely iodine deficient during pregnancy may exhibit cretinism, characterized by profound intellectual impairment, deaf-mutism, and motor rigidity. Low maternal T_4 concentration in the second trimester is the leading cause of preventable intellectual deficits worldwide. A recent randomized clinical trial demonstrated that in moderately to severely iodine-deficient areas without universal salt iodization, lactating women who receive one dose of 400 mg oral iodized oil after delivery can provide adequate iodine to their infants through breast milk for at least 6 months. Direct infant iodine supplementation was less effective at improving infant iodine status.

Diagnosis of Thyroid Disorders in Pregnancy

Levels of TSH and thyroid hormone are both used to diagnose thyroid disease in pregnancy. The first-line screening test to assess thyroid status should be measurement of the TSH level. TSH is the most reliable indicator of thyroid status because it indirectly reflects thyroid hormone levels as sensed by the pituitary gland.

When the TSH level is abnormally high or low, a follow-up study to measure the free T_4 level should be performed to determine if there is overt thyroid dysfunction. In cases of suspected hyperthyroidism, total T_3 is also measured. Total T_3 is used preferentially over free T_3 because assays for estimating free T_3 are less robust than those measuring free T_4. The level of free T_4 should be monitored in pregnant women being treated for hyperthyroidism, and the dose of antithyroid drug (ATD) (thioamide) should be adjusted accordingly to achieve a free T_4 at the upper end of the normal pregnancy range. Among women who also have T_3 thyrotoxicosis, total T_3 should be monitored with a goal level at the upper end of normal pregnancy range.

Whom to Test for Thyroid Disorders? (American Thyroid Association, 2017)

All patients seeking pregnancy, or newly pregnant, should undergo clinical evaluation. If any of the following risk factors are identified, testing for serum TSH is recommended:

- A history of hypothyroidism/hyperthyroidism or current symptoms/signs of thyroid dysfunction
- Known thyroid antibody positivity or presence of a goiter
- History of head or neck radiation or prior thyroid surgery
- Age >30 years
- Type 1 diabetes or other autoimmune disorders
- History of pregnancy loss, preterm delivery, or infertility
- Multiple prior pregnancies, more than 2
- Family history of autoimmune thyroid disease or thyroid dysfunction
- Morbid obesity [body mass index BMI 40 kg/m^2]
- Use of amiodarone or lithium, or recent administration of iodinated radiologic contrast
- Residing in an area of known moderate-to-severe iodine insufficiency.

■ HYPOTHYROIDISM

Hypothyroidism is the more prevalent thyroid disorder, present in up to 2-5% of pregnancies, while hyperthyroidism [usually Graves' disease (GD)] complicates another 0.2%.

The prevalence may be higher in areas of iodine insufficiency. When iodine nutrition is adequate, the most frequent cause of hypothyroidism is autoimmune thyroid disease (Hashimoto's thyroiditis). Therefore, not surprisingly, thyroid autoantibodies can be detected in approximately 30-60% of pregnant women with an elevated TSH concentration.

Classification

Overt Hypothyroidism
Overt hypothyroidism is defined as raised TSH above the upper limit of normal and a free T_4 below the lower limit of normal. The consensus from professional societies including ATA, Endocrine Society, and the American Association of Clinical Endocrinologist (AACE) is that any women with TSH >10 mIU even with normal free T_4 should be diagnosed as OH.

Subclinical Hypothyroidism
Subclinical hypothyroidism (SCH) is defined as an elevated serum TSH in the presence of a normal free T_4 level.

Isolated Hypothyroxinemia
Isolated hypothyroxinemia is typically defined as a FT_4 concentration in the lower 2.5th to 5th percentile of a given population in conjunction with a normal maternal TSH concentration.

■ OVERT HYPOTHYROIDISM
Overt hypothyroidism is the most prevalent thyroid dysfunction with prevalence: About 2–5% of women or 2–10/1,000 pregnancy.

Causes
- *Iodine deficiency:* In developing country, it is the most common cause.
- *Autoimmune, e.g., Hashimoto's thyroiditis:* Prominent in developed country and associated with thyroid peroxidase antibodies (TPO-Abs). There is association with other autoimmune diseases such as pernicious anemia, type 1 diabetes mellitus (DM), and vitiligo.
- *Iatrogenic:* Radioactive iodine ablation and thyroidectomy
- *Drugs:* Carbimazole, methimazole (MMI), propylthiouracil (PTU), amiodarone, and lithium
- *Transient thyroiditis:*
  - Subacute (de Quervain) thyroiditis
  - Postpartum thyroiditis.

Signs and Symptoms
Signs and symptoms may be masked by the hypermetabolic state of pregnancy. The discriminatory features are cold intolerance, bradycardia, and slow relaxation of deep tendon reflexes, particularly those of ankle. Other symptoms may include modest weight gain, constipation, hoarseness of voice, hair loss, brittle nails, and dry skin. Goiter may or may not be present and is more likely to occur in women who have Hashimoto thyroiditis (also known as Hashimoto disease) or who live in areas of endemic iodine deficiency. Hashimoto thyroiditis is the most common cause of hypothyroidism in pregnancy and is characterized by glandular destruction by autoantibodies, particularly antithyroid peroxidase (anti-TPO) antibodies.

Diagnosis
Laboratory confirmation is obtained from an elevated TSH, with or without a suppressed FT_4. Pregnant women with TSH >2.5 should be evaluated for TPO-Ab status (antithyroglobulin and anti-TPO-Ab). Patients may have macrocytic or normocytic normochromic anemia. Other laboratory abnormalities include elevated creatine phosphokinase, cholesterol, carotene, and liver function abnormality. Where origin of hypothyroid is autoimmune, there are association of other autoimmune diseases.

Ideally pregnancy-specific reference ranges for each trimester should be used and it should be defined by provider's institute/laboratory and should represent the typical population for whom care is provided. Reference range should be defined in healthy TPO-Ab negative pregnant women with optimal iodine intake and without thyroid illness. If pregnancy-specific TSH reference ranges are not available, an upper reference limit of *4 mIU/L* may be used (ATA, 2017) **(Table 1)**.

Maternal Risk
Severe or untreated hypothyroidism is associated with increased risk of spontaneous abortion, preeclampsia, preterm birth, abruptio placentae, and stillbirth. Patients may develop postpartum hemorrhage (PPH), anemia, and cardiac ventricular dysfunction. Adequate thyroid hormone replacement minimizes the risk of adverse outcomes.

Most serious consequence of untreated hypothyroidism is myxedema coma, which is rare but a medical emergency with a 20% mortality rate. Clinical features of myxedema coma include hypothermia, bradycardia, decrease deep tendon reflex and altered consciousness, hyponatremia, hypoglycemia, hypoxia, and hypercapnia.

Fetal Risk
Fetal risk includes prematurity, low birthweight (LBW), neonatal respiratory distress, neurocognitive implications, lower intellectual and motor scores, and congenital hypothyroidism (CHT). Fetus requires maternal thyroxin/T_4

TABLE 1: Trimester-specific thyroid hormone level.

Trimester	TSH (mIU/L)	FT_4 (pmol/L)	FT_3 (pmol/L)
1st	0.1–2.5	10–16	3–7
2nd	0.2–3	9–15.5	3–5.5
3rd	0.3–3	8–14.5	2.5–5.5

(FT_3: free triiodothyronine; FT_4: free thyroxine; TSH: thyroid-stimulating hormone)

for normal brain development before 12 weeks. Inadequate replacement may lead to reduced neuropsychological development of the offspring. It is rare for maternal thyroid inhibitory antibodies to cross the placenta and cause fetal hypothyroidism. The prevalence of fetal hypothyroidism in the offspring of women with Hashimoto thyroiditis is estimated to be only 1 in 180,000 neonates.

In parallel to the treatment of hypothyroidism in a general population, it is reasonable to target a TSH in lower half of trimester-specific range but when this is not available, target TSH below 2.5 mIU/L. Women on adequate replacement therapy are euthyroid at onset of pregnancy and have good maternal and fetal outcomes.

Management of Overt Hypothyroidism

Prepregnancy

Patients with known hypothyroidism should be counseled to optimize medical therapy and delay pregnancy until TSH < 2.5 mIU/L before pregnancy. Levothyroxine (LT_4) dose is adjusted to achieve a value between the lower reference range limit and 2.5 mIU/L (ATA, 2017).

Patient receiving LT_4 with a suspected/confirmed pregnancy should independently adjust their dose of LT_4 by 20–30% and urgently notify their caregiver for prompt testing and further evaluation. One means of accomplishing this is to administer two additional tablets weekly of the patient's current daily LT_4 dose. Counsel patient regarding increased demand of LT_4 during pregnancy and to contact her physician immediately upon a confirmed or suspected pregnancy and reassure her about the safety of LT_4 during pregnancy.

Management during Pregnancy

Overt maternal hypothyroidism is known to have serious adverse effects on the fetus. If OH is diagnosed during pregnancy, TFTs should be normalized as rapidly as possible. L-thyroxin is the drug of choice and the dose should be adjusted so as to keep the serum TSH below 2.5 mIU/L in the first trimester or 3 mIU/L in second and third trimesters. The aim is to maintain FT_4 at the upper end of the normal range and TSH in the trimester-specific normal range. Clinical studies have confirmed that the increased requirement for T_4 (or exogenous LT_4) occurs as early as 4–6 weeks of pregnancy. Such requirements gradually increase through 16–20 weeks of pregnancy and plateau thereafter until the time of delivery.

For pregnant women with previously diagnosed hypothyroidism, serum TSH levels should be measured every 3–4 weeks during the first half of pregnancy and every 6–10 weeks thereafter. TSH and free T_4 levels should be measured 3–4 weeks after every dosage adjustment (*ATA*). Changes in LT_4 dose at <4 weeks intervals may lead to overtreatment (*Endocrine Society Guideline*).

Several recommendations as mentioned below are available and to be considered according to the specific situation that fits the scenario.

The *updated guidelines issued by the ATA in 2014* are as follows:
- Pregnant women with OH should receive LT_4 replacement therapy with the dose titrated to achieve a TSH concentration within the trimester-specific reference range.
- Serial serum TSH levels should be assessed every 4 weeks during the first half of pregnancy to adjust LT_4 dosing to maintain TSH within the trimester-specific range.
- Serum TSH should be reassessed during the second half of pregnancy.
- In women already taking LT_4, two additional doses per week of the current LT_4 dose, given as one extra dose twice weekly with several days' separation, may be started as soon as pregnancy is confirmed. **Flowchart 1** shows 2017 ATA guideline for diagnosis and management of thyroid disease in pregnancy and postpartum.

Autoimmune thyroid disease without OH has been associated with a higher miscarriage rate. Anti-TPO or anti-Tg thyroid autoantibodies are present in 2–17% of unselected pregnant women, the prevalence varies with ethnicity. A recent study from Belgium in women seeking fertility treatment showed that both TPO-Ab and thyroglobulin antibody (TgAb) were present in 8% of women, while 5% demonstrated isolated TgAbs and 4% demonstrated isolated TPO-Ab concentrations. Those women with isolated TgAb positivity had a significantly higher serum TSH than women without thyroid autoimmunity.

Negro et al. showed that euthyroid Caucasian women with positive anti-TPO antibodies who were treated with LT_4 during the first trimester had lower miscarriage rates than those who were not treated. These women also had lower rates of premature delivery, comparable to rates in women without thyroid antibodies.

Dose of levothyroxine: Abalovich et al. determined the specific LT_4 dosages required to return these patients to a euthyroid state. The investigators found that the most successful dosages, as follow, varied according to baseline levels of TSH:
- *SCH (TSH 4.2 mIU/L or less):* 1.2 µg/kg/day
- *SCH (TSH >4.2–10 mIU/L):* 1.42 µg/kg/day
- *OH:* 2.33 µg/kg/day

These dosages proved appropriate in 89% and 77% of patients with subclinical or overt hypothyroidism, respectively.

American College of Obstetricians and Gynecologists (ACOG) recommendation: Initial dose 1–2 µg/kg daily or 100 µg. Further adjustment is made according to TSH level as follows:
- If TSH level is elevated but <10 mIU/L, add 25–50 µg/day
- If TSH level is >10 mIU/L but <20 mIU/L, add 50–75 µg/day
- If TSH level is >20 mIU/L, then add 75–100 µg/day.

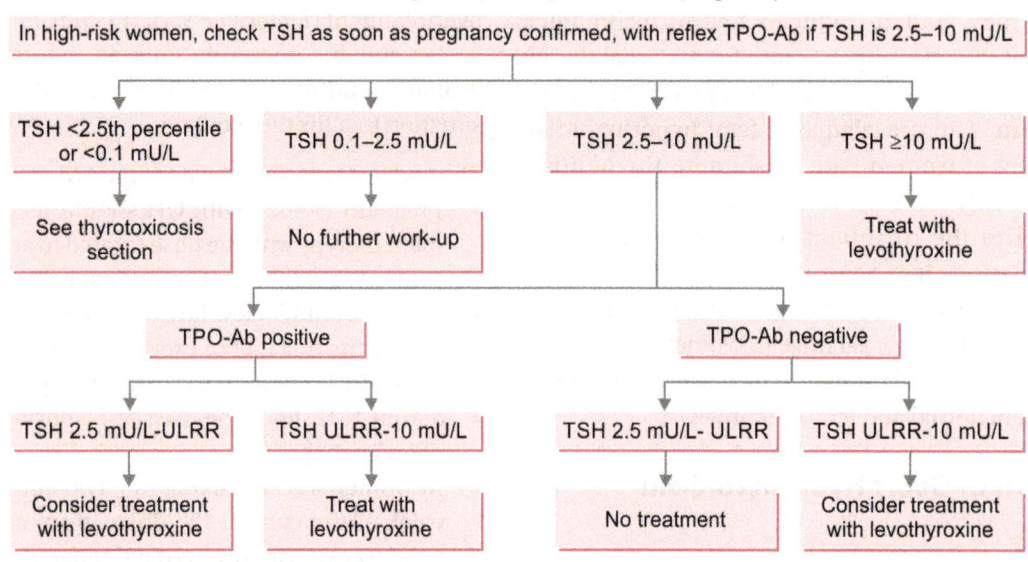

Flowchart 1: Testing for thyroid dysfunction in pregnancy.

(TPO-Ab: thyroid peroxidase antibody; TSH: thyroid-stimulating hormone; ULRR: upper limit of the reference range)
(*Source*: Alexander EK, Pearce EN, Brent GA, Brown RS, Chen H, Dosiou C, et al. 2017 Guidelines of the American Thyroid Association for the Diagnosis and Management of Thyroid Disease during Pregnancy and the Postpartum. Thyroid. 2017;27(3))

After the dose adjustment, TFT (TSH) should be checked in every trimester to maintain euthyroid. Women with thyroid autoimmunity who are euthyroid in the early stages of pregnancy are at risk of developing hypothyroidism and should be monitored every 4–6 weeks for elevation of TSH above the normal range for pregnancy.

Note: LT_4 should not be taken with prenatal iron, vitamins, or calcium supplements as these may reduce absorption and effectiveness.

Labor and delivery: No specific measures are necessary in well-controlled patients. Large maternal goiter may cause anesthetic complications if general anesthesia (GA) is needed.

Postnatal management: Reduce LT_4 dosage to prepregnancy regimen. Check TFTs at 6 weeks postpartum. Observe for signs of postpartum thyroiditis and screen for postpartum depression.

Neonatal Management (American Thyroid Association Guidelines, 2017)

- All newborns should be screened for congenital hypothyroidism (CHT) by blood spot analysis typically 2–5 days after birth in order to avoid confounding by the physiologic surge in neonatal TSH.
- Neonates with CHT, LT_4 should be started at a dose of 10–15 µg/day for a term baby depending on the severity of initial hypothyroidism. In a premature baby, lower dose is utilized. For optimal cognitive outcomes, therapy should be initiated within 2 weeks of life.

Newborn Screening and Treatment

A well-defined protocol given by *Indian Society for Pediatric and Adolescent Endocrinology (ISPAE)* for newborn screening is as follows:

- Screening should be done for every newborn using cord blood, or postnatal blood ideally at 48–72 hours of age.
- Neonates with screen TSH >20 mIU/L or >34 mIU/L for samples taken between 24 and 48 hours of age should be recalled for confirmation by venous blood.
- Venous confirmatory TSH >20 mIU/L before age 2 weeks and >10 mIU/L after age 2 weeks, with low T_4 (<10 µg/dL) or FT_4 (<1.17 ng/dL) *indicate primary CHT* and treatment should be initiated.
- LT_4 is commenced at 10–15 µg/kg in the neonatal period. Serum T_4/FT_4 is measured at 2 weeks and TSH and T_4/FT_4 at 1 month, then 2 monthly till 6 months, 3 monthly from 6 months to 3 years and every 3–6 months thereafter. Babies with the possibility of transient CHT should be re-evaluated at age 3 years, to assess the need for lifelong therapy.

■ SUBCLINICAL HYPOTHYROIDISM

Subclinical hypothyroidism describes a high TSH and normal T_4 concentration. The prevalence of SCH in pregnancy has been estimated to be 2–5%, more common in women particularly those who have thyroid antibodies. SCH is unlikely to progress to OH during pregnancy in otherwise healthy women but is increasingly being discussed as adverse maternal and fetal outcomes have been observed. Ultrasonography may have prognostic value in SCH. An Italian study found progression to OH occurred more often in patients whose ultrasonographic thyroid scan showed diffuse hypoechogenicity (an indication of chronic thyroiditis).

Significant controversy persists regarding the treatment of patients with mild hypothyroidism. Some have argued that treatment of these patients improves symptoms, prevents progression to OH, and may have cardioprotective benefits. Reviews by the US Preventive Services Task Force found inconclusive evidence to recommend aggressive treatment of patients with TSH levels of 4.5–10 mIU/L. The Endocrine Society recommends T_4 replacement in pregnant women with SCH. The ACOG does not recommend it as a routine measure.

A large randomized controlled trial published in 2012, the Controlled Antenatal Thyroid Screening (known as CATS) trial, and the Maternal–Fetal Medicine Units Network's Randomized Trial of Thyroxine Therapy for Subclinical Hypothyroidism or Hypothyroxinemia Diagnosed During Pregnancy published in 2017 demonstrated no difference in neurocognitive development in offspring through age 5 years who were born to women screened and treated for SCH. Moreover, follow-up of children from the CATS study through age 9 years confirmed that there was no neurodevelopmental improvement in offspring of treated women.

Diagnosis is essentially a biochemical one as symptoms may be mild, nonspecific, or even absent. In pregnancy, its diagnosis is often incidental. Higher TSH and higher SCH prevalence level are consistently seen in those who are TPO-Ab or TgAb positive.

Maternal and fetal risk: In some studies, maternal SCH has been shown to be associated with higher incidences of preterm birth, abruptio placentae, admission of infants to the intensive care nursery, preeclampsia with severe features, and gestational diabetes. However, other studies have not identified a link between maternal SCH and these adverse obstetric outcomes. Currently, there is no evidence that identification and treatment of SCH during pregnancy improve these outcomes.

HYPERTHYROIDISM

Introduction

Hyperthyroidism is characterized by a decreased TSH level and an increased free T_4 level. It occurs in 0.2–0.7% of pregnancies, hyperthyroidism can be overt (suppressed TSH and elevated T_3 and/or T_4) or subclinical (suppressed TSH and normal T_3 and T_4).

Causes of Hyperthyroidism in Pregnancy

- Graves' disease
- Toxic nodular goiter and toxic adenoma
- Subacute thyroiditis (De Quervain or postpartum)
- Gestational transient thyrotoxicosis and trophoblastic disease
- *Others:* Overtreatment of hypothyroidism, amiodarone treatment, lithium therapy, hyperfunctioning teratoma (struma ovarii), and TSH-secreting pituitary adenoma.

Graves' disease is the most common cause of hyperthyroidism in pregnancy, accounts for 95% of all cases. GD is an autoimmune disease in which there is production of autoantibodies directed against the TSH receptor that stimulates the thyroid gland to an increased production of thyroid hormone. Biochemically, increased serum levels of TSH receptor antibodies (TRAb) are detectable in 95% of patients with GD. Hyperthyroidism caused by multinodular toxic goiter or toxic solitary adenoma is not considered of autoimmune origin, but develops from thyroid autonomy, where the synthesis of thyroid hormone occurs independently of regulation by TSH. Such thyroid autonomy is often seen as a late consequence of iodine deficiency.

Signs and Symptoms

Most women are diagnosed before pregnancy and may be on treatment. The signs and symptoms of inadequately treated maternal thyrotoxicosis include nervousness, tremors, heat intolerance, weight loss or failure to gain weight, excessive sweating, palpitations, and hypertension.

Distinctive features of GD are ophthalmopathy (signs include lid lag and lid retraction), dermopathy (signs include localized or pretibial myxedema), and goiter. Another sign commonly seen is atrial fibrillation on electrocardiogram (ECG). Some symptoms of hyperthyroidism are similar to normal symptoms of pregnancy or some nonthyroid associated diseases, the results of serum TFTs differentiate thyroid disease from these other possibilities.

Effects of Thyrotoxicosis on Pregnancy

Pregnancy outcome depends on whether metabolic control is achieved before and during pregnancy. Maternal and fetal outcome is generally good if hyperthyroidism is controlled before pregnancy. Untreated or poorly controlled thyrotoxicosis is associated with subfertility, increased risk of miscarriage, intrauterine growth restriction (IUGR), and premature delivery, placental abruption, pregnancy-induced hypertension, pulmonary embolism (PE), infection, and increased perinatal mortality. Both early and late (still birth) loss have been reported. Inadequately treated maternal thyrotoxicosis is also associated with a greater risk of preeclampsia with severe features, maternal heart failure, and thyroid storm than treated.

Fetus and Neonatal Effects

Uncontrolled maternal hyperthyroidism has been associated with fetal tachycardia, small for gestational age babies, prematurity, stillbirths, and congenital malformations.

Fetal and neonatal risks associated with GD are related either to the disease itself or to thioamide (PTU or MMI) treatment. Because a large proportion of thyroid disease in women is mediated by antibodies (thyroid-stimulating immunoglobulin and TSH-binding inhibitory immunoglobulins also known as thyrotropin-binding inhibitory immunoglobulins) that cross the placenta, there is risk of development of immune-mediated hyperthyroidism and hypothyroidism in the neonates.

About 1-5% of these neonates have hyperthyroidism or neonatal GD. Fetal thyrotoxicosis may be suspected in a fetus with persistent tachycardia (>160 beats/minute), a goiter or growth restriction. Fetal thyrotoxicosis may result in preterm delivery, development of fetal craniosynostosis, heart failure (hydrops fetalis), hepatosplenomegaly, thrombocytopenia, exophthalmos, and goiter. Additional neonatal features include jaundice, poor feeding, poor weight gain, and irritability.

Thyrotoxicosis presenting in neonatal period is usually transient lasting only 2-3 months after delivery. Presentation may be delayed (2 weeks) postnatally if mother was on medication at the time of delivery. Effect on maternal antithyroid medication usually cleared quickly from neonatal circulation, but the thyroid stimulating antibodies are cleared at a slower rate, neonates should be monitored accordingly.

Management

Preconception

Conception should be avoided until 6 months after radioiodine therapy and woman on ATDs should be euthyroid for 3 months prior to conception. Patient should be counseled regarding the risk of birth defects with antithyroid dugs (ATDs) as well need for continuation of treatment.

Prenatal Period

Autoimmune hyperthyroidism may improve as pregnancy advances with fall of antibody. Mild hyperthyroidism (slightly elevated thyroid hormone levels, minimal symptoms) often is monitored closely without therapy as long as both the mother and the baby are doing well.

When hyperthyroidism is severe enough to require therapy, antithyroid medications are the treatment of choice, with propylthiouracil (PTU) being preferred in the first trimester. Pregnancy-specific reference range should be used when interpreting thyroid function result and therapy continued with the aim to keep free T_4 in the high-normal to mildly elevated range with the lowest dose of antithyroid medication to minimize the development of hypothyroidism or goiter in the baby. Titration is done based on the FT_4 levels and not the TSH as the TSH may take multiple weeks to return back to its reference range. TFTs should be checked once in every 3-4 weeks at the starting of the treatment.

Patients on methimazole (MMI) before pregnancy should be switched to PTU as early as possible. When shifting from MMI to PTU, a dose ratio of approximately 1:20 should be used (e.g., MMI 5 mg/D = PTU 50 mg twice daily). PTU can be switched to CBZ (carbimazole) or MMI in the second trimester. Women on ATD, FT_4/TT_4, and TSH should be monitored approximately every 4 weeks.

Antithyroid medicaion requirement often decreases during late gestation and in some, it may be discontinued toward the end of pregnancy. Following cessation, maternal thyroid testing and clinical examination should be done every 1-2 weeks. If remains euthyroid, the test interval can be extended to 2-4 weeks.

Patients with past history of GD or taking ATD for GD, serum TRAb (TSH receptor autoantibody) testing is recommended at first prenatal visit. If TRAb is high (more than three times of upper reference range), fetus is carefully monitored for hypothyroidism throughout pregnancy even if mother is euthyroid after thyroidectomy. Repeat testing should be done at 18-22 weeks. If TRAb is elevated and mother is taking ATD in the third trimester, a TRAb should be performed in late pregnancy at 30-34 weeks to evaluate the need for neonatal and postnatal monitoring. High TRAb in the last trimester is a risk factor for fetal thyrotoxicosis. Treat fetal thyrotoxicosis with increased doses of maternal hypothyroid treatment.

Ultrasound monitoring of fetal growth, goiter, and fetal heart rate is recommended if TRAb levels are more than three times the above upper reference limit. Serial growth monitoring if fetal growth restriction is suspected.

Drug Treatment with Dose

Propylthiouracil: Initial dose 50-150 mg is administered orally three times a day. Maintenance dose: 50 mg to be administered orally twice or three times a day. MMI: Initial dose: 10-20 mg/day to be administered orally once a day. Maintenance dose to be changed as per the reduction in TFTs.

Side Effects of Antithyroid Drugs

Side effects include simple rash, fever, urticaria to severe hepatitis or liver toxicity, systemic lupus erythematosus (SLE)-like syndrome, and agranulocytosis.

Antithyroid drugs MMI or PTU cross the placenta and can potentially impair the baby's thyroid function and cause fetal goiter. Use of either drug in the first trimester of pregnancy has been associated with birth defects, although the defects associated with PTU are less frequent and less severe. MMI embryopathy includes aplasia cutis, upper airway atresia, esophageal and other gastrointestinal atresias, abdominal wall defects, and ventricular septal defects. The types of birth defects after PTU exposure are less severe. Current international guidelines recommend the use of PTU in the first trimester of pregnancy and to consider shifting from PTU to MMI/CMZ after the first trimester considering risk of liver failure associated with the use of PTU.

Patients who cannot be adequately treated with antithyroid medications (i.e., those who develop an allergic reaction to the drugs), surgery is an acceptable alternative. Surgical removal of the thyroid gland is safest in the second trimester. Radioiodine is contraindicated to treat hyperthyroidism during pregnancy since it readily crosses the placenta, can cause destruction of fetal thyroid gland, and result in permanent hypothyroidism.

β-blockers: β-blockers can be used during pregnancy to treat significant palpitations and tremor due to hyperthyroidism. Propranolol is commonly used at a dose of 20-40 mg two-three times daily, it inhibits T_4-T_3 conversion. Alternatively other β-blockers may be used except atenolol, which is pregnancy category D. They should be used sparingly due to reports of impaired fetal growth associated with long-term use. Typically, these drugs are only required until the hyperthyroidism is controlled with antithyroid medications.

Labor and Delivery

With the stress of infection, labor or operative delivery a "thyroid storm" can occur in poorly controlled patient. This is a medical emergency, characterized by pyrexia, confusion, and cardiac failure.

Management includes:
- Decrease T_3/T_4 production with MMI/CBZ or PTU
- Potassium iodide 8 hourly 1-2 hours after thionamides
- Supportive therapy (maintain blood volume, glycemic and temperature control, and restore electrolyte balance)
- Propranolol.

Postpartum

Graves' disease typically worsens in the postpartum period or may occur for the first time in the postpartum. When new hyperthyroidism occurs in the first months after delivery, the cause may be either GD or postpartum thyroiditis and testing with careful follow-up is needed to distinguish between the two. Higher doses of antithyroid medications may be required during this time and close monitoring of TFTs is necessary. Test thyroid function of the baby on days 3-4 and 7-10 days of life.

With high TRAb titer in late pregnancy, there is risk of neonatal thyrotoxicosis; treatment with ATDs may be necessary for few days. If mother has been on high dose of antithyroid medication, treatment with LT_4 supplementation may be necessary for few days.

Although very small quantities of both PTU and MMI are transferred into breast milk, total daily doses of up to 20 mg MMI or 450 mg PTU are considered safe and monitoring of the breastfed infants' thyroid status is not required. Relapse of GD is seen in a large number of females within 3 months of their delivery. This may be due to the disappearance of immunosuppression of pregnancy. TSH and FT_4 values need to be monitored at 6 weeks and then at 12 weeks' interval.

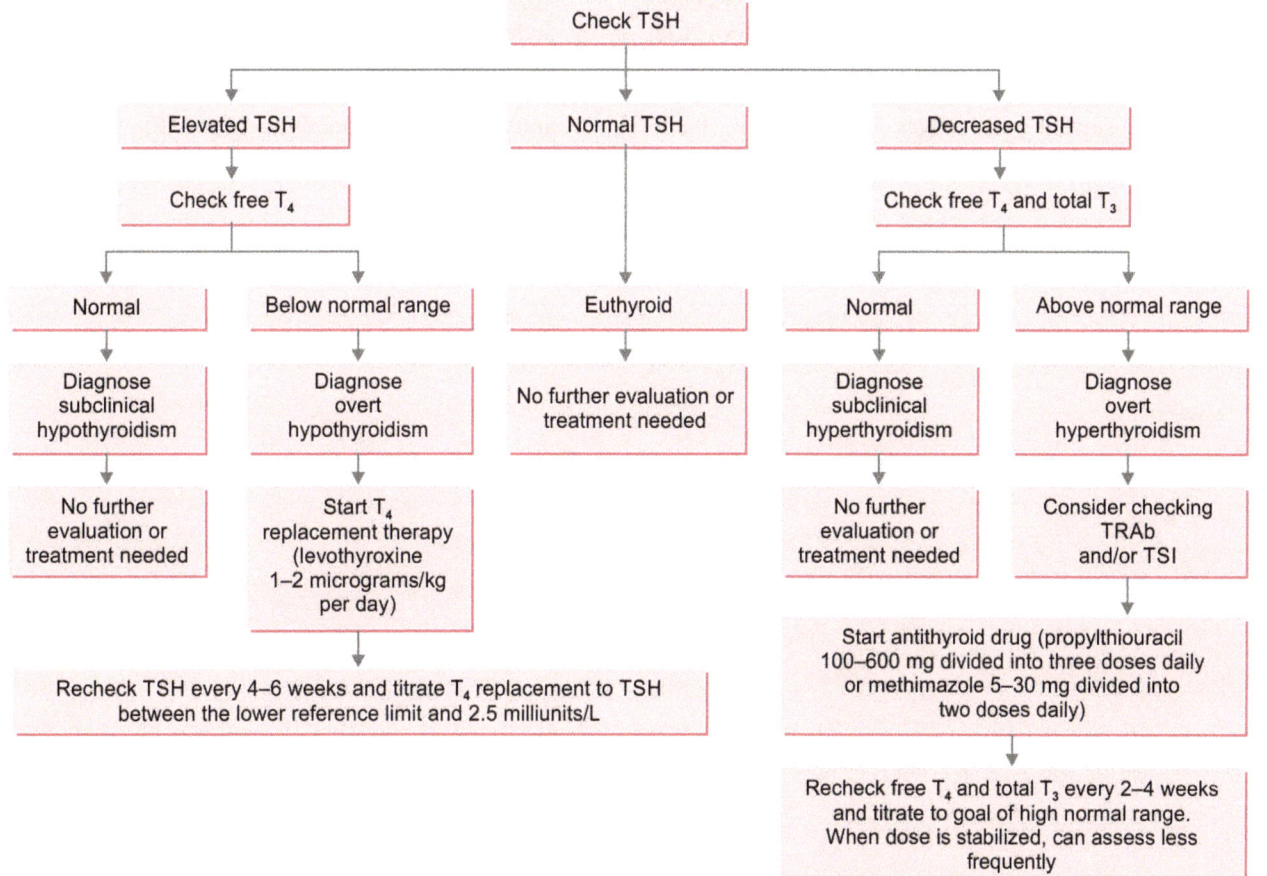

Summary: Management of thyroid dysfunction according to thyroid-stimulating hormone (TSH) level.

(T_3: triiodothyronine; T_4: thyroxine; TRAb: TSH receptor antibody; TSI: thyroid stimulating immunoglobulin)
Source: ACOG Practice Bulletin, Number 223, June 2020

SUBCLINICAL HYPERTHYROIDISM

Subclinical hyperthyroidism, reported in 0.8–1.7% of pregnant women, is characterized by an abnormally low serum TSH concentration with free T_4 levels within the normal reference range. It has not been associated with adverse pregnancy outcome. Treatment of pregnant women with subclinical hyperthyroidism is not recommended because there is no demonstrated benefit to the mother or the fetus. In addition, there are theoretical risks to the fetus because antithyroid medications cross the placenta and may adversely affect fetal thyroid function.

SUGGESTED READING

1. Abalovich M, Vazquez A, Alcaraz G, Kitaigrodsky A, Szuman G, Calabrese C, et al. Adequate levothyroxine doses for the treatment of hypothyroidism newly discovered during pregnancy. Thyroid. 2013;23(11):1479-83.
2. ACOG Update. Thyroid disease in pregnancy. 2020. [online] Available from: https://www.obgproject.com/2020/06/22/acog-update-thyroid-disease-in-pregnancy. [Last accessed April 2022].
3. Alexander EK, Pearceet EN, Brent GA, Brown RS, Chen H, Dosiou C, et al. 2017 Guidelines of the American Thyroid Association for the diagnosis and management of thyroid disease during pregnancy and the postpartum. Thyroid. 2017;27(3):315-89.
4. American Thyroid Association. Hyperthyroidism in Pregnancy. [online] Available from: https://www.thyroid.org/hyperthyroidism-in-pregnancy/. [Last accessed April 2022]. www.thyroid.org,2019.
5. Andersen S, Laurberg P. Managing hyperthyroidism in pregnancy: current perspectives. Int J Womens Health. 2016;8:497-504.
6. Casey BM, Metz TD. Thyroid disease in pregnancy. ACOG Practice Bulletin No. 223. American College of Obstetricians and Gynecologists. Obstet Gynecol. 2020;135(6):e261-74.
7. FOGSI Medical Disorders in Pregnancy Committee. Thyroid Update in Pregnancy. 2021. [online] Available from: https://www.fogsi.org/wp-content/uploads/committee-2020-activities/thyroid-update-in-pregnancy.pdf. [Last accessed April 2022].
8. Jarvis S, Nelson-Piercy C. Thyroid disease in pregnancy. In: James D, Steer PJ, Weiner CP, Gonik B, Robson SC (Eds). High-risk Pregnancy: Management Options, 5th edition. Cambridge: Cambridge University Press; 2018. pp. 1192-217.
9. Jonklaas J, Bianco AC, Bauer AJ, Burman KD, Cappola AR, Celi FS, et al. Updated guidelines issued by the American Thyroid Association in 2014. Prepared by the American Thyroid Association Task Force on thyroid hormone replacement. Thyroid. 2014;24(12):1670-751.
10. Lazarus J, Brown RS, Daumerie C, Hubalewska-Dydejczyk A, Negro R, Vaidya B. 2014 European thyroid association guidelines for the management of subclinical hypothyroidism in pregnancy and in children. Eur Thyroid J. 2014;3(2):76-94.
11. Orlander PR. (2021). Hypothyroidism Treatment and Management. Practice Essentials. [online] Available from: https://emedicine.medscape.com/article/122393-overview. [Last accessed April 2022].
12. Singh S, Sandhu S. Thyroid disease and Pregnancy. In: Lockwood CJ, Moore T, Copel J, Silver RM, Resnik R (Eds). Creasy and Resniks Maternal Fetal Medicine. 8th edition. Amsterdam: Elsevier; 2018.
13. Sudhanshu S, Riaz I, Sharma R, Desai MP, Parikh R, Bhatia V. Newborn screening guidelines for congenital hypothyroidism in India: Recommendations of the Indian Society for Pediatric and Adolescent Endocrinology (ISPAE) - Part II: Imaging, treatment and follow-up. Indian J Pediatr. 2018;85(6):448-53.

CHAPTER 14

Systemic Lupus Erythematosus in Pregnancy

■ INTRODUCTION

Systemic lupus erythematosus (SLE) is an autoimmune disease in which the body's immune system mistakenly attacks healthy tissue in many parts of the body with persistent autoantibody production. It is a chronic inflammatory disease with multiorgan involvement including the joints, skin, kidney, serous membrane, hematological and nervous system. There are periods of illness, called flares, and periods of remission during which there are few symptoms. The disease has several phenotypes, with varying clinical presentation ranging from mild mucocutaneous manifestations to multiorgan and severe central nervous system involvement.

Systemic lupus erythematosus predominantly affects women of childbearing age, therefore, common in pregnancy.

Pregnancy with SLE carries a higher maternal and fetal risk compared with pregnancy in healthy women. The prognosis for both the mother and the child is best when the disease has been quiescent for at least 6 months prior to the pregnancy. Disease flare during pregnancy poses challenges with respect to distinguishing physiologic changes related to pregnancy from disease-related manifestations. Thus, a multidisciplinary approach with close medical, obstetric, and neonatal monitoring is necessary to optimize both maternal and fetal outcomes.

■ EPIDEMIOLOGY

Global incidence and prevalence of SLE vary widely, owing to inherent variation in population demographics, environmental exposures, and socioeconomic factors. The prevalence of SLE in the United States is 14.6–50.8 cases per 100,000 population. In Europe, the incidence is 0.3–5.1 per 100,000 per year and a prevalence of 6.5–85 per 100,000. The incidence is dramatically higher in women than in men, the female-to-male ratio is about 9:1. The incidence peaks between ages 15 and 45 years and decreases after menopause, although still is twice as high in women compared to men. SLE may affect 1:1,000 women during pregnancy.

Certain ethnic groups are more vulnerable than others to developing SLE and experience increased morbidity and mortality. The race and sex-specific incidence of SLE per 100,000 persons are 0.4 in white males, 3.5 in white females, 0.7 in African American males, and 9.2 in African American females. Evidence suggests that SLE is more common in African American and Hispanic groups than in whites. When the prevalence of SLE is stratified by race, the prevalence among African Caribbean individuals was approximately five times the rate observed in people of white descent. In the United States, the prevalence of SLE in female African Americans ranges from 17.9 to 283 cases per 100,000. A West Indian study of female patients with SLE reported a prevalence of 83.8 cases per 100,000.

■ ETIOLOGY

Systemic lupus erythematosus is a multifactorial disease with unknown exact etiology, however, several genetic, immunological, endocrine, and environmental factors play a role in the etiopathogenesis of SLE. Postulated that environmental and infectious factors trigger the onset of disease in genetically susceptible individuals.

Genetic Factors

More than 50 genes or genomic loci have been identified to be associated with SLE. Normal variations (polymorphisms) in many genes can affect the risk of developing SLE, and in most cases, multiple genetic factors are thought to be involved. In rare cases, SLE is caused by mutations in single genes. The most important genes involved in the pathogenesis of SLE include human leukocyte antigen-DR2 (HLA-DR2), HLA-DR3, HLA class 3, C1q, and interferon (IFN) regulatory factor 5. Variations in these genes likely affect proper targeting and control of the immune response. Familial segregation and high concordance rates in identical twins suggest a strong genetic contribution in SLE but the inheritance pattern is usually unknown. The concordance in monozygotic twin is 25–50%, while it is 2–5% in dizygotic twin, and 10% patients with SLE have an affected relative.

Hormone

Systemic lupus erythematosus affects women more than men, androgens are considered protective. The use of estrogen-containing contraceptives and postmenopausal hormone replacement therapy can cause flares in patients with SLE. Women with SLE experience more severe symptoms during pregnancy and during reproductive periods. Both of these observations have led to believe that the female hormone estrogen may play a role in causing SLE. Estrogens and prolactin promote autoimmunity and increase the B-cell activation factor production and modulate lymphocyte and plasmacytoid dendritic cell (pDC) activation. Estrogen-mediated decrease in suppressor cell function upregulates T cell response with production of proinflammatory cytokines interleukin (IL)-1, 2, 6, and tumor necrosis factor alpha (TNF-α) that may lead to disease activity.

Environmental Factors

A variety of environmental factors including viral infections, diet, stress, chemical exposures, and sunlight are thought to play a role in triggering this complex disorder.

About 10% of SLE cases are thought to be triggered by drug exposure. While procainamide and hydralazine have the highest incidence of causing drug-induced lupus, >100 drugs have been associated with drug-induced lupus. Sulfa-drugs are well known to cause flares in patients with SLE, others include hydralazine, isoniazid, quinidine, and chlorpromazine.

Ultraviolet rays and sun exposure leads to increased cell apoptosis and is one of the well-known triggers for SLE. Several viral infections have been implicated, antibodies against Epstein–Barr virus (EBV) are more prevalent in children and adults with SLE compared to the general population. Smoking is also thought to be a risk, with a dose–response manner. Other potential risk factors include silica exposure, vitamin D deficiency, alfalfa sprouts, and foods-containing canavanine.

■ PATHOPHYSIOLOGY (HYPOTHESIS) (FIG. 1)

The pathophysiology of SLE is constantly evolving.

A break in the tolerance in genetically susceptible individuals, on exposure to environmental factors, leads to the activation of autoimmunity. The pathophysiology

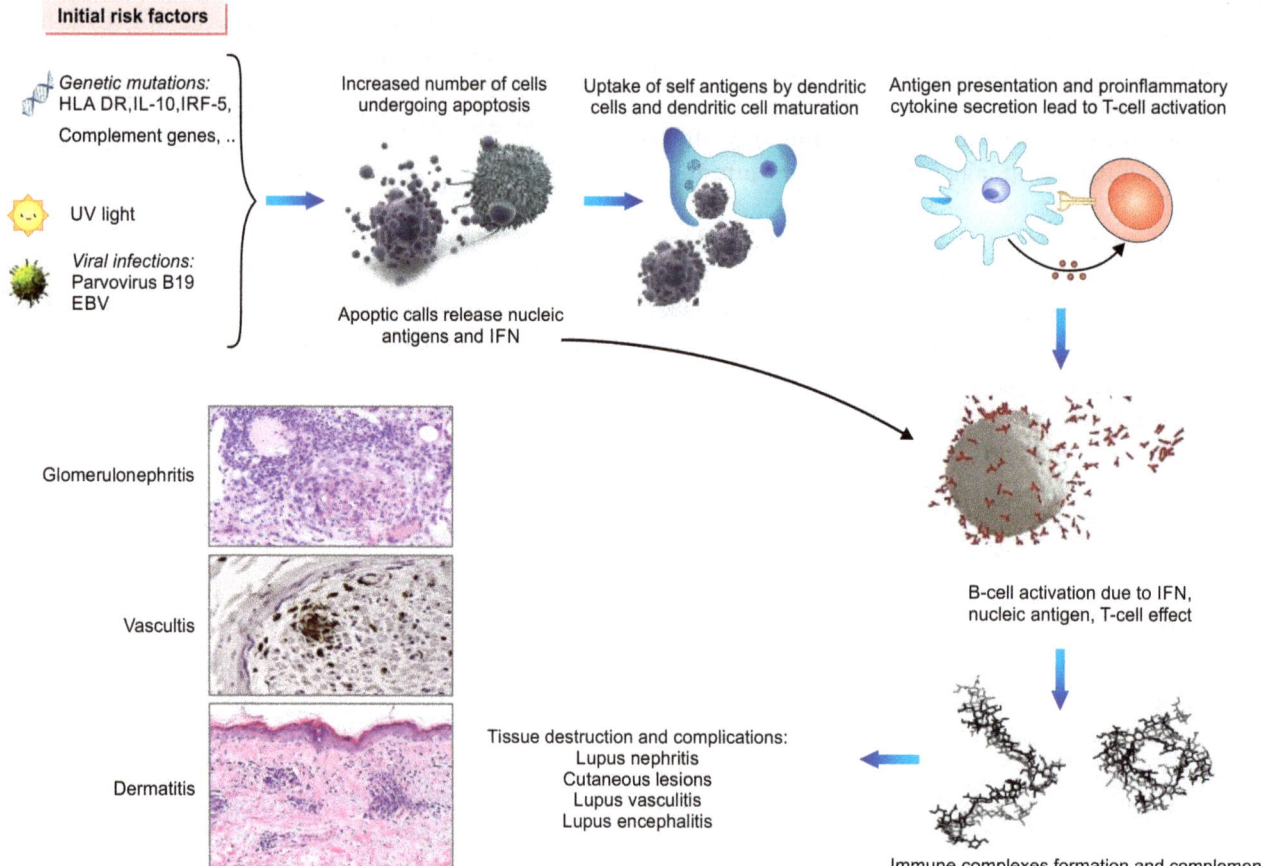

Fig. 1: Pathophysiology of SLE.
(EBV: Epstein–Barr virus; HLA-DR: human leukocyte antigen-DR; IFN: interferon; IL: interleukin; IRF: interferon regulatory factor 5; SLE: systemic lupus erythematosus; UV: ultraviolet)
Source: wikidoc.org.

involves overproduction of autoantibodies directed against various nuclear components as well as cell-surface antigens and deposition of immune complexes in different organs of the body. Aberrant innate immune responses play a significant role in the pathogenesis of SLE, contributing both to tissue injury via release of inflammatory cytokines and to aberrant activation of T and B cells, with the latter leading to pathogenic autoantibody production and resultant end-organ injury.

Nearly all of the pathological manifestations of SLE occur due to antibody formation and the creation and deposition of immune complexes in different organs of the body which may lead to complement activation and more organ damage.

DIAGNOSIS

There is no single diagnostic marker, the disease is identified through a combination of clinical and laboratory criteria. Initial presentation includes varying combination of polyarthralgia, fatigue, photosensitive skin rash, and serositis to life-threatening renal, hematologic, or central nervous system involvement. Up to half of all patients present with evidence of lupus nephritis (LN). The classic presentation of a triad of fever, joint pain, and rash in a woman of childbearing age should prompt investigation into the diagnosis of SLE.

SYMPTOMS

Symptoms of SLE vary from person to person and they may come and go and change over time. Lupus shares symptoms with other diseases, which can make it difficult to diagnose. Constitutional symptoms: Fatigue, malaise, fever, anorexia, and weight loss is common and are seen in >90% of patients with SLE and are often the initial presenting feature.

Mucocutaneous Manifestations

More than 80% of patients with SLE suffer from mucocutaneous involvement. Lupus-specific lesions include acute cutaneous lupus erythematosus (ACLE), subacute cutaneous lupus erythematosus (SCLE), and chronic cutaneous lupus erythematosus (CCLE).

The hallmark ACLE lesion is the malar rash or the butterfly rash, which is an erythematous raised pruritic rash involving the cheeks and nasal bridge. The rash may be macular or papular and spares the nasolabial folds (photoprotected). It usually has an acute onset, but may last several weeks, and may cause induration and scaling. The malar rash may fluctuate with lupus activity **(Fig. 2A)**.

Subacute cutaneous lupus erythematosus rash is a photosensitive, widespread, nonscarring, nonindurated rash. SCLE may be either papulosquamous resembling

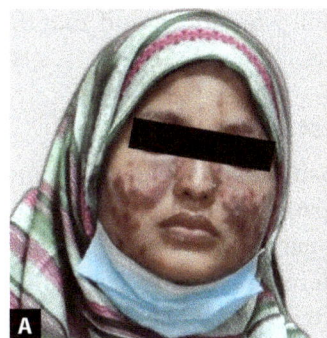 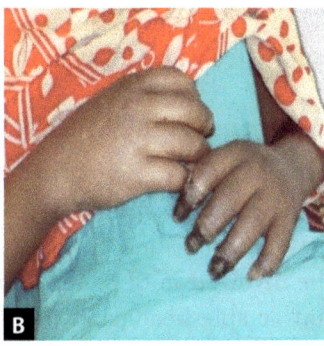

Figs. 2A and B: (A) Malar rash in SLE; (B) Raynaud's phenomenon in SLE.

psoriasis or an annular/polycystic lesion with central clearing and peripheral scaling. SCLE lesions may last several months but usually, heal without scarring. SCLE rash is seen in patients with a positive Anti-Ro (SSA) antibody in up to 90% of the cases. SCLE can also be caused by some drugs such as hydrochlorothiazide.

Discoid lupus erythematosus (DLE) is the most common form of CCLE. The lesions are disk-shaped erythematous papules or plaques with adherent scaling and central clearing. DLE heals with scarring, and when present on the scalp, can be associated with permanent alopecia.

Oral and nasal ulcers are common in SLE, often are painless. They may present as gradual onset erythema, macule, petechiae, erosions, or ulcers involving any part of the oral cavity with most common locations being the hard palate, the buccal mucosa, and the vermilion border.

Musculoskeletal Manifestations

Approximately 80–90% of patients with SLE suffer from musculoskeletal involvement at some point during their disease course which may range from mild arthralgias to deforming arthritis. Lupus arthritis is typically a nonerosive, symmetrical inflammatory polyarthritis affecting predominantly the small joints of the hands, knees, and wrists, although any joint can be involved. Avascular necrosis (with or without steroid use) can occur in up to 10% of patients with SLE and is usually bilateral and involves the hip joints.

Hematologic and Reticuloendothelial Manifestations

Anemia is present in >50% of patients with SLE and most commonly is anemia of chronic disease. Other causes of anemia may include iron deficiency anemia, Coombs' positive autoimmune hemolytic anemia, red blood cell aplasia, and microangiopathic hemolytic anemia, which may be associated with antiphospholipid antibody (APLA) syndrome. Leukopenia secondary to neutropenia or lymphopenia is also very frequent and can be severe.

Thrombocytopenia can be mild or severe and may be associated with APLA syndrome.

Neuropsychiatric Manifestations

Neurologic and psychiatric manifestation known as lupus cerebritis develops in 10–35% patients. Both central nervous system (CNS) and peripheral nervous systems (PNS) may be involved in SLE, most common CNS manifestation is intractable headaches, reported in >50% cases. Focal or generalized seizures may be seen, and are associated with disease activity, although they carry a favorable prognosis. Other CNS manifestations include aseptic meningitis, demyelinating syndrome including optic neuritis and myelitis, and movement disorders such as chorea and cognitive dysfunction. Patients with SLE are also at high risk for ischemic strokes. Cranial and peripheral neuropathies and syndromes mimicking Guillain–Barré syndrome and myasthenia gravis are the peripheral nervous system manifestations. Psychiatric manifestations are especially difficult to diagnose and may range from depression and anxiety to Frank psychosis.

Lupus Nephritis

Lupus nephritis can involve the glomeruli, the interstitium, tubules, and the vessels with immune complex deposition in all four compartments. Lupus nephritis occurs in about two-third of patients with SLE, proteinuria is present in 75% cases, hematuria or pyuria in 40%, and cellular cast in 33% cases. Renal biopsy is necessary to confirm the diagnosis of LN and determine the histologic type. Biopsy is the key to understand prognosis and provide direction for appropriate treatment. Women with active LN should be encouraged to delay pregnancy until the disease is inactive for at least 6 months to optimize maternal outcomes.

There are four basic histologic and clinical categories of LN: Diffuse proliferative glomerulonephritis (DPGN), focal proliferative glomerulonephritis (GN), membranous GN, and mesangial GN:

1. *DPGN:* Most common (40%) and most severe, 10 years survival around 60%. Typical presentation of DPGN is moderate to heavy proteinuria, nephrotic syndrome, hematuria, pyuria, cast, low complement, and circulating immune complex.
2. *Focal proliferative GN:* Patients have mild hypertension (HTN) and proteinuria, serious renal insufficiency is uncommon.
3. *Membranous GN:* Have moderate to heavy proteinuria, no active urinary sediment, no renal insufficiency
4. *Mesangial GN:* Least clinically severe, best long-term prognosis

Classification Criteria

American College of Rheumatology (ACR) first developed the SLE classification criteria in 1971 and revised them in 1982 and 1997. The 1997 ACR criteria were further revised by the Systemic Lupus International Collaborating Clinics (SLICC) group in 2012.

Revised American College of Rheumatology Classification (Table 1)

Systemic lupus erythematosus can be said to be present if four or more of the following criteria are present simultaneously or serially.

The SLICC criteria made some notable changes to the 1997 ACR to improve clinical relevance. It requires at least one of the four criteria to be clinical and at least one of the four criteria to be immunologic. Further, patients with biopsy-proven nephritis and positive antinuclear antibody (ANA) or anti-double-stranded DNA (anti-ds DNA) could be directly classified as SLE even if they lacked any other criteria. Compared to the 1997 ACR criteria, the SLICC criteria have an improvement in the sensitivity and are considered to be more valid and clinically relevant.

EULAR/ACR Criteria (European League Against Rheumatism/American College of Rheumatology Classification) for Systemic Lupus Erythematosus, 2019

The EULAR and the ACR have jointly developed new classification criteria for SLE; prompted by the need for criteria that were both highly sensitive and specific. The new 2019 EULAR/ACR classification criteria for SLE requires a positive ANA as obligatory entry criterion. Other criteria were chosen from seven clinical (constitutional, hematologic, neuropsychiatric, mucocutaneous, serosal, musculoskeletal, and renal) and three immunologic (APLAs, complement proteins, SLE-specific antibodies) categories, and weighted from 2 to 10. Patients with ≥10 points are classified as having SLE. In the validation cohort, the new criteria had a sensitivity of 96.1% and specificity of 93.4%, compared with 82.8% sensitivity and 93.4% specificity of the ACR 1997 and 96.7% sensitivity and 83.7% specificity of the SLICC 2012 criteria. **Flowchart 1** outlines the weighted point system used to classify a patient as SLE.

DIAGNOSIS OF SYSTEMIC LUPUS ERYTHEMATOSUS

The diagnosis of SLE can be challenging, and no single clinical feature or laboratory abnormality can confirm a diagnosis of SLE. SLE is diagnosed based on the constellation of signs, symptoms, and appropriate laboratory

TABLE 1: ACR Classification criteria for SLE.	
Criteria	**Definition**
Malar rash	Fixed erythema, flat or raised, over the malar eminences, tending to spare the nasolabial folds
Discoid rash	Erythematous raised patches with adherent keratotic scaling and follicular plugging; atrophic scarring possible in older lesions
Photosensitivity	Skin rash as a result of unusual reaction to sunlight, by patient history or physician observation
Oral ulcers	Oral or nasopharyngeal ulceration, usually painless
Arthritis	Nonerosive arthritis involving two or more peripheral joints, characterized by tenderness, swelling, or effusion
Serositis	• *Pleuritis:* Convincing history of pleuritic pain or rubbing heard by a physician, or evidence of pleural effusion • *Pericarditis:* Documented by electrocardiogram (ECG) or rub or evidence of effusion
Renal	• Persistent proteinuria >0.5 g/day or >3+ if quantitation not performed • *Cellular casts:* Red cell, hemoglobin, granular, tubular, or mixed
Neurologic	• *Seizures:* In the absence of offending drugs or known metabolic derangements (e.g., uremia, ketoacidosis, or electrolyte imbalance) • *Psychosis:* In the absence of drugs or metabolic derangements
Hematologic	• Hemolytic anemia with reticulocytosis • *Leukopenia:* <4,000/μL on two or more occasions • *Lymphopenia:* <1500/μL on two or more occasions • *Thrombocytopenia:* <100,000/μL in absence of drugs

Immunologic	• *Anti-DNA:* Antibody to native DNA in abnormal titer
	• *Anti-Sm:* Presence of antibody to Sm nuclear antigen
	• *Antiphospholipid antibodies:* Positive finding of based on:
	  – An abnormal S. level of immunoglobulin G (IgG) or IgM anticardiolipin antibodies
	  – A positive test result for lupus anticoagulant using a standard method
	  – A false-positive serologic test for syphilis for 6 months

Antinuclear antibody (ANA)	An abnormal ANA titer by immunofluorescence or an equivalent assay at any time and in the absence of drugs known to be associated with "drug-induced lupus" syndrome

workup. Imaging and histopathology may play a crucial role as well.

Diagnosis Based on Serological Markers

Antinuclear Antibody

Antinuclear antibody serves as a screening test. Elevated titer to 1:40 or higher is most sensitive. >99% of patients with SLE have an elevated titer, may be present in other autoimmune disease, weakly present in about 20–40% of healthy women.

Antinuclear Antibody Subtypes

Anti-ds DNA: More specific for SLE. Present in more than three-fourth of untreated patients at the time of presentation. Titer is related to disease activity specially LN. Increased levels have been shown to correlate with disease exacerbation and prematurity in pregnancy.

Anti-Sm antibodies: Present in about 30–40% of patients with SLE. Highly specific for disease at high titer but sensitivity low.

Anti-Ro (Anti-SSA) antibodies: Positive in 33% of patients, associated with congenital complete heart block (CCHB) and neonatal lupus (NL) syndrome.

Anti-La (Anti-SSB) antibodies: Positive in 50% patient with anti-Ro antibodies. Of particular importance, it is associated with NL.

Antibodies to RNP (ribonucleoprotein): Positive in 20–40% patients with SLE. Found in a number of other connective tissue disease.

Antiphospholipid Antibodies

Lupus anticoagulant (LAC) and anticardiolipin antibody (ACA) are present in 25–50% patients with SLE. APLA is linked with recurrent miscarriage, other pregnancy complication, and thromboembolic manifestation.

Other Tests

Complements

Patients with SLE have low levels of complements (C_3, C_4, and CH50). SLE exacerbation is signaled by decline of C_3 and C_4 level during pregnancy.

Flowchart 1: EULAR/ACR SLE classification criteria (2019).

```
┌─────────────────────────────────────────────────────────────────┐
│                        Entry criterion                          │
│ Antinuclear antibodies (ANA) at a titer of ≥1:80 on HEp-2 cells │
│              or an equivalent positive test (ever)              │
└─────────────────────────────────────────────────────────────────┘
                                ↓
┌─────────────────────────────────────────────────────────────────┐
│               If absent, do not classify as SLE                 │
│               If present, apply additive criteria               │
└─────────────────────────────────────────────────────────────────┘
                                ↓
```

Additive criteria
Do not count a criterion if there is a more likely explanation than SLE.
Occurrence of a criterion on at least one occasion is sufficient.
SLE classification requires at least one clinical criterion and ≥10 points.
Criteria need not occur simultaneously.
Within each domain, only the highest weighted criterion is counted toward the total scores.

Clinical domains and criteria	Weight	Immunology domains and criteria	Weight
Constitutional Fever	2	**Antiphospholipid antibodies** • Anti-cardiolipin antibodies OR • Anti-β2-GP1 antibodies OR • Lupus anticoagulant	2
Hematologic • Leukopenia • Thrombocytopenia • Autoimmune hemolysis	3 4 4	**Complement proteins** • Low C3 OR low C4 • Low C3 and low C4	3 4
Neuropsychiatric • Delirium • Psychosis • Seizure	2 3 5	**SLE-specific antibodies** • Anti-dsDNA antibody* OR • Anti-Smith antibody	6
Mucocutaneous • Nonscarring alopecia • Oral ulcers • Subacute cutaneous OR discoid lupus • Acute cutaneous lupus	2 2 4 6		
Serosal • Pleural or pericardial effusion • Acute pericarditis	5 6		
Musculoskeletal Joint involvement	6		
Renal • Proteinuria >0.5 g/24 h • Renal biopsy class II or V lupus nephritis • Renal biopsy Class III or IV lupus nephritis	4 8 10		
Total score:			

↓

Classify as Systemic Lupus Erythematosus with a score of 10 or more if entry criterion fulfilled

Blood Picture

Lower level of RBC (red blood cell) due to hemolytic anemia with reticulocytosis. There is leukopenia (<4,000/cumm of blood), lymphopenia (<1,500/cumm), and thrombocytopenia (platelet <100,000/cumm). In addition, there will be elevated erythrocyte sedimentation rate (ESR) and elevated C-reactive protein (CRP).

Tests for Serious Complications

- *Renal function test:* High level of serum creatinine and blood urea nitrogen (BUN).
- *Urine analysis:* Protein and cellular cast, if present distinguish between pre-eclampsia and LN.
- *Renal biopsy:* To detect histological categories of LN.
- *Liver function test:* Elevated serum glutamic pyruvic transaminase (SGPT), serum glutamic-oxaloacetic transaminase (SGOT), and low serum albumin.

DIAGNOSIS OF DISEASE ACTIVITY

The clinical course of SLE is variable and may be characterized by active disease, unpredictable disease flares, and remissions.

Active Disease

Systemic lupus erythematosus is considered active if two or more of the following criteria are present:
- Acute synovitis
- Pleurisy or pericarditis
- Psychiatric or CNS manifestation
- Thrombocytopenia, leukopenia, Coombs' positive hemolytic anemia
- Active skin or mucous membrane lesion
- Fever without infection
- Low serum complement
- Active renal disease—abnormal urine analysis (proteinuria).

Remission

Patients are said to be in remission if no symptom, have normal hemoglobin (Hb) and WBC (white blood cell), anti-Ds DNA antibody normal, normal C_3, C_4 level, maintenance therapy with hydroxychloroquine (HCQ), and prednisolone <7.5 mg/day.

Systemic Lupus Erythematosus Flare

There is no consensus on what constitutes a disease flare, but most definitions have incorporated a combination of results from serologic measures and disease activity indices. Flares are generally categorized by severity, with moderate or severe flares being the most clinically significant. Flare is indicated by onset of new signs of disease in a previously normal organ system, e.g., extreme fatigue, skin lesion, arthritis, anemia, lymphopenia, rising anti-Ds DNA antibody titer, increased proteinuria, and active urinary sediment.

Flares can occur during any trimester, but are more likely to occur in the second half of pregnancy and the early postpartum period. The frequency of exacerbation or persistently active disease varies with disease activity at conception. Rates range from 7 to 33% in women who have been in remission for at least 6 months to 61–67% in women who have active disease at the time of conception. Renal disease flare is the most common exacerbation seen. Serositis with pleural and pericardial effusions is noted in up to 10% of these patients.

Mild Systemic Lupus Erythematosus Flare

Mild SLE flare is said when a patient with SLE develops new onset low-grade fever, malar rash, and arthralgias, and feels increasingly fatigued. Laboratory evaluation is notable for a mild leukopenia. This patient may require no treatment. Alternatively, the patient may require the addition of HCQ or the equivalent of prednisone 7.5 mg/day or less.

Moderate Systemic Lupus Erythematosus Flare

A patient with SLE who develops pleuritic chest pain and a swelling of the wrists. Laboratory evaluation reveals elevated acute phase reactants. A chest radiograph is notable for a right-sided pleural effusion. The patient may require a short course of prednisone.

Severe Systemic Lupus Erythematosus Flare

A patient with SLE who develops new-onset renal insufficiency and significant proteinuria due to LN. Laboratory evaluation is notable for a low C_3, C_4, elevated dsDNA antibodies, and elevated acute phase reactants. The patient may require high doses of glucocorticoids (e.g., 1–2 mg/kg/day of prednisone or equivalent or intermittent intravenous "pulses" of methylprednisolone), additional immunosuppressive therapy (e.g., cyclophosphamide, azathioprine, or mycophenolate mofetil), and/or hospitalization.

■ MANAGEMENT

Preconceptional Evaluation

Active SLE at the time of conception is a strong predictor of adverse maternal and obstetrical outcomes. The preconception evaluation in women with SLE includes assessment of disease activity, major organ involvement, and determine whether pregnancy may pose an unacceptably high maternal or fetal risk as well as hypercoagulability or concurrent medical disorders that may impact pregnancy. Previous obstetric outcomes should be reviewed, with particular attention to history of small for gestational age fetus, preeclampsia, stillbirth, miscarriage, and preterm birth. Preconception assessment should include medication review and adjust to achieve optimal control on safe drugs before conception that are least harmful to the fetus and patient education about their role in disease management.

Disease Activity

If active disease initiate intervention to optimize disease activity and defer pregnancy, obtain autoantibody for risk evaluation, especially antiphospholipid and anti-Ro antibody. Assess major organ function—advice against pregnancy if severe dysfunction. Patients with evidence of active SLE, especially LN, should be advised to defer pregnancy until the disease is well controlled for at least 6 months. For those with renal insufficiency, counseling should include an assessment of the risk of temporary or permanent decline in renal function.

Recent history of stroke, cardiac involvement, pulmonary HTN, severe interstitial lung disease, and advanced renal insufficiency can result in poor pregnancy outcome for both the mother and the fetus. Women with these or other worrisome medical conditions should be counseled carefully as to their individual risk profile, with clear discussion of the morbidity and mortality risks to both the mother and the fetus associated with pregnancy.

Counsel about potential obstetric problems such as pregnancy loss, preterm birth, gestational HTN/pulmonary embolism (PE), intrauterine growth restriction (IUGR), SLE flare, and NL syndrome.

Contraindications to Pregnancy

Maternal risk factors where pregnancy should be avoided include severe manifestation of cardiomyopathy, cardiac valve disease, pulmonary HTN, interstitial lung disease, and serious neurological manifestation. Moderate to severe renal insufficiency may put a woman at risk of organ failure. Pregnancy is contraindicated in severe pulmonary HTN [systolic pulmonary artery pressure (PAP) >50 mm Hg], severe restrictive lung disease (vital capacity <1 L), advanced renal insufficiency (creatinine >2.8 mg/dL), previous severe PE, or HELLP (Hemolysis, Elevated Liver enzymes and Low Platelets) despite therapy.

Pregnancy should be deferred in cases of severe disease flare within last 6 months, active LN, stroke within the previous 6 months. Significant lupus activity within 6 months prior to conception is associated with fourfold increased risk of fetal loss and more than fourfold increased risk of flare. Patients can plan pregnancy if in remission for 6 months prior to conception preferably >1 year, cytotoxic drug stopped for >6 months, maintenance therapy with HCQ or glucocorticoid (<7.5 mg/day). Ideally pregnancy is undertaken without immunosuppressive therapy or steroid, reduced anti-HTN to an acceptable level.

Specific Laboratory Testing

In addition to routine tests, following special tests should be done in the preconception period:
- Anti-Ro/SSA and anti-La/SSB antibodies
- Renal function (creatinine, urinalysis with urine sediment, spot urine protein/creatinine ratio)
- Complete blood count (CBC)
- Liver function tests
- Anti-ds DNA antibodies
- Complement (CH50, or C_3 and C_4)

Consider testing for APLAs [LAC, immunoglobulin G (IgG) and IgM ACAs, and IgG and IgM anti-β2-glycoprotein (GP) antibodies] in women with prior poor obstetric performance.

Management in Pregnancy

Management of pregnant women with SLE should involve close collaboration between a rheumatologist and an obstetrician experienced in caring for high-risk mothers, may need consultation from nephrologist and hematologist. Patients should be seen at 2–4 weeks' interval, with assessment of maternal blood pressure, proteinuria, and SLE symptoms at each visit. Routine testing of serologies and complement levels in each trimester may be of value in identifying the asymptomatic patient before a clinically recognizable flare in disease activity.

Monitoring Systemic Lupus Erythematosus Activity

Women should be assessed by a rheumatologist for disease activity at least once each trimester, and more frequently if she has active SLE. The schedule for monitoring includes the following mentioned below.

Initial evaluation: At the first visit after (or at which) pregnancy is confirmed, the following investigations are recommended:
- Physical examination, including blood pressure
- Renal function (creatinine, urinalysis, spot urine protein/creatinine ratio)
- CBC
- Liver function tests
- Anti-Ro/SSA and anti-La/SSB antibodies
- LAC and anticardiolipin antibody assays
- Anti-ds DNA antibodies
- Complement (CH50, or C_3 and C_4)
- Serum uric acid

Some physiological changes of pregnancy may overlap with features of active SLE, making differentiation difficult; symptoms of extreme fatigue, fever, myalgia, and arthralgia are diagnostic of SLE. Laboratory findings that may be present during a normal pregnancy include mild anemia, elevated ESR, and mild proteinuria; proteinuria should remain below 300 mg/24 hours. A baseline 24-hour urine collection can be helpful to distinguish lupus flare from preeclampsia and normal changes later in pregnancy. Also, during normal pregnancy, complement levels may rise by 10–50%, and may appear to remain normal despite active SLE. Thus, the trend of complement levels is generally more informative than the actual value.

Differentiate pre-eclampsia (PE) and SLE: Laboratory testing must be interpreted in the clinical context and women who show evidence of increased serologic activity but who remain asymptomatic should be monitored more closely **(Table 2)**. The following laboratory tests are recommended at regular intervals during pregnancy:
- CBC
- Creatinine
- Urinalysis with examination of urinary sediment
- Spot urine protein/creatinine ratio or 24-hour urine collection.

The anti-ds DNA antibodies and complement (CH50, or C_3 and C_4) should be performed, rising anti-ds DNA titers or decreasing levels of C_3 or C_4 are suggestive of disease activation. Additional laboratory tests such as liver function tests and serum uric acid should be guided by the clinical presentation. The frequency of laboratory testing is individualized and varies with disease activity. Patients with stable disease should ideally undergo laboratory testing each trimester, but those with active lupus will require more frequent testing.

Pregnancy with SLE is associated with higher risk of complications compared to normal, many fold increased risk of maternal death, preeclampsia, preterm labor, thrombosis, infection, and hematologic complications. PE complicates 16–30% of SLE, eclampsia—four times more common. About 10% of women with SLE have hypothyroidism. Autoimmune thyroid tests should be checked in addition to free thyroxine (fT_4) and thyroid-stimulating hormone (TSH).

Maternal-fetal monitoring: The optimal monitoring schedule to ensure maternal and fetal health during pregnancy is not known. Women with risk factors or poor prognostic indicators will require more frequent monitoring. In addition to routine prenatal care, monitoring for women with SLE includes the following mentioned in **Table 3**.

TABLE 2: Laboratory criteria to differentiate pre-eclampsia from SLE.

Test	Pre-eclampsia	SLE
Serologic		
Decreased complement	++	+++
Anti-ds DNA	–	+++
Antithrombin III deficiency	++	+
Hematologic		
Microangiopathic hemolytic anemia	++	–
Coombs' positive hemolytic anemia	–	++
Thrombocytopenia	+	++
Leukopenia	+	+++
Renal		
Hematuria	–	+++
Cellular casts	+	++
Elevated serum creatinine	+	++
Elevated BUN/creatinine	+	++
Hypocalciuria	++	+
Liver transaminases	++	+

(PE: pulmonary embolism; SLE: systemic lupus erythematosus)

Drug Treatment

The treatment of active SLE during pregnancy is guided by the severity and degree of organ involvement, similar to the approach for patients in the nonpregnant state. Some medications used to treat SLE may cross the placenta and cause fetal harm. Thus, the risks and benefits of treatment during pregnancy must be weighed against the risk of SLE activity having a deleterious effect on the mother and the fetus.

Four main groups of useful drugs prescribed in SLE include nonsteroidal anti-inflammatory drugs (NSAIDs), antimalarials, corticosteroid, and cytotoxic drugs. Other treatment options are plasma exchange and intravenous immunoglobulin (IVIg).

The ACR guideline recommends that all women with SLE take HCQ during pregnancy, if possible. If a patient is already taking HCQ, continuing it during pregnancy is strongly recommended; if she is not taking HCQ, starting it if there is no contraindication. The ACR also conditionally recommends treating SLE patients with low-dose aspirin (81 or 100 mg daily), beginning in the first trimester.

EULAR guidelines recommend HCQ be taken preconceptionally and throughout pregnancy to control disease activity. HCQ, oral glucocorticoids, azathioprine, cyclosporine, and tacrolimus can be used to prevent or manage SLE flares during pregnancy. Moderate-to-severe flares can be managed with additional strategies, including glucocorticoids intravenous pulse therapy, IVIg, and plasmapheresis. Mycophenolic acid, cyclophosphamide, leflunomide, and methotrexate should be avoided.

Hydroxychloroquine

Hydroxychloroquine is an antimalarial drug that inhibits toll-like receptors 7 and 9. These are potent drivers of type 1 interferon production. HCQ is useful in both cutaneous and systemic lupus. Approximately half of patients with cutaneous lupus fail to respond to standard doses (200 mg daily) and may benefit from higher doses (400 mg daily). In addition to improving skin symptoms, HCQ reduces

TABLE 3: Antenatal care in SLE.

Clinical review	Investigations	Specific monitoring
• *Rheumatologist*: 4–6 weekly, more frequent if active disease or flare • *Obstetrician*: Monthly till week 20, then 2 weekly till week 28, and weekly thereafter	• *Each visit*: Blood count, serum uric acid, urea, creatinine, electrolyte levels, liver function tests, urinalysis, spot urine protein/creatinine ratio, complement levels, and ds DNA antibodies • *Ultrasound*: Early pregnancy for gestational dating, between weeks 16 and 20 screen for fetal anomalies 4 weekly, thereafter, to monitor growth • *Fetal surveillance tests (FSTs)*: Weekly from 26th week	• *Positive anti-Ro antibodies*: Fetal echocardiography, weekly from 16 to 26 and biweekly thereafter, continuing till delivery • *Pre-eclampsia*: Uterine artery Doppler (week 20 and 4 weekly thereafter) • Umbilical artery Doppler (weekly from 26 onward) • *IUGR*: frequency of growth monitoring by USG and FST

(IUGR: intrauterine growth restriction)

flares of systemic lupus and LN. It also lowers cholesterol and thromboembolic risk in patients with APLAs, therapy minimizes glucocorticoid-induced osteoporosis, and improves overall survival. The major complications of HCQ therapy are ocular-transient and reversible corneal deposits occur in about 10% cases.

Hydroxychloroquine is safe in pregnancy. Most pregnant women with SLE are advised to continue HCQ to reduce the risk of SLE flares and prevent damage. Several studies have demonstrated fewer disease flares and better outcomes in patients continuing HCQ during pregnancy. A large prospective study, with 257 pregnancies in 197 women, found that discontinuation of HCQ during pregnancy was associated with a higher rate of flare, compared with women who either continued HCQ during pregnancy or never took it. Dose is <6.5 mg/kg/day in mild lupus.

Glucocorticoids

Control of disease with the lowest possible dose of prednisone, ideally <10 mg/day; <7.5 mg/day in mild lupus, higher dose >0.5 mg/kg/day in moderate case to prevent flare. While there are some reports of glucocorticoid use during the first trimester being associated with cleft lip, with and without cleft palate, subsequent studies have failed to consistently demonstrate an increased risk of this malformation. Chronic use may cause PE, uteroplacental insufficiency, IUGR, and glucose intolerance. Screening for gestational diabetes mellitus (GDM) should be done at 22–24 weeks, 28–30 weeks, and 32–34 weeks in women on glucocorticoids.

Nonsteroidal Anti-inflammatory Drugs (Aspirin, Ibuprofen, and Indomethacin)

There is conflicting evidence as to whether exposure to NSAIDs during the first trimester increases the risk of spontaneous abortion. There is a small increased risk of oligohydramnios when NSAIDs are used beyond 20 weeks; the US Food and Drug Administration (FDA) recommends that the lowest dose and shortest duration of NSAID be used between 20 and 30 weeks of gestation. Use of NSAIDs after 30 weeks of gestation may cause premature closure of the ductus arteriosus, as well as other complications, and should be avoided altogether from the third trimester onward. Long-term use cause oligohydramnios, intraventricular hemorrhage (IVH), and neonatal renal insufficiency.

Antiproliferative Drugs

Three antiproliferative immunosuppressants are primarily used in systemic lupus—azathioprine, methotrexate, and mycophenolate. Among these three, methotrexate and mycophenolate are teratogenic and contraindicated in pregnancy.

Azathioprine

Azathioprine is compatible with pregnancy, but doses should not exceed 2 mg/kg/day. It is nonteratogenic, use if steroid is ineffective, may cause IUGR.

Tacrolimus

Tacrolimus, a calcineurin inhibitor that is 100 times more potent in vitro compared with cyclosporine, has been used as induction and maintenance therapy in SLE nephritis. A small case series of nine pregnant lupus patients reported successful disease maintenance or control of LN flares with tacrolimus. A subsequent series of 54 deliveries in 40 patients found that pregnancy outcomes were similar between tacrolimus versus non-tacrolimus exposure. A causal relationship between tacrolimus and birth defects has not been found.

Biologic Medications

Data regarding the use of biologic medications such as the B-cell depleting antibody, *rituximab*, or the B-cell activating factor (BAFF) inhibitor, *belimumab*, during pregnancy are limited. Given that IgG does not cross the placenta in significant amounts until 12 weeks of gestation, these medications can be continued through conception.

Intravenous Immunoglobulin

Prepared from the plasma of thousands of blood donors, therapeutic IVIg mostly consists of human polyspecific IgG. The use of IVIg in SLE is still considered experimental without any clear indications. Several anecdotal reports and a few studies have shown promising results on the effectiveness of IVIg in the treatment of SLE particularly with LN and in case of recurrent pregnancy loss (RPL) with APLA. A daily infusion of 400 mg immunoglobulins per kg body weight was given during five consecutive days every month to a patient with RPL resulted in successful pregnancy, with no adverse effect on pregnancy.

Drugs Contraindicated in Pregnancy

- *Methotrexate:* Methotrexate is teratogenic and should not be used during pregnancy.
- *Mycophenolate mofetil:* Mycophenolate is effective in nonrenal disease that is refractory to corticosteroids and is superior to azathioprine. However, it is contraindicated in pregnancy. Congenital anomalies (external ear anomaly, cleft lip, palate, distal limb, heart, esophagus, kidney anomaly) have been reported in infants exposed to mycophenolate mofetil during pregnancy. Use in the first trimester cause pregnancy loss.
- *Cyclophosphamide:* Cyclophosphamide is associated with congenital malformations and should be avoided during the first trimester, use only in severe cases

as DPGN. In life-threatening clinical situations, this medication has been used in late pregnancy.

Adjunctive therapies: In vitamin D insufficiency and deficiency, supplementation may decrease disease activity and improve fatigue. Supplementation may improve endothelial function, which may reduce cardiovascular disease.

Presence of Antiphospholipid Antibodies

Antiphospholipid antibodies are present in about a quarter to a half of patients with SLE; however, few patients develop thrombotic or obstetric complications related to antiphospholipid syndrome (APS). Pregnant women with SLE who have an obstetric history suggestive of APS (fetal death after 10 weeks or three or more consecutive miscarriages, or premature birth <34 weeks due to preeclampsia or placental insufficiency) or unexplained venous or arterial thrombotic event, should be tested for the presence of APLAs (i.e., LAC, IgG and IgM ACAs; and IgG and IgM anti-β2-GP).

Antiphospholipid antibody is associated with significant risk of pregnancy morbidity and loss. Antiphospholipid antibody increases the risk of PE, placental insufficiency, IUGR, and preterm delivery. Management strategies differ, based on the risk profile of each pregnancy. Low-dose aspirin as antiplatelet agent is safe in pregnancy, generally recommended alone for asymptomatic women with only persistently positive APLA and no prior event. Aspirin in combination with prophylactic doses of heparin significantly reduces the risk of pregnancy loss in obstetric APS and is the current treatment of choice. Low-dose aspirin starting from approximately 12 weeks of gestation, to reduce the risk of preeclampsia and its sequelae (e.g., fetal growth restriction), regardless of the presence of APLAs, is the recommendation by the United States Preventive Services Task Force.

Low Molecular Weight Heparin/Unfractionated Heparin

Heparin does not cross the placenta and is the anticoagulant of choice during pregnancy. Low molecular weight heparin (LMWH) has similar efficacy and safety to unfractionated heparin (UFH). The ease of administration, higher antithrombotic to anticoagulant ratio, and predictable bioavailability have led to widespread use of LMWH instead of UFH. LMWH must be transitioned to UFH prior to delivery. Heparin treatment needs to be continued up to 6 weeks postpartum. Patients with prior systemic thrombosis should receive full therapeutic doses of heparin throughout pregnancy.

Labor and Delivery

Deliver at term, avoid postdate, continuous fetal heart rate (FHR) monitoring in labor. Stress dose of glucocorticoid, during labor or lower segment caesarean section (LSCS), to all patients who has been treated with chronic steroid within previous year. Dose: Intravenous (IV) hydrocortisone in three doses of 100 mg every 8 hours.

Postnatal Management

Check neonate for NL manifestation. Breastfeeding is feasible. Some women will experience exacerbations of SLE in the postpartum period, rate of SLE flares ranges from 13 to 70%; but the majority of flares are mild.

Restart maintenance therapy in postpartum. Women who have had active disease at conception and those with significant end-organ damage are at greater risk of disease flares in the postpartum period compared with women with inactive disease. Thus, periodic assessment of disease activity is warranted.

Recommended laboratory tests in postpartum: The following laboratory tests are recommended at 1 month following an uncomplicated delivery:
- Urinalysis, urine protein/urine creatinine ratio
- Renal function if the urinalysis is abnormal
- CBC

Additionally, the following laboratory tests in patients with severe disease or in those in whom the anti-ds DNA and complement levels correlate well with disease activity:
- Anti-ds DNA
- Complement (CH50, or C_3 and C_4)

Maternal Complications

Pregnancy in the setting of SLE is associated with a higher risk of complications compared with healthy women. Several predictors of adverse pregnancy outcomes among women with SLE have been identified and include active disease, use of antihypertensives, prior LN, the presence of APLAs, and thrombocytopenia.

The largest study to evaluate maternal and pregnancy complications associated with SLE included 13,555 pregnancies, found women with SLE had a two- to fourfold increased rate of obstetric complications including preterm labor, unplanned cesarean delivery, fetal growth restriction, preeclampsia, and eclampsia. Patients with SLE also had a significantly higher risk of thrombosis, infection, thrombocytopenia, and transfusion. This study also reported that maternal mortality was 20-fold higher among women with SLE. A large population-based study suggested that pregnancy complications including mortality rates are decreasing in the recent years, although still higher compared with those without SLE.

Preeclampsia: It is one of the most frequent complications of pregnancy in SLE, occurring in 16–30% of women with SLE, compared with 4.6% in the general obstetric population. While preeclampsia presenting later in pregnancy can often be managed expectantly, in pre- and periviable gestations, delivery is indicated to prevent catastrophic maternal complications. In women at elevated risk of PE, low-dose aspirin has been shown to reduce the absolute risk of disease by approximately 2–5% when initiated between 12 and 16 weeks of gestation.

Preterm birth: Rates of preterm birth from 15 to 50% have been reported, compared to 12% of normal pregnancies in the United States obstetric population, with increased incidence in women with LN or high disease activity. The majority of preterm births are medically indicated due to preeclampsia or maternal SLE activity. The presence of LN and active disease are the strongest predictors for early delivery.

Risk of SLE flare: Flares can occur in any trimester, >50% SLE exacerbation in pregnancy occur in the first trimester, rate of flare highest who discontinued their prepregnancy HCQ.

Lupus nephritis exacerbation: Transient deterioration of renal function occurs in 17% cases, permanent deterioration of renal function in 8% case. Sole predictor for flare-serum creatinine >1.2 mg/dL or proteinuria >500 mg in 24 hours urine collection. Outlook for pregnant women with nephropathy is favorable if disease is well-controlled and renal function preserved. Studies showed women who began pregnancy with nephrotic syndrome, went on renal failure after delivery, while women with inactive LN prior to conception rarely suffer permanent deterioration during pregnancy.

Fetal and Neonatal Risks

Fetal complications in patients with SLE include miscarriage and stillbirth (20%), growth restriction, NL syndromes, and complications of prematurity. Women with SLE are at increased risk of fetal death beyond 10 weeks, particularly in the presence of active SLE, LN, and APS. Proteinuria, HTN, thrombocytopenia, and APLA are negative predictors for fetal survival.

Fetal growth restriction: About 10–30% of pregnancies in women with SLE are complicated by fetal growth restriction and small-for-gestational-age babies compared with about 10% of pregnancies in the general obstetric population. As with other complications, the risk is higher in the presence of active disease, HTN, and LN.

NL: NL is a passively transferred autoimmune disease that occurs in some babies born to mothers with anti-Ro/SSA or anti-La/SSB antibodies, who may or may not carry the diagnosis of SLE or Sjögren. The major manifestations of NL are either cutaneous or cardiac, other manifestations include hematologic and hepatic abnormalities. <5% develop NL; risk 15% with positive anti-SSA, anti-SSB antibody.

Dermatologic manifestation: Neonatal lupus erythematosus (NLE) lesions are typically annular erythematous plaques with a slight scale, which appear predominately on the scalp, neck, or face (typically periorbital in distribution), but similar plaques may appear on the trunk or extremities. Usually appear in the first week of life, may last up to 6 months.

Hematologic manifestations: Rare, include autoimmune hemolytic anemia, neutropenia, profound thrombocytopenia, may occur in the first 2 weeks of life.

CCHB: The most serious complication in the neonate is CCHB which occurs in 2% cases. There is permanent damage to the fetal cardiac conduction system, especially in area of atrioventricular (AV) node by passively acquired fetal autoimmunity from maternal antibodies, anti-Ro, and anti-La antibodies. In women who have had a child with CCHB, the risk of complete heart block increases to approximately 16–18% for subsequent pregnancies, or 10–15% when a previous infant had cutaneous NL.

Diagnosis is made between 18 and 24 weeks, when fetal bradycardia (60–80 beats/minute) detected during a routine ANV. Fetal echocardiography reveals complete AV dissociation with a structurally normal heart. In less severe cases, there is a role of pacemaker. Sequelae in most severe cases—cardiac failure-nonimmune fetal hydrops (NIFH)-fetal death. Maternal administration of fluorinated corticosteroids has shown fetal survival benefit in some studies, majority of survivors require pacemakers.

Hepatosplenomegaly: Neonate may have hepatosplenomegaly. The clinical spectrum of associated hepatobiliary disease ranges from mild elevations of aminotransferase levels to conjugated hyperbilirubinemia with normal or slightly elevated aminotransferase levels.

Neurologic involvement: may also be seen in NLE and may manifest as hydrocephalus and/or macrocephaly.

■ SUGGESTED READING

1. Aringer M, Costenbader K, Daikh D, Brinks R, Mosca M, Ramsey-Goldman R, et al. 2019 European League Against Rheumatism/American College of Rheumatology classification criteria for systemic lupus erythematosus. Ann Rheum Dis. 2019;78(9):1151-9.
2. Arnout J, Spitz B, Wittevrongel C, Vanrusselt M. High-dose intravenous immunoglobulin treatment of a pregnant patient with an antiphospholipid syndrome: immunological changes associated with a successful outcome. Thromb Haemost. 1994;71(6):741-7.
3. Barber MRW, Drenkard C. Global epidemiology of systemic lupus erythematosus. Nat Rev Rheumatol. 2021;17(9):515-32.
4. Bermas BL, Smith NA. Pregnancy in women with systemic lupus erythematosus. UpToDate. 2021.
5. Buyon JP, Kim MY, Guerra MM, Laskin CA, Petri M, Lockshin MD, et al. Predictors of pregnancy outcomes in patients with lupus: A cohort study. Ann Intern Med. 2015;163(3):153.

6. Cush J. (2019). New EULAR /ACR classification criteria for SLE. [online] Available from: rheumnow.com/. [Last accessed April 2022].
7. Eudy AM, Siega-Riz AM, Engel SM, Franceschini N, Howard AG, Clowse MEB, et al. Effect of pregnancy on disease flares in patients with systemic lupus erythematosus. Ann Rheum Dis. 2018;77(6):855-60.
8. Gibson CM, Mir M. (2020). Systemic lupus erythematosus pathophysiology. Wiki Doc. [online] Available from: https://www.wikidoc.org/index.php/Systemic_lupus_erythematosus_overview#:~:text=The%20pathophysiology%20of%20systemic%20lupus,UV)%20light%20and%20certain%20infections. [Last accessed April 2022].
9. Khurana R. (2020). Systemic Lupus Erythematosus and Pregnancy. [online] Available from: https://emedicine.medscape.com/article/335055-overview#:~:text=Pregnancy%20in%20women%20with%20lupus,severe%20renal%20exacerbations%20are%20possible. [Last accessed April 2022].
10. Lateef A, Petri M. Managing lupus patients during pregnancy. Best Pract Res Clin Rheumatol. 2013;27(3):10.1016/j.berh.2013.07.005.
11. McKeon KP, Jiang SH. Treatment of systemic lupus erythematosus. Aust Prescr. 2020;43(3):85-90.
12. Mehta B, Luo Y, Xu J, Sammaritano L, Salmon J, Lockshin M, et al. Trends in maternal and fetal outcomes among pregnant women with systemic lupus erythematosus in the United States: A cross-sectional analysis. Ann Intern Med. 2019;171(3):164-71.
13. Peaceman A, Ramsey-Goldman R. Autoimmune connective tissue disease in pregnancy. Glob Libr women Med. 2008.
14. Sammaritano LR, Salmon JE. Pregnancy and rheumatic disease. In: Creasy and Resnik's Maternal Fetal Medicine, 8th edition. Amsterdam: Elsevier; 2019.
15. The American College of Obstetricians and Gynaecologists. (2020). Systemic Lupus Erythematosus. [online] Available from: https://www.acog.org/clinical/journals-and-publications/clinical-updates/2020/07/systemic-lupus-erythematosus. [Last accessed April 2022].
16. Vaillant AAJ, Goya A. Systemic Lupus Erythematosus. Treasure Island (FL): StatPearls Publishing; 2022.
17. Wallace DJ, Pisetsky DS. Overview of the management and prognosis of systemic lupus erythematosus in adults. UpToDate. 2021.
18. Wenderfer SE, Thacker T. Intravenous immunoglobulin in the management of lupus nephritis. Autoimmune Dis. 2012; 2012:589359.
19. Yang H, Liu H, Xu D, Zhao L, Wang Q, Leng X, et al. Pregnancy-related systemic lupus erythematosus: clinical features, outcome and risk factors of disease flares—a case control study. PLoS One. 2014;9(8):e104375.

CHAPTER 15

Recurrent Pregnancy Loss

DEFINITION

Spontaneous pregnancy loss is a surprisingly common occurrence, occurs in approximately 15-25% of all pregnancies. Indeed, the risk of loss is between 9 and 12% in women aged ≤35 years, increases to 50% in women aged >40 years. The risk of miscarriage after two consecutive losses is 17-25% and the risk after three consecutive losses is between 25 and 46% and the risk gets worse with increasing maternal age and an increasing number of miscarriages. Recurrent pregnancy loss (RPL) is defined as two or more pregnancy losses occurring prior to 20 weeks of gestation. The definition of RPL has long been debated, there is lack of consensus among international societies regarding the number of miscarriages required for defining recurrent miscarriage (RM).

- American Society for Reproductive Medicine (ASRM) has defined RPL as two or more failed clinical pregnancies (pregnancy in this case requiring ultrasound or histological confirmation), thereby excluding biochemical pregnancies but requiring only two losses.
- European Society of Human Reproduction and Embryology (ESHRE) defines diagnosis of RPL after the loss of two or more pregnancies. This definition includes pregnancy losses both after spontaneous conception and assisted reproductive technology (ART), but excludes ectopic and molar pregnancies (if identified as such) and implantation failure.
- Royal College of Obstetricians and Gynaecologists (RCOG) defined RPL as three or more consecutive pregnancy losses at <20 weeks of gestation including nonvisualized ones (biochemical pregnancy).
- The German, Austrian, and Swiss Societies of Gynecology and Obstetrics (DGGG/OEGGG/SGGG) also consider RM as ≥3 consecutive losses.
- International Committee for Monitoring Assisted Reproductive Technology; World Health Organization (ICMART) defined the loss of an embryo/fetus of <400 g if gestational age is unknown.

Recurrent early pregnancy loss (REPL) or embryonic loss is defined as the loss of two or more pregnancies occurring before 10 weeks of gestation and fetal loss when it occurs after 10 gestational weeks, factors associated with each may differ. Primary RPL refers to multiple losses in a woman with no previous viable infants, whereas secondary RPL refers to multiple losses in a woman who has already had a pregnancy beyond 20 gestational weeks.

PREVALENCE

The incidence of RPL varies widely between reports because of the differences in the definitions and criteria used, as well as the populations' characteristics but most studies report that RPL affects 1-2% of women, if preclinical pregnancies are included, the prevalence can be high as 3% and only 1% experience three or more loss (ASRM, 2012).

ETIOLOGY

Common established causes of RPL include genetics, age, antiphospholipid syndrome (APS), uterine anomalies, and hormonal or metabolic disorders. Other etiologies have been proposed but are still considered controversial and include inherited thrombophilia, infection, alloimmunity, sperm quality, and lifestyle issues. In almost 50% cases, the cause remains unknown **(Fig. 1)**.

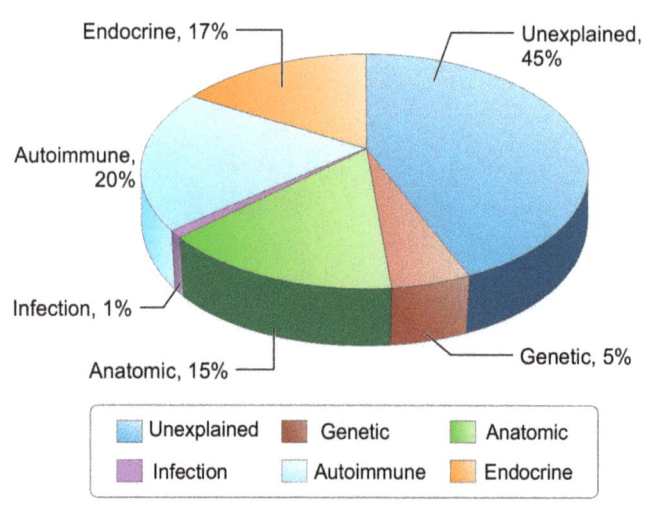

Fig. 1: Causes of RPL.

Age and Pregnancy Loss

Spontaneous miscarriage occurs in 10–15% of clinically recognized pregnancies, the major underlying cause being embryonic aneuploidy. Since meiotic chromosome segregation errors in oocytes account for majority of embryonic aneuploidies which increase with age, the risk of having a miscarriage is strongly influenced by female age. The background risk of having three miscarriages for women <25 years is around 0.13% but 100 times more likely (~13%) if over 40 years. A large prospective study reported the age-related risk of miscarriage in recognized pregnancies to be: 12–19 years, 13%; 20–24 years, 11%; 25–29 years, 12%; 30–34 years, 15%; 35–39 years, 25%; 40–44 years, 51%; and ≥45 years, 93%. Advanced paternal age has also been identified a risk factor for miscarriage. The risk of miscarriage is highest among couples where the woman is ≥35 years and the man ≥40 years of age.

Chromosomal Abnormality

The vast majority (50–60%) of early pregnancy losses are the consequence of chromosomal abnormalities **(Fig. 2A)**, which can be of parental origin, or arise de novo in the gametes prior to fertilization due to maternal nondisjunction of meiosis 1 or after fertilization from parents with normal chromosomes. Most miscarriages with aneuploidies arise de novo and the risk increases with maternal age. Less frequently the miscarriage is a result of a gamete with an unbalanced chromosomal translocation inherited from a parent carrying a balanced chromosome rearrangement, some may be due to submicroscopic chromosomal changes.

Numerical abnormalities account for ~95% of all abnormalities seen in miscarriages, these include autosomal trisomy involving chromosomes 16, 21, 22, 13, and 18 (with 47 chromosomes rather than 46), sex chromosome trisomy (47, XXY), or monosomy (45X). Single-gene, X-linked, or polygenic/multifactorial disorders can also result in sporadic or RM. Parental chromosomal anomalies **(Fig. 2B)** account for 2–5% of RPL, translocations are the most common aberrations, followed by inversions, insertions, and mosaicism in light of its frequency and causality. Translocations may be reciprocal (~60%), involving the exchange of genetic material from one chromosome to another, or Robertsonian (~40%), where the long arms of two acrocentric chromosomes incorrectly share a centrosome.

Although carriers of a balanced reciprocal translocation are usually phenotypically normal, their pregnancies are at increased risk of miscarriage (50%), compared to noncarrier couples with RPL (30%). The risk of miscarriage is influenced by the size and the genetic content of the rearranged chromosomal segments. Reciprocal translocation may result in a live birth with multiple congenital malformation and/or mental disability secondary to an unbalanced chromosomal arrangement; chance of having a live birth with an unbalanced chromosome complement is 1–15%.

Robertsonian translocation involves the acrocentric chromosomes (13, 14, 15, 21, and 22), which fuse near the centromere region with loss of short arms. Individual with Robertsonian translocations has 45 chromosomes. Since only the satellite material is lost, no phenotype is associated with a Robertsonian translocation, but when these individuals have children, there is risk of both Robertsonian and one of the normal homologous chromosomes being inherited from the parent, resulting in trisomy. One common Robertsonian translocation involves chromosomes 14 and 21, with the risk of child with trisomy 21 (Down syndrome)—"translocation Down syndrome."

Uterine Factors

Anatomic Defects

Uterine anomalies are reportedly found in up to ~16.7% in RPL as compared with ~6.7% in the general population and

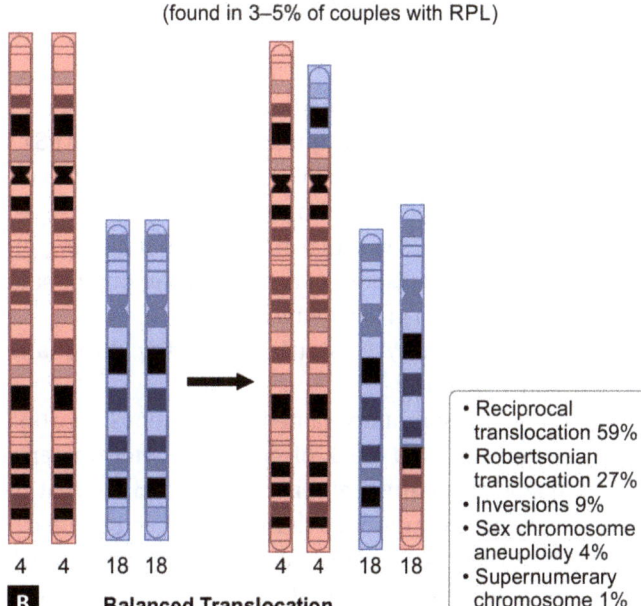

Figs. 2A and B: (A) Different types structural chromosomal defect; (B) Balanced reciprocal traslocation between chromosome 4 & 18. (RPL: recurrent pregnancy loss)
Source: Figure (A) Slide Serve; Figure (B) Wikipedia.

can be classified as acquired or congenital. According to the American Fertility Society (AFS)/*ASRM* and the European Society for Human Reproduction and Embryology/European Society for Gynecological Endoscopy classification, congenital uterine anomalies are found in 8.4–12.6% of women with RPL, which is seven to eight times higher than the general population.

Congenital Müllerian tract malformations include septate uterus, bicornuate uterus, didelphic uterus, and unicornuate uterus. Septate uterus is the most common congenital uterine abnormality associated with spontaneous miscarriage identified in ~5% of women with RM in one series, reported incidence varies from 1.8 to 37%. It has been reported that women with arcuate uterus tend to miscarry in the second trimester, while women with septate uterus are more likely to miscarry in the first trimester. Acquired abnormalities include intrauterine adhesions, myomas, and endometrial polyps. Submucosal myomas are reportedly found in 4.5% of women with RPL, polyps are found in 2-3% of women with RPL.

Cervical weakness is a recognized cause of second-trimester miscarriage, but the true incidence is unknown. There is currently no satisfactory objective test that can identify women with cervical weakness in the nonpregnant state. The diagnosis is usually based on a history of second-trimester miscarriage preceded by spontaneous rupture of membranes or painless cervical dilatation.

Antiphospholipid Syndrome

Antiphospholipid syndrome is characterized by the presence of antiphospholipid antibodies (aPL) and has long been associated with RPL. The prevalence of APS in women with RPL varies according to studies, from as low as 6% to as high as 42%, but generally accepted to be 5–20%.

According to international consensus classification criteria, antiphospholipid antibody syndrome (APS) is present, if at least one of the following clinical criteria and one of the laboratory criteria are met:
- *Clinical criteria 1:* Vascular thrombosis including one or more clinical episodes of an arterial, venous, or small vessel thrombosis in any tissue or organ
- *Clinical criteria 2:* Obstetric morbidity. Pregnancy morbidity includes:
  - Three or more unexplained spontaneous abortions before the 10th week of gestation when maternal anatomic or hormonal abnormalities and paternal and maternal chromosomal causes have been excluded.
  - One or more unexplained deaths of a morphologically normal fetus at or beyond the 10th week of gestation.
  - One or more preterm births of a morphologically normal fetus before the 34th week of gestation because of eclampsia or severe pre-eclampsia or recognized features of placental insufficiency.

Laboratory criteria include either:
- Lupus anticoagulant (LA) present in plasma, on two or more occasions at least 12 weeks apart
- *Anticardiolipin (aCL):* Immunoglobulin G (IgG) and/or IgM isotype in serum or plasma, present in medium or high titer [i.e., >40 GPL units or MPL units, or >99th percentile], on two or more occasions, at least 12 weeks apart
- Anti-β2-glycoprotein I antibody of IgG and/or IgM isotype in serum or plasma (in titer >99th percentile), present on two or more occasions at least 12 weeks apart

Mechanism of Pregnancy Loss

Antiphospholipid antibodies are thought to impair pregnancy through various mechanisms, including inhibition of villous cytotrophoblast differentiation and extravillous cytotrophoblast invasion into the decidua, thrombosis of the uteroplacental vasculature, and initiation of a local inflammatory response via complement activation at the maternal-fetal interface. Inappropriate secretion of human chorionic gonadotropin and growth factor, and induction of syncytiotrophoblast apoptosis may also play a role in pregnancy failure.

Hormonal and Metabolic Factors

It is generally agreed that maternal endocrine disorders (e.g., diabetes and thyroid dysfunction) should be evaluated and treated.

Diabetes

Uncontrolled diabetes is associated with increased pregnancy loss. The increased risk in poorly controlled diabetic women is believed to be secondary to hyperglycemia, maternal vascular disease, and possibly immunologic factors. There is no increased risk of miscarriage in women with well-controlled diabetes mellitus (DM).

Thyroid Dysfunction

Poorly controlled thyroid disease (hypo- or hyperthyroidism) is associated with infertility and pregnancy loss. While miscarriage is increased with overt hypothyroidism, the association between subclinical hypothyroidism (SCH) and pregnancy loss is less clear. Thyroid autoimmunity has been related to unexplained infertility and implantation failure, however, direct evidence is still lacking. ESHRE guideline recommends thyroid screening [TSH and thyroid peroxidase (TPO)-antibodies] in women with RPL. Abnormal TSH and TPO antibody levels should be followed up by T_4 testing.

Hyperprolactinemia is associated with infertility and miscarriage by altering the hypothalamic–pituitary–ovarian axis, thus leading to impaired folliculogenesis and anovulation. Serum prolactin testing is not recommended by ESHRE in women with RPL in the absence of clinical symptoms of hyperprolactinemia (oligo/amenorrhea).

Polycystic ovarian syndrome (PCOS) is associated with an increased risk of miscarriage. Many mechanisms are thought to be involved, including insulin resistance and hyperinsulinemia, hyperandrogenemia, or increased plasminogen activator inhibitor-1 activity. Lifestyle modifications, including weight reduction and exercise, improve insulin resistance and could thus decrease the risk of miscarriage.

Assessment of PCOS, fasting insulin, and fasting glucose is not recommended by ESHRE in women with RPL to improve next pregnancy prognosis. An elevated androgen index appears to be a prognostic factor for a subsequent miscarriage in women with RM.

Luteal phase defect: A 2015 Committee Opinion released by the *ASRM* concluded that "there is no reproducible, pathophysiologically relevant and clinically practical standard to diagnose luteal phase deficiency and distinguish fertile from infertile women." ESHRE and ASRM does not recommend performing luteal phase testing. Administration of progesterone to women with sporadic miscarriages is ineffective. However, in patients with three or more consecutive miscarriages, empiric progestogen administration may be of some potential benefit. A large UK-based randomized controlled trial (RCT) [Progesterone in Recurrent Miscarriage (PROMISE) Trial 2015] failed to show a benefit with progesterone replacement.

Inherited Thrombophilia

Inherited thrombophilia is a genetic predisposition increasing the tendency to develop venous thrombosis and has been evaluated as a potential cause of pregnancy loss. The most common thrombophilia factors are factor V Leiden, prothrombin gene mutation, protein C and protein S deficiency, antithrombin III deficiency and methyltetrahydrofolate reductase (MTHFR) mutation. Combined prevalence of inherited thrombophilia in the general population is ~5%.

A meta-analysis of retrospective studies reported strong association between second-trimester miscarriage and inherited thrombophilia. Screening for inherited thrombophilia is recommended in pregnant women with a history of venous thromboembolism, however, the association with RPL remains controversial. RCOG advises testing for thrombophilia after second-trimester loss, not for recurrent early pregnancy loss (REPL). Routine testing of women with RPL for inherited thrombophilia is not currently recommended by ESHRE.

Alloimmune Factors

Allogeneic factors may cause RPL by a mechanism similar to that of graft rejection in transplant recipients, an abnormal maternal immune response to fetus or placenta.

Some authorities have suggested that idiopathic RPL is alloimmune in nature. Suggested mechanisms include the presence of cytotoxic antibodies, absence of maternal blocking antibodies, human leukocyte antigen (HLA) compatibility of the couple, inappropriate sharing of HLAs, and disturbances in natural killer (NK) cell function, and distribution.

Dysregulation of the normal immune mechanism probably operates at the maternal–fetal interface and may involve increased activity of uterine natural killer (uNK) cells, which appear to regulate placental and trophoblast growth, local immunomodulation, and control of trophoblast invasion, in addition, being an important component of the local maternal immune response to pathogens.

In contrast, more recent studies have shown no relationship between the risk of pregnancy loss and the presence or absence of HLA compatibility, absence of maternal leukocytotoxic antibodies, blocking antibodies, or elevated NK cell activity. At this point, the role of alloimmunity in the mechanism of RPL is unclear, so the treatment of these problems is still speculative and investigational.

Cytokines

Cytokines are immune molecules that control both immune and other cells. Cytokine responses are generally characterized either as T-helper-1 (Th-1) type, with production of the proinflammatory cytokines—interleukin 2, interferon, and tumor necrosis factor alpha (TNF-α) or as T-helper-2 (Th-2) type, with production of the anti-inflammatory cytokines interleukins 4, 6, and 10. It has been suggested that normal pregnancy might be the result of a predominantly Th-2 cytokine response, whereas women with RM have a bias toward mounting a Th-1 cytokine response. A meta-analysis concluded that the available data are not consistent with more than modest associations between cytokine polymorphisms and RM.

Infection

Ureaplasma urealyticum, Mycoplasma hominis, chlamydia, *Listeria monocytogenes, Toxoplasma gondii*, rubella, cytomegalovirus, herpes virus, and other less frequent pathogens have been identified more frequently in vaginal and cervical cultures and serum from women with sporadic miscarriages. Any severe infection that leads to bacteremia or viremia can cause sporadic miscarriage. There are no convincing data that infections cause RPL. For an infective agent to be implicated in the etiology of repeated pregnancy loss, it must be capable of persisting in the genital tract avoiding detection or must cause insufficient symptoms to disturb the woman. As *Toxoplasma*, rubella, cytomegalovirus, herpes, and *Listeria* infections do not fulfil these criteria, routine TORCH screening should be abandoned. The presence of bacterial vaginosis (BV) in the first trimester of pregnancy has been reported as a risk factor for second-trimester miscarriage and preterm delivery, but the evidence for an association with first-trimester miscarriage is inconsistent.

Male Factors

Sperm aneuploidy and DNA fragmentation have been studied in couples with RPL. Abnormal DNA fragmentation may be seen in the setting of advanced paternal age or may result from correctable environmental factors, such as exogenous heat, toxic exposures, varicoceles, or increased reactive oxygen species in semen. There are contradictory data regarding a causal effect between pregnancy loss and fragmentation of sperm DNA in in-vitro fertilization (IVF) cycles. Currently, routine testing for sperm ploidy [e.g., fluorescence in situ hybridization (FISH) or DNA fragmentation] is not recommended. It is suggested to assess lifestyle factors (smoking, alcohol consumption, exercise pattern, and body weight). Assessing sperm DNA fragmentation in couples with RPL can be considered for explanatory purposes in IVF cycles, based on indirect evidence (ESHRE).

Lifestyle, Environmental, Occupational Factors

Numerous exogenous agents have been implicated in fetal losses including maternal alcohol (>5 units a week), cocaine abuse, excessive coffee (>3-4 cups/day), and smoking.

Alcohol consumption should be avoided during pregnancy for many reasons. Some authors found only a slightly increased risk for abortion in women who drank in the first trimester, whereas others found alcohol consumption to be nearly identical in women who did and did not experience abortion. Armstrong et al. found the odds ratio (OR) to be 1.82 with 20 drinks or more per week.

Caffeine

Maternal caffeine consumption has been associated with an increased risk of spontaneous miscarriage in a dose-dependent manner. Mills et al. showed that the OR for association between pregnancy loss and caffeine (coffee and other dietary forms) is only 1.15 [95% confidence interval (CI) 0.89-1.49]. Women exposed to much higher levels may, however, be at greater risk. Klebanoff et al. reported an association between pregnancy losses and caffeine ingestion >300 mg daily (1.9-fold increase).

Cigarette Smoking

Active and passive maternal smoking is damaging in every trimester of human pregnancy. Cigarette smoke contains numerous toxins which exert a direct effect on the placental and fetal cell proliferation and differentiation and can explain the increased risk of miscarriage, fetal growth restriction (FGR), stillbirth, preterm birth, and placental abruption, reported by epidemiological studies. Harlap and Shiona reported nonsignificant risks of both first and second trimester losses (1.01 first trimester; 1.21 second trimester) with smoking.

X-ray Irradiation and Chemotherapeutic Agents

Irradiation and antineoplastic agents in high doses are acknowledged abortifacients. Diagnostic X-rays, even pelvic X-rays, rarely result in exposures to a level that places a woman at increased risk. The exposure is usually to doses that are far less (1-2 rad or 0.01-0.02 Gy), with 10 rads (0.1 Gy) considered the lowest level of significance. It is prudent for pregnant hospital workers to avoid handling chemotherapeutic agents and to minimize exposures during diagnostic imaging.

Chemicals

Many chemical agents have been claimed to be associated with fetal losses, but only a few are accepted as potentially causative. These include anesthetic gases, arsenic, aniline dyes, benzene, solvents, ethylene oxide, formaldehyde, pesticides, and certain divalent cations (lead, mercury, and cadmium). Workers in rubber industries, battery factories, and chemical production plants are among those at potential risk.

Psychological Factors

Impaired psychological well-being predisposes to early fetal losses has been claimed but never proved. Although data to support a psychological role in the etiology of RPL are inconclusive, it is clearly advisable to offer these patients psychological support and counseling. Studies have reported a beneficial effect of psychological well-being.

■ INVESTIGATIONS AND MANAGEMENT

Recurrent pregnancy loss is a distressing and frustrating condition for both clinicians and patients as, despite intensive workup, no clear underlying pathology is found in at least 50% of couples, thus remaining unexplained. Potentially treatable maternal causes that will be found in about 40% of cases as recognized by RCOG, ASRM, or ESHRE include uterine abnormalities, APS, thyroid, and prolactin endocrine disorders. Therefore, particular sensitivity is required in assessing and counseling couples with RM. Ideally, the couple should be seen together at a dedicated RM clinic.

Evaluation

After three losses, couples have traditionally been directed to formal evaluation. Although this lacks firm scientific basis for waiting until three losses, but this is the benchmark for the RCOG and the ESHRE. The American College of Obstetricians and Gynecologists (ACOG) defines recurrent loss as either two or three consecutive losses and ASRM as two losses. Neither ACOG nor ASRM consider it relevant whether losses are consecutive or not. A couple experiencing a single loss should be counseled and provide recurrence risk rates. Infertile couples in their fourth decade may choose to be evaluated formally after only two losses.

If the threshold number of miscarriages required for making the diagnosis of RM is set too low, many women who have an otherwise good prognosis would be subjected to unnecessary investigations, whereas setting it too high will risk avoidable pregnancy losses in patients with rectifiable pathology. Setting the threshold depends on the background risk for miscarriage and this risk is closely correlated with female age. Another consideration is whether biochemical or only clinically recognized pregnancies are included since the background risk of losing three clinical pregnancies is low compared to losing three biochemical pregnancies (0.3 vs. 22%).

Royal College of Obstetricians and Gynaecologists Green-top Guideline on RM in 2011 "Best practices" included referral of patients to a specialist clinic and an ultrasound for evaluation of the uterus. Grade D recommendations included testing for APS and genetic testing of products of conception (POC) after the third and subsequent loss. The 2012 ASRM assessment of RPL includes analyzing parental karyotypes, evaluating uterine anatomy and screening for APS, thyroid, and prolactin abnormalities. Karyotype analysis of POC should only be used in the setting of ongoing therapy for RPL.

Chromosomal Abnormalities

Vast majority of early pregnancy losses are the consequence of chromosomal abnormalities, specifically, trisomy, monosomy, and polyploidy. A recent meta-analysis by Smith, et al., including 55 published studies, performed a comprehensive and up-to-date review on genetic analysis of miscarriage tissue from women with a single or RPL. In this study, the chromosomal abnormalities most frequently detected in POC were trisomies (58-61%), followed by monosomies X (8-13%), structural anomalies (7-9%), and polyploidies (2-9%). In this systematic review, the detected prevalence of chromosomal abnormalities was comparable between conventional karyotyping (47%; 95% CI 43-51%), array comparative genomic hybridization (aCGH) (48%; 95% CI 39-57%), and single nucleotide polymorphism (SNP) microarray (60%; 95% CI 58-63%).

When assessing a new patient with two or more spontaneous losses, it is important to obtain POC karyotype for genetic analysis in subsequent loss. This allows the practitioner to determine more precisely whether a diagnostic work-up for RPL is indicated or not. Structural chromosomal abnormalities are found in 2-5% of RM couples. RCOG in 2011 issued a Grade D recommendation to obtain cytogenetic analysis on POC after the third or subsequent consecutive miscarriage. They stated that knowledge of the POC karyotype provides prognostic value to the clinician in counseling the couple on subsequent successful pregnancies. Parental peripheral blood karyotyping of both partners should be performed in couples with RM and referral of the couple for genetic counseling where testing of POC reports an unbalanced structural chromosomal abnormality. ESHRE recommends testing only in couples at an increased risk, evidenced by a prior child with congenital abnormalities, offspring with unbalanced chromosomes, or a translocation in POC. The ASRM Practice Committee recommends against the use of karyotype analysis of the POC except in the setting of ongoing therapy for RPL. According to the committee, "if the evaluation identifies a remediable cause, cytogenetic analysis of subsequent losses can be employed to evaluate whether the event was random and not a treatment failure per se".

The ASRM and RCOG positions on POC genetic testing for RPL were based on the then current standard of conventional G-banding karyotype analysis. Up to 50% of "46, XX normal" reports from POC testing result from maternal cell contamination. Therefore, ESHRE recommends chromosomal microarray analysis (CMA) as the preferred modality for POC genetic testing because it is not limited by tissue culture failure or false negative results secondary to maternal cell contamination; limitations of CMA technology include the inability to detect balanced structural chromosomal rearrangements and low-level mosaicism. The 2017 ESHRE Guidelines issued a conditional recommendation against the routine use of POC genetic analysis but issued a strong recommendation in favor of using microarray CMA whenever genetic analysis was performed on POC for explanatory purposes. ESHRE recognized that the "genetic analysis of pregnancy tissue has the benefit of providing the patient with a reason for the pregnancy loss and may help to determine whether further investigations or treatments are required." If the POC CMA reveals an unbalanced translocation or an inversion, then a karyotype analysis of both parents should be performed. In addition to genetic counseling, expectant management versus IVF with preimplantation genetic testing (PGT) should be considered and discussed.

Genetic counseling is important when a structural genetic factor is identified. It offers the couple a prognosis of future pregnancies with an unbalanced chromosome complements and the opportunity for familial chromosome studies. The likelihood of a subsequent healthy live birth depends on the chromosome(s) involved and the type of rearrangement. When one of the partners has a structural genetic abnormality, preimplantation genetic diagnosis (PGD) for specific translocations, with transfer of unaffected embryos, or the use of donor gametes may be offered. Amniocentesis or chorionic villus sampling are other options to detect the genetic abnormality in the offspring.

Anatomical Abnormalities

Women with recurrent first-trimester miscarriage and all women with one or more second-trimester miscarriages should have a pelvic ultrasound to assess uterine anatomy. Suspected uterine anomalies may require further investigations to confirm the diagnosis, using hysteroscopy, laparoscopy, or three-dimensional (3D) pelvic ultrasound.

Two-dimensional ultrasonography with or without saline infusion [sonohysterography (SHG)] usually constitutes the first-line investigations. The Thessaloniki ESHRE/ESGE consensus group recommended 3D ultrasonography for investigating uterine anomalies in high-risk patients, and magnetic resonance imaging and endoscopic examinations for suspected complex malformations or diagnostic difficulties. An ESHRE committee concluded that 3D ultrasound technology has an accuracy of 97.6% (CI 94.3–100) for the diagnosis of female genital tract anomalies when compared with hysteroscopy ± laparoscopy. SHG is more accurate than hysterosalpingography (HSG) in diagnosing uterine malformations. It can be used to evaluate uterine morphology when three-dimensional ultrasound (3D US) is not available, or when tubal patency has to be investigated (ESHRE).

Women with a history of second-trimester miscarriage and suspected cervical weakness who have not undergone a history-indicated cerclage may be offered serial cervical sonographic surveillance. In women with a singleton pregnancy and a history of one second-trimester miscarriage attributable to cervical factors, an ultrasound-indicated cerclage should be offered if a cervical length of 25 mm or less, detected by transvaginal scan before 24 weeks of gestation. A meta-analysis of individual patient-level data from four RCTs reported that in women with singleton pregnancies, a short cervix (<25 mm), and previous second-trimester miscarriage, cerclage may reduce the incidence of preterm birth before 35 weeks of gestation [relative risk (RR) 0.57, 95% CI 0.33–99].

In their recent guidelines for managing uterine septa, the ASRM recommended that "it is reasonable to consider septum incision, a view supported by the DGGG/OEGGG/SGGG. Until gold-standard RCT-quality evidence emerges, the growing consensus supports septal resection. A large retrospective study found that, following hysteroscopic septal resection, miscarriage decreased from 41.7 to 11.9%. In another study involving 361 patients, the miscarriage rate decreased from 94.3 to 16.1% and livebirth rate increased from 2.4 to 75%.

An earlier systematic review found an association between fibroids and higher miscarriage rates but robust prospective evidence that myomectomy reduces miscarriage is lacking. Until better quality evidence emerges, the ASRM and DGGG/OEGGG/SGGG propose that it is reasonable to undertake surgical correction in cases of uterine cavity defects associated with fibroids, polyps, and adhesions. Surgical removal of intramural fibroids in women with RPL is not recommended by ESHRE. Metroplasty is also not recommended for bicornuate uterus with normal cervix. There is insufficient evidence in favor of metroplasty in women with bicorporeal uterus and double cervix (former AFS classification didelphic uterus) and RPL.

Antiphospholipid antibody syndrome: RCOG, ESHRE, and ASRM recommend testing for APS using LA and aCL antibody, in all patients with RPL. RCOG recommends all women with recurrent first-trimester miscarriage and all women with one or more second-trimester miscarriage should be screened before next pregnancy for aPL. ESHRE recommends screening for aPL [LA, and anticardiolipin antibodies (ACA IgG and IgM)] after two pregnancy losses.

For women who fulfil the laboratory criteria of APS, ESHRE recommends administration of low-dose aspirin (LDA) (75–100 mg/day), starting before conception and a prophylactic dose of twice daily unfractionated heparin (UFH) or low molecular weight heparin (LMWH) starting at date of a positive pregnancy test, and continuing till delivery *to prevent further miscarriage*. LMWH is as safe as UFH and has potential advantages during pregnancy, since it causes less heparin-induced thrombocytopenia, can be administered once daily, and is associated with a lower risk of heparin-induced osteoporosis.

The combination of twice daily UFH and LDA appears to confer a significant benefit in pregnancies with aPLs and otherwise unexplained RPL; comparable efficacy of low molecular weight heparin has not been established (ASRM).

Endocrine Problems

DM: Women with diabetes who have high hemoglobin A1c levels in the first trimester are at risk of miscarriage and fetal malformation, well-controlled DM is not a risk. Tight control of blood glucose, and optimal weight is recommended in women with DM and pregnancy loss.

PCOS: A meta-analysis of 17 RCTs of metformin in women with PCOS and infertility showed that metformin has no effect on the sporadic miscarriage risk when administered prepregnancy. Uncontrolled small studies have shown that use of metformin during pregnancy is associated with a reduction in the miscarriage rate in women with RM and PCOS.

Thyroid disease: Overt hypothyroidism before conception or during early gestation should be treated with levothyroxine in women with RPL. While miscarriage is increased with overt hypothyroidism, there is conflicting evidence regarding treatment of women with SCH. Treatment of women with SCH may reduce the risk of miscarriage, but the potential benefit of treatment should be balanced against the risks. A recent large retrospective cohort study involving 5,405 pregnant women with SCH, T4 replacement was associated with reduced miscarriage only in those with TSH >4 mIU/L and not if TSH was 2.5–4 mIU/L.

Another uncertainty pertains to the significance of thyroid autoimmunity [antibodies to TPO and/or thyroglobulin (Tg)], which is present in ~14% of reproductive women. The Endocrine Society Clinical Practice Guideline (2012) on the management of thyroid dysfunction during pregnancy and postpartum acknowledged an association of SCH (women with TSH >2.5 mIU/L and normal T_4) with adverse pregnancy outcome, and thyroid replacement considered especially in women with TPO antibodies. American Thyroid Association (ATA) has given a strong recommendation for T_4 use with combined autoimmunity and TSH >4 mIU/L and a weak recommendation to consider T_4 with autoimmunity and TSH >2.5 mIU/L. Current recommendations support ATA recommendation—T_4 for TSH >4 mIU/L but not at TSH of 2.5–4 mIU/L in the absence of thyroid antibodies.

Hyperprolactinemia: Hyperprolactinemia may be associated with RPL through alterations in the hypothalamic–pituitary–ovarian axis, resulting in impaired folliculogenesis and oocyte maturation, and/or a short luteal phase. Normalization of prolactin levels with a dopamine agonist improved subsequent pregnancy outcomes in patients with RPL. In one study, treatment resulted in an 85.7% liveborn rate, whereas the untreated cohort had a 52.4% liveborn outcome.

Progesterone therapy: Progesterone is necessary for successful implantation and the maintenance of pregnancy. This benefit of progesterone could be explained by its immunomodulatory actions in inducing a pregnancy protective shift from proinflammatory Th-1 cytokine responses to a more favorable anti-inflammatory Th-2 cytokine response. It has been suggested that normal pregnancy might be the result of a predominantly Th-2 cytokine response, whereas women with RM have a bias toward mounting a Th-1 cytokine response. Administration of progesterone to women with sporadic miscarriages is ineffective. However, in patients with three or more consecutive miscarriages immediately preceding their current pregnancy, empiric progestogen administration may be of some potential benefit (ASRM Practice Committee 2012).

The Progesterone in Recurrent Miscarriage (PROMISE) trial involved 836 women with idiopathic RM randomized to receive either 400 mg of vaginal micronized progesterone (Utrogestan®) twice daily or placebo from the time of positive pregnancy test up to 12 weeks of gestation. There was no difference between the two groups in miscarriage or live birth rates. In contrast, another RCT involving 700 women were tested whether the same dose of vaginally administered natural progesterone (Prontogest®) would benefit unexplained RM patients, but unlike the PROMISE trial, that trial commenced treatment in the luteal phase immediately after documentation of ovulation using either ultrasound or luteinizing hormone (LH) kits and continued until 28 weeks of gestation. This Egyptian trial found significantly lower miscarriage rates (12.4 vs. 23.3%) and higher live birth rates (92 vs. 77%) in the treated group. These data suggest that progesterone is likely to be beneficial in unexplained RM. Natural progesterone may be beneficial but should be started in the luteal phase with consideration given to continuing beyond the first trimester.

Infections

Some infections, such as *L. monocytogenes*, *T. gondii*, cytomegalovirus, and primary genital herpes, are known to cause sporadic pregnancy loss, but there are no convincing data that infections cause RPL. So, there is no clear indication for screening for vaginal infection in these women (ASRM). BV is associated with second-trimester miscarriage but prospective evidence linking BV or other infective agents with REPL is lacking. A randomized placebo-controlled trial reported that treatment of BV early in the second trimester with oral clindamycin significantly reduces the incidence of second-trimester miscarriage and preterm birth in the general population.

Inherited Thrombophilia

Although an association between hereditary thrombophilia and fetal loss has been suggested, prospective cohort studies have failed to confirm this. According to the British Committee for Standards in Haematology (BSSH), antithrombotic therapy should not be offered to pregnant women based on tests for heritable thrombophilia to prevent pregnancy-related complications. Testing for thrombophilia (specifically, factor V Leiden and the prothrombin gene mutations, protein C, protein S, and antithrombin deficiencies) may be offered to women with a personal history of unprovoked thrombosis or provoked with a minor risk factor like travel, and those who have a family history of thrombosis associated with high-risk thrombophilia, (antithrombin deficiency or protein C or protein S deficiency) but testing women with a family history of low-risk thrombophilia (heterogeneous factor V Leiden) is not indicated. Asymptomatic women with a family history of venous thrombosis should be tested if an event in a first-degree relative was unprovoked, or provoked by pregnancy. Screening for inherited thrombophilia is clinically justified when a patient has a personal history of venous thromboembolism in the setting of a nonrecurrent risk factor (such as surgery), routine testing of women with RPL for inherited thrombophilia is not currently recommended (ESHRE).

The efficacy of thromboprophylaxis during pregnancy in women with recurrent first-trimester miscarriage who have inherited thrombophilias, but who are otherwise asymptomatic, has not been assessed in prospective RCTs. Cohort studies have suggested that heparin therapy may improve the live birth rate for these women. A meta-analysis of eight trials involving 483 patients with previous late (≥10 weeks) or recurrent early losses found no benefit with LMWH. However, one prospective randomized trial demonstrated the efficacy of LMWH (enoxaparin) for the treatment of women with a history of a single late miscarriage after 10 weeks of gestation who carry the factor V Leiden or prothrombin gene mutation or have protein S deficiency, live-birth rate of women treated with enoxaparin was 86% compared with 29% in women taking LDA alone (OR 15.5, 95% CI 7–34).

Alloimmune Factors

Immunotherapy

There is inconsistent data regarding role of immunotherapy in RPL. An RCOG Scientific Impact Paper devoted entirely to NK cells concluded that measurement of peripheral blood NK cells "are of limited value in aiding our understanding of the role of uterine NK cells in reproductive failure." Treatment with intravenous immunoglobulin (IVIg) has been proposed, however, several trials and meta-analyses concluded that IVIg is ineffective for primary RPL; their use may provoke significant maternal and fetal morbidity.

Intralipid is a fat emulsion used for parenteral nutrition. It has been proposed that intralipid might benefit RM by reducing peripheral blood NK cell activity and suppressing proinflammatory cytokines. Intralipid has been evaluated in only one RCT that tested whether a 250 mL infusion on the day of oocyte retrieval (with further infusions if there was a positive pregnancy test) could increase chemical pregnancy rates in RM patients with elevated peripheral blood NK cells (>12%) undergoing IVF. No benefit was found for the primary outcome, i.e., chemical pregnancy, although increased rates of ongoing pregnancies and live birth rates were observed. The authors concluded this requires further investigation by appropriately powered studies.

Tumor Necrosis Factor-α

Tumor necrosis factor-α is a proinflammatory cytokine produced by T-helper 1 cells and can be neutralized using anti-TNF-α drugs such as adalimumab (Humira®). One small retrospective study found improved live birth rates when anti-TNF-α was combined with other regimes that included heparin, LDA, and/or IVIg.

Granulocyte Colony-Stimulating Factor

Granulocyte colony-stimulating factor (G-CSF) is a cytokine produced by decidual cells that stimulate granulocyte proliferation and differentiation. One small RCT of 68 women with unexplained RM found that G-CSF treatment (administered subcutaneously from the sixth day after ovulation to the ninth week of gestation) increased live birth rates from 48% in the placebo group to 83% in the treatment group.

Homocysteinemia

Hyperhomocysteinemia therapy includes dietary interventions, high-dose folic acid (5 mg/day), vitamin B_{12} (0.5 mg), and prophylactic LMWH, monitor homocysteine level.

Vitamin D

Deficiency has been shown to be associated with several obstetric complications including miscarriage. ESHRE issued a recommendation to consider vitamin D supplementation for all cases of RPL as part of preconception counseling.

Lifestyle Modification

Epidemiological studies suggest that lifestyle modifications can increase fertility potential, although these have not been definitively tested in randomized trials. Modifications including eliminating use of tobacco products, alcohol, and caffeine and reduction in body mass index (for obese women) would benefit not only miscarriage but also the risk profile for later pregnancy. Antioxidants for men have not been shown to improve the chance of a live birth.

■ NEWER TREATMENT OPTIONS

Sitagliptin

One proposed mechanism for RPL is impaired decidualization due to low endometrial mesenchymal stem-like progenitor cell (eMSC) colony counts. In a small randomized trial of patients with at least three prior miscarriages, sitagliptin (a dipeptidyl peptidase-4 inhibitor used for treatment of type 2 diabetes) increased eMSC colony counts compared with placebo. However, the trial did not assess the clinically important outcomes of pregnancy or live birth rates. While sitagliptin may be a promising future treatment of RPL, adequately powered clinical trials are needed before prescribing it for this indication (UpToDate, January 2020).

Combined Medical Therapy

An observational study compared 50 pregnant women who were treated before and during pregnancy with a combination of prednisone (20 mg/day), progesterone (20 mg/day), aspirin (100 mg/day), and folate (5 mg every second day) with 52 women who were not treated during the same observation period. The first-trimester miscarriage rate was 19% in the treated group and 63% in the control group; this difference was not statistically significant. The live birth rates in the treated group and control groups were 77 and 35%, respectively ($p = 0.04$). With combined treatment of four agents, it is unclear which of the treatments was beneficial.

UNEXPLAINED RECURRENT MISCARRIAGE

A significant proportion of cases of RM remain unexplained despite detailed investigation. ESHRE does not recommend lymphocyte immunization therapy/IVIg/glucocorticoids as a treatment of unexplained RPL or RPL with selected immunological biomarkers. There is insufficient evidence to recommend intralipid therapy or G-CSF for improving live birth rate in women with unexplained RPL.

Women with unexplained RM have an excellent prognosis for future pregnancy outcome without pharmacological intervention if supportive care offered alone in the setting of a dedicated early pregnancy assessment unit. These women can be reassured that the prognosis for a successful future pregnancy with supportive care alone is in the region of 75%.

CONCLUSION

Recurrent miscarriage is a complex condition requiring consideration of multiple factors for appropriate workup and management. A particular individual's prognosis will depend on both the underlying cause for pregnancy losses and the number of prior losses. The decision to intervene depends on the benefit-to-risk ratio of proposed treatment. Correction of endocrine disorders, APLA, and anatomic anomalies have the highest success rates, approximately 60–90%. Patients with a cytogenetic basis for loss experience a wide range of success (20–80%) that depends on the type of abnormality present. Overall, the prognosis for RPL is encouraging. Even with the diagnosis of RPL and as many as four to five prior losses, a patient is more likely to carry her next pregnancy to term than to have another loss.

SUGGESTED READING

1. American College of Obstetricians and Gynecologists Women's Health Care Physicians ACOG Practice Bulletin No. 138: inherited thrombophilias in pregnancy. Obstet Gynecol. 2013;122(3):706-17.
2. Christiansen OB, Andersen A-MN, Bosch E, Daya S, Delves PJ, Hviid TV, et al. Evidence-based investigations and treatments of recurrent pregnancy loss. Fert Steril. 2005;83: 821-39.
3. de la Rochebrochard E, Thonneau P. Paternal age and maternal age are risk factors for miscarriage; results of a multicentre European study. Hum Reprod. 2002;17(6):1649-56.
4. ESHRE Early Pregnancy Guideline Development Group. (2017). Recurrent Pregnancy loss. [online] Available from: https://www.eshre.eu/Guidelines-and-Legal/Guidelines/Recurrent-pregnancy-loss. [Last accessed April 2022].
5. ESHRE Guideline Group on RPL; Atik RB, Christiansen OB, Elson J, Kolte AM, Lewis S, et al. ESHRE guideline: recurrent pregnancy loss. Human Reprod Open. 2018:1-12.
6. Hachem HE. Recurrent pregnancy loss: current perspectives. Int J Womens Health. 2017;9:331-45.
7. Homer HA. Modern management of recurrent miscarriage. Aust NZJ Obstet Gynaecol. 2019;59(1):36-44.
8. Hyde KJ, Schust DJ. Genetic considerations in recurrent pregnancy loss. Cold Spring Harb Perspect Med. 2015; 5(3):a023119.
9. Ismail AM, Abbas AM, Ali MK, Amin AF. Peri-conceptional progesterone treatment in women with unexplained recurrent miscarriage: a randomized double-blind placebo-controlled trial. J Matern Fetal Neonatal Med. 2018;31(3): 388-94.
10. Jauniaux E, Farquharson RG, Christiansen OB, Exalto N. Evidence based guidelines for the investigation and medical treatment of recurrent miscarriage. Human Reprod. 2006; 21(9):2216-2.
11. Karata S, Aydin Y, Ocer F, Buyru A, Balci H. Hereditary thrombophilia, anti-beta2 glycoprotein 1 IgM, and anti-annexin V antibodies in recurrent pregnancy loss. Am J Reprod Immunol. 2012;67(3):251-5.
12. Papas, Ralph S. Kutteh, William H. A new algorithm for the evaluation of recurrent pregnancy loss redefining unexplained miscarriage: review of current guidelines. Curr Opin Obstet Gynecol. 2020;32(5):371-9.
13. Practice Committee of the American Society for Reproductive Medicine. Evaluation and treatment of recurrent pregnancy loss: a committee opinion. Fertil Steril. 2012;98(5): 1103-11.
14. Royal College of Obstetricians and Gynecologists. The investigation and treatment of couples with recurrent first-trimester and second-trimester miscarriage. Green-top guideline no 17. London, UK: Royal College of Obstetricians and Gynecologists; 2011.
15. Rull K, Nagirnaja L, Laan M. Genetics of recurrent miscarriage: challenges, current knowledge, future directions. Front Genet. 2012;3:34.
16. Simpson J, Carson S. Genetic and nongenetic causes of pregnancy loss. Glob Libr Women Med. 2013;10.3843/GLOWM.10319.

17. Tewary S, Lucas ES, Fujihara R, Kimani PK, Polanco A, Brighton PJ, et al. Impact of sitagliptin on endometrial mesenchymal stem-like progenitor cells: A randomised, double-blind placebo-controlled feasibility trial. EBioMedicine. 2020;51:102597.
18. The Practice Committee of the American Society for Reproductive Medicine. Etiology of recurrent pregnancy loss. Fertil Steril, 2012.
19. Toth B, Würfel W, Bohlmann M, Zschocke J, Rudnik-Schöneborn S, Nawroth F, et al. Recurrent miscarriage: diagnostic and therapeutic procedures. Guideline of the DGGG, OEGGG and SGGG (S2k-Level, AWMF Registry Number 015/050). Geburtshilfe Frauenheilkd. 2018;78(4):364-81.
20. Tulandi T, Al-Fozan HM. Recurrent pregnancy loss: Management. UpToDate. 2020.
21. Van Dijk MM, Kolte AM, Limpens J, Kirk E, Quenby S, van Wely M, et al. Recurrent pregnancy loss: diagnostic workup after two or three pregnancy losses? A systematic review of the literature and meta-analysis. Hum Reprod Update. 2020;26(3):356-67.
22. Zegers-Hochschild F, Adamson GD, de Mouzon J, Ishihara O, Mansour R, Nygren K, et al. International Committee for Monitoring Assisted Reproductive Technology; World Health Organization. International Committee for Monitoring Assisted Reproductive Technology (ICMART) and the World Health Organization (WHO) revised glossary of ART terminology, 2009. Fertil Steril. 2009;92(5):1520-4.

CHAPTER 16

Multiple Gestation

INTRODUCTION

The term multifetal gestation includes twins, triplets, and higher-order multiples. Multiple births account for a large proportion of neonatal morbidity and mortality. Prematurity, monochorionicity, and growth restriction pose the main risks to the fetus and neonates in multiple pregnancy. Multiple gestations are more likely to have complications of preterm labor, preterm premature rupture of the membranes, pre-eclampsia, pyelonephritis, placental abruption, and postpartum hemorrhage. Gestational diabetes is higher in twin and triplet pregnancies compared to singleton pregnancy. Congenital abnormalities are also increasing in multiple pregnancies particularly in monochorionic gestation, making management decision more challenging for the obstetrician because the fate of the sibling fetus is also linked. Neurodevelopment may be impacted in multiple gestations as well. In the French EPIPAGE study, a population-based cohort study on very preterm birth (PTB) (gestational age <32 weeks), adjusted analysis of 5-year follow-up data showed that children from twin births compared with those from singleton births, had a lower survival rate [adjusted odds ratio (OR) 1.3; 95% confidence interval (CI) 11–1.5] and a lower score on mental processing composite testing without severe neurodevelopmental impairment (mean difference, 2.4; 95% CI 4.8–0.01).

In a multicenter study on PTBs (27 weeks) from Australia and New Zealand, the mortality rate for multiples was higher than for singleton (24.7 vs. 21.9%). In the USA, studies showed stillbirth rate increased from 5.6/1,000 for singleton to 14.1/1,000 for twin to 30.5/1,000 for triplets. The excess perinatal mortality and morbidity is higher in monochorionic than dichorionic twin pregnancy. Though perinatal deaths have decreased over time, the risk of prematurity has not changed significantly, while only 2% of singletons are born at a gestational age <33 weeks, 14% of twins are premature. The mean duration of gestation is 35.1 weeks for twin pregnancy, 31.9 weeks for triplet pregnancy, and 29.5 weeks for quadruplet pregnancy with increased risk of perinatal complications. Intensive antenatal surveillance lowers the risk of stillbirth.

INCIDENCE

The incidence of multiple pregnancies has been on the rise over the last 20 years. The overall incidence continues to increase worldwide because of the widespread use of assisted reproductive technologies and increasing maternal age at childbirth. The incidence is >3% of all live births in the United States.

CLASSIFICATION OF TWINS (FIG. 1)

Twin pregnancies are commonly divided according to zygosity or chorionicity as these have important implications for pregnancy and infant outcome. Chorionicity should be established as soon as possible during pregnancy because it can affect future management decisions. The optimal time for diagnosis is in the first trimester or early second trimester.

- According to zygosity, twin may be dizygotic or monozygotic
- According to chorionicity, it may be dichorionic or monochorionic.
- Monochorionic twin again may be subdivided into diamniotic and monoamniotic.

Dizygotic Twins

Among all twins 70–90% result from simultaneous maturation of two oocytes and fertilization by different spermatozoa (dizygotic twin). Two zygotes have different genetic constitutions. Each zygotes implant individually within the uterus. Each develops its own placenta, amnion, and chorionic sac. Sometimes, two placentas may fuse to form a single placenta.

Monozygotic Twins

Monozygotic twins develop from single fertilized ovum and result from splitting of the zygote at various

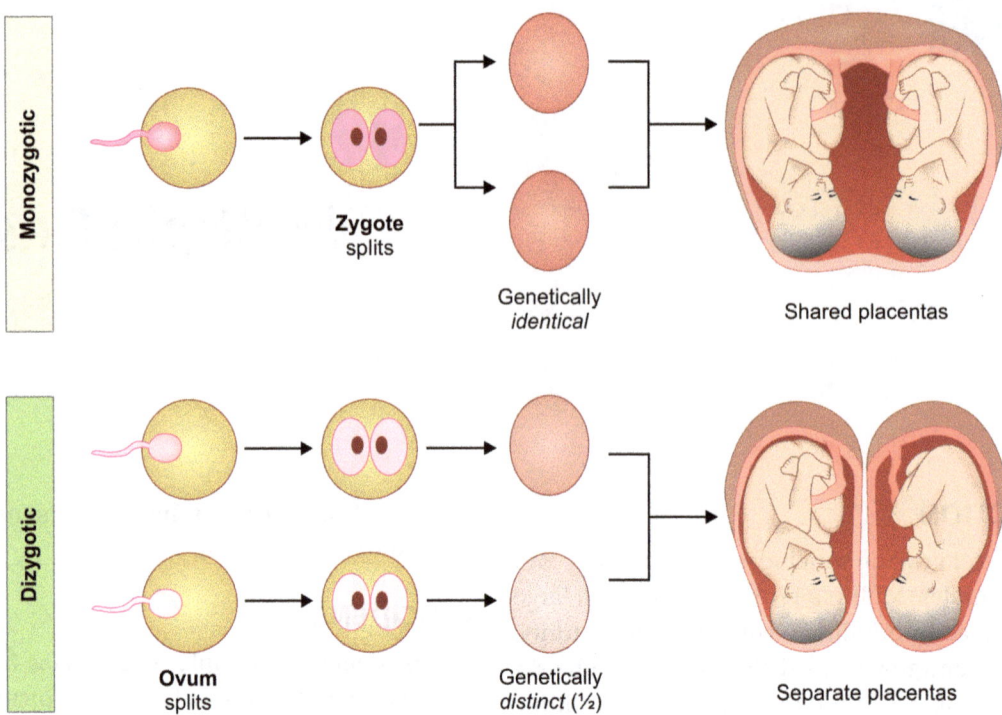

Fig. 1: Classification of twins.

stages of development. Incidence of monozygotic twin is 3–4 per 1,000 live births. The chorionicity and amnionicity of monozygotic twins are determined by the time at which the zygote splits or cleaves.

Diamniotic Dichorionic

Diamniotic dichorionic constitutes 30% of monozygotic twin, results from cleavage of the embryo at two-cell stage (shortly after fertilization); two separate zygotes develop. Blastocysts implant separately and each embryo has its own placenta and chorionic sac, resulting in dichorionic-diamniotic (Di-Di) twins **(Fig. 2)**.

Monochorionic Diamniotic

In approximately 75% of monozygotic twins, cleavage occurs after day 3, when the blastocyst has already formed. Inner cell mass splits into two separate groups of cells within the same blastocyst cavity, this results in a monochorionic diamniotic (Mo-Di) pregnancy. A monochorionic pregnancy has one placenta, shared by both twins. As long as the cleavage occurs between days 4 and 8 (which is usually the case), each twin will form an amnion but be surrounded by one outer sac (chorion) **(Fig. 3)**.

Monochorionic monoamniotic (Mo-Mo) twin: This is rare (approximately 1%). When the cleavage occurs at the bilaminar germ disk stage (9th to 13th day), it results in two embryos having a common single placenta, single chorionic, and amniotic cavity. This is a very high-risk situation with a high mortality rate for both twins due to umbilical cord entanglement **(Fig. 3)**.

Conjoined twin: In rare instances, cleavage occurs after day 13. This produces twins that are monoamniotic-monochorionic. In these cases, the embryos themselves have not had time to completely separate, partial splitting of the primitive node and streak results in formation of conjoined twin **(Fig. 4)**.

Diagnosis of Chorionicity

Ultrasound examination remains the most reliable method for diagnosis of multiple gestations. Ultrasonography (USG) prior to 14 weeks has 100% sensitivity and 99% specificity for detection of chorionicity. The most reliable predictor of a dichorionic gestation is the presence of two separate placentas.

Visualization of a triangular projection of placenta between the layers of the dividing membrane is known as twin peak or lambda (λ) sign, twin-peak sign is suggestive of dichorionic, diamniotic gestation. A Mo-Di gestation can have the presence of a "T" sign, which is the appearance of the amnion as it comes off the placenta at a 90° angle. The λ sign is virtually diagnostic of dichorionicity, λ sign may disappear after 16 weeks. Absence of λ sign or presence of T sign is used for monochorionicity **(Fig.5A and B)**.

Before 8 Weeks' Gestation (Figs. 6A to C)

Two separate gestational sacs surrounded by a thick echogenic ring are suggestive of dichorionicity. If separate echogenic rings are not visible, monochorionicity is likely. Two fetal poles with two yolk sacs in a monochorionic gestation suggest diamniocity. Presence of two fetal poles with only one yolk sac suggests monoamniotic gestation.

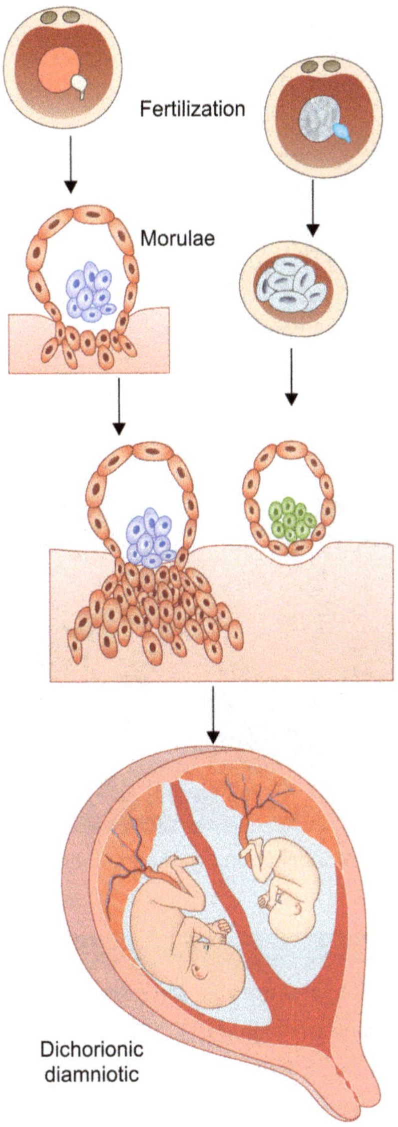

Fig. 2: Dizygotic twin.

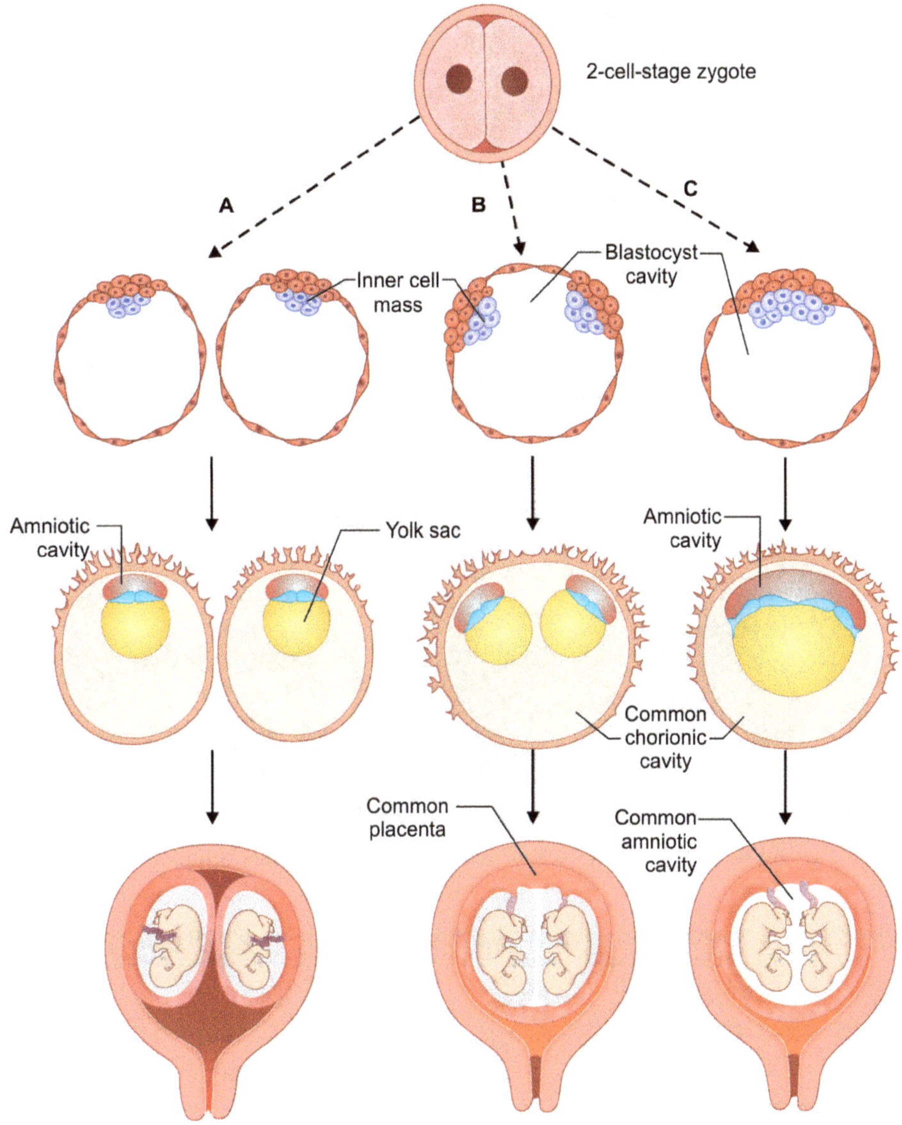

Fig. 3: Monozygotic twin.

Between 9th and 14th Weeks
Chorionicity is determined simply by counting the layers of dividing membrane near its insertion. Presence of three or four layers suggests dichorionicity (positive predictive value 100%), whereas only two layers suggest monochorionicity. Maximum thickness of dividing membrane of 2 mm is also used for diagnosis of monochorionicity (accuracy 90%).

MATERNAL AND FETAL RISKS OF MULTIPLE PREGNANCY
Table 1 as show maternal and fetal risks of multiple pregnancy.

MANAGEMENT OF MULTIPLE PREGNANCY
Counseling
Patient including husband should be counseled about complications of twin pregnancy, particularly problem of monochorionicity, the increased risk of miscarriage, aneuploidy, structural abnormalities, anemia, PTB, growth disorders, venous thromboembolism, cesarean section, and postpartum hemorrhage. Mode of delivery, timing and

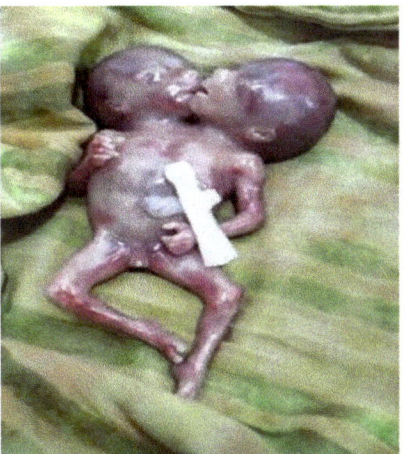

Fig. 4: Conjoint twin.

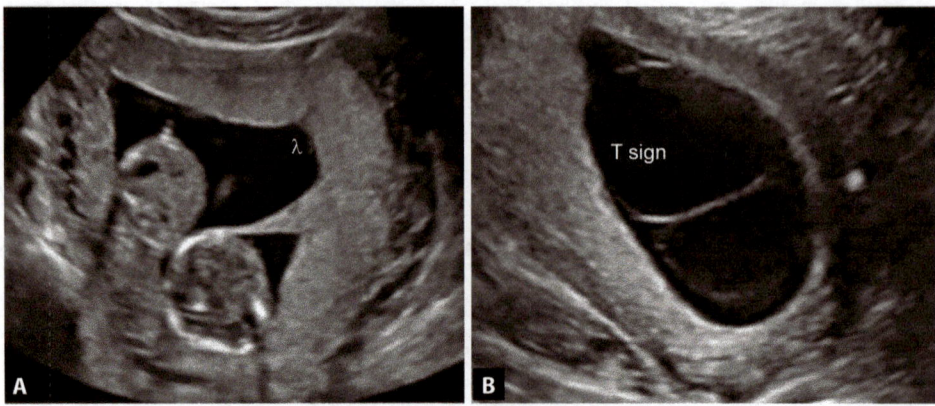

Figs. 5A and B: Image of lambda (λ) and T sign.

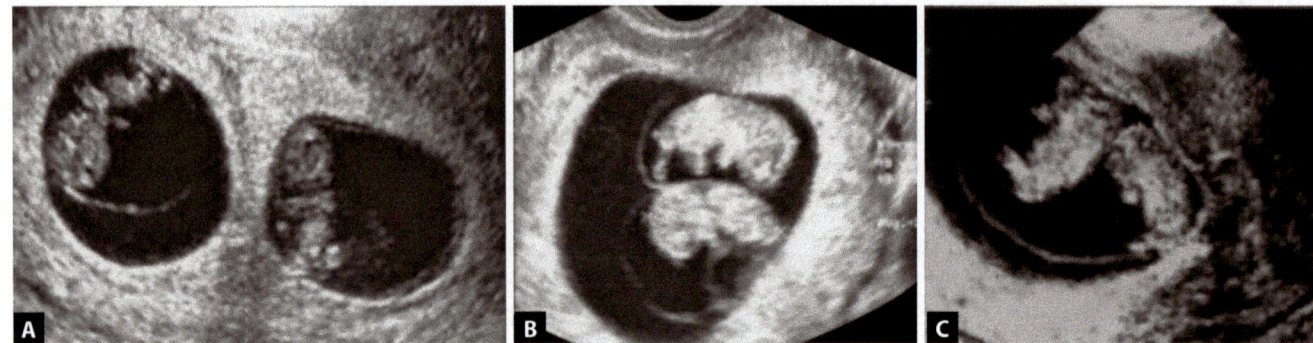

Figs. 6A to C: (A) Di-Di: Dichorionic-diamniotic; (B) Mo-Di: Monochorionic diamniotic; (C) Mo-Mo: Monochorionic monoamniotic.

TABLE 1: Maternal and fetal risks of multiple pregnancy.		
Maternal risk	**Fetal risk**	**Fetal risk—specific to monochorionic multiples**
Hyperemesis gravidarum	Miscarriage	Twin-to-twin transfusion syndrome (TTTS)
Anemia	Congenital anomalies	Twin reversed arterial perfusion sequence (TRAP)
Urinary tract infection	Single fetal demise	Twin anemia polycythemia sequence
Hypertension	Preterm birth	Selective growth restriction
Preeclampsia/eclampsia	PROM	Cord entanglement
Gestation diabetes	Cord prolapse	Conjoined twin
Obstetric cholestasis	Twin entrapment	
Acute fatty liver of pregnancy	Perinatal mortality	
Hemorrhage (both APH and PPH)	Stillbirth	
Polyhydramnios	Fetal growth restriction	
Preterm labor/PROM	Discordant growth	
Operative vaginal delivery		
Cesarean section		
Maternal mortality		

(APH: antepartum hemorrhage; PPH: postpartum hemorrhage; PROM: premature rupture of membranes)

place of delivery, and need for early delivery should also be discussed.

Antenatal Management

Women with a twin pregnancy should be cared for by an experienced multidisciplinary team in a specialized twin clinic. Twins that develop complications, and all Mo-Mo twins, should be referred to a tertiary center. The National Institute for Health and Care Excellence advises women with a twin pregnancy to take 75 mg of aspirin daily from 12 weeks until birth if they have an additional risk factor for preeclampsia. Hemoglobin concentration should be checked at 20–24 weeks' gestation, as well as at the usual 28 and 34 weeks. No evidence for prophylactic progesterone, tocolytic, or cervical cerclage.

Antenatal Visit (National Institute for Health and Care Excellence Guideline, 2019)

- *Eight visits for dichorionic diamniotic twin:*
  - Six visits with USG scan: At 11^{+2} to 14^{+1}, 20, 24, 28, 32, and 36 weeks
  - Additional two visits (without scan) at 16 and 34 weeks
- *11 visits for uncomplicated Mo-Di twin:* All with USG scan at 11^{+2} to 14^{+1}, 16, 18, 20, 22, 24, 26, 28, 30, 32, and 34 weeks in order to detect twin-to-twin transfusion
- *Nine visits for trichorionic triamniotic triplet:*
  - Eight visits with USG scan: At 11^{+2} to 14^{+1}, 20, 24, 26, 28, 30, 32, and 34 weeks
  - An additional visit (without scan) at 16 weeks
- *11 visits for dichorionic triamniotic or monochorionic triamniotic triplet:*
  - All with USG scan: At 11^{+2} to 14^{+1}, 16, 18, 20, 22, 24, 26, 28, 30, 32, and 34 weeks.

At each ultrasound, fetal biometry (head circumference, abdominal circumference, and femur length), amniotic fluid volume, and estimated fetal weight (EFW) should be assessed for both twins. If discordance in growth or fluid is noted, then umbilical artery (UA) Doppler assessment should be performed. In Mo-Di twins, assessment for twin-to-twin transfusion syndrome (TTTS) at each scan will include measurement of the deepest vertical pocket of amniotic fluid. In monochorionic twins, the middle cerebral artery (MCA) peak systolic velocity (PSV) should be considered from 20 weeks' gestation onward to screen for twin anemia polycythemia sequence. In all twin pregnancies, the 20th week anatomy scan should include measurement of cervical length (CL) to identify women at increased risk of extreme prematurity, a CL threshold of 20 mm or less should be used.

International Federation of Gynecology and Obstetrics Recommendation on Ultrasonogram

- *First USG:* 11^{+0} to 13^{+6}:
  - For dating of pregnancy
  - Fetal viability
  - Determination of chorionicity and amnionicity
  - Exclusion of aneuploidy
- *Repeat USG:*
  - *Anomaly scan* at 18^{+0} to 20^{+6} weeks
  - *Screening for PTB:* CL measurement by transvaginal ultrasound scan (TVS) at 16, 18, 20, and 24 weeks. CL <20 mm is associated with a 10-fold positive likelihood ratio for PTB before 32 weeks of gestation.
  - *At each USG:* Estimation of fetal biometry, amniotic fluid volume, and fetal weight. *If discordance in growth or fluid:* UA Doppler velocimetry should be done.
  - *MCA PSV* from 20 weeks' onward to screen for "anemia-polycythemia sequence" in monochorionic twins
  - *At 34 weeks:* To determine presentation of the leading twin to determine the mode of delivery

Patients presenting later than 14 weeks' gestation should be dated according to the head circumference of the larger twin. During the prenatal scans, each twin should be labeled and described using as many features as possible, for example: "Twin A (female) is on the maternal left and closer to the cervix with an anterior placenta."

Management of Problems

Screening, Diagnosis, and Management of Fetal Growth Restriction

Doppler assessment of the UA for each fetus, at least weekly, if:

- There is an EFW discordance of 20% or more
- The EFW of any of fetus is below 10th centile for gestational age

Twin pregnancies complicated by selective fetal growth restriction (sFGR) (EFW discordance of 25% or more and/or the EFW of any of fetus below 10th centile for gestational age) should be followed up in a specialist center with serial ultrasound scans. Dichorionic twin with sFGR the timing of delivery can be decided based on the risk-benefit assessment, as in singletons. Classification of sFGR in monochorionic twins is complex. There is little evidence to guide the management of monochorionic twins affected by sFGR, but options include early delivery, laser ablation, or cord occlusion of the growth restricted fetus. Monitoring should be at least every 2 weeks with fetal Dopplers. If there is a real risk of demise of one twin very early (e.g., before 26 weeks' gestation), selective laser photocoagulation of the communicating vessels or selective termination should be considered.

Management of Single In Utero Death

When death of one of a monochorionic twin pair is diagnosed, the urge to swiftly deliver the other should be resisted. This is because, if that twin is going to suffer damage, it is likely to have already occurred by the time the death of its co-twin is diagnosed. The live twin should initially be assessed for immediate compromise using cardiotocography (CTG) or MCA Doppler to assess for fetal anemia. Immediate delivery seems reasonable if the death occurs later in the third trimester; otherwise, immediate delivery that puts the surviving twin at risk of the complications of prematurity is not justified.

Multifetal Reduction

Given the risks that multiple gestations confer, some women elect for fetal reduction, especially in the setting of higher order multiples. This is typically performed by potassium chloride injection into the selected fetus. The overall postprocedure pregnancy loss rate is estimated at approximately 6–12%, depending on gestational age. The ongoing early preterm delivery (between 24 and 28 weeks' gestation) risk is approximately 4.5%. In monochorionic twins, feticide is performed by cord occlusion, radiofrequency ablation, or laser ablation of the cord of the affected twin after counseling the parents of the potential risks to the surviving co-twin. The procedure causes demise of the affected twin and also isolates its circulation from that of its co-twin. Survival of the co-twin is around 80%, but there is an increased risk of adverse neurological sequelae. Therefore, multifetal reduction in a monochorionic twin setting is typically not recommended.

Improved pregnancy outcomes have been reported from multifetal reduction of triplets to twins and particularly in those with reduction from triplets to singleton gestations. However, the rates of pregnancy loss before 24 weeks and preterm delivery before 32–34 weeks' gestation were similar in the twin and singleton pregnancies, and the prevalence of gestational diabetes and gestational hypertension was not significantly different between the groups with triplet reduction to twin and triplet reduction to singleton gestations.

Indications for Referral to a Tertiary Center (National Institute for Health and Care Excellence Guideline, 2019)

- Monochorionic monoamniotic twins
- Dichorionic diamniotic triplets
- Monochorionic diamniotic triplets
- Monochorionic monoamniotic triplets
- Conjoined twin and triplets
- Any complications associated with Monochorionic twin
- Fetal weight discordance (of 25% or more) and an EFW of any of the babies below 10th centile for GA.

Timing of Delivery in Uncomplicated Twin and Triplet

Multiple pregnancy has a higher risk for PTB. Around 60% of twins will deliver spontaneously before 37^{+0} weeks of gestation. Women carrying dichorionic twins or Mo-Di twins should be offered elective delivery (either by induction of labor or caesarean section) from 37^{+0} and 36 weeks' gestation, respectively.

National Institute for Health and Care Excellence Recommendation on Delivery

Dichorionic Twin Pregnancies

Elective birth from 37^{+0} to 37^{+6} weeks' gestation. When appropriate obstetric experience is available, vaginal birth is the preferred mode of birth for all twin pregnancies that meet the following criteria:

- Twins must be diamniotic
- Twin 1 cephalic
- Twin 2 is not >500 g heavier than twin I
- Neither twin has any evidence of fetal compromise requiring caesarean section.

Monochorionic Diamniotic Twin Pregnancies

Elective birth from 36^{+0} to 36^{+6} weeks gestation after a course of prophylactic corticosteroids has been offered. In many countries, Mo-Di twins will commonly be delivered by cesarean section; however, when uncomplicated, the option of vaginal birth could be offered to the parents. There is a possible risk of acute TTTS occurring during labor, although the risk of this appears to be small.

Uncomplicated Monoamniotic Twin

Monochorionic monoamniotic twin pregnancies carry a high perinatal loss rate of up to 50% before 16 weeks' gestation. The incidence of TTTS in Mo-Mo twin is 6%, with cerebral injury of 5%. The timing of delivery is elective cesarean delivery at 32^{+0} to 33^{+6} weeks' gestation (after administration of corticosteroid).

Triplet Pregnancy

Uncomplicated trichorionic triamniotic or dichorionic triamniotic triplet—elective birth from 35 weeks 0 days after a course of antenatal corticosteroids has been offered. Monochorionic triamniotic triplet pregnancy or a triplet pregnancy with shared amnion—the timing of birth will be decided individually.

▪ INTRAPARTUM MANAGEMENT

Preparation and Monitoring

Management should be multidisciplinary with adequate obstetric and nursing staff, anesthesiologist, and neonatologist. Consider prostaglandin/oxytocin for induction or oxytocin for augmentation. Offer continuous CTG using dual channel monitoring in established labor to allow simultaneous monitoring of both fetal hearts. Ideally, after membrane rupture, first twin should be monitored by fetal scalp electrode and using an external monitor for the second twin. If facilities available and if necessary, perform a portable USG to confirm presentation of each twin and locate the fetal hearts in labor room.

Ensure that oxytocin infusion is available to be used after the first twin is delivered. Withhold the intramuscular (IM) oxytocin after the birth of the first twin. Clamp and cut the umbilical cord after the birth of the first twin. Consider the commencement of an oxytocin infusion in consultation with the obstetric staff for the prevention of uterine inertia. 10 IU of oxytocin in 500 mL of Hartmann's or normal saline commencing at 6 mL/hour. Conduct the delivery of the first twin, if it is a cephalic presentation, as for a normal birth.

Delivery of the Second Twin

Perform an abdominal palpation and vaginal examination immediately after delivery of twin 1. This allows determination of the lie and presentation and position of twin 2 and excludes cord presentation/prolapse. Confirm fetal presentation by portable ultrasound as required. External cephalic version or internal podalic manipulation of the fetus may be required for malpresentation. Perform an artificial rupture of membranes (ARM) when clinically appropriate. Withhold the third stage oxytocin until after delivery of the second twin. Continuous intrapartum fetal heart monitoring is recommended. Delivery of the second twin usually occurs within 30 minutes of the first twin but may be prolonged if the fetal heart rate is normal. Active management of the delivery of the second twin is recommended to avoid prolonged interval. Collect cord blood from both twins after the birth of twin 2.

Postnatal Care

Counseling regarding breastfeeding and need for extra support. As there is threefold increase in the risk of postnatal depression, if it develops, early referral to psychiatrists is recommended.

■ MONOCHORIONIC TWINS

About 20% of twins are monochorionic, monochorionic twins are monozygotic; that is, they arise from one fertilized ovum and commonly have a shared placenta with vascular anastomoses between the two fetal circulations and are associated with higher risk of complications. Monochorionic twins are usually diamniotic, with each twin in a separate amniotic sac. Rarely, the twins may be in a single sac (monoamniotic) or even conjoined. Monoamniotic twin historically carries a higher risk of perinatal morbidity and mortality than diamniotic twin, with a perinatal mortality >50%. These configurations depend upon the stage of development at which the inner cell mass divides.

Ultrasonography Assessment

Following an ultrasound scan at 11–14 weeks for assessment of chorionicity, nuchal translucency, and early anatomy, ultrasound should be performed every 2 weeks from 16 weeks' gestation. Ultrasound should be undertaken by a center with sufficient experience to recognize complication and refer appropriately if they occur. International Society of Ultrasound in Obstetrics and Gynecology (ISUOG) recommends all women with monochorionic pregnancies should receive 2 weekly ultrasound surveillance from 16 weeks onward, this has been shown to reduce the incidence of "late stage" TTTS diagnosis. Early-stage diagnosis and earlier intervention are likely to improve the outcome.

Complications of Monochorionic Twin

Perinatal Loss

Perinatal mortality of monochorionic twins is nearly twice than dichorionic twins (2.8 vs. 1.6%) and four times as high as singletons (2.8 vs. 0.7%). There is sixfold higher fetal loss rate (12 vs. 2%) than that of dichorionic twins and singletons prior to viability (between 10 and 24 weeks).

Vascular Anastomoses

Vascular anastomoses present in (96%) monochorionic twin with increased morbidity and mortality related to the angioarchitecture of monochorionic placenta. Anastomoses can cause significant blood volume shifts between the fetuses, leading to unique complications such as:
- *TTTS:* 15%
- Twin reversed arterial perfusion (TRAP)
- Acute fetofetal transfusion after single fetal demise
- Selective intrauterine growth restriction (IUGR), commonly due to unequal placental sharing and velamentous cord insertion

All of these conditions contribute to an overall higher perinatal mortality of monochorionic, when compared to dichorionic twin.

■ TWIN–TWIN TRANSFUSION SYNDROME (FIGS. 7A AND B)

Twin-to-twin transfusion syndrome is a unique complication of monochorionic multiple pregnancies, resulting from imbalanced blood flow through the vascular anastomoses in the placenta. In most monochorionic twins, interfetal transfusion across the anastomoses is a balanced phenomenon. In 10–15% cases, imbalance in net blood flow develops, resulting in TTTS.

Twin-to-twin transfusion syndrome may take one of two forms:
1. *TOPS (twin oligohydramnios/polyhydramnios sequence):* It affects approximately 10% of monochorionic twins, and is most commonly seen in the mid-trimester (15–26 weeks). This is recognized as "classical" TTTS, with oligohydramnios, poor growth, and abnormal UA Dopplers in the donor, and polyhydramnios progressing

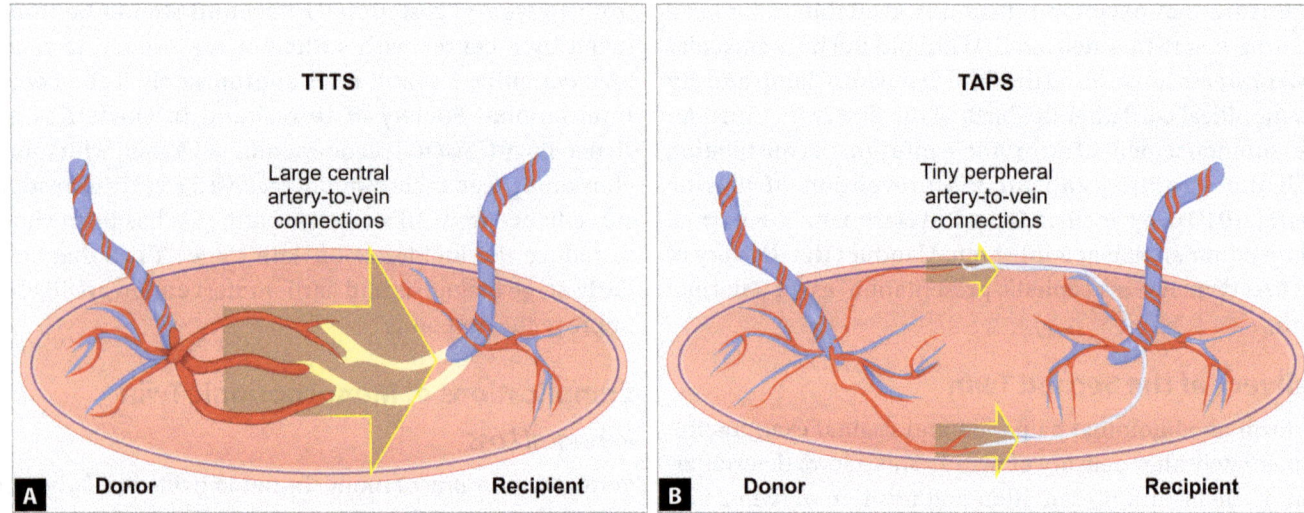

Figs. 7A and B: Mechanism of development of TTTS and TAPS.

to cardiac dysfunction and cardiac failure in the recipient.

2. *TAPS (twin anemia/polycythemia sequence):* It affects up to 5% of monochorionic twins, and 10% of twins that have undergone laser therapy for TOPS. TAPS results in very slow transfusion (5–15 mL/24 hours) from donor to recipient, characterized by presence of only few tiny (≤1 mm) unidirectional arteriovenous (AV) anastomoses without a compensating arterioarterial (AA) anastomosis. So, is not characterized by extreme amniotic fluid discordance and cardiac dysfunction, but by significantly discordant MCA peak systolic velocities, reflecting anemia and polycythemia in the donor and recipient, respectively. It is more common in later pregnancy, and is often recognized as "neonatal TTTS" when very discordant hemoglobin levels are recognized at birth. Nevertheless, TAPS can also be associated with significant fetal anemia and in utero compromise requiring treatment. For this reason, ultrasound examination in monochorionic twins should include growth, amniotic fluid volume in each sac, bladder volume, UA, and (after 20 weeks) MCA Doppler wave forms.

Sonographic Diagnosis of Twin-to-twin Transfusion Syndrome

Hydramnios in the recipient sac (defined as deepest vertical pocket of ≥8 cm prior to 20 weeks and ≥10 cm after 20 weeks) secondary to polyuria. Oligohydramnios in the donor's sac (deepest vertical pocket ≤2 cm) secondary to oliguria.

Other typical sonographic criteria include presence of a single placenta, sex concordance, significant growth discordance (approximately 20%), discrepancy in size of umbilical cords, presence of fetal hydrops or cardiac dysfunction, abnormal UA Doppler findings, such as absent end-diastolic flow in the donor fetus.

Clinical Features

The donor fetus is relatively hypoperfused, demonstrating signs of IUGR and oligohydramnios. Eventually, anhydramnios leading to typical stuck twin appearance because of inability to visualize the dividing membrane separate from the fetal body. The donor fetus has a significantly lower hematocrit than the recipient fetus (36 vs. 47%). The recipient fetus is hyperperfused, becomes hypertensive, and develops biventricular hypertrophy and diastolic dysfunction, which tends to be progressive without definitive therapy, ultimately leads to cardiac failure. Significant polyhydramnios increases intrauterine pressure leading to increased rates of preterm labor or preterm premature rupture of the membranes (pPROM).

Diagnosis

Twin-to-twin transfusion syndrome is a diagnosis of exclusion, management involves exclusion of other causes of significant growth discordance such as stuck twin phenomenon, fetal anomalies including chromosomal defect, fetal infection, placental insufficiency, and abnormal cord insertion. Diagnosis requires careful sonographic assessment of fetal anatomy, color Doppler studies, and fetal echocardiogram.

Quintero Staging

Quintero staging system has been developed for categorizing disease severity and standardizing comparison of different treatment results.
- *Stage I:* There is oligohydramnios, but the bladder of the donor twin is still visible.

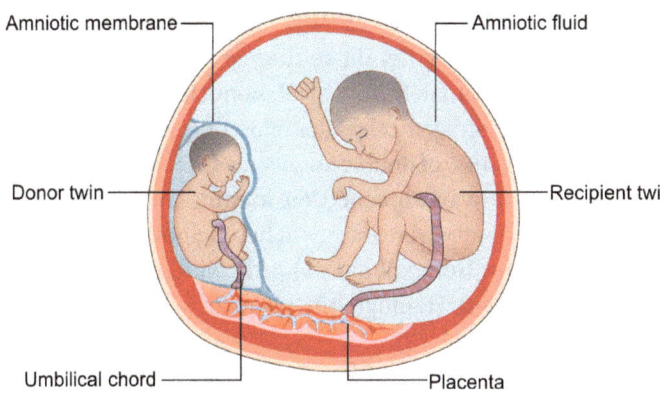

Fig. 8: Twin oligohydramnios/polyhydramnios sequence (TOPS).

- *Stage II:* The bladder of the donor twin is no longer visible, after an hour of observation; fetal Doppler values remains normal.
- *Stage III:* Abnormal Doppler studies are evident (i.e., absent/reversed end-diastolic velocity in the UA, reversed flow in the ductus venosus or pulsatile flow in the umbilical vein).
- *Stage IV:* One or both twins show signs of heart failure, such as hydrops
- *Stage V:* Intrauterine death of one or both fetuses

Most stage I TTTS do not require treatment, approximately 75% remain stable or regress. For stages ≥III, prognosis is particularly poor, with a reported perinatal loss rate of 70–100%.

Management

Expectant Management

Aggressive invasive fetal therapy is controversial in early-stage disease as almost 70% stage I TTTS remain stable or regress. Expectant management for severe TTTS is associated with high rates of perinatal mortality, as high as 80–100%. Patients with early-onset TTTS may be offered for selective termination of one twin (usually the donor) or termination of the entire pregnancy. Some severe cases may be managed by cord ligation of one twin, particularly if there is a fetal anomaly in one twin. If TTTS develops later in pregnancy, treatment may be less aggressive depending on the disease severity and gestational age.

Medical Treatment

Medical treatment includes maternal administration of sulindac, a prostaglandin inhibitor that results in decreased amniotic fluid, which may in turn, stabilize fetal lie and theoretically reduce risk of cord entanglement. Other medications that are used include digoxin and nifedipine but are not very effective.

Mild TTTS (e.g., Stage I), or late gestation disease (after >26 weeks), may occasionally be managed expectantly or by serial amnioreduction, with or without preterm delivery. Other management approaches include amniotic septostomy and fetoscopic laser coagulation of placental anastomoses.

Laser Ablation

Laser ablation is considered to be the best first-line treatment for severe TTTS. It is the only therapy that directly treats the underlying pathophysiology of TTTS. It should be performed in fetal medicine centers experienced in dealing with such cases, having a minimum two experienced operators and at least 15 procedures performed per year (rolling 3-year average) to maximize perinatal outcomes and minimize long-term morbidity. Amnioreduction prior to laser surgery may lead to increased membrane separation and make subsequent laser treatment more difficult.

Fetal Surveillance after Twin-to-twin Transfusion Syndrome Treatment

Weekly sonographic evaluation including Doppler study in the first month and two-weekly Doppler thereafter. USG evaluation should include fetal brain, heart, and limbs. Doppler should include umbilical artery pulsatility index (UAPI), MCA PSV, and ductus venosus Doppler velocities. Fetal growth monitoring (by calculating EFW) and fetal echocardiogram to exclude functional heart abnormalities and right ventricular outflow tract obstruction. Demonstration of bladder filling and increasing amniotic fluid in the donor is a sign of TTTS resolution. A routine magnetic resonance imaging (MRI) at around 30 weeks can detect more subtle brain lesions.

After successful procedures, there is usually a decrease in discordancy and more than half of the donors show catch-up growth, ultimately resulting in a normal birth weight. If complete laser separation of shared vessels has been confidently achieved, and if TTTS features resolve, then maintain the pregnancy until 37 weeks. If that all placental anastomoses have been ablated is not confirmed, elective delivery of TTTS cases at 34 weeks is recommended. Delivery of pregnancy complicated by TTTS and those treated, should be between 34^{+0} and 36^{+6} weeks of gestation (RCOG Green-top Guideline No. 51). Two neonatal resuscitation teams should be present at delivery.

Complications Following Laser Treatment

Preterm Premature Rupture of the Membranes

Preterm premature rupture of the membranes remains the most important complication, incidence prior to 34 weeks is 28%. In 12% cases, occurs within 3 weeks after the procedure.

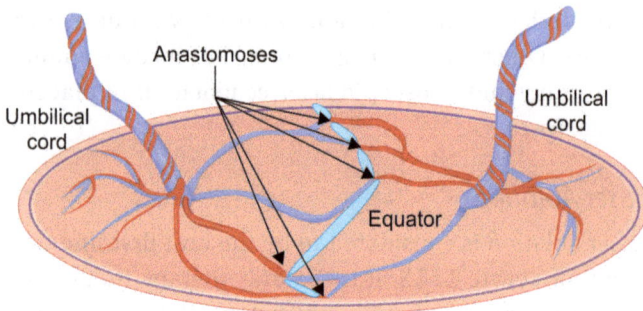

Fig. 9: Equatorial zone.

Cause may be:
- Iatrogenic membrane defect.
- An inflammatory response leading to activation of enzymatic cascade that degrades the membrane, and eventually leads to pPROM.

Preterm Birth
About 20% between 24 and 32 weeks of gestation.

Demise of One or Both Fetuses
60% of intrauterine deaths with laser occur within 48 hours and 75% within 1 week after the procedure.

Persistent Twin-to-twin Transfusion Syndrome
Up to one-third of cases of laser ablation, one or more anastomoses are missed during the procedure. Missed large anastomoses may result in intrauterine fetal demise (IUFD) or persistent TTTS, development of TAPS, other fetal complications (uncommon) include limb reduction deformities, cerebral anomalies, intestinal atresia, and congenital skin loss.

Modification of the primary fetoscopic laser technique by "equatorial laser dichorionization" (the Solomon technique) has been reported to reduce, but not ameliorate, the risk of postlaser TAPS **(Fig. 9)**.

Maternal Complications
Transient maternal mirror or Ballantyne's syndrome (pulmonary edema, placental abruption, chorioamnionitis and bleeding requiring transfusion) has been reported.

Outcome of Severe TTTS after Fetoscopic Laser Ablation
Quintero stage III or IV: At least one survivor in 73-74% of pregnancies. Overall survival rate is 55-57%. Mean gestational age at delivery for the survivors 32.2 weeks. Studies found 96% of the survivors develop normally at mean age of 35.8 months. Rate of neurological handicap was 4% in one study, 9-11% in some other studies.

Twin Anemia Polycythemia Sequence
Twin anemia polycythemia sequence may occur spontaneously in approximately 3.5% of all monochorionic twins, but may also result iatrogenically after fetoscopic laser photocoagulation in up to 16% of double survivors. TAPS may be responsible for previously unexplained late intrauterine deaths. There will be chronic and severe intertwin hemoglobin discordancy:
- *In the donor:* Hemoglobin ≤11 g/dL with reticulocytosis
- *In the recipient:* Hemoglobin ≥20 g/dL

Iatrogenic Twin Anemia Polycythemia Sequence
Iatrogenic twin anemia polycythemia swquence (TAPS) is diagnosed antenatally by MCA Doppler velocimetry in the absence of the significant oligohydramnios/polyhydramnios. PSV of the MCA above 1.5 multiples of median (MoM), suggestive of fetal anemia in the donor. A decreased MCA PSV <1 MoM, suggestive of polycythemia in recipient twin.

Spontaneous Twin Anemia Polycythemia Sequence
Usually occurs after 30 weeks especially in pairs with progressive discordant growth after 26 weeks. Placentas of spontaneous TAPS and iatrogenic TAPS show striking similarity, characterized by presence of only few tiny (≤1 mm) unidirectional AV anastomoses without a compensating AA anastomoses. These allow a slow transfusion of blood from the donor to the recipient. The very slow intertwin transfusion allows more time for hemodynamic compensatory mechanisms to take place.

Fetal Risk
Severe anemia may result in hydrops and intrauterine death of the donor. Severe polycythemia may cause cardiac failure or vascular accidents and death of the recipient. TAPS usually occurs in the third trimester and severe polyhydramnios is unusual.

Management options: Include:
- Expectant management
- Delivery
- Intrauterine blood transfusion (intravenous and/or intraperitoneal, with or without partial exchange)
- Selective feticide
- Fetoscopic laser surgery

Perinatal Outcome
Perinatal outcome varies according to severity, range from double intrauterine demise to the birth of two healthy neonates with significant hemoglobin discordance. Donor twin may be severely anemic and require blood transfusion, whereas recipient twin may be severely polycythemic requiring partial exchange transfusion. Severe cerebral injury in TAPS has also been described.

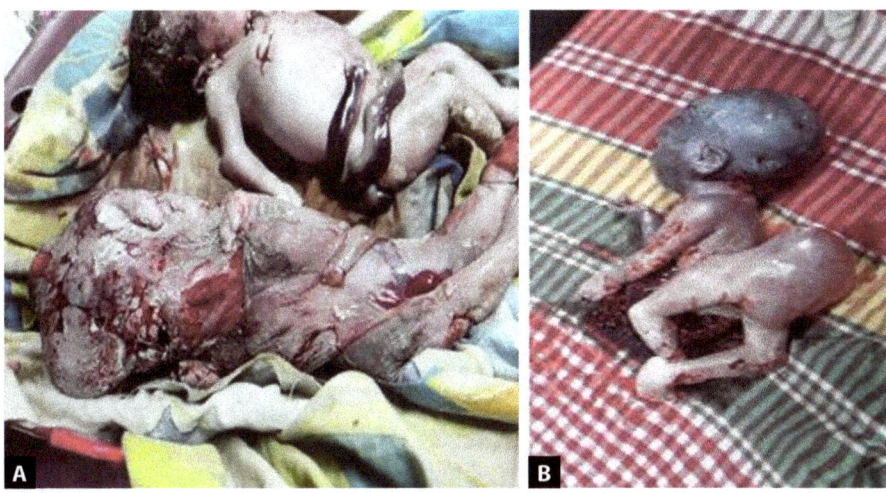

Figs. 10A and B: (A) Monochorionic twin (TTTS)(Both dead); (B) Monochorionic twin (TRAP) sequence.

TWIN REVERSED ARTERIAL PERFUSION SEQUENCE

In TRAP, one twin has an absent, rudimentary, or nonfunctioning heart (acardiac twin) and the other twin is normal (pump twin). Incidence of TRAP is about 1% among monozygotic twins or 1 in 35,000 to 50,000 births.

Pathophysiology

Recipient or perfused twin develops early first-trimester circulatory failure. Development of AA anastomoses results in a profoundly abnormal twin mass. Reversal of blood flow in the UA brings deoxygenated blood from the co-twin to the acardiac twin. Perfusion is asymmetric in the recipient twin with relative hypoperfusion of the upper part of the body resulting in significant structural anomalies including anencephaly, holoprosencephaly, absent limbs, absent lungs, intestinal atresia, abdominal wall defects and absent liver, spleen, or kidneys.

Donor, or "pump twin": Usually structurally normal (aneuploidy in 9%). Provides circulation for itself and for the recipient through a direct umbilical arterial-to-arterial anastomosis, is at risk for development of hydrops or congestive cardiac failure.

Prenatal Diagnosis

Based on USG, one normal-appearing fetus and another, profoundly abnormal appearing fetus or amorphous mass of tissue in a monochorionic twin pregnancy. The placentation is most commonly Mo-Di (74%). Monoamniotic is present in only 24% of cases. Up to one-third of fetuses have abnormal karyotype.

Doppler Velocimetry

Doppler velocimetry will demonstrate reversed direction of flow in the UA of acardiac twin. Other associated findings are polyhydramnios, single UA, velamentous, or conjoined insertion of cord.

Antepartum Management

The goal is to maximize the outcome for the structurally normal pump twin.

Criteria for Intervention

Twin reversed arterial perfusion has increased risk for congestive cardiac failure. When the ratio of the weight of the perfused twin to the weight of the pump twin is >0.7, the chance of congestive cardiac failure is 30%. Other criteria for interventions include abdominal circumference in the acardiac twin greater than or equal to the pump twin, polyhydramnios with maximum vertical fluid pocket >8 cm, abnormal Doppler studies, hydrops in the pump twin or TRAP in the setting of monoamniocity. If any of these are noted before 32–34 weeks of gestation, antenatal intervention should be considered.

Expectant Management

With absence of above features, expectant management is done, which includes serial sonographic evaluation, serial weekly echocardiography, and antenatal corticosteroid before delivery. Sign of cardiac decompensation after 32–34 weeks should prompt consideration for delivery.

Invasive procedures to interrupt vascular supply to the acardiac mass: Includes:
- Fetoscopy (with bipolar cord coagulation or laser ablation)
- Radiofrequency thermoablation
- Thermocoagulation
- Harmonic ultrasound scalpel to the acardiac twin's cord
- Injection of thrombogenic coil into recipients' umbilical cord

Radiofrequency ablation is useful in presence of significant oligohydramnios that limits fetoscopic visualization.

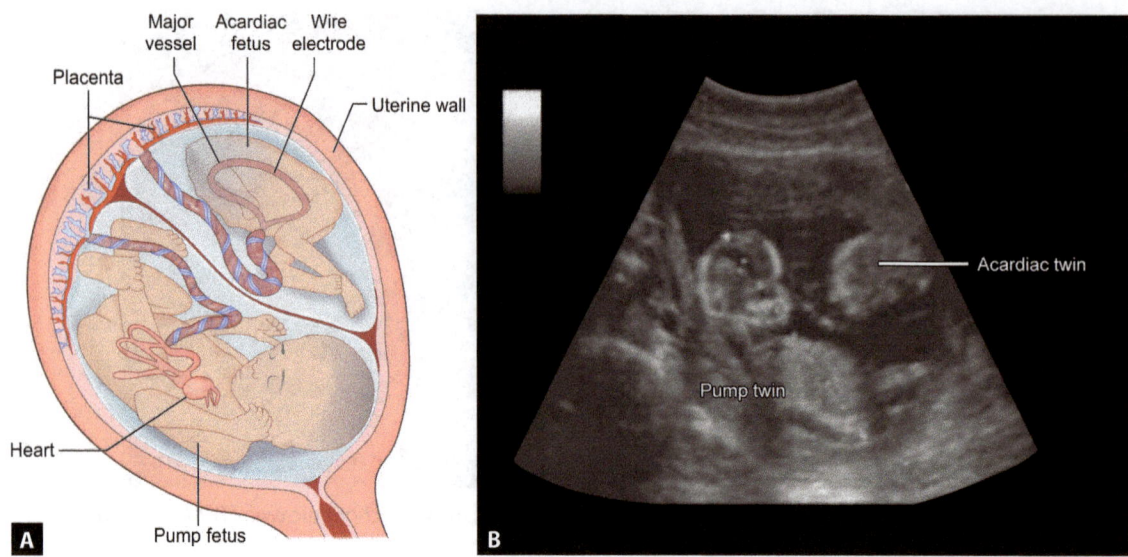

Figs. 11A and B: (A) Diagrammatic image; (B) USG image of acardiac twin.

Outcome

Overall perinatal mortality of the pump twin ranges from 50 to 75%. Polyhydramnios leading to prematurity is the major factor determining prognosis. Survival rates for cord coagulation and radiofrequency ablation are similar, ranges from 70 to 80%.

Outcome of the newborn: Main problems include complications of prematurity and congestive cardiac failure. Other problems are massive hepatosplenomegaly, ascites with hypoplasia of abdominal musculature, edema, and hypoalbuminemia due to inadequate liver synthesis of albumin. Respiratory assistance as well as support of myocardial function with inotropic medication may be required. Surfactant therapy may be needed when delivery occurs at <30 weeks. Postnatal consultation with pediatric cardiologist and echocardiography are recommended.

INTRAUTERINE DEMISE OF ONE FETUS

Intrauterine fetal demise of one twin occurs most commonly during the first trimester—known as vanishing twin. The prognosis of the surviving twin is excellent. In the second and third trimesters, it is more often associated with monochorionic placentation and may be related with worse outcome of surviving co-twin. Incidence of single fetal demise is 21% in first trimester, while 2–5% of twin pregnancies and 14–17% of triplet pregnancies may demise in the second and third trimesters.

A systematic review of studies that evaluated the prognosis of the co-twin following a single twin death after 14 weeks in monochorionic and dichorionic twin (monoamniotic twins were excluded) has shown the rates of fetal demise of the co-twin were 41 and 22%, respectively (comparing monochorionic versus dichorionic: OR 2.06, 95% CI 1.14–3.71) and the rates of PTBs were 59 and 54%, respectively (comparing monochorionic versus dichorionic: OR 1.42, 95% CI 0.67–2.99). In monochorionic pregnancies, 20% of co-twin survivors had abnormal antenatal cranial imaging.

The rates of abnormal postnatal cranial imaging were 43 and 12%, respectively (comparing monochorionic versus dichorionic: OR 5.41, 95% CI 1.03–28.56), the rates of neurodevelopmental impairment of the co-twin were 29 and 10%, respectively (comparing monochorionic versus dichorionic: OR 3.06, 95% CI 0.88–10.61) and the rates of neonatal death of the co-twin were 28 and 21%, respectively (comparing monochorionic versus dichorionic: OR 1.95, 95% CI 1.00–3.79). In addition, in monochorionic twins, a single fetal death before 28 weeks of gestation increased the risk for co-twin fetal and neonatal death compared with single fetal death after 28 weeks.

Etiology

Etiology often remains elusive, similar to singletons including genetic and structural abnormalities, abruption and placental insufficiency, cord abnormalities such as velamentous cord insertion, infection, and maternal disease, e.g., diabetes and hypertension. Etiology unique to the twining process—TTTS, acute fetofetal transfusion, cord entanglement.

Single fetal damage adversely affects the surviving fetus or fetuses in two ways:
1. Multiorgan damage including multicystic encephalomalacia in monochorionic pregnancies
2. Preterm labor and delivery

Multicystic Encephalomalacia

Incidence 20% among the surviving co-twin in a monochorionic pregnancy. Here, cystic lesions occur in the cerebral white matter distributed in areas supplied by the anterior and MCAs, associated with profound neurological handicap.

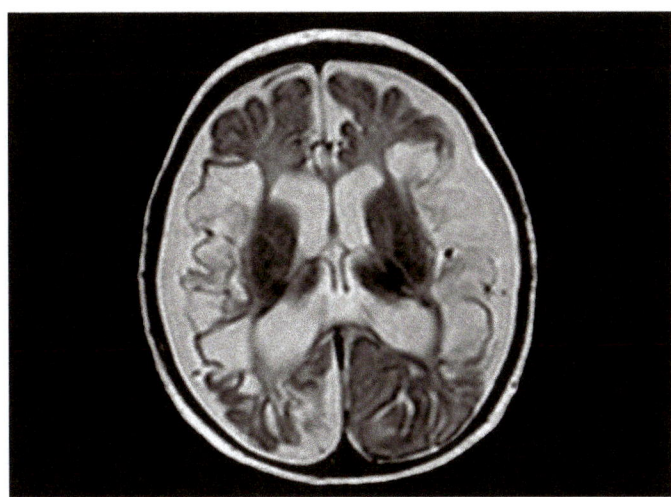

Fig. 12: Image of multicystic encephalomalacia.

Pathophysiology of multicystic encephalomalacia: Death of one twin in a monochorionic pair may result in death or neurological disability in the survivor. These events occur around the time of the fetal death, postulated due to agonal hypotension as the blood volume of the survivor is "dumped" precipitously into the body of the co-twin through shared vascular communications, or possibly due to the release of thromboplastins from the deceased twin into the shared circulation, resulting in disseminated intravascular coagulation (DIC). This leads to infarction and cystic damage of multiple organ systems including kidneys, lungs, spleen, liver, and brain.

The current widely acceptable theory—blood from the surviving twin may rapidly "back-bleed" into the demised twin through placental anastomoses—acute fetofetal transfusion. The demised twin may become congested and surviving twin may become anemic. Significant hypotension will lead to ischemic damage to the vital organ in the surviving twin.

Management of Pregnancy with Single Fetal Demise

To identify the cause of death, a complete biometric and anatomic assessment of both dead and surviving twins, amniotic fluid volume, any evidence of IUGR, and evaluation of cord insertion sites is needed. Determination of chorionicity—if not detected earlier. Woman should be managed in a tertiary care center. Management depends on gestational age, fetal lung maturity, and detection of in utero compromise of the surviving twin. Once viability has been achieved management is similar for both dichorionic and monochorionic pregnancies. A single course of antenatal corticosteroids should be administered.

Patients with monochorionic pregnancies should be counseled about the risk including multicystic encephalomalacia but no interventions are available to reduce the risk. Surviving fetus should be monitored by weekly USG including Doppler, biophysical profiles (BPPs), and nonstress tests (NSTs). If any abnormalities such as IUGR or oligohydramnios detected, fetal testing should be intensified. MCA surveillance should be offered to the surviving twin, and intrauterine transfusion offered if the survivor has evidence of severe anemia. USG of the fetal brain may be suggestive of multicystic encephalomalacia but cannot make a definitive diagnosis. MRI should be done after approximately 2–3 weeks to diagnose neurological damage secondary to hypovolemia. As the injury seems to occur at the time of demise, so immediate delivery of the co-twin following single IUFD, does not improve outcome, rather adds to the risk of prematurity. Delivery of the survivor at a preterm gestation will not prevent further damage unless there is evidence of CTG abnormalities or significant fetal anemia.

Demise Before the Age of Viability

Dichorionic Pregnancy

Managed expectantly until 37 weeks of gestation. Fetal surveillance and a single course of antenatal steroids considered once viability is reached. In a dichorionic pregnancy, multicystic encephalomalacia sequence is not a concern since there are no placental vascular anastomoses; however, death of one twin may reflect an adverse intrauterine environment that could also place the co-twin at risk for morbidity or mortality.

Monochorionic Pregnancy

The patient should be counseled regarding the risk of multiorgan injury including multicystic encephalomalacia. USG and fetal MRI may be helpful. Some patients may opt to termination of the entire pregnancy. If patient desires expectant management, treatment is same as dichorionic pregnancy once the co-twin reaches the viability.

Maternal Risk of Single Fetal Demise

Disseminated intravascular coagulopathy was once estimated as 25% following single fetal demise. But no clinical cases of DIC were noted from recent reviews of spontaneous single IUFD and selective terminations in multiple gestations. Maternal hypofibrinogenemia or DIC following death of one fetus of a multiple gestation has been described in only a few case reports. So, it is not necessary to monitor for maternal coagulopathy in these cases since it is rare. Although some experts have treated these patients with a short course of heparin, spontaneous resolution of hypofibrinogenemia occurs without therapy. Consider heparin therapy if there is active hypofibrinogenemia-related bleeding, hypofibrinogenemia in a patient at high risk of hemorrhage such as with placental previa or abruptio placentae, or if there are thrombotic complications.

Maternal Monitoring

Baseline hematological parameters including prothrombin time, activated partial thromboplastin time (APTT), fibrinogen level, and platelet count, if these values are within normal limits, further laboratory surveillance is not needed.

Elective Delivery

At approximately 37 weeks or earlier, if fetal status is nonreassuring. At delivery, cord blood gas and hematocrit measurements should be performed. Autopsy of dead fetus and placental histological examination is recommended.

Fetal Intervention

In known monochorionic pregnancies with impending death of one twin, preterm delivery may be indicated to prevent neurologic injury of the survivor or to save both twins. Selective termination may be considered during impending death in an effort to protect the healthy co-fetus or fetuses. Intracardiac potassium chloride (KCL) injection is contraindicated in monochorionic pregnancies. Cord occlusive methods such as fetoscopic cord ligation, fetoscopic ablation of communicating placental vessels, or radiofrequency cord ablation can be considered. Intrauterine transfusion may be considered when MCA Doppler shows fetal anemia. This may increase survival of severely handicapped infants.

Treatment of the Newborn

Surviving infants should be evaluated postnatally for neurological injury. A thorough neurological assessment and assessment of other organs such as kidneys, liver, spleen, etc., is needed. Follow-up assessment for growth and development is also important.

SELECTIVE INTRAUTERINE GROWTH RESTRICTION

The management of growth restriction and/or discordance depends on chorionicity.

Monochorionic Twins

The goal of managing pregnancies with sFGR is to identify those that can be safely managed conservatively versus those that might benefit from fetal intervention. In a high proportion of cases, sFGR coexists with TTTS, twin anemia-polycythemia sequence (TAPS), or discordant fetal anomalies. Due to substantial overlap between these disorders, a systematic approach to evaluation is required to arrive at the correct diagnosis and initiate management planning.

Dichorionic Twins

Growth restriction is generally managed as in singletons: Determination of the cause, serial ultrasound assessment of fetal growth, ongoing evaluation of fetal well-being (BPP or NST with assessment of amniotic fluid volume, and Doppler velocimetry), and timely delivery based on combination of factors (gestational age, UA Doppler, BPP score, ductus venosus Doppler, and the presence or absence of risk factors for, or signs of, uteroplacental insufficiency).

In dichorionic twins, a systematic review found that the risk of fetal demise increased with increasing discordance: ≥15% (OR 9.8, 95% CI 3.9–29.4), ≥20% (OR 7.0, 95% CI 4.15–11.8), ≥25% (OR 17.4, 95% CI 8.3–36.7), ≥30% (OR 22.9, 95% CI 10.2–51.6) compared with no discordance. The smaller twin was at higher risk of fetal demise than the larger twin. The risk of fetal demise was not increased when the weights of the discordant twins remained appropriate for gestational age (AGA), the small number of cases in the study may have underestimated this association.

MALFORMATIONS IN TWINS

Congenital malformations occur more commonly in twins as compared to singletons. It is more common in monozygotic than dizygotic twin pregnancies. The diagnosis of congenital anomaly in one twin is especially problematic since decisions regarding monitoring, therapy, and delivery affect both fetuses. Expectant management, in utero therapy, pregnancy termination, and selective feticide should all be discussed, if appropriate for the type of abnormality and gestational age. Patients who choose to continue the pregnancy should understand how the anomalous fetus might affect the co-twin's outcome (e.g., PTB and organ damage), including the role of chorionicity.

Incidence

Overall incidence is about 6%.

Management

When both fetuses in a twin pregnancy are concordant for malformations, management is straightforward and include usual obstetric management of twin gestations and required intervention of that particular malformation. When one twin has a congenital malformation but the co-twin is normal, management decision depends on the type of abnormality and prognosis, gestational age at diagnosis, chorionicity of the pregnancy, effect of the anomalous fetus on normal co-twin, and ethical beliefs of the parents.

Options include:
- Expectant management
- Selective termination of anomalous fetus and
- Termination of the entire pregnancy.

Dichorionic Twins

In dichorionic twins, selective termination of the anomalous fetus is a safe and effective option in expert hands, although there is 20% risk of miscarriage or preterm delivery of the co-twin. Because of these risks, expectant management may be a safer option if the twin with the anomaly is not expected to have prolonged survival or a favorable outcome (e.g., trisomy 18). Anencephaly is an exception since it is associated with polyhydramnios and PTB. Karyotyping for twin with malformation is recommended. Serial amnioreduction, if there is significant polyhydramnios to reduce the risk of prematurity.

Monochorionic Twins

In monochorionic twins, selective feticide can be performed but the technique is different from that in dichorionic twins and is more challenging. It necessitates obstructing one umbilical cord (e.g., radiofrequency or laser ablation, bipolar coagulation, and ligation) rather than intravascular injection of potassium chloride or digoxin in order to reduce risk to the co-twin associated with shared circulations.

Delivery

At 37 weeks or after lung maturity. Mode of delivery determined by obstetric indication applied for normal twin gestations, individual malformation, and fetal prognosis.

SUGGESTED READING

1. Benirschke K. Multiple gestation: The biology of twinning. In: Creasy RK, Resnik R, Iams JD, Lockwood CJ, Moore TR, Greene MF (Eds). Creasy and Resnik's Maternal-Fetal Medicine Principles and Practice, 7th edition. Philadelphia: Elsevier; 2014.
2. Bianchi DW, Crombleholme TM, D'Alton ME, Malone FD. Conjoined twins. In: Fetology Diagnosis and Management of Fetal Patient, 2nd edition. New York: McGraw-Hill; 2010.
3. Bianchi DW, Crombleholme TM, D'Alton ME, Malone FD. Fetology Diagnosis and Management of Fetal Patient, 2nd edition. New York: McGraw-Hill; 2010.
4. Bianchi DW, Crombleholme TM, D'Alton ME, Malone FD. Intrauterine death of one twin. In: Fetology Diagnosis and Management of Fetal Patient, 2nd edition. New York: McGraw-Hill; 2010. pp. 810-17.
5. Bianchi DW, Crombleholme TM, D'Alton ME, Malone FD. Malformations in twins. In: Fetology Diagnosis and Management of Fetal Patient, 2nd edition. New York: McGraw-Hill; 2010. pp. 803-09.
6. Bianchi DW, Crombleholme TM, D'Alton ME, Malone FD. Monoamniotic twin. In: Fetology Diagnosis and Management of Fetal Patient, 2nd edition. New York: McGraw-Hill; 2010. pp. 818-34.
7. Bianchi DW, Crombleholme TM, D'Alton ME, Malone FD. Twin reversed arterial perfusion sequence. In: Fetology diagnosis and Management of Fetal Patient, 2nd edition. New York: McGraw-Hill; 2010. pp. 835-42.
8. Chasen ST. Twin pregnancy: Management of pregnancy complications. UpToDate. 2021.
9. Dodd JM, Grivell RM, Crowther CA. Multiple pregnancy. In: James D, Steer PJ, Weiner CP, Gonik B (Eds). High-risk Pregnancy Management Options, 4th edition. Missouri: Elsevier; 2011.
10. FIGO Working Group on Good Clinical Practice in Maternal-Fetal Medicine, Good clinical practice advice: Management of twin pregnancy. Int J Gynecol Obstet. 2019;144:330-7.
11. Fox TB. (2006). Multiple Pregnancies: Determining Chorionicity and Amnionicity. Department of Radiologic Sciences Faculty Papers. Paper 1. [online] Available from: https://jdc.jefferson.edu/rsfp/1. [Last accessed April 2022].
12. Kilby MD, Bricker L. Management of monochorionic twin pregnancy. BJOG. 2016;I24:e1-45.
13. Lewi L, Deprest J. Fetal problems in multiple pregnancy. In: James D, Steer PJ, Weiner CP, Gonik B (Eds). High-risk Pregnancy Management Options, 4th edition. Missouri: Elsevier; 2011.
14. Malone FD, D'Alton ME. Multiple gestation: clinical characteristics and management. In: Creasy RK, Resnik R, Iams JD, Lockwood CJ, Moore TR, Greene MF (Eds). Creasy and Resnik's Maternal-Fetal Medicine Principles and Practice, 7th edition. Philadelphia: Elsevier; 2014.
15. National Institute for Health and Care Excellence. Twin and triplet pregnancy. NICE guideline. [online] Available from: www.nice.org.uk/guidance/ng137. [Last accessed April 2022].
16. Sadler TW. Third month to birth: the fetus and placenta. Langman's Medical Embryology, 14th edition. Philadelphia: Wolters Kluwer; 2019. pp. 121-5.
17. Tamblyn J, Moris RK. Multiple pregnancy. In: James D, Steer PJ, Weiner CP, Gonik B, Robson SC (Eds). High-risk Pregnancy Management Options, 5th edition. London: Cambridge University Press; 2017.
18. The Royal Australian and New Zealand College of Obstetricians and Gynaecologists. Management of monochorionic twin pregnancy. [online] Available from: https://obgyn.onlinelibrary.wiley.com/doi/10.1111/1471-0528.14188. [Last accessed April 2022].

CHAPTER 17

Rhesus Alloimmunization

■ INTRODUCTION

Alloimmunization refers to an immune response to foreign antigens, encountered through exposure to the cells or tissue from a genetically different members of the same species. Red cell alloimmunization in pregnancy is the formation of antibodies in the mother to fetal red cell antigens, where the mother is exposed to a mismatch of paternally derived red blood cell (RBC) antigens from the fetus, after a sensitizing event during pregnancy. The maternal generation of antibodies capable of placental transfer, target fetal RBCs containing such antigens for destruction, the effect can range from very mild, with minimal to no fetal effects, to very severe *hemolytic disease* of the fetus and the newborn requiring fetal therapy.

Advances in the prevention and treatment of Rh D-alloimmunization have been one of the great success stories of modern obstetrics. Implementation of programs for antenatal and postnatal *anti-D immune globulin* prophylaxis has led to a significant reduction in the frequency of D alloimmunization and associated fetal/neonatal complications. The postpartum administration of Rh D immune globulin introduced since 1970s has reduced the rate of alloimmunization in at-risk pregnancies from approximately 13–16% to approximately 0.5–1.8%. The risk was further reduced to 0.14–0.2% with the addition of routine antepartum administration of anti-D immunoglobulin. D alloimmunization with serious sequelae in offspring still occurs, particularly in resource-limited countries where anti-D immune globulin is not widely available. Again, despite considerable proof of efficacy, there are still a large number of cases of Rh D-alloimmunization because of failure to follow established protocols. Estimated that approximately 50% of children with untreated hemolytic disease of the newborn (HDN) will die of the disease or develop brain damage; with appropriate monitoring and intervention hemolytic disease of the fetus and newborn (HDFN) can be treated successfully in most cases.

■ EPIDEMIOLOGY

There is wide variation in prevalence rates of Rh D-negative individuals between regions. The frequency of the Rh D-negative phenotype is most common in individuals of European and North American descent (15–17%), comparatively less in the regions of Africa and India (3–8%), and is rarest in Asia (0.1–0.3%). About 15% of white European and 5% of African and Indian ancestral groups lack the D antigen (Rh-negative) on their RBCs, while East Asian women are almost always Rh-positive. In Bangladesh, 3.95% of total population is Rh negative.

High birth rates in low prevalence areas mean Rh HDN is still an important cause of morbidity and mortality in countries without prophylaxis programs. In such countries, 14% of affected fetuses are stillborn and of the survivors, 30% have severe disease almost certainly fatal without treatment, while an additional 30% having moderate disease which would manifest as severe hyperbilirubinemia that untreated may result in brain damage and/or death, 40% of cases would require no treatment.

■ GENETICS

The Rh blood group system consists of over 50 antigens present in about 1 in 80 pregnant women, which cause HDFN in 1 in 300–600 live births. Most common antigens inducing antibodies D, C, c, E, and e. There is no "d" antigen, but C and c and E and e are alternate alleles with codominant expression. Some combination of DCE is inherited as a haplotype from each parent. A pregnant woman who is Rh D-negative can form anti-C, -c, -E, and/or -e antibodies if exposed to fetal red cells with C, c, E, and/or e antigens inherited from the father that the mother does not share. Although an Rh D-negative mother may have received prophylactic anti-D immune globulin, this would not prevent alloimmunization to other Rh antigens (c, C, E, and e).

Approximately 97% of all cases of erythroblastosis fetalis are caused by maternal antibody directed against Rh D antigen present on fetal RBC. A small percentage may be caused by immunization against another rhesus antigen, (mainly C and E) or non-rhesus antigen (notably Kell). Maternal alloimmunization may also be the result of transfusion of Rh-positive blood to Rh-negative woman. Other antibody groups capable of causing HDFN (more commonly neonatal jaundice) include the Fy, Jk, and MNS systems.

Cell-free Fetal DNA Testing for Rhesus and Non-rhesus Red Cell Antigen

Cell-free fetal DNA (cffDNA) testing from maternal blood allows noninvasive identification of fetal RBC antigens, including D, c, C, e, E, and Kell. Rhesus D, c, C, and e are detectable from 16 weeks of gestation and Kell from 20 weeks.

Blood is routinely tested for ABO and rhesus group, but no screening or immune prophylaxis program is available for non-rhesus and other atypical antigens. As a result, a significant number of new immunizations are due to non-D red cell antigen. In the USA, two-third women with positive Kell antibody gives history of previous blood transfusion. This can be prevented by giving Kell negative blood for transfusion in adolescent girls and women of reproductive age.

Three antibodies commonly associated with severe hemolytic disease are anti-D, anti-c, and anti-Kell antibody. In terms of prevalence, the E and C antigens are the most frequent cause of alloimmunization after D and Kell. Anti-c antibodies are equivalent to anti-D antibodies in their need for neonatal exchange transfusion, E antigen has traditionally been regarded as less antigenic than D and cause less severe hemolytic disease of the newborn.

Cell-free fetal DNA testing is available in Europe for the C, c, E, and Kell antigen but not yet available in the USA. Currently, in the UK, routine screening for atypical antibodies are carried out at booking and this is repeated at 28 weeks. Treatment is like Rh D alloimmune women and involves monitoring of maternal antibody titer and fetal assessment of anemia using middle cerebral artery (MCA)-Doppler. With alloimmunization to c, E, and C antigens, assessment with ultrasonography (USG) should be started early because fetal anemia may occur at a lower antibody level than with rhesus-D antibody. Anti-Kell antibody attacks and destroys fetal erythroid precursor cells with low hematocrit and anemia without any accompanying increase in bilirubin breakdown products. However, MCA peak systolic velocity (PSV) can reliably predict fetal anemia in these fetuses.

■ RISK OF DEVELOPMENT OF FETAL RH DISEASE

Risk of development of fetal Rh disease depends on:
- ABO incompatibility
- Husbands genotype and phenotype
- Volume of fetomaternal hemorrhage (FMH)
- Degree of maternal immune response [related to antigenicity of fetal RBCs and type of immunoglobulin G (IgG)]
- The antigen load and frequency of exposure.

ABO Blood Group Status

With an ABO-compatible fetus, the overall risk of alloimmunization if not treated with anti-D Ig is approximately 16%. However, if ABO incompatibility exists, the risk is only 1.5–2%. The protective effect conferred by ABO incompatibility is believed to be due to maternal destruction and subsequent clearance of the ABO-incompatible fetal erythrocytes before Rh sensitization occurs.

Husbands Genotype and Phenotype

Forty percent (40%) of Rh +ve men are homozygous and 60% are heterozygous; in a homozygous father, all babies will be positive; in a heterozygous father, 50% of babies will be positive and 50% negative **(Figs. 1A and B)**.

Volume of Fetomaternal Hemorrhage

As little as 0.1 mL FMH can cause alloimmunization. About 15–50% of births produce sufficient volumes of hemorrhage to cause alloimmunization.

Nonresponders

Less than 20% of Rh D incompatible pregnancies actually lead to maternal alloimmunization depending on the maternal immune response; as many as 30% of Rh D-negative individuals have been demonstrated not to become alloimmunized even when challenged with large volumes of Rh D-positive blood (nonresponders).

Fetal Sex

Fetal sex may play an important role in fetal response. Studies have shown hydrops fetalis was increased 13-fold in Rh +ve male fetus compared to female fetus.

■ PATHOGENESIS OF RH ALLOIMMUNIZATION

Rh D alloimmunization occurs when an Rh D-negative woman is exposed to red cells expressing the Rh D antigen. Although the fetal and maternal circulations are separate, the fetal maternal interface is not an absolute barrier, there is considerable trafficking of many types of cells between mother and fetus throughout gestation. Events such as miscarriage, ectopic pregnancy, antenatal bleeding, and delivery, as well as procedures such as chorionic villus sampling, amniocentesis, pregnancy-related uterine curettage, and surgical treatment of ectopic pregnancy can lead to maternal exposure to fetal RBCs and, consequently, Rh D alloimmunization.

The volume leading to Rh D-alloimmunization can be as small as 0.1 mL or as large as 30 mL.

Response to Antigenic Stimulus (Flowchart 1)

Primary response is a slow response, takes 5–16 weeks after the sensitizing events. The antibody produced—IgM

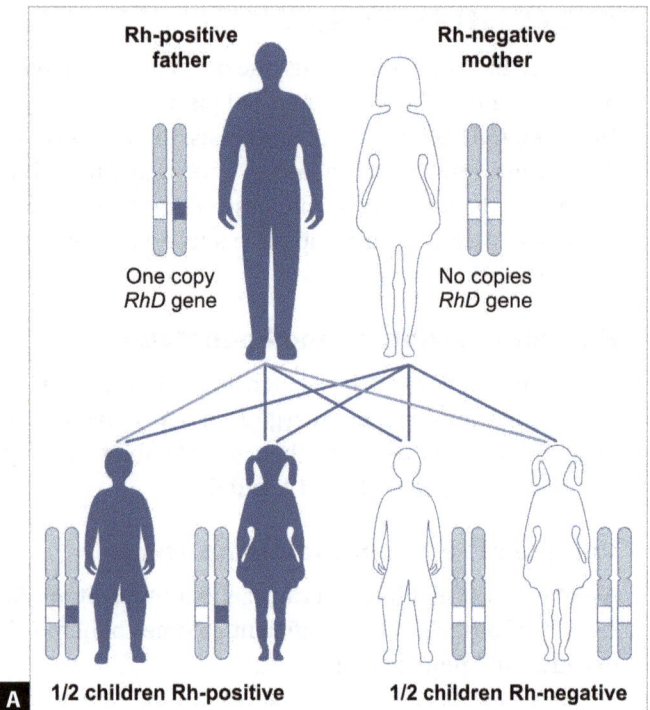
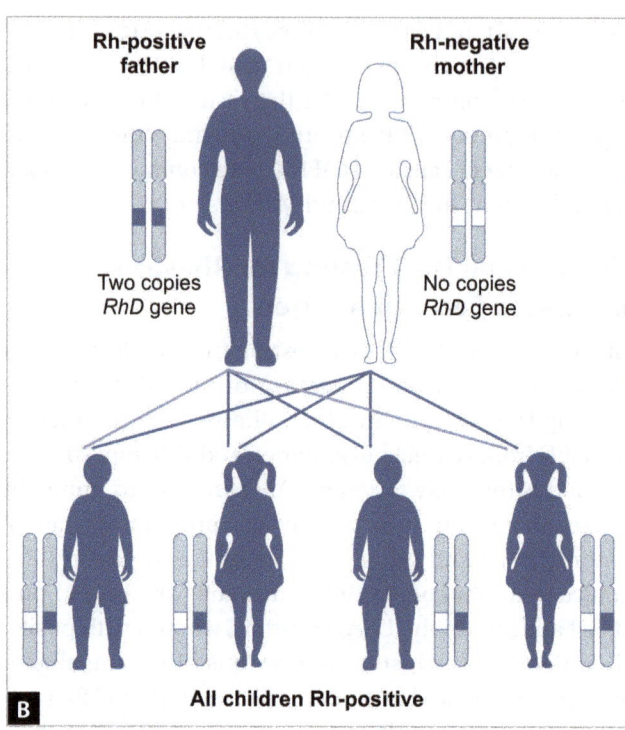

Figs. 1A and B: Genetic basis of Rh-sensitization.
(*Source:* US National Library of Medicine. Modified by Focus IT)

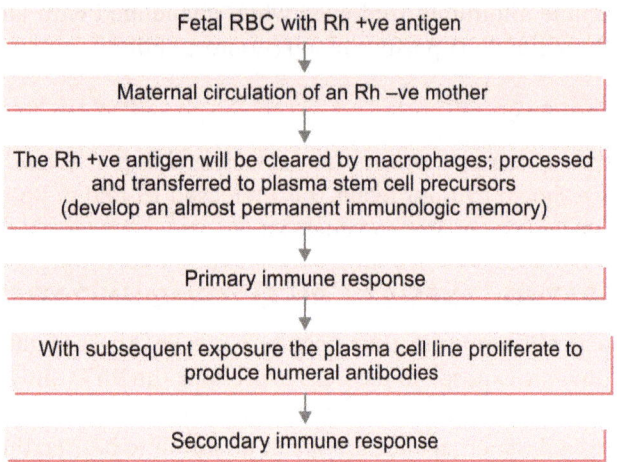

Flowchart 1: The mechanism of development of the Rh immune response.

antibody, having molecular weight 900,000 that does not cross the placenta. Secondary response—a rapid response, IgG antibody is produced, molecular weight 160.000 that can cross the placenta.

After the initial exposure, memory B lymphocytes await the appearance of red cells containing the same antigen in a subsequent pregnancy. Once stimulated by fetal erythrocytes, these B lymphocytes differentiate into plasma cells that can rapidly proliferate and produce IgG antibody which increases maternal antibody titer. Maternal IgG cross the placenta, attach to fetal erythrocytes that have paternal antigen. These cells are then sequestered by the macrophage in the fetal liver and spleen, where they undergo extravascular hemolysis, producing fetal anemia—may lead to fetal heart failure, massive edema (hydrops), and intrauterine fetal demise (IUFD). Extravascular hemolysis may also cause enlargement of the newborn's liver and spleen and varied degree of neonatal hyperbilirubinemia. HDFN may also be associated with thrombocytopenia and neutropenia. The risk increases with increasingly severe anemia and is most common in hydropic fetuses.

Physiological Response of Fetus to Anemia

Enhanced bone marrow production of reticulocytes when fetal hemoglobin (Hb) deficit exceeds 2 g/dL compared to normal, erythroblasts appear in fetal liver at an Hb deficit of 7 g/dL and cardiac output increases. Hydrops fetalis, collection of fluid in at least in two serous compartments, ascites, plural, or pericardial effusion indicating end-stage disease, occurs with Hb deficit of 7 g/dL or more.

Neonatal hyperbilirubinemia results from excessive destruction of RBCs in the absence of placental clearance and inability of immature liver to conjugate bilirubin.

Pregnancies designated as high risk of excessive fetal–maternal hemorrhage, including cases of abruptio placentae, placenta previa, intrauterine manipulation, or fetal death, require additional anti-D immune globulin. It is recommended that all Rh D-negative women giving birth to Rh D-positive infants undergo additional testing initially with a qualitative screening test (such as the rosette assay) and, if indicated, quantitative testing (such as the Kleihauer–Betke test) to determine the number of doses of Rh D immune globulin required to prevent alloimmunization.

DIAGNOSIS OF MATERNAL ALLOIMMUNIZATION

Antibody Titer in Saline

Rh-positive cells suspended in saline solutions are agglutinated by IgM anti-D antibody but not by IgG anti-D antibody. This test measures IgM or recent antibody production.

Antibody Titer in Albumin

Antibody titer in albumin reflects the presence of any antibody IgG or IgM in maternal sera.

Indirect Coombs' Test

- *First step:* Known Rh-positive RBCs are suspended with maternal serum, anti-D antibody present in maternal sera will adhere to the RBCs.
- *Second step:* The RBCs are then washed and suspended with antihuman globulin Coombs' serum. Red cell coated with maternal anti-Rh-D will be agglutinated by the Coombs serum.

Direct Coombs' Test

Direct Coombs' test performed on the neonate's RBCs to detect the presence of maternal antibody on the RBC. Fetal RBC is put in Coombs' serum; if the cells are agglutinated, it indicates maternal antibody is present.

DETECTION AND ESTIMATION OF FETAL BLOOD IN MATERNAL CIRCULATION

Rosette Screening Test (Figs. 2A to C)

Is a sensitive, qualitative test, can detect up to 10 mL of fetal blood in the maternal circulation. Incubate a maternal 3–5% red cell suspension with IgG anti-D at 37°C. The anti-D will bind to any fetal D+ cells that are present. After washing to remove unbound anti-D, add indicator red cells. Indicator cells are ficin-treated R_2R_2 cells that will bind to the antibody-coated fetal RBCs causing agglutination ("rosettes") that can be detected by light microscopy. A specified number of agglutinates (e.g., 3 or more in 10 fields *or* 7 or more in 5 fields) is designated a positive and suggests a significant FMH (>30 mL) requiring more Rh Ig. A positive rosette test should be followed with a method to determine the percentage of fetal RBCs in maternal circulation, such as the Kleihauer–Betke test or flow cytometry.

Kleihauer–Betke Test (Fig. 3)

The Kleihauer–Betke test is employed to quantify the volume of hemorrhage so that appropriate dose of anti-D Ig can be administered. The Kleihauer–Betke acid elution test relies on the principle that fetal RBCs contain mostly fetal HbF, which is resistant to acid elution, whereas adult Hb is acid sensitive. Up to 0.3% of women have a FMH >15 mL, which will not be adequately covered by 1,500 IU (300 µg) of anti-D antibody, needs Kleihauer test to quantify FMH.

Procedure

Maternal blood is fixed on a slide with ethanol 80%. Citrate phosphate buffer is added to remove adult Hb. Stained with hematoxylin–eosin, the fetal RBCs are left rose-pink in color,

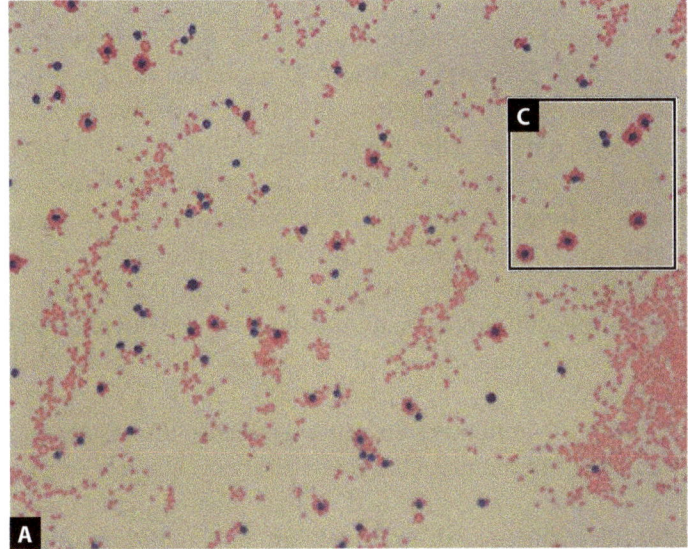
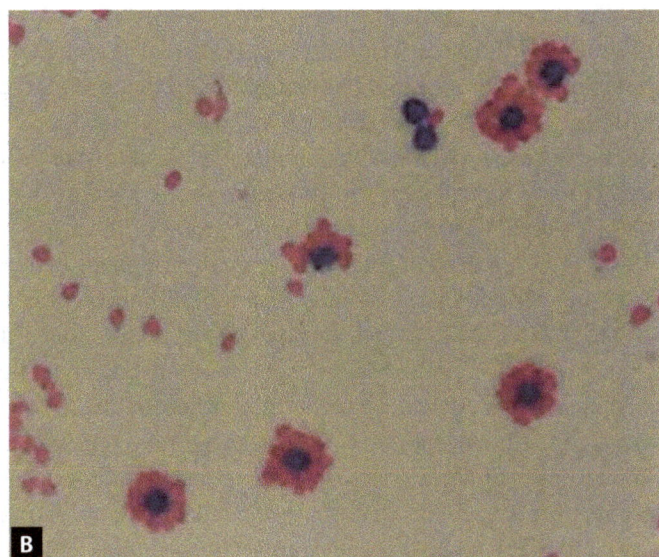

Figs. 2A to C: Rosette screening test.

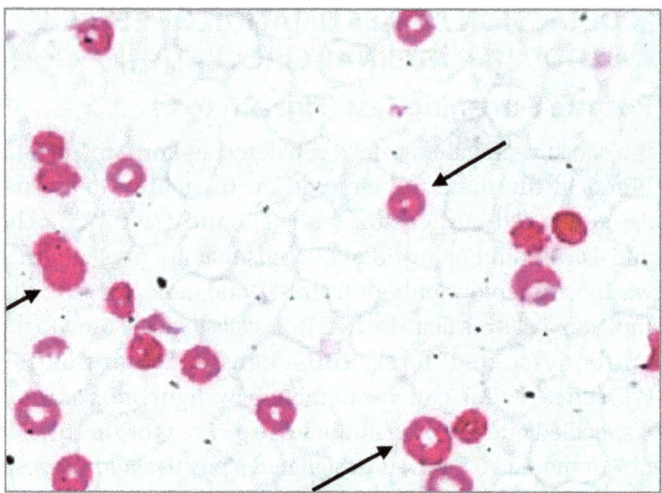

Fig. 3: Kleihauer–Betke test.

and the maternal cells appear "ghost-like" due to the absence of staining.

Fetal cells are counted by the formula:

$$\frac{\text{Fetal volume}}{\text{Maternal blood volume}} = \frac{\text{Number of fetal cells counted}}{\text{Number of maternal cells counted}}$$

Flow Cytometry (Fig. 4)

Flow cytometry is a specialized technique that is an alternative method available in some hospitals for quantification of fetal–maternal hemorrhage, although its use is limited by equipment and staffing costs. It uses monoclonal antibodies to HbF or the Rh D antigen with quantification of fluorescence, and is highly sensitive and accurate in identifying fetal red cells in maternal blood although its use is limited.

■ PREVENTION OF RH ALLOIMMUNIZARTION

At the booking appointment, the woman should be offered ABO and Rh blood typing. If patient is negative, husband's ABO and Rh blood typing should be done. If the husband is negative, no extra care is needed.

If the husband is positive, Rh genotyping of husband. If husband heterozygous, the rhesus-negative woman can be offered cffDNA test to know blood group of the fetus at 15–16 weeks' gestation (blood must not be obtained before 12 completed weeks' gestation, as the result will be inaccurate). If cell-free DNA (cfDNA) results on maternal plasma, suggest that the fetus is male and D-negative, then prophylactic antenatal anti-D immune globulin can be omitted [*Royal College of Obstetricians and Gynaecologists (RCOG) guideline*]. However, if the fetus is female and D-negative on cfDNA testing, the possibility that the result reflects the maternal rather than the fetal *RhD* gene cannot be excluded without incorporating single nucleotide polymorphisms (SNPs) to verify the presence of fetal DNA in the maternal sample [American College of Obstetricians and Gynecologists (ACOG)].

Benefits of Cell Free DNA Testing

Because of limited availability of anti-D and rare but harmful effects such as virus transmission, is a reason for introduction of noninvasive RhD screening. Additionally exposing approximately 40% of women (who do not carry RhD-positive fetuses) to a blood product they do not need has been described as ethically unacceptable when a fetal RhD genotyping test exists.

American College of Obstetricians and Gynecologists does not recommend the use of cffDNA for fetal *RhD* testing. In several other countries (e.g., Denmark, Netherlands, Sweden, England, France, and Finland), fetal *RhD* determination is performed routinely and administration of antenatal anti-D immune globulin is avoided when an *RhD*-negative fetus is identified.

A meta-analysis of 30 studies of cfDNA for *RhD* determination (n = 10,290 tests) found sensitivity of 99.3% [95% confidence interval (CI) 98.2–99.7] and specificity was 98.4% (95% CI 96.4–99.3) for pregnancies tested in the first (after 11 weeks) and second trimesters; sensitivity with real-time quantitative polymerase chain reaction (PCR) was higher than with conventional PCR. If antepartum prophylaxis is based on cfDNA results, it has been estimated that 1:86,000 D-negative women would have a future pregnancy affected by HDFN that could have been prevented by universal antepartum prophylaxis.

Antibody Screening

Antibody screening should be done in all Rh -ve women at booking visit including who have received anti-D immunoglobulin in previous pregnancy as administration of anti-D immunoglobulin does not guarantee 100% prevention. If anti-D antibody is identified, further history should be obtained and investigation undertaken to determine whether this is immune mediated or passive (as a result of previous injection of anti-D immune globulin). If it is clear that the origin of the anti-D antibodies detected is a previous routine antenatal anti-D immune globulin prophylaxis or anti-D immune globulin given for a potentially sensitizing event, then the woman should continue to be offered anti-D prophylaxis.

If Rh D-antibodies are present because of sensitization, anti-D immune globulin is not effective, will not prevent a rise in maternal titer, and management should proceed in accordance with protocols for Rh D-alloimmunized pregnancies. Ab screening should be done specially for

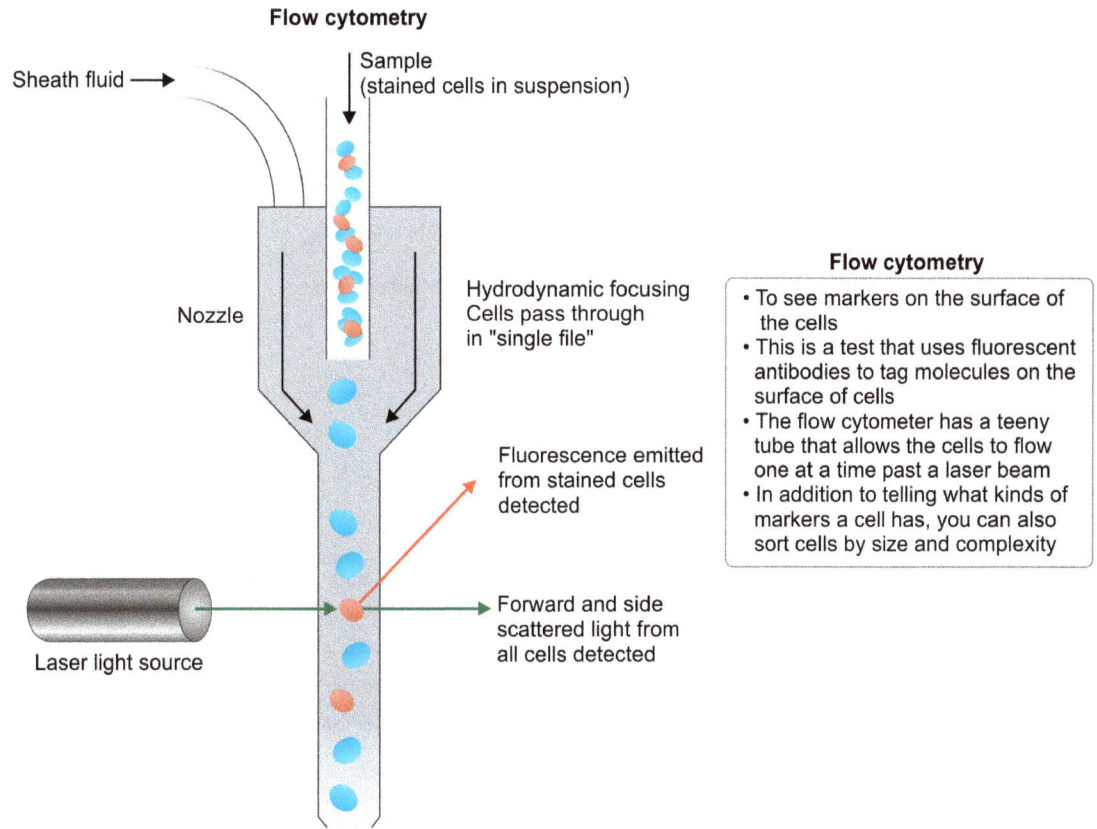

Fig. 4: Flow cytometry.

women who had history of blood transfusion, unexplained fetal death, or jaundice.

Antenatal Anti-D Prophylaxis

Exogenous administration of a dose of anti-D Ig is sufficient to suppress an antibody-mediated immune suppression (AMIS). The ideal time to administer anti-D immune globulin is within 72 hours of a potentially sensitizing event but it has been suggested that a patient may still receive some benefit from anti-D immune globulin as late as 28 days' postpartum.

Mechanism of AMIS: The most likely mechanism is rapid macrophage-mediated clearance of anti-D-coated red cells and/or downregulation of antigen-specific B cells before an immune response occurs, thereby suppressing the primary immune response. Additionally, these antigen-antibody complexes stimulate the release of cytokines by immune effector cells that inhibit the proliferation of antigen-specific B cells. Routine antenatal anti-D prophylaxis (RAADP) to all Rh D-negative pregnant women can reduce the Rh D immunization to 0.2–0.4%.

Current practice in USA is administration of a single dose of 300 µg of anti-D immunoglobulin at 28 weeks followed by a second dose after birth if newborn's Rh D typing is positive. In the UK, recommendations using different doses given as two injections at 28 weeks and at 34 weeks, or as a single administration at 28 weeks.

In the past, some authorities advised giving a second dose of Rh D immune globulin in women who have not given birth 12 weeks after receiving their antenatal dose. However, the vast majority of women who give birth >12 weeks after receiving antenatal Rh D immune globulin do not become alloimmunized. Most guidelines do not recommend a second dose of anti-D immune globulin until after delivery when newborn Rh D typing becomes available.

Prophylaxis after Pregnancy Complications

Prophylactic anti-D immune globulin should be given to any D-negative nonalloimmunized pregnant woman who has an event potentially associated with placental trauma or disruption of the fetomaternal interface and whose fetus is or may be D-positive. These include the following mentioned in **Flowchart 2**.

Threatened abortion: The D antigen is detectable on embryonic red cells by 38 days after conception (i.e., 7 + 3 weeks of gestation); fetal–maternal hemorrhage, although rare, has been documented in 3–11% of women with threatened abortion between 7 and 13 weeks of gestation. Several national guidelines (including RCOG) recommend against giving anti-D immune globulin to women with threatened abortion, with a viable fetus, particularly if

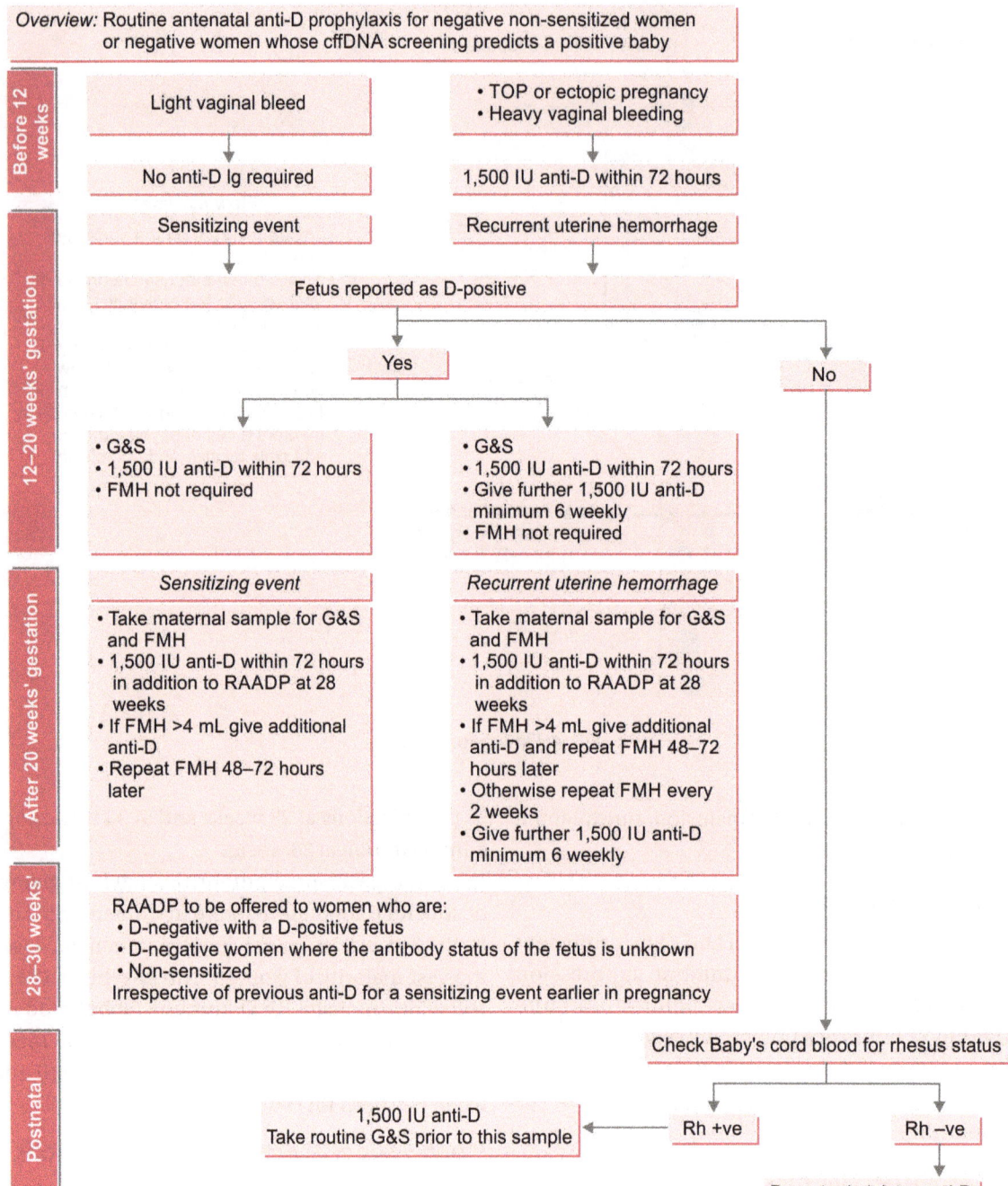

Flowchart 2: Algorithm of anti-D prophylaxis.

(cffDNA: cell-free fetal DNA; FMH: fetomaternal hemorrhage; G&S: group & screen; RAADP: routine antenatal anti-D prophylaxis)

bleeding stops before 12 weeks of gestation. The mean red cell volume at 8 and 12 weeks is 0.33 and 1.5 mL, respectively. Because of the theoretic risk of alloimmunization, anti-D immune globulin at a dose of 50 µg can be used for first-trimester events which protect against a fetomaternal bleed of 2.5 mL red cells; however, there is no harm in giving the standard 300 µg (1,500 IU) dose, which is more readily available. An incidental finding of a subchorionic hematoma on ultrasound examination is not an indication for antepartum prophylaxis in the absence of vaginal bleeding.

Spontaneous or induced abortion: At 12 weeks of gestation, the total fetal-placental blood volume is 3 mL or 1.5 mL of fetal red cells. This volume is adequate to sensitize some patients, and the risk of Rh D alloimmunization is estimated to be 1.5–2% in susceptible women after spontaneous miscarriage and 4–5% after dilation and curettage. Some groups do not recommend prophylactic anti-D immune globulin after a complete spontaneous miscarriage before 12 weeks of gestation if the uterus is not instrumented, but do recommend prophylaxis (300 μg) when curettage is performed because the procedure increases the chances of fetomaternal bleeding (*ACOG*).

Ectopic pregnancy: Alloimmunization has been reported to occur in 24% of women with a ruptured tubal pregnancy. It may be transplacental or may result from absorption of fetal blood by the maternal peritoneum.

Hydatidiform mole: A complete mole does not contain fetal red cells, but prophylaxis after evacuation is suggested because fetal red cells are present in partial molar pregnancies.

Invasive prenatal diagnostic or therapeutic procedures: Chorionic villus sampling, amniocentesis/amnioinfusion, fetal blood sampling, fetoscopy/fetoscopic surgery, and multifetal reduction are associated with fetomaternal bleeding. Chorionic villus sampling has been estimated to carry a 14% risk of fetal–maternal hemorrhage of 0.6 mL or more. Traditionally, rate of fetal–maternal hemorrhage after amniocentesis was thought to be 2–6% even if the placenta was not traversed. Recent studies suggest the rate of fetal–maternal hemorrhage may be lower than previously thought but not negligible and alloimmunization is possible. Similarly, other invasive procedures such as cordocentesis also can cause fetal–maternal hemorrhage and warrant anti-D immune globulin prophylaxis. Administration of Rh D immune globulin is recommended with all invasive diagnostic procedures, when the fetuses could be Rh D positive. Doses from 50 to 120 μg have been recommended before 12 weeks of gestational age. For chorionic villus sampling and amniocentesis performed after 12 weeks of gestation, 125 or 300 μg is recommended.

Blunt abdominal trauma and external cephalic version: Blunt abdominal trauma (e.g., fall, intimate partner violence, and motor vehicle crash) or external cephalic version may result in fetomaternal bleeding, possibly related to clinical or subclinical placental abruption. Although not invasive, external cephalic version (regardless of success) is associated with a 2–6% risk of fetal–maternal hemorrhage and anti-D immune globulin is indicated for unsensitized Rh D-negative patients.

Recurrent bleeding, monitoring, and repeat dosing: As the half-life of anti-D immune globulin is approximately 3 weeks, *ACOG recommends* to monitor the maternal antibody titer every 3 weeks in women with recurrent antepartum bleeding who have received prophylaxis. If the result is positive, indicating that anti-D immune globulin from the previous dose of prophylaxis is still present, no additional treatment is necessary. If the result is negative, then the woman may not be protected. In these cases, a test to evaluate the volume of fetal RBCs in the maternal circulation is obtained by Klehaur test and a repeat dose 300 μg of anti-D immune globulin is administered, with additional dosing as indicated by the results of testing for fetomaternal bleeding.

Royal College of Obstetricians and Gynaecologists recommendation on recurrent bleeding: Between 12 and 20 weeks' gestation 1,500 IU anti-D Ig at a minimum of 6 weekly intervals in recurrent bleeding. At and after 20 weeks' gestation, a 1,500 IU anti-D Ig should be given at 6 weekly intervals. FMH should be estimated when anti-D is first given and thereafter every 2 weeks. If positive, additional anti-D Ig should be given to cover the volume of fetal red cells, FMH should be retested after 48–72 hours. At or after 28 weeks, gestation, for any potentially sensitizing event 1,500 IU anti-D Ig should be given within 72 hours of the event even if the woman has received RAADP at 28 weeks. FMH should be retested after 48–72 hours. Thereafter, for recurrent bleeding, 1,500 IU anti-D Ig should be given at 6 weeks intervals, FMH should be estimated every 2 weeks. Additional anti-D will be necessary if the volume of FMH exceeds that covered by the standard anti-D dose.

Additional Anti-D Dose Calculation

A dose of 1,500 IU IM is sufficient to treat a FMH of up to 15 mL fetal red cells, give additional doses of anti-D Ig using the following dose calculations: Rhophylac: 100 iu anti-D per 1 mL fetal red cells administered IM or IV.

Fetal death in the second or third trimester: Fetal death occurs in fetal–maternal hemorrhage in up to 13% of cases in which no obvious other cause is found (e.g., hypertensive disease and fetal anomalies). Fetal demise can be an immunizing event when caused by massive FMH or occult abruption. Therefore, anti-D immune globulin should be administered to Rh D-negative women who experience fetal death in the second or third trimester after calculation of FMH.

Women undergoing postpartum sterilization procedures: Whether anti-D immune globulin should be administered to women undergoing a postpartum sterilization procedure is controversial. Some of these women will subsequently become pregnant as a result of a failed procedure, reanastomosis of the fallopian tubes, or in vitro fertilization. Even if the patient does not become pregnant, if alloimmunization occurs, it will limit the availability of compatible red cell units if she requires an emergency blood transfusion later in life.

Prophylaxis after delivery: Following delivery, a cord sample should be taken to test the ABO and D group of the baby for all Rh D-negative women, even those who have been previously screened for cffDNA, as there is a 0.1% chance that the predicted blood group is incorrect.

An appropriate dose of anti-D immune globulin should be administered to nonalloimmunized D-negative women within 72 hours of delivery of a D-positive newborn. If the pregnancy is nonviable and no sample obtained from the baby, prophylactic anti-D Ig should be administered to D-negative nonsensitized women. The 300 µg dose of anti-D immune globulin is adequate to protect against maternal alloimmunization from as much as 15 mL fetal red cells (30 mL D-positive fetal whole blood), given before 72 hours. The longer prophylaxis is delayed, the less it will be protective, but it has been suggested that a patient may still receive some benefit given as late as 10 days postpartum.

Screening for FMH: The incidence of fetomaternal bleeding >20–30 mL at delivery is estimated to be approximately 1 in 200–300 deliveries, bleeding >80 mL and >150 mL occurs in 1 in 1,000 deliveries and 1 in 5,000 deliveries, respectively (e.g., cesarean delivery). For this reason, Rh D-negative women who give birth to Rh D-positive infants should undergo additional testing to assess the volume of fetal–maternal hemorrhage and guide the amount of Rh D immune globulin required to prevent alloimmunization. It is advised that all women undergo such screening after delivery because a policy of only screening with high-risk conditions for excess fetal–maternal hemorrhage, such as abruptio placentae or manual removal of the placenta, will fail to identify a large number of cases requiring more than the standard postpartum dose of Rh D immune globulin.

The rosette test is a qualitative, yet sensitive test for fetomaternal bleeding, performing this test as an initial screen. The test is designed to give a negative result when the amount of fetomaternal bleeding is small (<2 mL or 0.04% fetal cells). A standard dose of anti-D immune globulin is given to patients with a negative test. When the rosette test is positive, a Kleihauer–Betke test or flow cytometry is recommended to determine the percentage of fetal RBCs in the maternal blood to determine the dose of anti D.

Note: Maternal samples for FMH should be collected within 2 hours but no earlier than 30 minutes postdelivery to allow any FMH to be dispersed in the maternal circulation.

Calculation of Dose of Anti-D

The percentage of fetal RBCs is multiplied by 50 to estimate the volume of the fetomaternal bleeding (50 is the factor used to represent the average maternal blood volume of 5 liters). This is then divided by 30 (the amount of fetomaternal bleeding covered by one vial of 300 µg of anti-D immune globulin) to determine the number of vials of anti-D immune globulin that should be administered.

For example, a patient with a Kleihauer–Betke result of 1.5% fetal cells would be assumed to have had 85 mL FMH. The 85 mL total FMH volume is divided by 30 mL (the amount of fetomaternal bleeding covered by one vial of 300 µg of anti-D immune globulin) yielding a need for 2.8 vials of anti-D immune globulin. The 2.8 vial is rounded up to 3 vials and then an extra vial is added; thus, the recommended dose in this case would be a total of 4 vials (1,200 µg).

No more than five 300 µg doses should be administered intramuscularly in a 24-hour period. However, large doses, if indicated, can be given using an intravenous preparation (WinRho SDF, Rhophylac). In these cases, no more than 600 µg should be given every 8 hours intravenously until the total calculated dose is achieved *(ACOG)*.

RCOG recommendation on postnatal anti-D: The minimum dose to be administered should be calculated as 100 IU for each additional milliliter of fetal cells.

Note: Anti-D injection to be given in deltoid muscle, if given to gluteal region, it often reaches the subcutaneous tissue and absorption may be delayed.

Positive titer at delivery: Routine administration of antepartum and postpartum anti-D immune globulin has reduced the prevalence of D alloimmunization to 0.1–0.3% of D-negative pregnant women. Some women who receive anti-D immune globulin at 28 weeks will still have a low antibody titer at term (≤4). Anti-D immune globulin should be given to these women if they deliver a D-positive infant unless alloimmunization is proven as indicated by an anti-D titer >1:4.

FAILURE TO PREVENT RH D-ALLOIMMUNIZATION

In spite of recommendations for immunoprophylaxis, approximately 0.1–0.4% of women at risk become sensitized during pregnancy. This might be because of a failure of administering antenatal prophylaxis in the third trimester of pregnancy, insufficient dosage or failure of timely administration (within 72 hours) of anti-D immune globulin after a known sensitizing event during pregnancy (or after birth), or an unrecognized fetal–maternal hemorrhage at some point in the pregnancy.

A recent retrospective study from New Zealand identified reasons for continued cases of sensitization–omission of immune globulin after a recognized sensitizing event in 41% of cases and administration outside of recommended guidelines in 13% of cases. An additional reason for Rh D alloimmunization is the small rate (0.1–0.2%) of spontaneous immunization despite adherence to the recommended prophylaxis protocol, in other words, prophylaxis is not 100% effective.

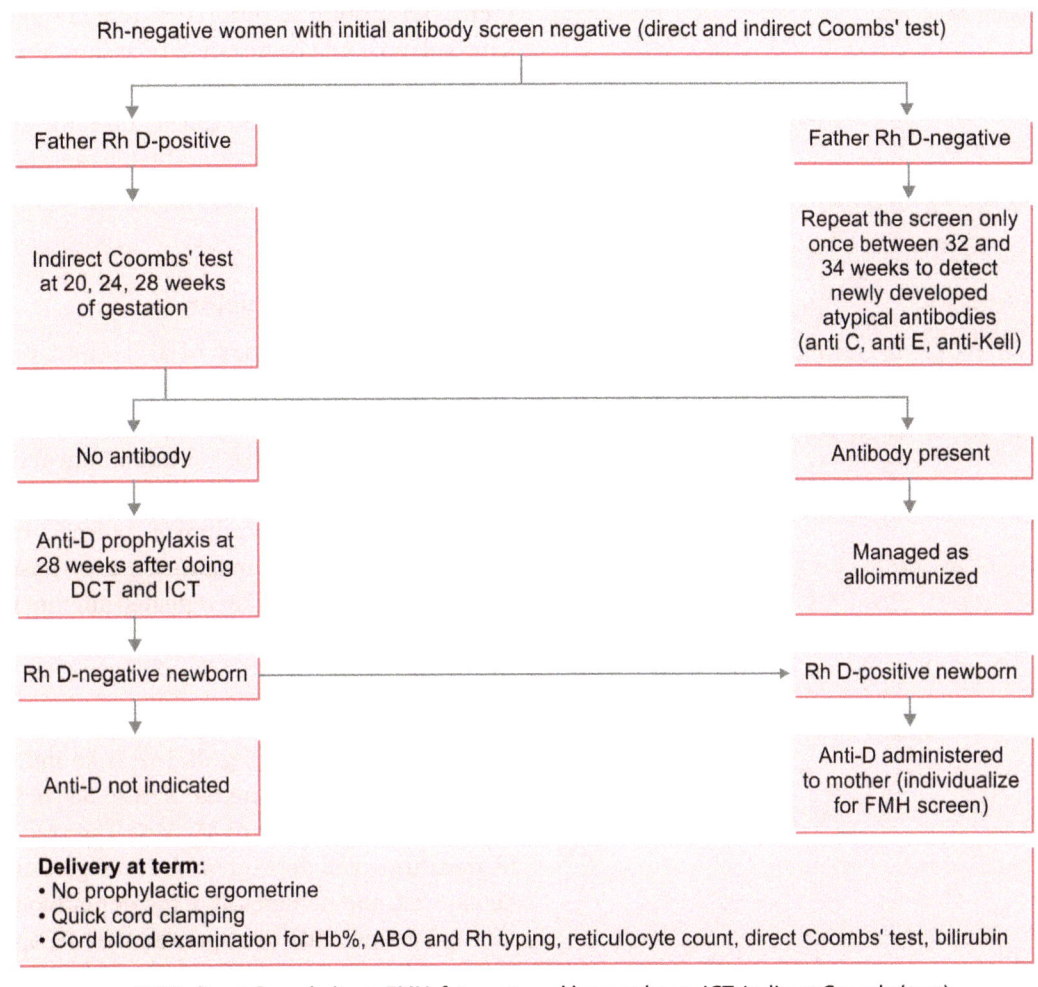

Flowchart 3: Management of Rh-negative non-immunized pregnancy.

(DCT: direct Coombs' test; FMH: fetomaternal hemorrhage; ICT: indirect Coombs' test)

Management of Rh-negative Pregnancy

Rh-negative women can be categorized in two groups:
1. Rh-negative nonimmunized women **(Flowchart 3)**
2. Rh-negative immunized women.

Rh-negative Nonimmunized Women

All women should have their antibody status determined (indirect and direct Coombs' test) at their first antenatal visit (RCOG, 2014). Management is shown in **Flowchart 3**.

Management of Rh-negative Immunized Pregnancy

Maternal antibody titer is most useful in assessing the risk of fetal anemia during a first affected pregnancy. The correlation between antibody titer and transfer of fetal cells into maternal circulation that exists in first affected pregnancy is lost in subsequent pregnancy.

First step of management is determination of paternal zygosity, if father is heterozygous, fetus has 50% chance of being Rh negative, cffDNA should be used to determine fetal RHD status. In case of other red cell antigens, amniocentesis can be carried out after 15 weeks or cffDNA test (if available).

In a first affected pregnancy, fetal effects of alloimmunization tend to be less severe, but worsen with every subsequent pregnancy. Ab screening done at first prenatal visit, once an antibody reported to cause HDFN has been detected, a titer should be obtained to see if it is below a critical value. A critical titer is defined as the titer associated with significant risk for fetal hydrops (32 for anti-D Ab, and most other antibodies, 8 for anti-Kell). If titer below critical value, repeat titer monthly till 24 weeks and 2 weekly thereafter.

Serial amniocentesis for estimation of bilirubin in amniotic fluid: Serial amniocentesis every 1–2 weeks, initiated as early as 16 weeks. Spectrophotometry analysis of bilirubin in amniotic fluid is done and optical density of the fluid at wavelength 450 nm is plotted in Liley's chart/Queenan curve. The deviation bulge obtained is directly proportion to the severity **(Figs. 5 and 6)**.

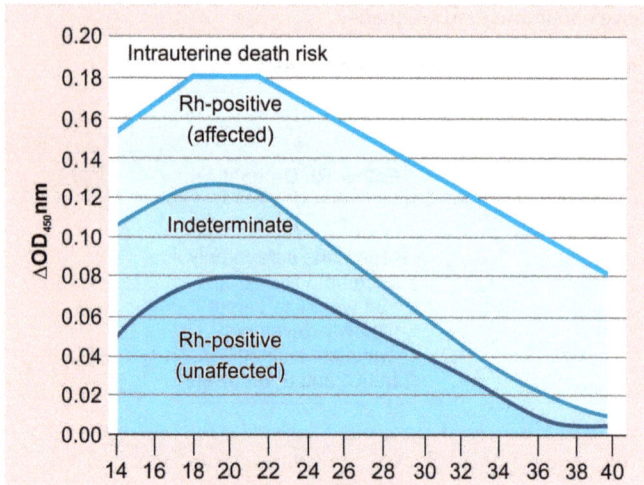

Fig. 5: Queenan curve.

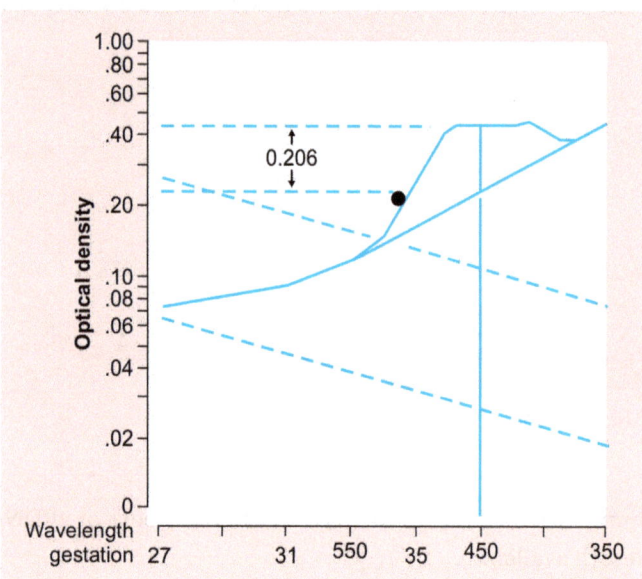

Fig. 6: Liley's chart.

Doppler of MCA: Performed serially every 1–2 weeks starting at 24 weeks. If titer has increased, but MCA-PSV is <1.5 multiples of median (MoM), patient is still managed with weekly MCA-PSV measurement. Antenatal testing of nonstress test (NST) or biophysical profile (BPP) should be initiated at 32 weeks. Cases where MCA-PSV has reached 1.5 MoM level, MCA-PSV is repeated after 1 week and if it remains at this level or rises, is an indication for cordocentesis for determination of fetal hematocrit, direct Coombs' test, Hb, and need for intrauterine transfusion (IUT). Using cut-off of 1.5 MoM, fetuses with moderate-to-severe anemia are identified with a positive predictive value of 65%, negative predictive value of 100%, and false positive rate of 12%. Hydrops is normally not observed until an HbF deficit of at least 7 g/dL below the mean for gestational age.

Other USG features of severe anemia are cardiomegaly, increased umbilical vein (UV) diameter, enlargement of liver, spleen, and visualization of ascites. Prospective study found MCA Doppler velocity is superior to measurement of optical density at 450 nm using both Liley curve and Queenan curve in detection of fetal anemia. The accuracy of MCA Doppler 85% compared to 76% for Liley curve and 81% for Queenan curve.

Intrauterine Transfusion

- There are two types of IUT—intraperitoneal and intravascular.
- Until direct intravascular transfusion (IVT) was introduced in mid-1980, intraperitoneal transfusion was the method of IUT for >20 years.
- Direct IVT is the procedure of choice nowadays.
- In difficult situation, maternal obesity, posterior placenta, failure to get blood after repeated attempt intraperitoneal transfusion (IPT) given.

Direct Intravascular Transfusion

A hematocrit of <30% (8 g/dL Hb) is an indication for IUT. The aim is to increase hematocrit to 35–40% in early mid-trimester and after that to 45–55%. The volume of blood to be transfused will depend on the fetal gestation, initial fetal hematocrit, and hematocrit of the donor blood. If the donor unit has hematocrit of approximately 75%, the estimated fetal weight in gram using USG is multiplied by a factor of 0.02 to determine the volume of red cell to be transfused to achieve a hematocrit increase of 10%. It may also be calculated by using the formula:

Volume of blood to be transfused

$$= \frac{\text{Desired hematocrit} - \text{Fetal hematocrit}}{\text{Donor hematocrit} - \text{Desired hematocrit}} \times \text{Fetoplacental blood volume}$$

Procedure

Maternal sedation: If mother is apprehensive, she can be given sedative such as tablet lorazepam, 2 mg 1 hour before the procedure. Under continuous high-resolution ultrasound guidance, procedure is performed using free-hand technique. Three trained persons are required—one to perform the procedure, second person for withdrawing and pushing the blood, and third person getting the fetal hematocrit and for the estimation of blood to be transfused.

Site of puncture: When the placenta is anterior, 22 G spinal needle is traversed through placenta and needle is guided in the umbilical vein near its insertion. Once the needle tip is seen in the umbilical vein, 1 mL of blood is withdrawn.

Blood is immediately checked for fetal blood group, Rh status, Hb, and hematocrit by using automatic analyzer. Preliminary calculation for amount of blood transfusion is kept ready on a paper and as soon as fetal hematocrit value is available, third person can quickly do the final calculation. The needle is attached to three-way connector which, in turn, is connected to the donor blood bag. Blood is slowly pushed at a rate of 10 mL/min. Once the total desired amount is transfused, 1 mL blood is collected for checking post-transfusion hematocrit.

In the extremely anemic fetus, do not increase the initial hematocrit to by more than fourfold to allow fetal cardiovascular system to compensate for the acute change in viscosity. A repeat procedure can be done after 48 hours to normalize fetal hematocrit. Subsequent transfusion is given at an interval of 2–3 weeks. Hydrops typically reverses after 1–2 transfusion, placentomegaly is the last feature to reverse. Cordocentesis requires a degree of expertise, and has the potential for serious complication including bleeding, FMH, fetal loss (1–2% after 24 weeks, may be as high as 5% before this), placental abruption, thrombosis of the vessel, fetal distress, and amnionitis. After the procedure, cardiotocography (CTG) tracings are taken and monitored for at least half an hour for any fetal heart decelerations.

Intraperitoneal transfusion: If the placenta is posterior, approach to placenta may be difficult, in such case, there is an option of using a free loop of umbilical cord, hepatic vein, or to perform IPT. Formula for calculating IPT vol—subtracting 20 from gestational age in weeks and multiply by 10. Blood in the peritoneal cavity is expected to be absorbed in 7–10 days.

Note: In all cases, the donor cell should be rigorously tested for infection, CMV -ve, packed to final hematocrit 75–85%, leukocyte reduced by using special micropore and irradiated by 25 Gy to prevent graft versus host reaction.

Timing of Delivery

Most experienced center perform IUT till 35 weeks with delivery at 37–38 weeks, administration of oral phenobarbitone to mother for 7–10 days helps in fetal hepatic maturity to allow improved conjugation of bilirubin. If delivery occurs before 36 weeks, steroids are given to ensure lung maturity and deliver 24 hours after second dose of betamethasone.

Things to follow during delivery:
- No prophylactic ergometrine
- Quick cord clamping
- Cord blood examination for Hb%, ABO and Rh typing, reticulocyte count, direct Coombs test, and bilirubin
- Rh -ve blood (0 -ve) should be kept ready before delivery of alloimmunized pregnancies for neonatal exchanged transfusion.

Management of Previously Affected Fetus (Flowchart 4)

If the patient has a history of previous perinatal loss due to HDFN, a previous need for IUT, or previous need for neonatal exchange transfusion, fetus is more likely to develop severe anemia at an earlier gestation. Assessment of fetal anemia should be carried out 10 weeks prior to gestational age at which the previous pregnancy was affected. Patient should be referred to perinatal center with experience in managing severe alloimmunized pregnancies. Maternal titer should not be used for deciding when to initiate fetal surveillance. In case of antigen positive fetus detected by cffDNA or amniocentesis, serial MCA Doppler is initiated as early as 16 weeks. Detection of an extremely elevated titer at the start of pregnancy may warrant consideration for immunomodulation.

History of Severely Anemic Early Second Trimester Fetus in a Previous Pregnancy—Plasmapheresis: A Newer Option

This costly procedure is indicated only when there is an H/O hydrops prior to 20–22 weeks and father is homozygous. It reduces antibody concentration by 80% but decline is transient, can delay the need for fetal transfusion by several weeks. Potential adverse effects relate to maternal morbidity (e.g., infection, hematoma formation) and altered maternal and fetal hemodynamics, as well as the loss of systemically important proteins.

Single volume of plasmapheresis done every other day for three procedures in the 12th week of gestation with 5% albumin used for volume replacement. The patients IG pool replaced after third procedure by administering 1 g/kg of intravenous immunoglobulin (IVIg) diluted in normal saline, a second dose given on the following day and then weekly 1 g/kg till 20 weeks and then IUT. IVIgs given at high doses may block the transport of alloantibodies across the placenta by competitive inhibition, can reduce maternal alloantibody production, and delay clinically significant anemia until IUT is more feasible.

Immunomodulatory therapies, e.g., azathioprine, promethazine, and prednisolone, may prevent alloimmunization in high-risk women prior to RBC antigen exposure but current evidence is limited to case series. A second approach is biweekly IPT starting early in the second trimester (15 weeks), a volume of 5 mL is used up to 18 weeks and thereafter 10 mL vol is used.

Rhesus Alloimmunization

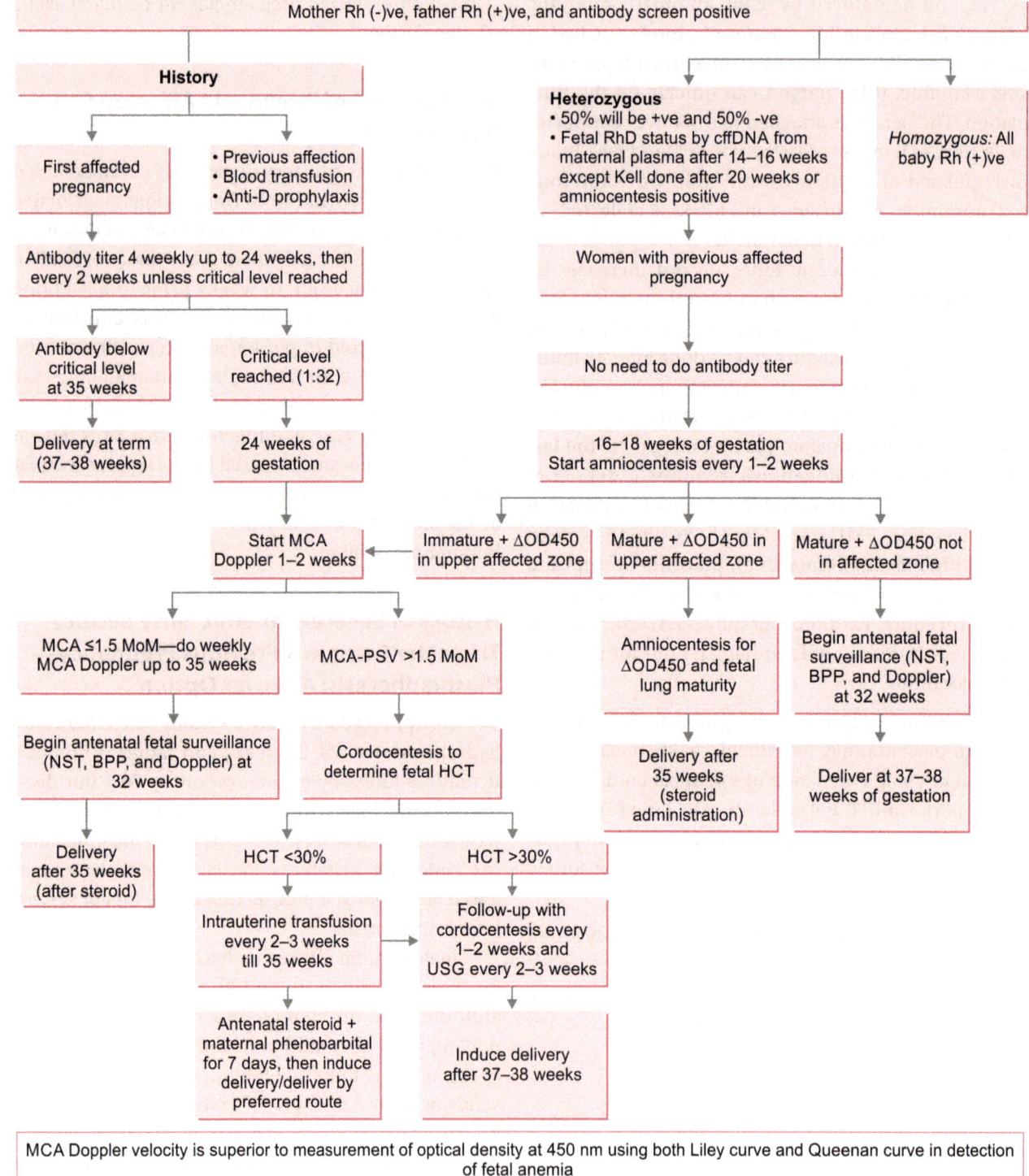

Flowchart 4: Management of Rh-negative immunized pregnancy.

MCA Doppler velocity is superior to measurement of optical density at 450 nm using both Liley curve and Queenan curve in detection of fetal anemia

(BPP: biophysical profile; cffDNA: cell-free fetal DNA; HCT: hematocrit; MCA-PSV: middle cerebral artery-peak systolic velocity; MoM: multiples of median; NST: nonstress test)

SUGGESTED READING

1. ABO and Rh blood type distribution by country (population averages). [online] Available from: https://rhesusnegative.net/themission/bloodtypefrequencies. [Last accessed April 2022].
2. ACOG Practice Bulletin No. 181: Prevention of Rh D alloimmunization. Obstetr Gynecol. 2017;130(2):e57-70.
3. Agarwal K. Treatment and prevention of Rh isoimmunization. J Fetal Med. 2014;1:81-8.
4. American College of Obstetricians and Gynecologists. ACOG practice bulletin no. 75: management of alloimmunization during pregnancy. Obstet Gynecol. 2006;108(2):457-64.
5. Castleman J, Gurney L. Identification and management of fetal anaemia: a practical guide. Obstetr Gynecol. 2021;23:196-205.

6. Chandra T, Gupta A. Prevalence of ABO and Rhesus blood groups in Northern India. J Blood Disord Transfus. 2012; 3:132.
7. Creasy RK, Resnik R, Iams JD, Lockwood CJ, Moore TR, Greene MF (Eds). Maternal-Fetal Medicine: Principles and Practice, 7th edition. eBook ISBN: Saunders; 2013.
8. Crowther C, Middleton P. Anti-D administration after childbirth for preventing Rhesus alloimmunisation. Cochrane Database Syst Rev. 2000;(2):CD000021.
9. Crowther CA, Keirse MJ. Anti-D administration in pregnancy for preventing rhesus alloimmunisation. Cochrane Database Syst Rev. 2000;(2):CD000020.
10. Guidelines for the use of Rh (D) Immunoglobulin (Anti-D) in obstetrics in Australia (C-Obs6). The Royal Australian and New Zealand College of Obstetricians and Gynaecologists. Victoria, Australia. 2011.
11. Harkness UF, Spinnato JA. Prevention and management of RhD isoimmunization. Clin Perinatol. 2004;31(4):721-42.
12. James D, Steer PJ, Weiner CP, Gonik B, Robson SC (Eds). High Risk Pregnancy, 5th edition. New Delhi: Cambridge University Press; 2018.
13. Krishna L. Obstetrics Protocols, 2nd edition. New Delhi: Jaypee Brothers Medical Publisher; 2016.
14. Mackie FL, Hemming K, Allen S, Morris RK, Kilby ME. The accuracy of cell-free fetal DNA-based non-invasive prenatal testing in singleton pregnancies: a systematic review and bivariate meta-analysis. BJOG. 2017;124:32.
15. Moise Jr KJ. RhD alloimmunization in pregnancy: overview. UpToDate. 2021.
16. Pirelli KJ, Pietz BC, Johnson ST, Pinder HL, Bellissimo DB. Molecular determination of RHD zygosity: predicting risk of hemolytic disease of the fetus and newborn related to anti-D. Prenat Diagn. 2010;30(12-13):1207-12.
17. Royal College of Obstetricians and Gynaecologist. The management of women with red cell antibodies during pregnancy. RCOG Green-top Guideline. 2014; 65, Edit 2020.
18. Sarkar RS, Philip J, Mallhi RS, Yadav P. Proportion of Rh phenotypes in voluntary blood donors. Med J Armed Forces India. 2013;69(4):330-4.
19. Timmins A, Evans K. Guidelines for the use of anti-D for the prevention of haemolytic disease of the fetus and newborn. NHS. 2019.

CHAPTER 18

Preterm Birth

INTRODUCTION

Preterm birth (PTB) is defined as birth between $20^{0/7}$ and $36^{6/7}$ weeks of gestation. An estimated 15 million babies are born too early every year, i.e., >1 in 10 babies and approximately 1 million children die due to complications of PTB. The risk of neonatal morbidity and mortality is inversely related to gestational age at delivery. PTBs account for approximately 70% of neonatal deaths and 36% of infant deaths. Babies who are born preterm often have short-term morbidities such as respiratory difficulties (respiratory distress syndrome), periventricular leukomalacia, intracranial hemorrhage, bronchopulmonary dysplasia, patent ductus arteriosus, necrotizing enterocolitis, retinopathy of prematurity, and infection. In the long term, many of these children suffer from neurological and developmental disabilities, 25–50% have visual and hearing problems. Apart from the medical sequela of PTB, prematurity also has large economic consequences. Accurate identification of women in true preterm labor (PTL) allows appropriate application of interventions that can improve neonatal outcome.

PREVALENCE

Preterm birth is truly a global problem. In the lower-income countries, on average, 12% of babies are born too early compared to 9% in higher-income countries. Within countries, poorer families are at higher risk. Global prevalence of PTB is 11%, of these about 80% PTBs occur in South Asia and sub-Saharan Africa. Bangladesh is in the 7th position among the top 10 countries with the largest number PTBs and deaths. Out of 3 million children born every year in Bangladesh, some 0.6 million are born premature, and 20,000 infants die (Report of The United Nations, 2019).

RISK FACTORS (FIG. 1)

Preterm birth is a complex syndrome in which various risk factors play an important role. Risk factors for PTB can be divided into following categories:

- *Maternal risk factors:* Extremes of age (<18 or >40 years), ethnicity, high or low maternal body mass index (BMI), smoking, and maternal infection
- *Maternal medical history:* Uterine abnormalities and prior excisional cervical procedures
- *Obstetric history:* Previous curettage, previous PTB
- *Current pregnancy:* Short pregnancy interval and multiple gestations

In addition to these risk factors, bacterial vaginosis, short cervical length, and positive fetal fibronectin (fFN) could be used as screening targets to identify women at risk for PTB.

Race and Ethnicity

There are ethnic disparities in the risk for PTB. A meta-analysis by Schaaf et al. indicated a higher risk of PTB among non-White women [odds ratio (OR) 2.0; 95% confidence interval (CI) 1.8–2.2] compared to Caucasian women.

Prepregnancy Body Mass Index

Women with both extremely low and high BMI are at risk of PTL. Women with extreme low BMI (<17 kg/m^2) have a significantly higher risk of spontaneous preterm birth (sPTB) (four times more risk). Similarly, those with an extremely high BMI (≥35 kg/m^2), the risk is increased due to a higher chance for premature rupture of the membranes (OR 1.6; 95% CI 1.1–2.3). It is hypothesized that higher number of circulating inflammatory agents in obese women contributes to a higher chance of premature rupture of the membranes.

Familial Risk Factors

1.8-fold increased risk of preterm labor (PTL) if sisters had PTL.

Bacterial Vaginosis

Bacterial vaginosis is an abnormal vaginal condition that results from overgrowth of *Gardnerella vaginalis*, *Mobiluncus*, *Bacteroides* spp., and *Mycoplasma hominis*, which replace the normal vaginal lactobacilli. Bacterial vaginosis is associated with an increased risk of PTB. A meta-analysis in

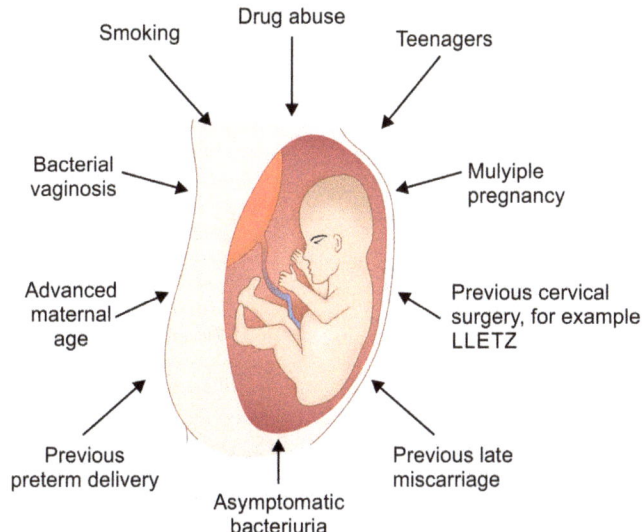

Fig. 1: Risk factors for preterm birth (PTB).
(LLETZ: large loop excision of the transformation zone)
Source: Sarah Vause, Tracey Johnston. Management of preterm labor. Arch Dis Child Fetal Neonatal Ed. 2000;83:F79-F85.

2007 by Leitich et al. in 30,518 women showed that bacterial vaginosis doubles the risk for sPTB in asymptomatic women (OR 2.16; 95% CI 1.56-3.00).

Genital and Extragenital Infection

Group B *Streptococcus* (GBS), sexually transmitted disease (STD), pyelonephritis, asymptomatic bacteriuria, appendicitis, and periodontal diseases are associated with PTL. Periodontal disease might trigger PTB because of hematogenous spread of pathogens, inflammatory cytokines, and organisms. It is hypothesized that treatment of periodontal disease during pregnancy might reduce PTB and improve perinatal outcomes.

Müllerian Duct Anomaly

Uterine anomalies such as uterine septum, unicornuate uterus, uterine didelphys, and bicornuate uterus are known to be associated with PTB. A retrospective cohort study comprising 203 singleton gestations in women with a uterine anomaly reported a significantly higher risk of sPTB (<37 weeks) compared to women with a normal anatomy (OR 5.9; 95% CI 4.3-8.1). A systematic review reported increased PTB rates before 37 weeks in women with septate uterus and unification defects (unicornuate, bicornuate, and didelphys uteri); risk ratio (RR 2.14, 95% CI 1.48-3.11; RR 2.97, 95% CI 2.08-4.23), respectively.

Cervical Factors

A short mid-pregnancy cervical length is associated with a high risk of sPTB. The relative risk of preterm delivery increases as the length of the cervix shortens. A cervical length <22 mm (fifth percentile) is associated with a relative risk of PTB of 9.49 (with a 95% CI of 5.95-15.15).

Cervical insufficiency refers to pathologic dilation and/or effacement of the uterine cervix in the absence of uterine contractions leading to previable pregnancy loss as well as sPTB. Cervical insufficiency due to intrinsic biochemical factors is probably a rare event (e.g., Ehlers-Danlos syndrome).

Cervical surgery, e.g., loop electrosurgical excision procedure (LEEP), cold knife conization, and LASER conization are associated with increased risk of PTL. Women who had a prior excisional procedure for cervical dysplasia have an overall (~13%) risk of sPTB before 35 weeks. Conner et al. performed a meta-analysis assessing the association between LEEP and PTB. They reported a higher risk of sPTB <37 weeks in the group that underwent a LEEP (pooled RR 1.60; 95% CI 0.99-2.55).

Prior Spontaneous Preterm Labor

Prior spontaneous preterm labor (sPTL) is the most significant nonmodifiable risk factor, recurrence risk twofold. The risk for a recurrent PTB increases if there is more than one PTB. Moreover, the risk is increased if the gestational age of the previous PTB was lower. Recurrence risk of a preterm singleton delivery before 37 weeks of gestation ranges from 15.8 to 30.2%. In women with previous preterm twins, recurrence risk in a following singleton gestation is ~10%. For a following twin gestation after a previous preterm singleton delivery, the recurrence risk is 57% (95% CI 51.9-61.9).

History of Curettage

Women with a previous pregnancy loss (either termination or miscarriage) managed by cervical dilatation and curettage are at higher risk for sPTB (OR 1.66; 95% CI 1.14-2.42). The risk increased twofold in women with two curettage procedures. Lemmers et al. performed a meta-analysis including 21 studies reporting on 1,853,017 women found women with a dilatation and curettage procedure had a higher risk of PTB before 37 weeks, compared to the group with no such history (OR 1.29; 95% CI 1.17-1.42), OR 1.69, 95% CI 1.20-2.38; for PTB <32 weeks. A more recent meta-analysis by Saccone et al. reported that a prior surgical management of either a spontaneous abortion (OR 1.19; 95% CI 1.03-1.37) or an indicated termination of pregnancy (OR 1.52; 95% CI 1.08-2.16) is an independent risk factor for a PTB. The exact mechanism that leads to the increased risk remains unclear, although mechanical damage to the cervix seems a logical explanation.

Pregnancy Interval

Both shorter and longer pregnancy intervals (<18 months and >60 months) have been associated with a higher risk of PTB. However, it is still unclear whether this association is the effect of confounding by other risk factors. So far, no causal effect between short or long pregnancy interval and adverse neonatal outcome has been determined. Women with a recent PTB should be counseled that a short pregnancy interval probably increases the risk of PTB.

Multiple Gestations

Women with a multiple gestation are known to be at increased risk of PTB. In 2013, the twin birth rate in the US was 33.7 per 1,000 births, 57% of twin gestation delivered before 37 weeks, of which 11% delivered very premature (before 32 weeks). In the Netherlands, a single-embryo transfer policy with assisted reproductive technology (ART) procedures has resulted in an impressive decrease of multiple pregnancies. In 2014, 3.8% of the pregnancies as a result of ART were a multiple gestation, compared to 22.2% in 2003. Global PTB rates can be further reduced by extensive implementation of single-embryo transfer.

Decidual Hemorrhage

Decidual hemorrhage (placental abruption) presents clinically as vaginal bleeding or retroplacental hematoma formation is associated with a high risk of PTL and preterm premature rupture of membranes (pPROM).

Lifestyle Factors

Smoking, heavy alcohol, stress, depression, strenuous physical activity are independent risk factors for PRL.

■ PATHOGENESIS

The pathophysiology of PTL involves at least four primary pathogenic processes that result in a final common pathway ending in spontaneous PTL and delivery:
1. Premature activation of the maternal or fetal hypothalamic–pituitary–adrenal (HPA) axis
2. Infection and inflammation
3. Decidual hemorrhage
4. Pathological uterine distention

Psychosocial Stress (Flowchart 1)

Major maternal psychosocial stress (e.g., depression, posttraumatic stress disorder, and anxiety) can activate maternal HPA axis and has been associated with a small (generally less than twofold) increased risk of sPTB. Stress increases placental production and release of corticotropin-releasing hormone (CRH) which appears to program a "placental clock" for earlier labor and delivery. Placental CRH stimulates fetal pituitary and adrenal to release cortisol, also stimulates the amniochorion and decidua to release prostaglandins, which further stimulate placental CRH release via a second positive feedback loop.

Placental CRH directly augments fetal adrenal dehydroepiandrosterone (DHEA) production. The placenta converts DHEA and DHEA-S to estrone (E1), estradiol (E2), and estriol (E3) which in the presence of estrogen receptor-alpha (ER-α)

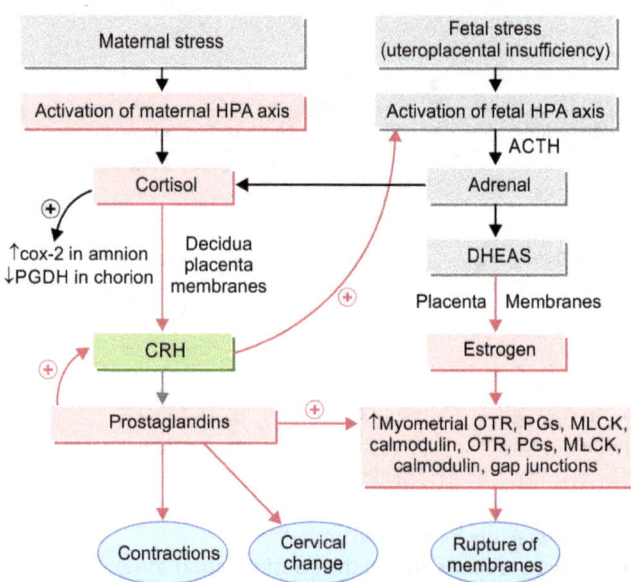

Flowchart 1: Mechanism of preterm labor in maternal stress.

(ACTH: adrenocorticotropic hormone; CRH: corticotrophin-releasing hormone; DHEAS: dehydroepiandrosterones; HPA: hypothalamic–pituitary–adrenal; MLCK: myosin light chain kinase; OTR: oxytocin receptor; PG: prostaglandin)

and reduced progesterone receptor (PR) action, increases gap junction formation, upregulation of oxytocin receptors, prostaglandin activity, and enzymes responsible for coordinated muscle contraction.

Bacterial Degradation of Membranes and Direct Uterotonic Effects

Bacteria may have a direct role in the pathogenesis of sPTB. Bacteria produce phospholipase A2 (which leads to prostaglandin synthesis) and endotoxin that stimulate uterine contractions and can cause PTL. Bacterial organisms (*Pseudomonas*, *Staphylococcus*, *Streptococcus*, *Bacteroides*, and *Enterobacter*) produce proteases, collagenases, and elastases that can degrade the fetal membranes, leading to pPROM (preterm PROM), subsequent spontaneous PTL.

Pathophysiology of Intrauterine Infection Causing Preterm Birth (Flowchart 2)

Bacterial ligands bind to toll-like receptors (TLRs) expressed on decidua, amnion, chorion, cervical, placental, and local leukocyte cell membranes. This induces the transcription factor NF-κB, which then triggers a maternal and/or fetal inflammatory response in susceptible individuals that is linked to sPTB. TLR-mediated response is ultimately characterized by the presence of activated neutrophils and, to a lesser extent, activated macrophages and various proinflammatory mediators [e.g., interleukin (IL) 1, 6, and 8; tumor necrosis factor (TNF), granulocyte colony-stimulating factor (G-CSF), and matrix metalloproteinases (MMPs)].

The key initial mediators IL-1β and TNF enhance prostaglandin production by inducing cyclooxygenase-2

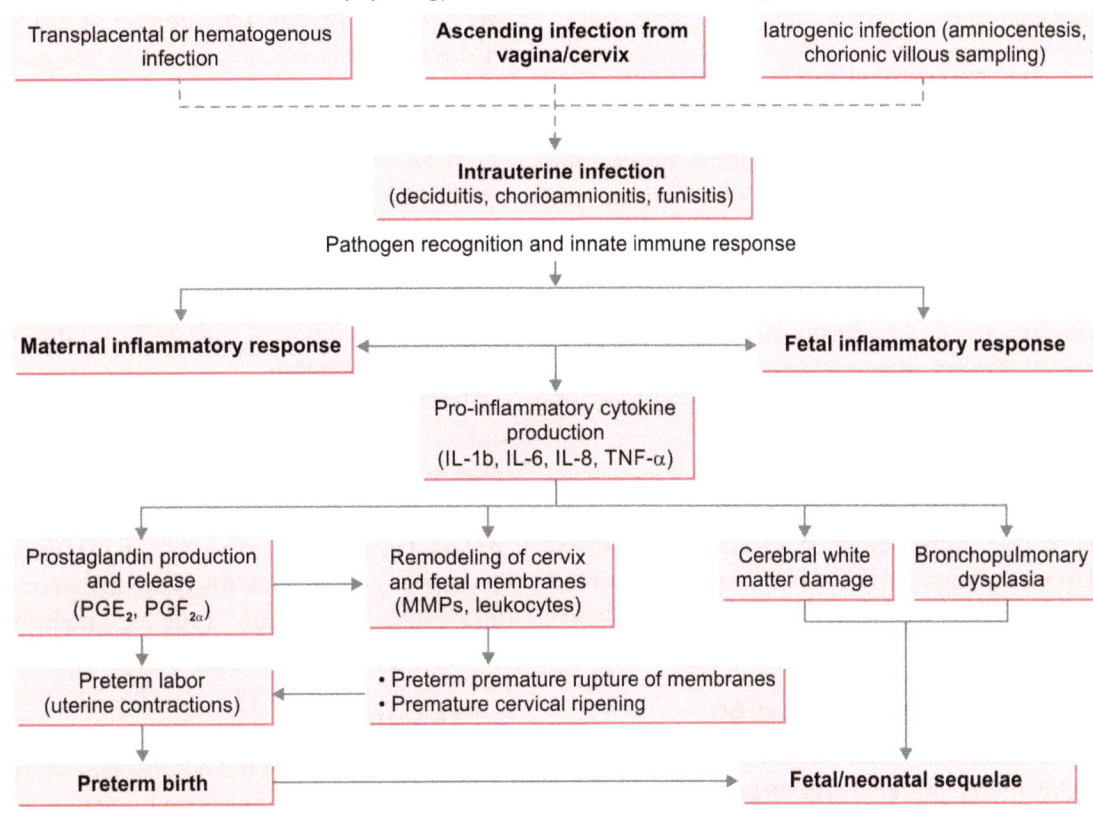

Flowchart 2: Pathophysiology of intrauterine infection causing preterm birth.

(IL: interleukin; MMP: matrix metalloproteinase; PGE: prostaglandin E)

(COX-2) expression in the amnion and decidua while inhibiting the prostaglandin-metabolizing enzyme, 15-hydroxyprostaglandin dehydrogenase (PGDH), in the chorion. IL-1β and/or TNF directly enhance the expression of various MMPs in the amniochorion, decidua, and cervix to degrade the extracellular matrix of the fetal membranes and cervix. Elevated proinflammatory mediator levels have been demonstrated in the amniotic fluid of women with PTL with intact membranes, and these levels correlated well with positive results from culture of the amniotic fluid and fetal membranes.

Pathologic Uterine Distention

Multiple gestation, polyhydramnios, and other causes of excessive uterine distention are well-described risk factors for sPTB. Enhanced stretching of the myometrium induces formation of gap junctions, upregulation of oxytocin receptors; production of inflammatory cytokines, prostaglandins, and myosin light chain kinase are critical events preceding uterine contractions and cervical dilation.

■ DIAGNOSTIC EVALUATION
History and Initial Examinations

Review patient's past and present obstetric and medical history, including risk factors for PTB. PTL may be triggered by an underlying obstetric complication (e.g., abruption) or medical/surgical disorder (e.g., appendicitis, bowel obstruction or strangulation, pyelonephritis, and acute cholecystitis) that requires specific intervention.

During initial examination, confirm gestational age, based on last menstrual period (LMP), and early ultrasound examination and record maternal vital signs (temperature, blood pressure, heart rate, respiratory rate) and fetal heart rate pattern.

Assessment of Contraction

Assess frequency, duration, and intensity of uterine contractions as well as cervical change. Examination of the uterus to assess firmness, tenderness, fetal size, and fetal position.

Prodromal Signs Symptoms of Labor

Prodromal signs symptoms of labor include menstrual-like cramping, mild, irregular contractions, low back ache, pressure sensation in the vagina or pelvis, vaginal discharge of mucus, which may be clear, pink, or slightly bloody (i.e., mucus plug, bloody show).

Speculum Examination

By wet nonlubricated speculum to assess cervical dilation (dilation ≥3 cm), any uterine bleeding (abruptio placentae or placenta previa), membrane status (intact or ruptured). Obtain a cervicovaginal fluid/specimen by rotating the swab in posterior fornix for 10 seconds for fFN testing (in suspicious cases).

Digital Cervical Examination

After exclusion of placenta previa and rupture of membranes from history, physical, laboratory, and ultrasound examinations as appropriate, assess cervical dilation and effacement. Distinguish between patients whose membranes have hour-glassed (prolapsed) through a mildly dilated and effaced cervix (suggestive of cervical insufficiency) and those who are in active labor with advanced cervical dilation and effacement. Transvaginal ultrasound (TVU) can help distinguish between the two entities when the diagnosis is uncertain.

Transvaginal Ultrasound Examination

A short cervix (<30 mm) before 34 weeks of gestation is predictive of an increased risk for PTB in all populations, while a long cervix (≥30 mm) has a high negative predictive value for PTB.

Obstetrical Ultrasound Examination

Obstetrical ultrasound examination provides useful information, including presence/absence of fetal, placental, and maternal anatomic abnormalities, confirmation of fetal presentation, assessment of amniotic fluid volume, and estimated fetal weight. This information may be used for counseling the patient regarding potential cause and outcome of PTB and determining the best route of delivery.

■ LABORATORY EVALUATION

- *Rectovaginal swab:* For GBS culture and antibiotic prophylaxis (if not done within the previous 5 weeks)
- *Urine culture:* Since asymptomatic bacteriuria is associated with an increased risk of PTL and birth
- *fFN test:* Should be performed (if gestational age <34 weeks, cervical dilation <3 cm, and cervical length 20–30 mm on TVU) to distinguish women in true PTL from those with false labor.

Fetal fibronectin is an extracellular matrix protein present at the decidual-chorionic interface. Disruption of this interface occurs due to subclinical infection or inflammation, abruption, or uterine contractions, which releases fFN into cervicovaginal secretions, this is the basis for its use as a marker for predicting sPTB. Qualitative fFN testing is increasingly used in Europe and North America to predict PTL in asymptomatic group during 24–34 weeks. A fixed threshold level of 50 ng/mL is considered as positive. Main benefit of qualitative fFN being its *high NPV (>96%)*. Validity of the test is 7–14 days.

Quantitative measurement of fFN appears to improve predictive value compared to use of the qualitative test using a 50 ng/mL threshold. In one prospective blinded study in symptomatic women, the positive predictive values of fFN thresholds of 10, 50, 200, and 500 ng/mL for PTB within 14 days were 11, 20, 37, and 46% respectively; for PTB <34 weeks, positive predictive values for the same thresholds were 19, 32, 61, and 75%, respectively.

National Institute for Healthcare and Excellence (NICE) recommends fFN testing for women with ≥30^{+0} weeks' gestation with threatened PTL if transvaginal cervical length (TVCL) is indicated but is not available or not acceptable. Combination of fFN and cervical length testing is advocated by some international bodies as predictive accuracy is superior to single test.

Testing for *sexually transmitted infections* (e.g., chlamydia and gonorrhea) depends on the patient's risk factors for these infections.

Other laboratory tests: Placental alpha-microglobulin-1 (PAMG-1) or phosphorylated insulin-like growth factor binding protein-1 (pIGFBP-1) in vaginal or cervical secretions suggest disruption of the fetal membranes (ROM or labor) and are potential markers of an increased risk of PTB.

■ DIAGNOSIS

Diagnosis is based on the clinical criteria of regular painful uterine contractions accompanied by cervical change (dilation and/or effacement).

- *Uterine contraction:* Regular painful uterine contractions (≥4 every 20 minutes or ≥8 in 60 minutes)
- *Cervical dilation and/or effacement:*
  - Cervical dilation ≥3 cm
  - Cervical length <20 mm (TVS)
  - Cervical length 20 to <30 mm (TVS) and positive fFN test.

Special Note

The positive predictive value of a positive fFN test result or a short cervix alone is poor and should not be used exclusively to direct management in the setting of acute symptoms.

■ MANAGEMENT

Guided by: Confirmation of diagnosis by *clinical criteria* of regular painful uterine contractions accompanied by cervical dilation and/or effacement and *gestational age*. Less than 10% of women with the clinical diagnosis of PTL actually give birth within 7 days of presentation.

Management Based on Cervical Length and Dilatation (Figs. 2A and B)

Symptomatic Women with Cervical Dilation <3 cm and Cervical Length 20 to <30 mm

Symptomatic women with cervical dilation <3 cm and cervical length 20 to <30 mm are at increased risk of PTB compared with women with longer cervical lengths, though most of these women do not deliver preterm; fFN test should

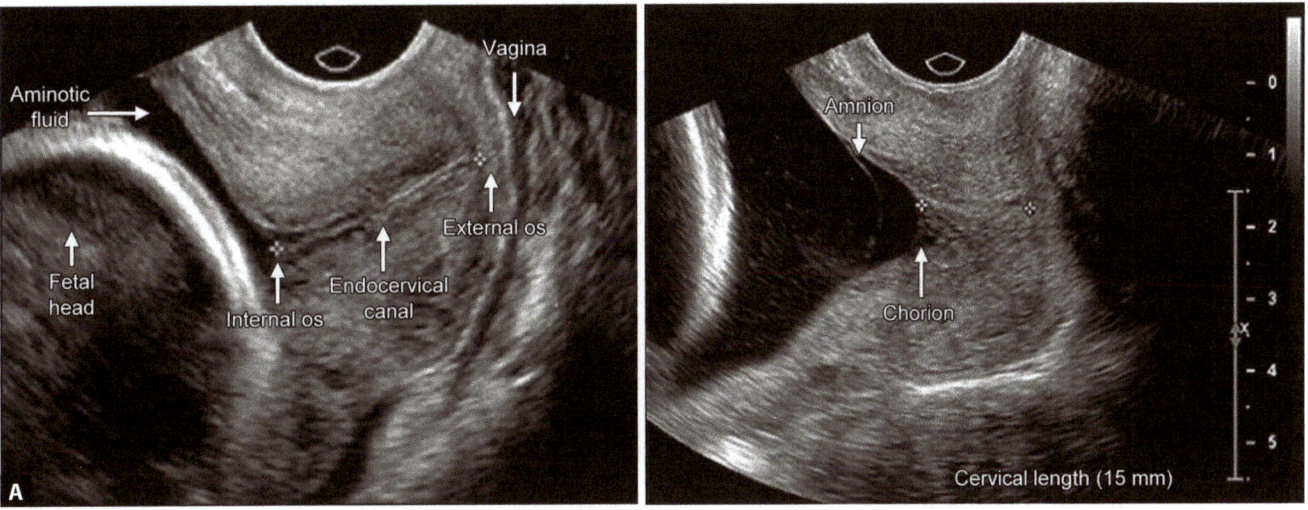

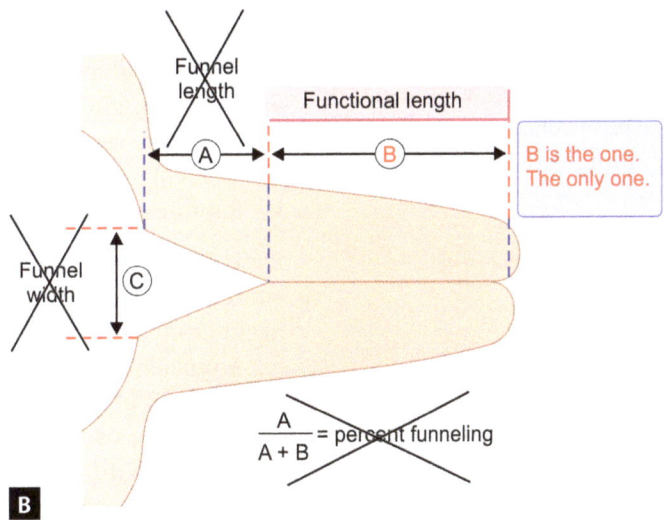

Figs. 2A and B: (A) TAS with normal Cx and short Cx with no funneling; (B) Diagrammatic features of funneled Cx.
(TAS: transabdominal sonography; TVS: transvaginal sonography)

be done in these cases. If the fFN test is positive, begin interventions to reduce morbidity associated with PTB. If the fFN test is negative, can discharge the patient after 6–12 hours of observation, given its high negative predictive value (98–100% for delivery within 7 or 14 days) after ensuring maternal and fetal well-being.

Cervical Length <20 mm

Symptomatic women with cervical length <20 mm are at high risk (>25%) of delivery within next 7 days; the addition of fFN testing does not significantly improve the predictive value of cervical length measurement alone, begin interventions to reduce morbidity associated with PTB.

Cervical Length ≥30 mm

Approximately 50% of women with symptoms of PTL have a TVU cervical length ≥30 mm and are at low risk (<5%) of delivery within next 7 days, regardless of fFN result; the addition of fFN testing will not significantly improve the predictive value of cervical length measurement alone.

Management Based on Gestational Age

Pregnancies ≥34 Weeks, Without Progressive Cervical Dilation and Effacement

Observe, if there is no progression of labor-can be discharged home, after 6–12 hours of observation as long as fetal well-being is confirmed (e.g., reactive nonstress test). Exclude obstetrical complications such as abruptio placentae, chorioamnionitis, and preterm rupture of membranes before discharge. If labor progresses, admit for delivery.

Gestational Age <34 Weeks

Pregnancies <34 weeks of gestation, cervical dilation <3 cm:
- TVU measurement of *cervical length* and laboratory analysis of cervicovaginal *fFN* help to support or exclude diagnosis of PTL.

- *Tocolytics:* For women diagnosed in PTL, administer tocolytic drugs for up to 48 hours (when safe to do so) so that antenatal corticosteroids (ACs) (primary or rescue) administered to the mother have time to achieve their maximum fetal/neonatal effects. Tocolytics provide time for safe transport of the mother, if indicated, to a facility that has an appropriate level of neonatal care if she delivers preterm. In utero, transport avoids the possibility that the mother and the infant will be separated in the first few hours/days of life.
- Antibiotics for group B streptococcal chemoprophylaxis (when appropriate)
- *Antenatal betamethasone:* Predelivery administration of betamethasone reduces the risk of neonatal death, respiratory distress syndrome, intraventricular hemorrhage, and necrotizing enterocolitis in preterm neonates.
- *Magnesium sulfate:* Administered for neuroprotection to pregnancies at 24–32 weeks of gestation. Results of the available clinical trials of magnesium sulfate for neuroprotection suggest that predelivery administration of magnesium sulfate reduces the occurrence of cerebral palsy when given with neuroprotective intent (RR, 0.71; 95% CI, 0.55–0.91).

TABLE 1: Management according to gestational age in women with preterm labor.

24^{+0} up to 32	32^{+0} to 33^{+6}	34^{+0} up
GBS prophylaxis	GBS prophylaxis	GBS prophylaxis
Steroids	Steroids	Steroids
Tocolysis through steroid window	Tocolysis through steroid window	
$MgSO_4$ for neuroprotection	$MgSO_4$ for neuroprotection	

(GBS: Group B *Streptococcus*)

Preterm Labor with Cervical Dilation ≥3 cm: Initiate Active Treatment

ACOG recommendations:
- *Betamethasone* to reduce neonatal morbidity and mortality
- *Tocolytic drugs* for up to 48 hours to delay delivery so that betamethasone given to the mother can achieve its maximum fetal effect
- *GBS chemoprophylaxis:* Continue until she delivers
- *Magnesium sulfate* for pregnancies between 24 and 32 weeks:
  - Women with preterm contractions without cervical change, especially those with cervical dilation of <2 cm, generally should not be treated with tocolytics.

Key Points in Management (Table 1 and Flowchart 3)

Group B Streptococcus Prophylaxis

Group B *Streptococcus* (GBS or *Streptococcus agalactiae*) is an encapsulated Gram-positive coccus that colonizes the gastrointestinal and genital tracts of 15–40% of pregnant women. Although GBS colonization is asymptomatic in these women, maternal colonization is a critical determinant of infection in neonates and young infants (<90 days of age), in whom GBS is the most common cause of bacterial infection. Vertical transmission primarily occurs when GBS passes from the vagina into the amniotic fluid after onset of labor or rupture of membranes but can also occur with intact membranes and during passage through the birth canal. Universal screening by rectovaginal culture during pregnancy is indicated between $36^{0/7}$ and $37^{6/7}$ weeks. In addition, GBS screening is indicated in the following conditions:
- Women with GBS bacteriuria any time in pregnancy or who had an infant with early-onset GBS infection in a previous pregnancy
- Women with positive rectovaginal culture for GBS
- Unknown antepartum culture status [culture not performed or result not found)/intrapartum fever ≥100.4°F (≥38°C)]
- Rupture of membranes ≥18 hours.

Dose: GBS is susceptible to penicillin G, ampicillin, cephalosporins, and vancomycin, but penicillin G is the most active agent in vitro.

Ampicillin 2 g IV stat and then 1 g every 4 hours. Since time of delivery cannot always be predicted, prophylaxis is begun at hospital admission for labor or rupture of membranes and continued every 4 hours until delivery. Treatment is most effective if administered at least 4 hours before delivery, oral treatment is not recommended. GBS chemoprophylaxis is recommended in active PTL, discontinued once the patient is no longer at imminent risk of PTB, even if the GBS rectovaginal culture is positive.

Antenatal Corticosteroid

- To all women at 24^{+0} to 33^{+6} weeks who are at increased risk of PTD
- Maximum efficacy occurs when delivery happens 2–7 days after administration of first dose of AC. Efficacy is incomplete before 24 hours from administration and appears to decline after 7 days.
- *World Health Organization (WHO) (2011) recommendation:* ACS between 24 and 34 weeks irrespective of whether a single or multiple birth, WHO does not recommend ACS after 34 weeks.
- Recent data indicate that betamethasone decreases newborn respiratory morbidity when given to women in the late preterm period between $34^{0/7}$ and $36^{6/7}$ weeks who are at risk of preterm delivery within 7 days and who have not previously received corticosteroids.

Flowchart 3: Management of preterm labor.

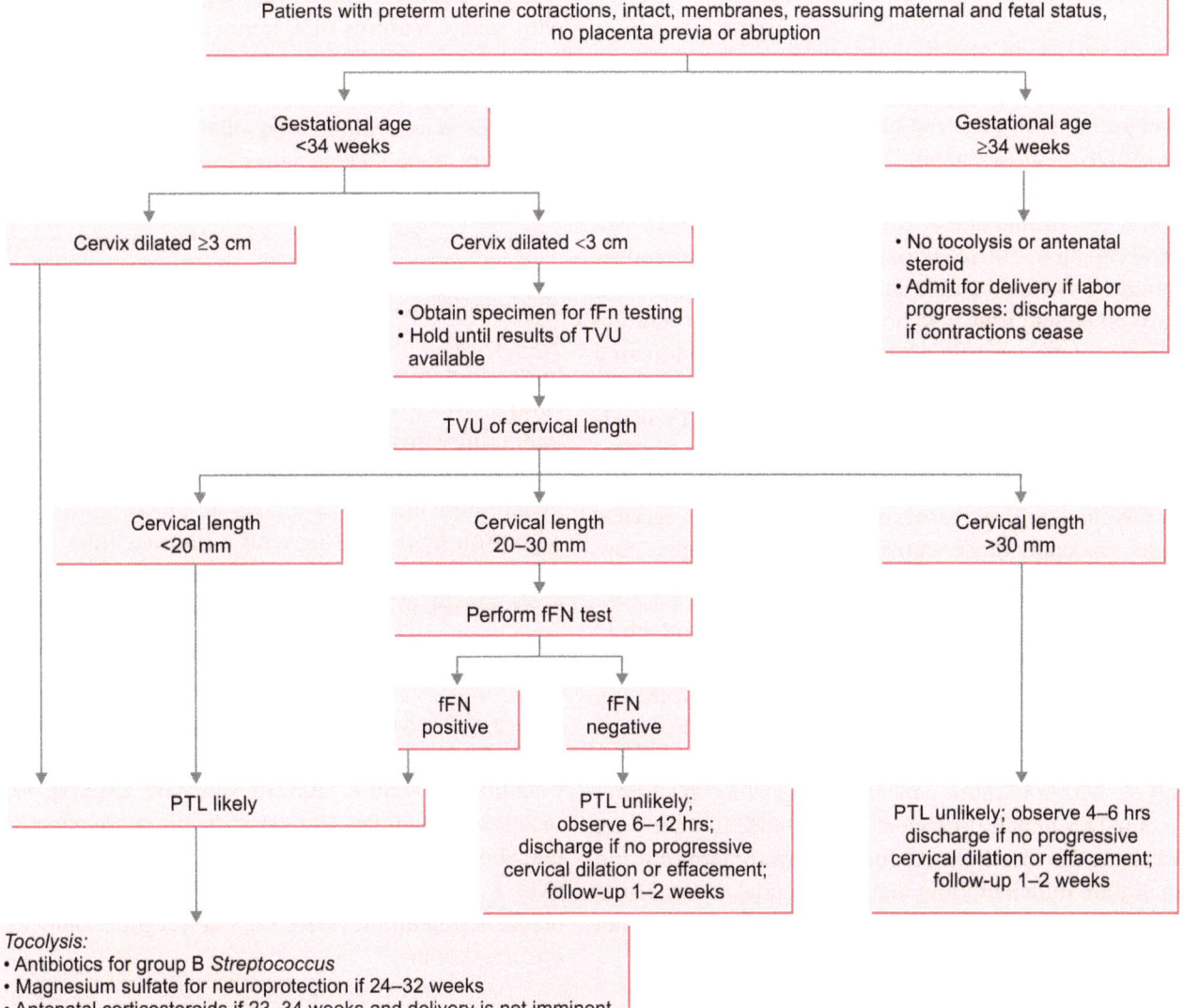

(IFN: indicates fetal fibronectin; PTL: preterm labor; TVU: transvaginat ultrasound)
Source: Adapted from Practice Bulletin No. 171: Management of Preterm Labor. Obstetrics & Gynecology: October 2016 - Volume 128 - Issue 4 - p e155-e164.

- Society for Maternal-Fetal Medicine (SMFM) recommends a two-dose course of ACS between 34^{+0} and 36^{+6} gestation with the following caveats:
    - Women with symptoms of PTL, cervical dilation ≥3 cm or effacement ≥75% before treatment
    - Tocolysis should not be used to delay delivery for completion of the course of steroids.
- The American College of Obstetricians and Gynecologists (ACOG) recommends administration of betamethasone at 34^{+0} to 36^{+6} weeks of gestation in women with singleton pregnancy, at imminent risk of PTB within 7 days, with the following caveats:
    - AC administration should not be administered to women with chorioamnionitis.
    - Tocolysis should not be used to delay delivery in women with symptoms of PTL to allow administration of ACs.
- Medically/obstetrically indicated preterm delivery should not be postponed for steroid administration.
- Newborns should be monitored for hypoglycemia.
- NICE (2019) recommends: ACS between 34^{+0} and 35^{+6} weeks who are in suspected, diagnosed, or established PTL, or are having a planned PTB or have pPROM.

Dose:
- *Dexamethasone:* Four doses of 6 mg 12 hours apart
- *Betamethasone:* Two doses of 12 mg 24 hours apart

Contraindications:
- Chorioamnionitis
- Cervical dilation ≥3 cm or effacement ≥75%

Side effects: Transient maternal hyperglycemia may occur approximately 12 hours after first dose and may last for 5 days. Leukocytosis in approximately 30% cases within

24 hours and lymphocyte count significantly decreases. These changes return to baseline within 3 days.

Tocolytics (Figs. 3A and B)

Approximately 30% of PTL spontaneously resolves and 50% of patients hospitalized for PTL actually give birth at term. *ACOG in 2016* opined "Interventions to reduce the likelihood of delivery should be reserved for women with PTL at a gestational age at which a delay in delivery will provide benefit to the newborn. Because tocolytic therapy is generally effective for up to 48 hours, only women with fetuses that would benefit from a 48 hours delay in delivery should receive tocolytic treatment". Tocolytics are not indicated before neonatal viability. Inhibition of acute PTL is less likely to be successful when cervical dilation is >3 cm. Tocolysis can still be effective in these cases, especially when the goal is to administer AC or safely transfer mother to a tertiary care center. Women with preterm contractions without cervical change, especially those with a cervical dilation of <2 cm, generally should not be treated with tocolytics.

Gestational Age Limit for Tocolysis: American College of Obstetricians and Gynecologists and SMFM recommend not to administer tocolysis before 24 weeks. In USA, a workshop in 2014, comprised of obstetric and pediatric experts, suggested 22^{+0} weeks as the lower limit for consideration tocolysis. There is more consensus regarding the upper gestational age limit for treatment, ACOG and SMFM consider 34 weeks as the threshold at which perinatal morbidity and mortality are sufficiently low, that the potential maternal and fetal complications and costs associated with inhibition of PTL and short-term delay of delivery are not justified.

Contraindications of tocolysis: Intrauterine fetal demise, lethal fetal anomaly, nonreassuring fetal status, preeclampsia with severe features or eclampsia, maternal hemorrhage with hemodynamic instability, intra-amniotic infection, pPROM, medical contraindications to tocolytic drug. Tocolysis is contraindicated when the maternal and fetal risks of prolonging pregnancy or the risks associated with these drugs are greater than the risks associated with PTB.

Mechanism of Action of Tocolysis: Myometrial contractility is a complex process, involves hormonal receptors, ions channels, intercellular gap junctions, and regulatory proteins such as oxytocin, endothelin, tachykinin, and angiotensin. Increase of intracellular Ca^{++} concentration is essential for contraction. Tocolytics causes uterine relaxation either by interfering with contractile protein synthesis or effect.

β-adrenergic receptor agonists, nitric oxide (NO) donors, magnesium, and calcium channel blockers cause uterine relaxation by interfering with an intracellular messenger responsible for contractile proteins effects. Atosiban, an oxytocin receptor antagonist, and prostaglandin-synthetase inhibitors cause uterine relaxation by interfering with endogenous myometrial stimulators.

Choice of Tocolytics: A meta-analysis of 95 randomized trials of all commonly used tocolytics found-COX-2 inhibitors, β-agonists, calcium channel blockers, $MgSO_4$, oxytocin receptor antagonists were statistically more effective than placebo/no tocolytic for delaying delivery for 48 hours. COX-2 inhibitors (indomethacin) and calcium channel blockers (nifedipine) have the highest probability of being the best therapy.

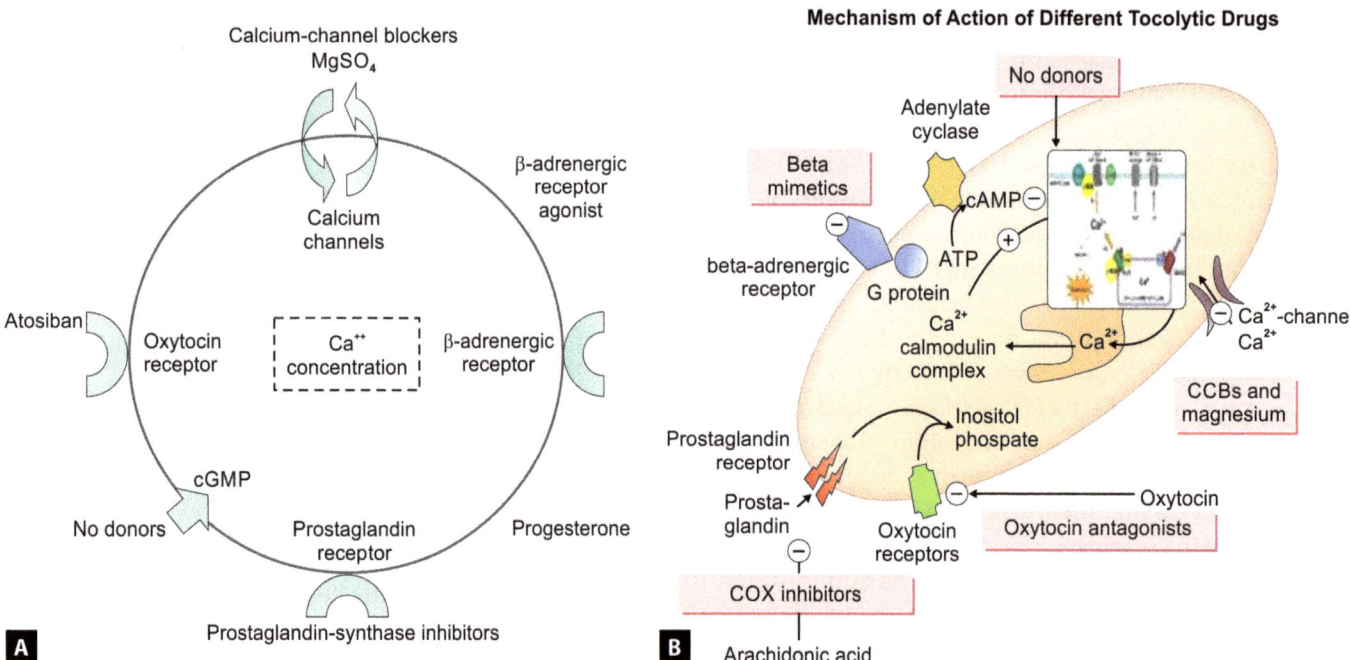

Figs. 3A and B: Tocolytics with mechanism of action.
Source: (A) National Institute of Health; (B) Slideshare.net.

First-line therapy

Between 24 and 32 weeks: Indomethacin is first-line therapy.

Dose: 50-100 mg loading dose (may be given orally or per rectum), followed by 25 mg orally every 4-6 hourly and should not be used >72 hours because of fetal risk of premature constriction of ductus arteriosus and oligohydramnios especially after 31-32 weeks.

Monitoring: If continued for >48 hours, weekly sonographic evaluation for oligohydramnios and narrowing of the ductus is warranted.

Contraindications: Maternal contraindications—platelet dysfunction or bleeding diathesis, hepatic dysfunction, gastrointestinal ulcerative disease, renal dysfunction, and asthma.

Between 32 and 34 weeks: Nifedipine is the first-line therapy.

Dose: Initial loading dose 20-30 mg orally, followed by an additional 10-20 mg orally every 3-8 hours up to 48 hours, maximum dose 180 mg/day.

Contraindications: Calcium channel blockers are contraindicated in hypotension, or preload-dependent cardiac lesions and should be used with caution in women with heart failure with reduced ejection fraction.

Second-line Therapy

If the first line drug does not inhibit contractions, begin therapy with another agent. As second line, use nifedipine at 24 and 32 weeks, and terbutaline at 32 and 34 weeks OR use terbutaline between 24 and 32 weeks as second line, who received nifedipine as first line.

Terbutaline: Selective β-2 agonists such as ritodrine and salbutamol have been used in clinical practice for PTL since the 1980s.

Dose: Administered as a continuous intravenous (IV) infusion, starting infusion at 2.5-5 µg/min and increasing by 2.5-5 µg/min every 20-30 minutes to a maximum of 25 µg/min, or until the contractions have abated. At this point, the infusion is reduced by decrements of 2.5-5 µg/min to the lowest dose that maintains uterine quiescence.

Maternal side effects: Tachycardia, hyperglycemia, and hypokalemia commonly occur.

Fetal side effects: Include fetal tachycardia, are analogous to the maternal effects. Neonatal hypoglycemia may result from fetal hyperinsulinemia in response to prolonged maternal hyperglycemia. Fetal acid/base status and neonatal well-being are not compromised by these agents. In the United States, the Food and Drug Administration (FDA) has warned that injectable terbutaline should not be used in pregnant women for prolonged (beyond 48-72 hours) period.

Atosiban: Atosiban is a selective oxytocin-vasopressin receptor antagonist. If nifedipine is contraindicated, offer oxytocin receptor antagonists (atosiban) for tocolysis, do not offer betamimetics (NICE). Atosiban competes with oxytocin for binding to its receptors in myometrium and decidua, prevents increase in intracellular free Ca^+ that happens when oxytocin binds. It is commonly used in Europe as first-line therapy.

Dose: Administered IV, begin with a bolus of 6.75 mg followed by a 300 µg/min infusion for 3 hours, and then 100 µg/min for up to 45 hours. Atosiban is the only tocolytic that has demonstrated superiority over placebo as maintenance therapy. Has low side effects profile, no absolute contraindications, seems to be safest choice in multiple pregnancy.

Magnesium Sulfate

Mechanism of action: The precise mechanism of magnesium's effects on uterine contractions has not been completely elucidated, despite >40 years of study. Magnesium probably competes with calcium at the level of the plasma membrane voltage-gated channels. It hyperpolarizes the plasma membrane and inhibits myosin light-chain kinase activity by competing with intracellular calcium at this site. Interference with the activity of myosin light-chain kinase reduces myometrial contractility. ACOG and the SMFM consider magnesium sulfate as an option for short-term prolongation of pregnancy (up to 48 hours) to allow administration of ACs to pregnant women at risk for preterm delivery within 7 days.

NICE 2015 recommendation: Women in established PTL or having a planned PTB within 24 hours:
- Offer $MgSO_4$ to mother between 24^{+0} and 29^{+6} weeks
- Consider $MgSO_4$ between 30^{+0} and 33^{+6} weeks

Dose: 4 g IV bolus over 15 minutes, followed by an infusion of 1 g per hour till birth or for 24 hours whichever is sooner (NICE).

WHO recommendation: $MgSO_4$ for women at risk of imminent PTB before 32 weeks for prevention of cerebral palsy. The minimum duration of administration for neuroprotection is not known but is <24 hours.

Maternal and fetal side effects: Magnesium sulfate causes fewer minor maternal side effects than β-agonists, but the risk of major adverse risk events is comparable. Diaphoresis and flushing are the most common side effects; magnesium toxicity is related to serum concentration. Maternal therapy causes a slight decrease in baseline fetal heart rate and fetal heart rate variability.

Contraindications: Magnesium sulfate tocolysis is contraindicated in women with myasthenia gravis.

Antibiotics

Although subclinical genital tract infection clearly contributes to the pathogenesis of PTB, there is no evidence-based role for antibiotic therapy in the prevention of prematurity in patients with acute PTL. There is no consensus whether women in acute PTL should be evaluated routinely for subclinical intra-amniotic infection. *WHO recommends antibiotic for women with pPROM but not for women with intact amniotic membrane and without clinical sign of infection.*

Afebrile patients with nonspecific laboratory or physical findings suggestive of infection, such as leukocytosis, unexplained maternal or fetal tachycardia, or uterine tenderness amniocentesis for Gram stain and glucose level before or just after administering first-line tocolysis. *Culture fluid for aerobes, anaerobes, Ureaplasma,* and *Mycoplasma.* Amniotic fluid cultures are positive in almost 65% women in whom tocolysis with a single agent is unsuccessful. Do not begin/continue tocolytic if the amniotic fluid tests are suggestive of subclinical infection.

Other Interventions

Maintenance tocolysis: It is ineffective, does not prolong pregnancy or prevent PTB, or improve neonatal outcome.

Initiation of progesterone supplementation: Women who were not on P4 before suspected PTL, do not begin P4 as an adjunct to tocolysis or as part of maintenance therapy, regardless of cervical length.

Rescue cerclage: Do not offer "rescue" cervical cerclage to women with signs of infection or active vaginal bleeding or uterine contractions. Cerclage may have a beneficial effect in preventing preterm delivery when there is a history of PTL and an objective decrease in cervical length or increased cervix dilatation in asymptomatic patients. Cerclage is indicated in women between 16^{+0} and 27^{+6} weeks with a dilated cervix and exposed, unruptured fetal membrane, after an acute episode. Benefits are likely to be greater for earlier gestations.

Prevention of Preterm Birth

TVCL in the second trimester has been shown to be one of the best predictors for PTB in singleton pregnancy. Several preventive measures have been examined over the past decades. Certain risk factors, such as sociodemographic factors, cannot be adjusted; however, this information can be used to determine women's individual risk profile. Clinical caregivers can inform patients on their risks. There are potential preventive interventions, including progesterone, cervical pessary, and cerclage, that have been studied in different patient populations.

General advice includes:
- *Birth spacing:* Advice for contraception (2 years)
- Stop smoking
- Nutritional support, and psychosocial support as needed
- Maintain ideal BMI (extremes of prepregnancy BMI are at higher risk for PTB)
- Counseling on prolonged work (>42 hours/week) or prolonged standing (>6 hours /day), night work has been linked to PTB.

Asymptomatic bacteriuria: Screening and treatment of asymptomatic bacteriuria.

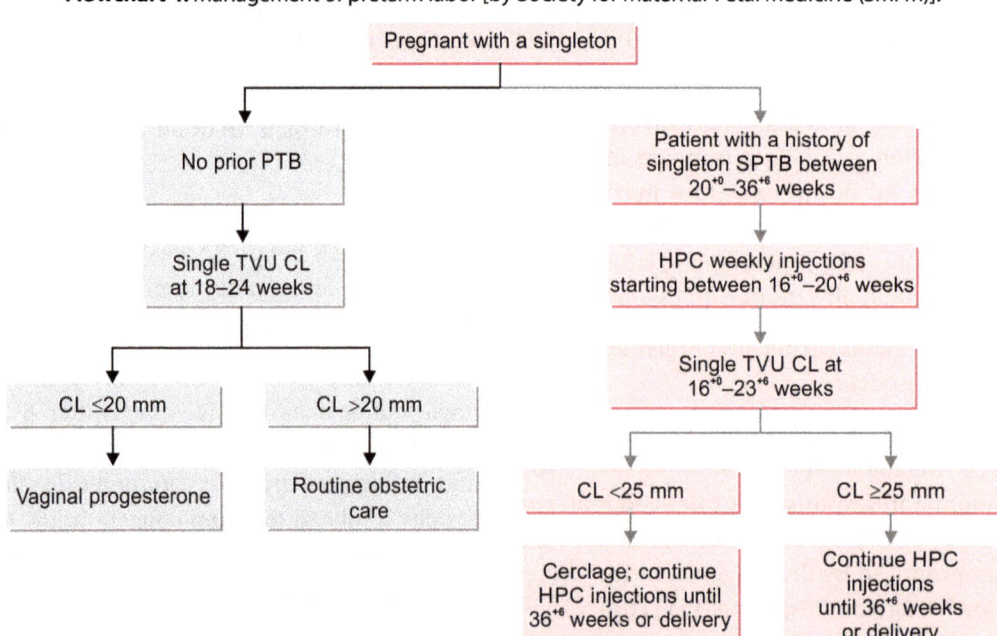

Flowchart 4: Management of preterm labor [by Society for Maternal-Fetal Medicine (SMFM)].

(CL: cervical length; HPC: hydroxyprogesterone caproate; PTB: preterm birth; sPTB: spontaneous preterm birth; TVU: transvaginal ultrasound)

Genital Infection

Consider treatment of bacterial vaginosis with clindamycin in women with a history of PTB.

Dose: 300 mm bd for 7 days or 2% cream (5 g) one full applicator at bed time 7 days or metronidazole 500 mg orally twice daily 7 days. For, *Ureaplasma* and *Mycoplasma* species—best is macrolide antibiotics, e.g., solithromycin.

Prophylactic Progesterone

Research has shown that progesterone could reduce recurrence rates of sPTB. In asymptomatic women presenting with prior history of PTB, early prophylaxis with either micronized P4 or 17 OHPC demonstrated to be efficacious in preventing recurrence. Prophylactic P4 has been approved by *ACOG*, *FDA*, and *NICE*.

In 2003, Meis et al. performed a double-blind placebo-controlled trial involving 463 women with a history of sPTB. They reported a significant reduction in recurrence rate of PTB before 37 weeks in the progesterone group (RR 0.66; 95% CI 0.54–0.81). In contrast, the recent OPPTIMUM study did not find a beneficial effect of vaginal progesterone in women with a previous PTB before 34 weeks in terms of reduction of PTB <34 weeks or fetal death (OR 0.82; 95% CI 0.58–1.16).

A Cochrane meta-analysis by Dodd et al. has shown that progesterone, in women with a past history of sPTB, significantly reduced PTB before 34 weeks when compared to the control group (RR 0.31; 95% CI 0.14–0.69). Moreover, there was an overall lower perinatal mortality (RR 0.50; 95% CI 0.33–0.75) in the progesterone group.

Choice of progesterone: So far, no difference in the effectiveness of both vaginal and intramuscular (17-OHPC) progesterone has been found. Vaginal progesterone rather than 17 OHPC appears to be a critical factor for preventing PTB with short cervix. NICE 2019 recommended prophylactic progesterone for women with H/O sPTB or mid-trimester loss (16^{+0} weeks onward) or TVS between 16^{+0} and 24^{+0} weeks showing cervical length of ≤25 mm. When using vaginal progesterone, "start treatment between 16^{+0} and 24^{+0} weeks of pregnancy and continue until at least 34 weeks" (2019).

Dose:
- *Short cervix:* Vaginal P4 8% gel or 100–400 mg micronized P4
- *Without short cervix:* 17 OHPC 250 mg IM weekly starting between 16 and 20 weeks till 36 weeks

Cervical Cerclage

Cerclage may have a beneficial effect in preventing preterm delivery when there is a history of PTL and an objective decrease in cervical length <25 mm or increase cervix dilatation in nonsymptomatic patients before 24 weeks. Success rate for cervical cerclage is approximately 80–90% for elective cerclages and 40–60% for emergency cerclage. It is not clear whether addition of 17 OHPC provides additional benefit to women with a cervical cerclage in place.

National Institute for Healthcare and Excellence recommends prophylactic cervical cerclage for women when transvaginal ultrasound between 16^{+0} and 24^{+0} weeks of pregnancy show a cervical length of 25 mm or less, and who have had either: pPROM in a previous pregnancy or a history of cervical trauma.

Pessary

The cervical pessary is a soft and flexible silicone device. It is folded and put around the cervix by a simple vaginal examination without causing any pain. Although the exact working mechanism is still unknown, pessaries may distribute the weight of the uterus on to the vaginal floor and relieve pressure on the internal os. Therefore, a pessary might prevent premature dilatation of the cervix and preterm rupture of the membranes. In addition, a pessary might support the immunological barrier between the chorion and vaginal microbiological flora, which helps to prevent PTB.

■ CONCLUSION

Prevention of PTB is one of the main obstetric goals. For an optimal prevention of PTB, risk stratification should be based on a combination of (maternal) risk factors, obstetric history, and screening tools. In singleton or multiple pregnancies with a short cervix, without previous PTB, a pessary or progesterone might prevent PTB. In women with a (recurrent) PTB in the past, progesterone and a cerclage may prevent recurrence. Accurate identification of women in true PTL allows appropriate application of interventions that can improve neonatal outcome on the contrary, accurate identification of women not actually in PTL avoids unnecessary and sometimes costly interventions in approximately 50% of patients with suspected PTL who subsequently deliver at term without tocolytic therapy.

■ SUGGESTED READING

1. American College of Obstetricians and Gynecologists and the Society for Maternal–Fetal Medicine; Ecker JL, Kaimal A, Mercer BM, Blackwell SC, deRegnier RA, et al. Periviable birth. American College of Obstetricians and Gynecologists and the Society for Maternal-Fetal Medicine. Am J Obstet Gynecol. 2015;215(2):B2-B12.e1.
2. American College of Obstetricians and Gynecologists' Committee on Practice Bulletins—Obstetrics. Practice Bulletin No. 171; Obstet Gynecol. 2016;128(4):e155-64.
3. American College of Obstetricians and Gynecologists' Committee on Practice Bulletins—Obstetrics. RCOG Practice Bulletin No. 171: Management of Preterm Labor. Obstet Gynecol. 2016;128(4):e155-64.
4. Berghella V, Palacio M, Ness A, Alfirevic Z, Nicolaides KH, Saccone G. Cervical length screening for prevention of preterm birth in singleton pregnancy with threatened

preterm labor: systematic review and meta-analysis of randomized controlled trials using individual patient-level data. Ultrasound Obstet Gynecol. 2017;49:322.
5. Berghella V, Saccone G. Fetal fibronectin testing for prevention of preterm birth in singleton pregnancies with threatened preterm labor: a systematic review and meta-analysis of randomized controlled trials. Am J Obstet Gynecol. 2016;215:431.
6. Crowther CA, Ashwood P, McPhee AJ, Flenady V, Tran T, Dodd JM, et al. Vaginal progesterone pessaries for pregnant women with a previous preterm birth to prevent neonatal respiratory distress syndrome (the PROGRESS Study): A multicentre, randomised, placebo-controlled trial. PLoS Med. 2017;14(9):e1002390.
7. Di Renzo GC, Roura LC, Facchinetti F, Antsaklis A, Breborowicz G, Gratacos E, et al. Guidelines for the management of spontaneous preterm labor: identification of spontaneous preterm labor, diagnosis of preterm premature rupture of membranes, and preventive tools for preterm birth. J Matern Fetal Neonatal Med. 2011;24(5).
8. Dodd JM, Jones L, Flenady V, Cincotta R, Crowther CA. Prenatal administration of progesterone for preventing preterm birth in women considered to be at risk of preterm birth. Cochrane Database Syst Rev. 2013;7:CD004947.
9. Haas DM, Caldwell DM, Kirkpatrick P, McIntosh JJ, Welton NJ. Tocolytic therapy for preterm delivery: systematic review and network meta-analysis. BMJ. 2012;345:e6226.
10. Hubinont C, Debieve F. Prevention of preterm labour: Update on Tocolysis. J Pregnancy. 2011;2011:941057.
11. Lee MJ, Guinn D. Antenatal corticosteroid therapy for reduction of neonatal respiratory morbidity and mortality from preterm delivery. UpToDate. 2019.
12. Lockwood CL. Preterm labor: Clinical findings, diagnostic evaluation, and initial treatment. UpToDate. 2019.
13. Lockwood CL. Spontaneous preterm birth: Pathogenesis. UpToDate. 2021.
14. National Collaborating Centre for Women's and Children's Health (UK). Preterm labour and birth. NICE guideline [NG25]. 2019.
15. Newnham JP, Dickinson JE, Hart RJ, Pennell CG, Arrese CA, Keelan JA. Strategies to prevent preterm birth. Front Immunol. 2014;5:584.
16. Norman JE, Marlow N, Messow CM, Shennan A, Bennett PR, Thornton S, et al. Vaginal progesterone prophylaxis for preterm birth (the OPPTIMUM study): a multicentre, randomised, double-blind trial. Lancet. 2016;387(10033):2106-16.
17. Raju TN, Mercer BM, Burchfield DJ, Joseph GF. Periviable birth: executive summary of a joint workshop by the Eunice Kennedy Shriver National Institute of Child Health and Human Development, Society for Maternal-Fetal Medicine, American Academy of Pediatrics, and American College of Obstetricians and Gynecologists. Am J Obstet Gynecol. 2014;210:406.
18. Simhan HN, Caritis M. Inhibition of acute preterm labor. UpToDate. 2020.
19. Society for Maternal Fetal Medicine Publications Committee. ACOG Committee Opinion number 419 October 2008 (replaces no. 291, November 2003). Use of progesterone to reduce preterm birth. Obstet Gynecol. 2008;112:963-5.
20. Sotiriadis A, Papatheodorou S, Kavvadias A, Makrydimas G. Transvaginal cervical length measurement for prediction of preterm birth in women with threatened preterm labor: a meta-analysis. Ultrasound Obstet Gynecol. 2010;35:5.
21. van Zijl MD, Koullali B, Ben WJ Mol, Pajkrt E, Oudijk MA. Prevention of preterm delivery: current challenges and future prospects. Int J Womens Health. 2016;8:633-45.
22. World Health Organization. WHO recommendations on interventions to improve preterm birth outcomes. Preterm Birth. Geneva: World Health Organization; 2018.

CHAPTER 19

Premature Rupture of Membranes

INTRODUCTION

Rupture of the fetal membranes is an integral part of the normal and abnormal parturition process. Spontaneous rupture of the membranes before the onset of labor is called premature rupture of membranes (PROM), complicates 6–19% of pregnancies with 3% of pregnant women having PROM before 37 weeks' gestation [preterm premature rupture of membranes (pPROM)]. Previable prelabor rupture of membrane occurs in <1% of pregnancies. pPROM is more likely to occur in populations of lower socioeconomic status and is responsible for, or associated with, approximately one-third of preterm births. It can lead to significant perinatal morbidity and mortality, primarily from prematurity, sepsis, cord prolapse, and pulmonary hypoplasia. In addition, there are risks associated with chorioamnionitis and placental abruption, the risk of which increases with the duration of membrane rupture.

Respiratory distress syndrome (RDS) is the most common complication after pPROM at any gestation. Serious perinatal morbidities that may lead to long-term sequelae or death are common when PROM leads to preterm birth remote from term. Acute neonatal morbidities such as necrotizing enterocolitis, intraventricular hemorrhage (IVH), and sepsis commonly complicate early preterm birth but are relatively uncommon near term. It has been established that preterm birth is a significant risk factor for long-term sequelae such as chronic lung disease, neurosensory impairment, cerebral palsy (CP), and developmental delay.

RISK FACTORS OF PRETERM PREMATURE RUPTURE OF MEMBRANES

Because the clinical course of pPROM is often unalterable once membrane rupture has occurred, it would be beneficial to identify women at risk and prevent membrane rupture from occurring. A number of risk factors have been identified, these include black race, low body mass index, low socioeconomic status, vaginal bleeding in the second and third trimester, cigarette smoking, illicit drug use, choriodecidual infection, or inflammation. Multiple gestation and polyhydramnios increase intrauterine pressure and may cause pPROM. A decrease in the collagen content of the membranes, e.g., Ehlers–Danlos syndrome, has been suggested to predispose patients to pPROM.

Women with a previous history of (H/O) pPROM have a 3.3-fold increased risk of preterm birth caused by pPROM (13.5 vs. 4.1%, $p < 0.01$) and a 14-fold higher risk of pPROM before 28 weeks (1.8 vs. 0.13%, $p < 0.01$) in a subsequent pregnancy.

A short cervix (<25 mm) by transvaginal ultrasonography (USG) has been associated with pPROM in both nulliparas and multiparas, and a positive fetal fibronectin (fFN) screen has also been associated with pPROM in multiparas. Nulliparas with a positive cervicovaginal fFN and a short cervix have been found to have a one-in-six risk (16.7%) of preterm birth caused by pPROM, whereas multiparas with a previous history, a short cervix, and a positive fFN have a 31-fold higher risk of PROM with delivery before 35 weeks than those without risk factors (25 vs. 0.8%, $p = 0.001$).

Women with H/O sexually transmitted infections, urinary tract infection (UTI) also have an increased risk of pPROM. Genital tract pathogens associated with PROM include Group B *Streptococcus* (GBS), *Escherichia coli*, *Neisseria gonorrhoeae*, *Chlamydia trachomatis*, *Bacteroides*, *Ureaplasma urealyticum*, *Mycoplasma hominis*, *Peptostreptococcus*, and *Gardnerella vaginalis*. Most commonly found bacterial isolates in acute chorioamnionitis are GBS and *E. coli* present in 20% cases but responsible for 67% cases of maternal and overwhelming fetal bacteremia. Bacterial vaginosis has been established as being associated with preterm birth and pPROM, it is unclear if this is a cause–effect relationship or if bacterial vaginosis only identifies those at risk for infection and inflammation.

PATHOPHYSIOLOGY

Although membrane rupture at term can result from a normal physiologic weakening of the membranes combined with shearing forces created by uterine contractions, pPROM can result from a wide array of pathologic mechanisms that act individually or in concert. These include intrinsic membrane weakness, mechanical stress, and ascending infection among others. Factors that could cause weakening of the fetal membranes and have been associated with PROM include local inflammation and infection, poor maternal nutrition, maternal smoking, and collagen deficiency syndromes. Choriodecidual inflammation plays an important role in pPROM, particularly when membrane rupture occurs remote from term. This is caused by an increase in local cytokines, an imbalance in the interaction between matrix metalloproteinases and tissue inhibitors of matrix metalloproteinases, increased collagenase, and protease activity.

The lower genital tract is a potential reservoir for bacteria that may ascend through the cervical canal and cause localized inflammation. Bacteria and maternal neutrophils are able to produce a number of proteolytic enzymes (e.g., collagenase, elastase, and gelatinase) that can cause local weakening of the membranes. Subsequent prostaglandin production resulting from localized inflammation can lead to occult contractions and increased shearing stress at the internal cervical os. Factors associated with mechanical distention of the membrane near the internal os include polyhydramnios, twin gestation, and incompetent cervix. Trauma may be associated with pPROM through an acute increase in intra-amniotic pressure or through the production of occult contractions. In many cases, the cause of premature membrane rupture remains unknown.

MATERNAL AND FETAL RISKS OF PRETERM PREMATURE RUPTURE OF MEMBRANES

Maternal risks of pPROM include chorioamnionitis (15-25%), postpartum infection (15-20%), abruptio placentae (4-12%), and postpartum hemorrhage (PPH). Although occurs infrequently, maternal sepsis has been reported in approximately 1% of cases, and isolated maternal deaths due to infection have also been reported.

Fetal risks result from complications of prematurity and include RDS (35%), sepsis, IVH, and necrotizing enterocolitis. *Neurodevelopmental impairment:* CP and periventricular leukomalacia have been linked to amnionitis, which is commonly seen after pPROM. CP may result from intrauterine inflammation associated with neonatal white matter damage. Elevated amniotic fluid cytokines and fetal systemic inflammation have been associated with pPROM and with periventricular leukomalacia. Umbilical cord accidents (1-2%) are associated with chance of fetal demise.

DIAGNOSIS OF PREMATURE RUPTURE OF MEMBRANES

The diagnosis of spontaneous rupture of the membranes is done from maternal history followed by a sterile speculum examination demonstrating liquor.

History

The woman will give H/O sudden gush of P/V watery discharge with continued leakage.

Per Abdominal Examination

Symphysio fundal height (SFH) does not correspond to the age of gestation. Uterus is full of fetus, fetal parts are easily felt, and fetal heart rate (FHR) is present.

Sterile Speculum Examination

Fluid is seen coming out of vagina or coming through cervix. If no fluid is coming out, ask the patient to cough or strain to see the fluid pooling in the vagina, or leaking from the cervical os. If pooling is observed, no further diagnostic test is needed.

Speculum examination should be performed in a manner that minimizes the risk of introducing infection. It provides an opportunity to inspect the cervix for umbilical cord prolapse or fetal parts prolapse, assess cervical dilatation and effacement, and obtain sample for culture as appropriate. During speculum examination, a cervical culture for Chlamydia and Gonorrhea should be performed, because women with these infections are seven times more likely to have PROM. After the speculum is removed, a vaginal and perianal (or anal) swab for GBS culture should be obtained.

Digital Cervical Examinations

Digital examinations generally should be avoided unless the patient appears to be in active labor or delivery seems imminent. Digital cervical examinations cause an average 9-day decrease in the latent period as it increases the risk of infection and add little to that available with speculum examination.

In diagnostic dilemma, the following tests are done:

- *Nitrazine paper test:* Hold a piece of nitrazine paper in a hemostat and touch it against the fluid on the speculum blade. A change in color from yellow to deep blue indicates PROM. The normal vaginal pH is between 4.5 and 6.0, whereas amniotic fluid is more alkaline, with a pH of 7.1-7.3. Nitrazine paper will turn blue when the pH is above 6.0. False-positive test results may occur in the presence of blood or semen, alkaline antiseptics, or bacterial vaginosis.
- *Fern test:* A separate swab should be used to obtain fluid from the posterior fornix or vaginal sidewalls. The fluid is dried on the slide, checked for ferning (arborization) under a low-power microscope. The presence of ferning indicates PROM, ferning has a sensitivity of approximately 90%. Vaginal blood may obscure the presence of ferns and mixture with cervical mucus can result in a false-positive result if the external cervical os has been swabbed.
- *fFN test:* fFN is a protein that functions as a "glue" attaching the amniotic sac to the uterine lining. The test measures the amount of fFN in vaginal secretions and

is performed like a Pap smear test. The detection of fFN in the vaginal fluid is a sign that a woman is at risk for preterm delivery, even if she is otherwise asymptomatic.

It is a simple bedside test, more sensitive, and specific than ferning and nitrazine tests, and can be used as complimentary test to confirm the clinical diagnosis of premature rupture of fetal membranes. It has high negative predictive value but positive result is not diagnostic.

- *AmniSure Rom test:* AmniSure (detecting placental alpha microglobulin-1 protein in vaginal fluid) may be used in diagnostic uncertainty. Amniotic protein test has high sensitivity for PROM but false positive rate may be as high as 19–30%. American College of Obstetricians and Gynecologists (ACOG) recommends that to reduce chance of adverse events in pPROM, AmniSure ROM tests should be part of overall standard method of diagnosis, including physical examination to detect leaking of amniotic fluid.

Limitations in ROM Test

A negative result does not assure the absence of membrane rupture.

False negatives may result if the amniotic sac has resealed or the position of the fetus has obstructed the rupture.

Presence of blood, meconium, antifungal creams or suppositories, or the use of lubricant with a vaginal examination may interfere with the device.

The test may not be accurate if sample collection and testing occurs after the timeframe recommended by the manufacturer.

- *Indigo-carmine dye:* If the diagnosis is still unclear, membrane rupture can be diagnosed unequivocally with ultrasonographically guided transabdominal instillation of indigo carmine dye, followed by the passage of blue-dyed fluid into the vagina, documented by a stained tampon or pad.
- *USG:* The role of ultrasound assessment of amniotic fluid volume is unclear.

MANAGEMENT

General Considerations

The management of PROM is among the most controversial issues in perinatal medicine. Management should be balanced by estimated risk for fetal and neonatal complications with immediate delivery against potential risk and benefits of conservative management. Regardless of obstetric management or clinical presentation, birth within 1 week of membrane rupture occurs in at least one half of patients with pPROM. In 35–50%, labor starts within 24 hours, in 70% within 72 hours, and 90% deliver within next 2 weeks. Spontaneous labor follows term PROM after 24, 48, and 96 hours in 70, 85, and 95% women, respectively.

The National Institute for Health and Care Excellence in England recommends expectant management in term PROM since spontaneous labor will start within 24 hours in 70–90% of cases. Norwegian guidelines suggest induction of labor 24 hours after PROM if there is no sign of infection and the cardiotocography (CTG) is reassuring. Other guidelines recommend induction of labor as soon as possible. In the latter recommendations, expectant management may still be considered acceptable in patients who decline induction of labor, provided the woman is appropriately counseled, and that the clinical condition of the woman and fetus is reassuring.

In all patients with PROM, gestational age, fetal presentation, and fetal well-being should be determined. Evaluation should include evidence of intrauterine infection, abruptio placentae, and fetal compromise. A combination of clinical assessment, maternal blood tests [C-reactive protein (CRP) and white cell count (WBC)], and FHR should be used to diagnose chorioamnionitis. Culture for GBS should be obtained when expectant management is being considered and GBS prophylaxis given based on prior culture results or intrapartum risk factors if cultures have not been performed previously.

Patients with pPROM should be admitted to hospital with periodic assessment for infection, placental abruption, umbilical cord compression, fetal well-being, and labor. Periodic ultrasound evaluation should be performed to monitor fetal growth as well as periodic FHR monitoring. Vital signs should be monitored and a rise in maternal temperature should raise suspicion for an intrauterine infection. Serial monitoring of leukocytes and inflammatory markers have not proved to be useful in diagnosing infection as they are found to be nonspecific if there is no clinical evidence of infection.

Immediate Delivery

Consider immediate delivery in the following conditions:
- Nonreassuring fetal status
- Chorioamnionitis
- Abruptio placentae—decision based on fetal status, the amount of bleeding, and gestational age
- Fetal death
- Advanced labor.

In absence of above indications management depends on gestational age:
- *Gestational age ≥ 37 weeks:* Delivery is recommended, however, short period of expectant management 12–14 hours may be "appropriately offered." If spontaneous onset of labor does not occur, induce labor with oxytocin, allow adequate time (12–18 hours) for latent phase to progress before performing a cesarean section for failed induction. Induction with prostaglandin is equally as effective as oxytocin but may have higher rates of chorioamnionitis. There is insufficient data to recommend for or against cervical ripening with mechanical methods such as a Foley balloon.

- *Late preterm ($34^{0/7}$ to $36^{6/7}$ weeks of gestation):* Either *expectant management or immediate delivery* is a reasonable option. Data suggests when comparing these two options, no difference in neonatal sepsis was found but there was an increased neonatal respiratory distress, mechanical ventilation, and intensive care unit (ICU) stay in the immediate delivery group. Maternal risk includes increased hemorrhage and infection in expectant management group.

  For both term and late pPROM, there is no substantial benefit in expectant management. Prolonging pregnancy after documentation of pulmonary maturity unnecessarily increases the likelihood of maternal amnionitis, umbilical cord compression, prolonged hospitalization, and neonatal infection, therefore, labor should be induced. Immediate management reduces the interval between rupture membrane and delivery, chorioamnionitis and postpartum febrile illness, reduce neonatal antibiotic therapy, and neonatal intensive care unit (NICU) admission. If expectant management is continued beyond $34^{0/7}$ weeks of gestation, the balance between benefit and risk should be carefully considered and discussed with patient. ACOG suggests either expectant management or immediate delivery for pregnancies with PROM at $34^{0/7th}$ to $36^{6/7th}$ weeks of gestation rather than routinely proceeding to delivery.

- *pPROM ($24^{0/7}$ to $33^{6/7}$ weeks of gestation):* In the absence of maternal or fetal contraindications, patients with PROM before $34^{0/7}$ weeks of gestation should be managed expectantly. Management includes hospital admission and monitoring for infection, hemorrhage (abruption), umbilical cord compression, fetal assessment, and evidence of labor.

  There is no consensus on the optimal frequency of assessment, but an acceptable strategy would include periodic ultrasonographic monitoring of fetal growth and periodic FHR monitoring. Observe closely for fetal or maternal tachycardia. A temperature elevation may indicate intrauterine infection. Prompt diagnosis of chorioamnionitis in preterm pregnancy requires a high index of suspicion because early sign symptoms may be subtle. In the absence of fever, regular contractions, uterine tenderness, or leukocytosis are possible indicators of amnionitis. Other criteria such as CRP and WBC count have variable sensitivity and specificity for diagnosing infection. Serial monitoring of leukocyte counts and other markers of inflammation have not been proved to be useful.

  Membranes may reseal spontaneously leading to good outcomes. Antibiotics is recommended to prolong latency (if no contraindications). A single-course of corticosteroids should be given. Obtain vaginal/rectal swab for GBS, and administer GBS prophylaxis as indicated. Patients with PROM before 32 weeks +0 days and imminent delivery are candidates for fetal neuroprotective treatment with magnesium sulfate (if no contraindications). In women with cerclage, it is unclear whether cerclage should be removed or retained but if retained, antibiotic therapy should not be extended beyond 7 days.

Delivery: Women whose pregnancy is complicated by pPROM after 24^{+0} weeks' gestation and who have no contraindications to continuing the pregnancy should be offered expectant management until 37^{+0} weeks; timing of birth should be discussed with each woman on an individual basis with careful consideration of patient preference and ongoing clinical assessment. [Royal College of Obstetricians and Gynaecologists (RCOG)—Grade A recommendation, 2019].

More recently, a Cochrane review of 3,617 women explored the effect of planned early delivery versus expectant management for women with pPROM. The authors conclude that in women with pPROM "with no contraindications to continuing the pregnancy, expectant management with careful monitoring is associated with better outcomes for the mother and baby." The Cochrane review found no differences between early birth and expectant management in neonatal sepsis or infection. Early delivery increased the incidence of RDS [relative risk (RR) 1.26, 95% confidence interval (CI) 1.05–1.53] and an increased rate of caesarean section (RR 1.26, 95% CI 1.11–1.44). There were no differences in overall perinatal mortality or intrauterine deaths when comparing early delivery with expectant management. Early birth was associated with a higher rate of neonatal death (RR 2.55, 95% CI 1.17–5.56) and need for ventilation (RR 1.27, 95% CI 1.02–1.58). The results and conclusions of this Cochrane review are influenced by those trials assessing "late" pPROM (34^{+0} to 36^{+6} weeks' gestation) such as the PPROMPT trial and it is less clear whether expectant management to 37^{+0} weeks' gestation is appropriate for women who experience pPROM at earlier gestations.

Adjunct Treatment

Adjunct management of pPROM includes considerations regarding tocolytics, corticosteroids, antibiotics, and magnesium sulfate.

Tocolysis

The use of tocolysis in pPROM is controversial and practice patterns vary widely among specialists. Tocolytic therapy may prolong the latent period but do not appear to improve neonatal outcomes. A meta-analysis of eight trials that included 408 women found use of tocolysis was associated with a longer latency period and a lower risk of delivery within 48 hours in women before $34^{0/7}$ weeks of gestation but was associated with a higher risk of chorioamnionitis.

A Cochrane review found that, compared with placebo, tocolysis in pPROM is associated with an average 73 hours longer latency of delivery (95% CI 20-126) and fewer births within 48 hours (RR 0.55, 95% CI 0.32-0.95). Tocolysis was associated with an increased risk of a 5-minute Apgar score of <7 and an increased need for ventilatory support. A retrospective case-control study in the contrary showed tocolysis after pPROM did not increase the interval between membrane rupture and delivery or reduced neonatal morbidity.

In the absence of clear evidence that tocolysis improves neonatal outcome following pPROM, it is reasonable not to use it. Additionally, it is possible that tocolysis could have adverse effects, such as delaying delivery from an infected environment, since there is an association between intrauterine infection, prostaglandin, and cytokine release and delivery. RCOG does not recommended tocolysis in women with pPROM because this treatment does not significantly improve perinatal outcome.

Indications for tocolysis: The principal indication for tocolysis in the setting of pPROM is to delay delivery for 48 hours to allow administration of a course of corticosteroids. As a general rule, tocolytics should not be administered for >48 hours. Tocolytics should not be administered to patients who are in advanced labor (>4 cm dilation) or who have any findings suggestive of subclinical or overt chorioamnionitis. Other potential contraindications include nonreassuring fetal testing (e.g., nonreactive non-stress test) and abruptio placentae.

Group B Streptococcus Prophylaxis

Revised guidelines from the Centers for Disease Control and Prevention (CDC) recommend that women with pPROM who are not in labor should receive intravenous GBS coverage for at least the first 48 hours of pPROM latency prophylaxis, until the GBS test results obtained on admission are available. The Society of Obstetricians and Gynaecologists of Canada (SOGC) and ACOG guidelines recommend 48 hours of GBS prophylaxis in addition to antibiotic therapy for latency for women with pPROM.

Supplemental Progesterone

A meta-analysis of randomized trials found initiation of progesterone supplementation after pPROM did not prolong the latency period or increase the gestational age at delivery. In women who were already on supplemental progesterone because of a prior pregnancy with preterm delivery related to preterm labor or pPROM, discontinue the medication upon diagnosis of pPROM. In particular, if the patient had been using vaginal progesterone, continuing vaginal administration may increase the risk for ascending infection.

Antenatal Corticosteroid

Antenatal corticosteroids (ACSs) reduce neonatal mortality, RDS, IVH, and necrotizing enterocolitis. ACSs are not associated with increased risks of maternal or neonatal infection regardless of gestational age and therefore should be given.

A single course should be considered between 24 and 34 weeks of gestation, may be given as early as 23 weeks in women with risk of delivery within next 7 days but should not be used in presence of frank infection. RCOG recommendation: "corticosteroids should be offered between 24^{+0} and 33^{+6} weeks" gestation; can be considered up to 35^{+6} weeks' gestation" (Grade A). Recent data indicates betamethasone in the late preterm period (between $34^{0/7}$ weeks and $36^{6/7}$ weeks) reduces respiratory morbidity in newborns. Weekly administration of ACS has been associated with a reduction in birth weight and head circumference and is not recommended.

Dose
- *Injection betamethasone:* 12 mg IM 24 hours apart for total two doses
- *Injection dexamethasone:* 6 mg IM 12 hourly for total four doses.

Antibiotics

Antibiotics prolong the latent period and improve outcomes, reduce maternal and neonatal infections, and gestational age-dependent morbidity, reduce the use of surfactant use before $34^{+0/7}$ weeks. A Cochrane review investigating the role of antibiotics for women with confirmed pPROM found that the use of antibiotics is associated with a statistically significant reduction in chorioamnionitis (RR 0.66, 95% CI 0.46-0.96). There was a significant reduction in the numbers of babies born within 48 hours (RR 0.71, 95% CI 0.58-0.87) and 7 days in the antibiotic group (RR 0.79, 95% CI 0.71-0.89). Neonatal infection, use of surfactant, oxygen therapy, and abnormal cerebral ultrasound prior to discharge from hospital was also reduced. It is advisable to administer appropriate antibiotics for intrapartum GBS prophylaxis to women who are carriers, even if these patients have previously received a course of antibiotics after pPROM.

Pharmacological agents and dose:
- Tablet erythromycin 250 mg 6 hourly for 10 days or until the woman is in established labor, whichever is sooner [National Institute for Healthcare and Excellence (NICE)]
- Intravenous ampicillin 2 g every 6 hours + tablet erythromycin 250 mg every 6 hours for 48 hours followed by oral amoxicillin 250 mg every 8 hours and erythromycin base 333 mg every 8 hours for 7 days (ACOG).

Magnesium Sulfate

Magnesium sulfate reduces the risk of CP and motor dysfunction. Women who have pPROM and are in established labor or having a planned preterm birth within 24 hours, intravenous magnesium sulfate should be offered between 24^{+0} and 29^{+6} weeks of gestation, can be considered between 30 and 33^{+6} weeks. Meta-analyses of randomized controlled trials have demonstrated that the administration of magnesium sulfate to women in established preterm labor or having a planned preterm birth in the following 24 hours, reduces CP (RR 0.69, 95% CI 0.55–0.88) and motor dysfunction in the offspring (RR 0.6, 95% CI 0.43–0.83). The benefit is greatest before 30^{+0} weeks of gestation.

- *Dose:* 4 g I/V bolus over 15 minutes followed by 1 g I/V per hour until birth or 24 hours (whichever is sooner)
- Monitor R/R, tendon reflex, urine output every 4 hourly.

Amnioinfusion

Amnioinfusion might improve neonatal outcomes in pPROM by preventing umbilical cord compression, postural deformities, pulmonary hypoplasia, and intrauterine infection. A Cochrane systematic review of five trials (using the data from four) found that amnioinfusion is associated with improved fetal umbilical artery pH at delivery, reduced variable decelerations in labor, neonatal death, neonatal sepsis, pulmonary hypoplasia, and puerperal sepsis. Another Cochrane review of one randomized controlled trial involving 66 women with spontaneous rupture of membranes between 26 and 35 weeks of gestation who received amnioinfusion during labor found no difference between amnioinfusion and no amnioinfusion for caesarean section, low Apgar scores, and neonatal death. Thus, there is insufficient evidence to recommend amnioinfusion in very pPROM as a method to prevent pulmonary hypoplasia.

Tissue sealants: A variety of tissue sealants (e.g., fibrin glue, gelatin sponge) have had some success in stopping leakage in case reports. Neither the safety nor the efficacy of these sealants has been established. There is insufficient evidence to recommend fibrin sealants as routine treatment for second-trimester oligohydramnios caused by pPROM.

Previable Premature Rupture of Membranes (<24 Weeks)

The probability of neonatal death and morbidity associated with previable PROM decreases with longer latency and advancing gestational age. About 40–50% patients with previable PROM give birth within the first week and approximately 70–80% will give birth 2–5 weeks after membrane rupture. The survival with PROM after 22 weeks is significantly higher (57.7%) than <22 weeks (14.4%). Women should be advised of, and observed for, symptoms of clinical chorioamnionitis (lower abdominal pain, abnormal vaginal discharge, fever, malaise, and reduced fetal movements). However, weekly high vaginal swab need not be performed. It is not necessary to carry out weekly maternal full blood count or CRP because the sensitivity of these tests in the detection of intrauterine infection is low (RCOG).

Patient needs counseling regarding the potential maternal, fetal, and neonatal risk following *expectant management/induction of labor*. Significant maternal complications that occur with previable PROM include intra-amniotic infection, endometritis, abruptio placentae, and retained placenta. Maternal sepsis risk is 1%.

Another concern of expectant management is that a long interval between PROM and delivery may increase the risk for perinatal infections in the offspring and associated severe neonatal morbidity and increased risk of perinatal death. Among survivors, a potential long-term outcome may be CP. The rate of pulmonary hypoplasia after PROM before 24 weeks of gestation is in the range of 10–20%. Pulmonary hypoplasia is associated with a high risk of mortality, but is rarely lethal with membrane rupture after 23–24 weeks of gestation. Early gestational age at membrane rupture and low residual amniotic fluid volume are the primary determinants of the incidence of pulmonary hypoplasia. Prolonged oligohydramnios also can result in fetal deformations, including Potter-like facies (e.g., low-set ears, recessed chin, and prominent bilateral epicanthal folds) and limb contractures or other positioning abnormalities. The reported frequency of skeletal deformations varies widely (1.5–38%) but many of these resolve with postnatal growth and physical therapy.

Management of previable PROM: Outpatient surveillance is an option following inpatient assessment. The decision to offer outpatient care depends on support at home. Distance from the hospital should be taken into account in discussion with the woman and markers of delivery latency should be assessed including presence of antepartum hemorrhage, amniotic fluid volume, gestational age at which pPROM occurred and clinical and laboratory markers of infection. Women should be advised to return to hospital immediately if sign symptoms of bleeding, labor, or infection (self-monitor temperature). Antibiotics may be considered as early as $20^{0/7}$ weeks of gestation. GBS prophylaxis, corticosteroids and tocolysis, and magnesium sulfate for neuroprotection are not recommended before viability **(Flowchart 1)**.

Management of Acute Chorioamnionitis

Diagnosis

Fever (>37.8°C or 100.4°F) and two or more of the following:
- Maternal pulse >100 bpm
- Uterine tenderness
- Fetal tachycardia >160 bpm

Flowchart 1: Management of patients with preterm premature rupture of membranes (pPROM).

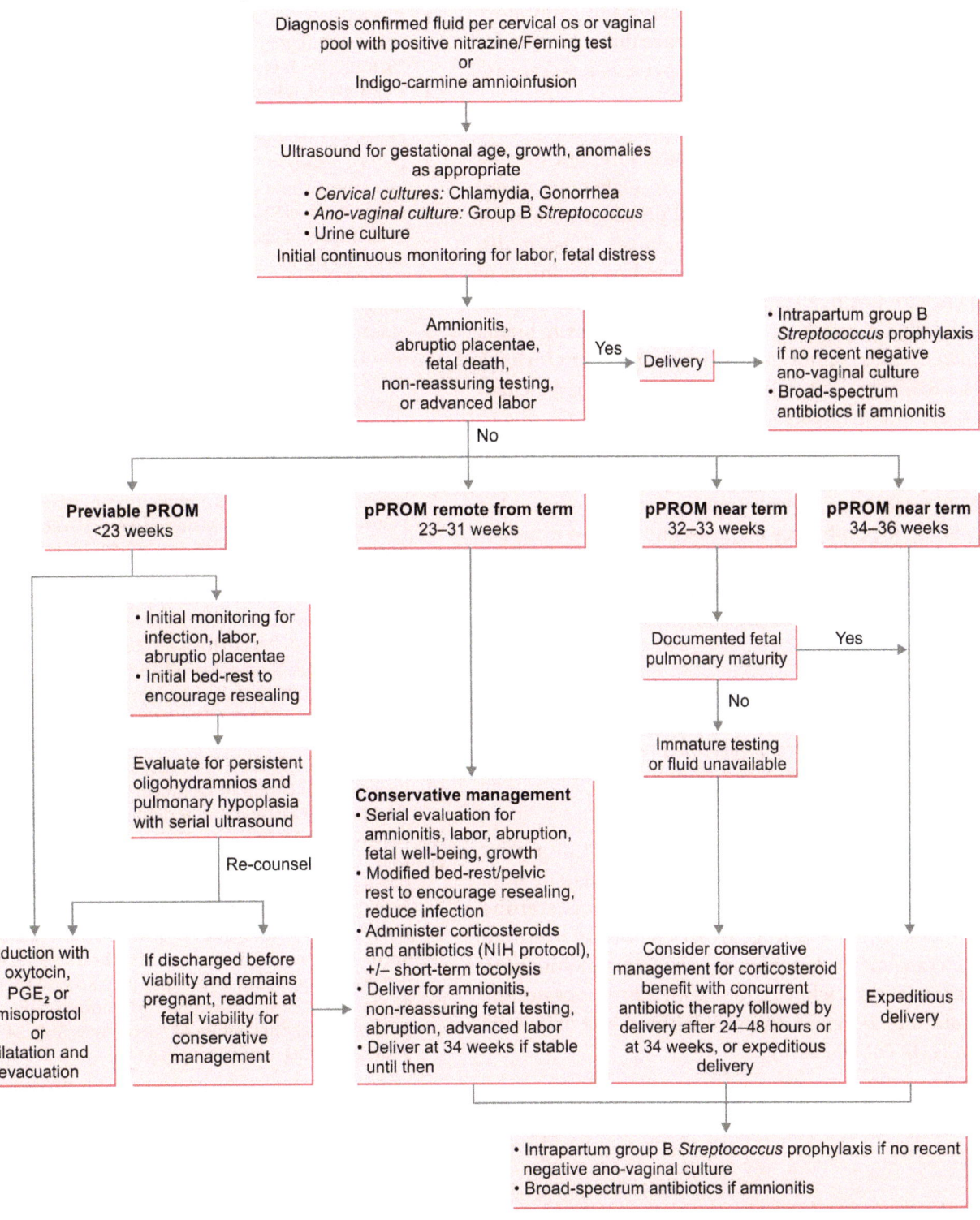

(NIH: National Institutes of Health; PGE$_2$: prostaglandin E2; PROM: premature rupture of membranes)
Source: Premature rupture of the membranes. Obstet Gynecol. 2003;101:178-93.

- Foul smelling vaginal discharge
- Leukocytosis >15,000 cumm
- CRP >2.7 mg/dL.

Management
Antibiotic treatment followed by expeditious delivery.

PREVENTION OF PREMATURE RUPTURE OF MEMBRANES IN FUTURE PREGNANCIES

Patients with prior pPROM have an increased risk of recurrent PROM and preterm birth. These women should be cared for by an obstetrician with an interest in preterm birth; ideally in a dedicated preterm labor clinic. Modifiable risk factors, such as smoking and respiratory diseases, should be addressed. Evidence that screening for lower genital tract infections and proper antenatal care are beneficial in preventing preterm birth.

Neither screening for asymptomatic infection with treatment of positive results nor empiric antibiotic therapy has been proven to prevent pPROM. A single randomized trial evaluated whether screening all pregnant women for genital tract infection (bacterial vaginosis, *T. vaginalis*, Candidiasis) before 20 weeks plus standard treatment of patients with positive results found that the intervention reduced the number of spontaneous preterm births compared with a control group (spontaneous preterm birth 3.0 vs. 5.3%, 95% CI 1.2–3.6). Limitations of this trial include that it did not distinguish between preterm births due to preterm labor versus pPROM and the authors used only Gram stain to diagnose infection.

A 2015 systematic review of randomized trials concluded that antibiotic prophylaxis in the second or third trimester did not reduce the risk of pPROM (RR 0.31, 95% CI 0.06–1.49; one trial, 229 women) or preterm birth (RR 0.85, 95% CI 0.64–1.14; five trials, 1,480 women); subsequent trials have also not shown a benefit.

Cervical cerclage: Serial transvaginal ultrasound scans to determine the cervical length and consider cerclage in the following situations: Current singleton pregnancy with prior spontaneous preterm birth before 34 weeks and cervical length <25 mm prior to 24 weeks.

Progesterone: Women who have had pPROM in a prior pregnancy with singleton pregnancy may benefit from progesterone supplementation. Offer progesterone supplementation starting at 16–24 weeks. Vaginal progesterone may help reduce the risk for premature birth with short cervix, while 17 alpha-hydroxyprogesterone caproate may be given to those without a short cervix (MARCH OF DIMES, 2020).

SUGGESTED READING

1. Committee on Practice Bulletins-Obstetrics. ACOG Practice Bulletin No 188. Prelabour Rupture of Membranes. 2018;131(1):e1-14.
2. Deborah M, Victoria MA. The prevention of early onset-neonatal group B streptococcal disease. SOGC Clinical Practice Guideline. 2016;l38(12).
3. Duff P, Lockwood CJ. Preterm prelabor rupture of membranes: management and outcome. UpToDate. 2021.
4. Lorthe E, Ancel PY, Torchin H, Kaminski M, Langer B, Subtil D, et al. Impact of latency duration on the prognosis of preterm infants after preterm premature rupture of membranes at 24 to 32 weeks' gestation: a national population-based cohort study. J Pediatr. 2017;182:47.
5. Mader J, Craig C. Management of Group B *Streptococcus*—positive women with preterm premature rupture of the membranes: still a therapeutic dilemma. J Obstetr Gynaecol Canada. 2018;40(12):1627-31.
6. Medina TM, Hill DA. Preterm premature rupture of membranes: diagnosis and management. Am Fam Physician. 2006;73(4):659-64.
7. Mercer BM, Edward KSC. Premature rupture of the membrane. In: Creasy and Resnik's Maternal-Fetal Medicine, 8th edition. Amsterdam: Elsevier; 2018. pp. 712-22.
8. Mercer BM. Preterm premature rupture of the membranes. GLOWN. 2008. [online] Available from: https://www.glowm.com/section-view/heading/Preterm%20Premature%20Rupture%20of%20the%20Membranes/item/120#.YmaqrdpByUk. [Last accessed April 2022].
9. Obgproject. (2017). ACOG Guidance Update: Diagnosis and Management of PROM (Prelabor Rupture of Membranes). [online] Available from: https://www.obgproject.com/2017/12/29/acog. [Last accessed April 2022].
10. Prevention of Group B Streptococcal Early-Onset Disease in Newborns, ACOG committee opinion No 797. Obstet Gynecol. 2020;135(2):e51-72.
11. RANZCOG. (2020). Term Prelabour Rupture of Membranes (Term PROM). [online] Available from: https://ranzcog.edu.au/RANZCOG_SITE/media/RANZCOG-MEDIA/Women%27s%20Health/Statement%20and%20guidelines/Clinical-Obstetrics/Term-Prelabour-Rupture-of-Membranes-(Term-Prom)-(C-Obs-36)-July-2021.pdf?ext=.pdf. [Last accessed April 2022].
12. Thomson AJ. Care of women presenting with suspected preterm prelabour rupture of membranes from 24^{+0} weeks of gestation. BJOG. 2019;126(9):e152-66.

CHAPTER 20

Amniotic Fluid Disorder

INTRODUCTION

Amniotic fluid (AF) is present from early in pregnancy and is produced almost exclusively by the fetus. It plays an important role in growth, development, and ultimately a good pregnancy outcome. It is usually well regulated in pregnancy. AF problems occur in about 7% of pregnancies. The main disorders associated with AF are:
- Excess fluid (polyhydramnios)
- Insufficient fluid (oligohydramnios).

Too much or too little AF is associated with increased maternal and perinatal complications. The perinatal mortality rate (PMR) approaches 90–100% with severe oligohydramnios in the second trimester and can exceed 50% with significant polyhydramnios in mid-pregnancy. Subjective or semiquantitative ultrasound measurement systems are used to identify and categorize disorders of amniotic fluid volume (AFV). Obstetric management is based on the underlying cause of the abnormal AFV.

PHYSIOLOGY OF AMNIOTIC FLUID SYNTHESIS

Amniotic fluid is produced from different sources through pregnancy. In early pregnancy, AF is a dialysate of maternal and fetal plasma, with water and solutes traversing the fetal skin bidirectionally. By the second trimester, when the fetal skin keratinizes and becomes impermeable to water, the AF becomes increasingly hypotonic and is derived predominantly from fetal urine and lung fluid. AF is removed mainly by fetal swallowing and absorption into fetal blood in the chorionic plate vessels (intramembranous pathway) and intravascular absorption. A fetus close to term produces between 500 and 1,200 mL urine and swallow between 210 and 760 mL of AF per day. This dynamic process of AF regulation results in a fairly stable volume of around 800 mL from 24 weeks' gestation until near term, when there is a decline (Figs. 1A and B). How this delicate balance is maintained is largely unknown; although the intramembranous pathway is currently believed to be the principal regulatory mechanism.

The relative attribution of each of these mechanisms varies over the course of the pregnancy. A disturbed equilibrium can be the result of compromised swallowing function or increased urination and can lead to polyhydramnios. Even small changes in this equilibrium can result in significant alterations in AF volume, which reflects the association between fetal gastrointestinal tract obstruction and severe cases of polyhydramnios.

Furthermore, uteroplacental unit function contributes to AF balance. If uteroplacental insufficiency occurs in association with fetal growth restriction, the fetus redistributes the blood flow to critical areas such as the heart, the brain, and the suprarenal glands, at the expense of renal perfusion. This reduced blood flow to the kidneys results in decreased renal output, leading to oligohydramnios.

Recently, a more modern concept recognizes that AF is dynamic and can rapidly change due to normal maternal physiological processes (hydration, activity and rest phase, position, etc.). It is unlikely that such factors would affect the ultrasound observations; however, they may alter the diagnosis near the upper and lower thresholds of normality.

POLYHYDRAMNIOS

Definition

Hydramnios, also called polyhydramnios, is a condition in which there is too much AF around the fetus. This assessment of polyhydramnios can be a subjective assessment or a quantitative estimation using the maximal vertical pocket (MVP), amniotic fluid index (AFI), two-diameter pocket or three-dimensional measurements. Currently, it is widely accepted that polyhydramnios is defined as an MVP >8 cm, or an AFI of 25 cm or greater. A reasonable working definition of polyhydramnios using current sonographic criteria is an AFI >95th centile for corresponding gestational age.

Incidence

Incidence varies between 0.1 and 3.0% in general obstetric population, as frequency depends upon criteria used for diagnosis.

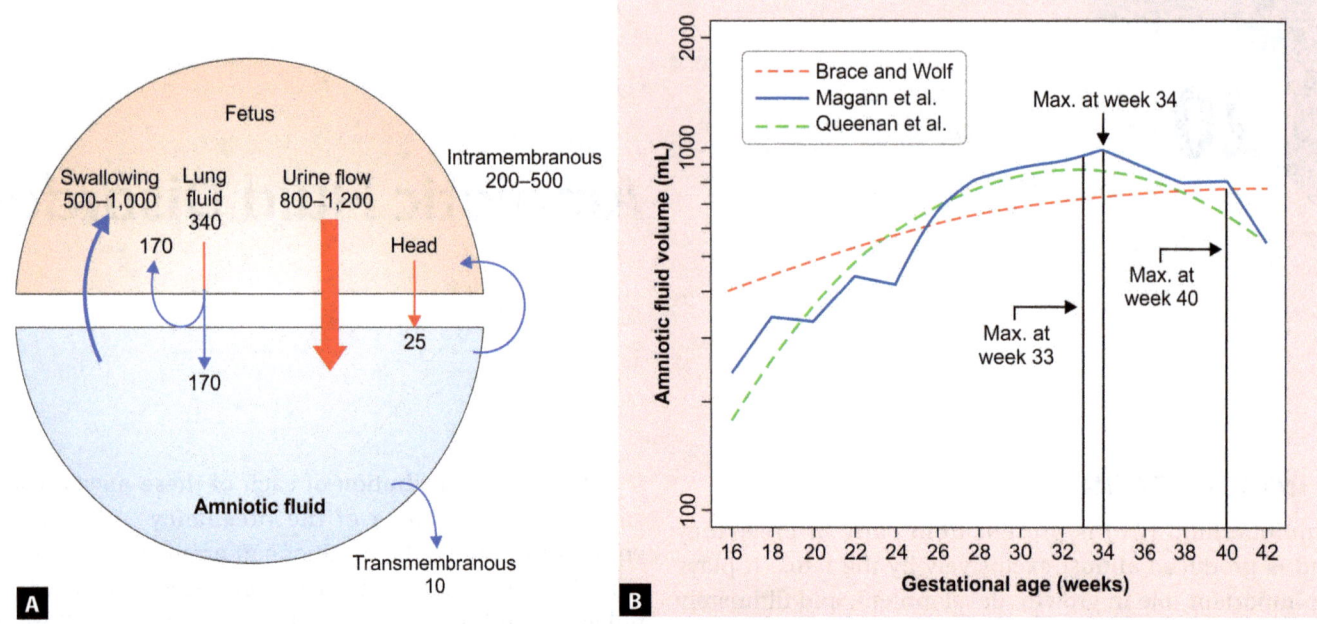

Figs. 1A and B: Amniotic fluid dynamics.
(Max.: maximum vertical pocket)

Classification

In about 80% of cases, the polyhydramnios is mild, in 15% moderate and in 5% severe.

- Based on AFI, polyhydramnios is classified as:
  - Mild (25–29 cm)
  - Moderate (30–34 cm)
  - Severe (>35 cm)
- Based on MVP, it can be classified as:
  - Mild (8–11 cm)
  - Moderate (12–15 cm)
  - Severe (>16 cm)

There is another classification depending on rapidity of onset. *Acute:* Rapid accumulation of AF within 1 week with severe abdominal pain and respiratory distress. *Subacute polyhydramnios* develops over a period of 2 weeks with less severe symptoms and *chronic hydramnios* is gradual accumulation with less maternal discomfort.

Etiology

Most cases of mild polyhydramnios are idiopathic, but most cases with moderate or severe polyhydramnios are due to maternal or fetal disorders. There are two major causes: (1) Reduced fetal swallowing and (2) increased fetal urination.

Reduced Fetal Swallowing

Due to brain abnormalities (e.g., anencephaly and Dandy–Walker malformation), facial tumors, gastrointestinal obstruction (e.g., esophageal or duodenal atresia, small bowel obstruction), compressive pulmonary disorders [e.g., pleural effusions, diaphragmatic hernia, congenital pulmonary airway malformation (CPAM), congenital high airway obstruction syndrome (CHAOS), narrow thoracic cage due to skeletal dysplasias], and fetal akinesia deformation sequence (due to neuromuscular impairment of fetal swallowing) may lead to polyhydramnios.

Increased Fetal Urination

From maternal diabetes mellitus and maternal uremia (increased glucose and urea cause osmotic diuresis), hyperdynamic fetal circulation due to fetal anemia (e.g., red blood cell isoimmunization or congenital infection), fetal and placental tumors (e.g., sacrococcygeal teratoma, placental chorioangioma), or twin-to-twin transfusion syndrome (TTTS) can also cause polyhydramnios.

Causes of Polyhydramnios

Table 1 shows the causes of polyhydramnios.

Clinical Presentation

In most cases, polyhydramnios develops late in the second or in the third trimester of pregnancy. Symptoms may include rapid growth of uterus and discomfort in the abdomen. Patients may suffer from difficulty in breathing or difficulty in lying down. Palpitation may also be a presenting complaint. Symptoms are mainly from mechanical stresses, patients may experience persistent shortness of breath, uterine irritability and contractions, and abdominal discomfort when uterine distention is severe. Symphysiofundal height is found more than the gestational age, abdomen is hugely enlarged, with fullness at the flanks. Abdominal skin tense and shiny; fetal lie and presentation unstable, fetal heart sounds not easily audible.

TABLE 1: Causes of polyhydramnios.	
Maternal	Rh-isoimmunization and uncontrolled diabetes
Placental	Chorioangioma, twin–twin transfusion syndrome, and circumvallate placenta
Fetal anomalies	
CNS	Anencephaly, meningomyelocele, holoprosencephaly, hydrocephalus, encephalocele, spina bifida, microcephaly, hydranencephaly, and DWM (Dandy–Walker Malformation)
Head and neck	Goiter, cystic hygroma, and cleft palate
Respiratory	Tracheal agenesis, CDH, congenital cystic adenomatoid malformation, bronchopulmonary dysplasia, and TOF
GIT	Esophageal atresia, duodenal or jejunal atresia, annular pancreas, midgut volvulus, omphalocele, and gastroschisis
Skeletal	Arthrogryposis multiplex, osteogenesis imperfecta, and thanatophoric dysplasia
Cardiac	Coarctation of aorta, fetal arrhythmias, and truncus arteriosus
Renal/endocrine	Bartter syndrome and vasopressin insufficiency
Fetal tumor	Sacrococcygeal teratoma, nephroma, and neuroblastoma
Genetic	Trisomy 13, 18, 21, monosomy, Pena–Shokeir syndrome, myotonia dystrophica, and Beckwith–Wiedemann syndrome
Intrauterine infection	Rubella, syphilis, toxoplasmosis, parvovirus, and CMV
Miscellaneous	Nonimmune hydrops fetalis, fetal retroperitoneal fibrosis
Idiopathic	50–60%

(CDH: congenital diaphragmatic hernia; CMV: cytomegalovirus; CNS: central nervous system; GIT: gastrointestinal tract; TOF: tetralogy of Fallot)

Diagnosis

Polyhydramnios is suspected if the uterus is large for gestational age (LGA) or if the fetus cannot be easily palpated or is ballotable.

Recognizing the importance of AF in obstetric outcomes—normal, increased, or decreased—the assessment of AFV for daily clinical practice has centered around ultrasound using either subjective or semiquantitative methodologies. Of the semiquantitative methodologies, only AFI and MVP are measured in routine clinical practice.

Subjective Assessment of AFV

The subjective assessment of AFV is a visual interpretation of AF using ultrasound examination without an objective measurement. There are limited data comparing the subjective evaluation of AFV with direct measures; however, the few publications available demonstrate a satisfactory correlation. For experienced sonographers, the subjective impression of normal compared with abnormal AFV may be used but is difficult to translate across users over time.

Semiquantitative Ultrasound Assessment of AFV

The two most common methods of objectively measuring the AFV are the *AFI and MVP* (also known as the single deepest vertical pocket).

The AFI is determined by summing four vertical quadrants with the transducer positioned in a sagittal plane perpendicular to the floor and was first introduced by Phelan and colleagues in 1987 for term pregnancies. This measurement system was subsequently expanded to include second and third trimester pregnancies (16–42 weeks' gestation), and gestation-specific normal ranges for AFI were developed.

The MVP technique is also widely used with a 2-cm cut-off being most widely clinically accepted as discriminating normal from low AF. The ultrasound threshold for low AFV is generally accepted as an AFI of 5 cm or less or a MVP of 2 cm or less as these values have been associated with an increased risk for adverse perinatal outcomes. Interestingly, the upper limit of AFI to define polyhydramnios is less well-defined but is typically >25 cm (or MVP > 8 cm) **(Figs. 2A and B)**.

Studies that have compared estimates of AFV by ultrasound (MVP and AFI) with actual measurements taken by the dye-dilution technique demonstrated that MVP and AFI measurements are poor predictors of actual AFV. Magann et al. reported a sensitivity of 10% (specificity 96%) for an AFI measurement of <5 cm and the sensitivity was 5% (specificity 98%) for MVP up to 2 cm for oligohydramnios. For cases of suspected polyhydramnios, an AFI >20 cm had a sensitivity of 29% (specificity 97%), as did an MVP of >8 cm (specificity 94%). The MVP method had fewer false-positive tests compared with the AFI. Based on these findings, the authors concluded that the MVP is superior to the AFI.

Most diagnoses of polyhydramnios are now based on sonographic findings. There is no consensus which one should be the method of choice. Due to asymmetric location of fetus within the uterus, the use of MVP technique may lead to an overdiagnosis of AF volume, therefore, AFI has been described as a more reliable means **(Fig. 3)**.

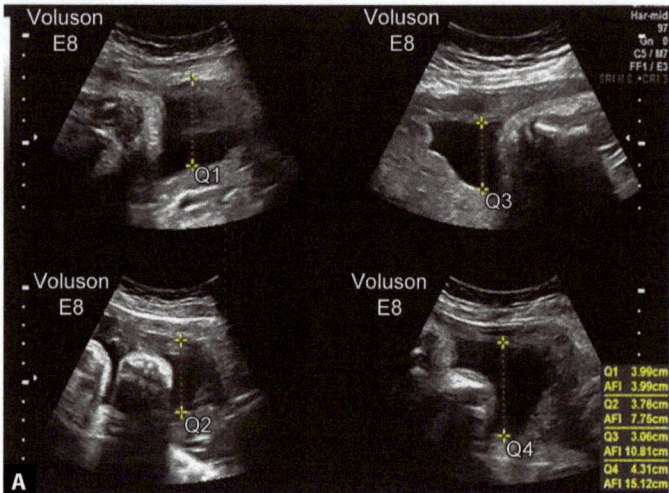 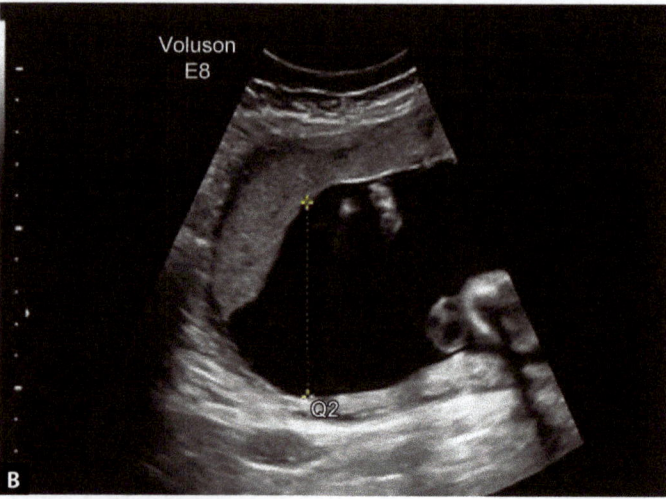

Figs. 2A and B: Ultrasound evaluation of amniotic fluid using the amniotic fluid index technique and the maximum vertical pocket technique.

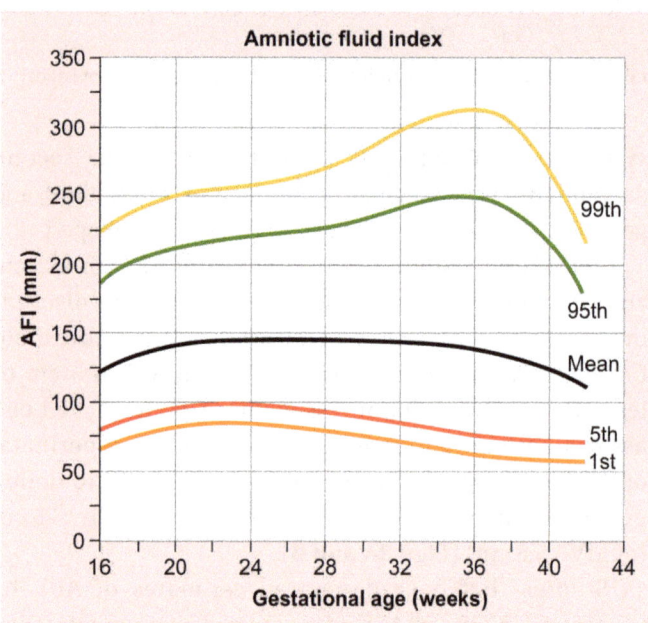

Fig. 3: Centile chart for amniotic fluid index.

Detailed Anomaly Scan

Detailed sonographic examination of fetus for any structural abnormality is the key to find out underlying cause of polyhydramnios. In spite of a normal sonographic evaluation, risk of a major anomaly is 1% with mild, 2% with moderate, and 11% with severe polyhydramnios. Small stomach or a nonvisualization of stomach, despite 45 minutes of scanning, is considered abnormal or suggestive of esophageal atresia. Evaluation of long bones and thorax will determine presence of a skeletal dysplasia. Assessment of fetal swallowing, movements, tone, and examination of joints are keys to diagnosis of neuromuscular abnormalities.

If fetal hydrops is identified, the next step is evaluation for an immune or nonimmune etiology. Evaluation of potential fetal anemia includes assessment of peak systolic velocity of the middle cerebral artery with a value >1.5 multiples of the median, suggesting moderate or severe anemia, irrespective of the cause. Work-up for fetal anemia includes testing for fetomaternal hemorrhage by Kleihauer–Betke test and screening for maternal antibodies to D, C, Kell, Duffy, and Kidd antigens to determine maternal antibody production against the fetal red blood cells. Fetal hydropic changes need testing for parvovirus infection.

Congenital cardiac disease found in ultrasonography (USG) demands fetal echocardiography for further evaluation. When evaluating significant ultrasound anomalies (placental calcifications, brain abnormality, etc.), fetal infections such as cytomegalovirus, toxoplasmosis, syphilis, and parvovirus B19 should be considered and testing for TORCH infection indicated.

In monochorionic multiple gestation, polyhydramnios in one of the twins may be a sequence suggestive of TTTS which entails a referral to fetal medicine specialist. Finally, assessment of cervical length to quantify the risk of preterm labor (PTL) is helpful in planning further management of pregnancy.

Search for Other Etiology

Search for other etiology—exclude diabetes mellitus
- Oral glucose tolerance test
- Glycosylated hemoglobin.

Genetic Analysis

In a fetus with no identifiable structural anomaly, role of karyotyping is controversial.

Amniocentesis must be offered in cases with identifiable structural anomaly on sonography, symmetric intrauterine growth restriction (IUGR), or when there is imperfect sonographic visualization of fetal anatomy. In severe polyhydramnios with a normal karyotype and ultrasound findings of anomalies, microarray or gene sequencing may detect a genetic abnormality of clinical significance. For example, 22q11.2 microdeletion syndrome is associated with polyhydramnios and hypoplastic thymus as the only sonographic findings. Noonan syndrome is often associated with polyhydramnios, as well as other abnormalities, and can be diagnosed by gene sequencing. Prenatal DNA testing should be considered for myotonic dystrophy mutation, if there is abnormal posturing of extremities on USG with relevant family history.

Complications of Polyhydramnios

- *Maternal:* Malpresentation, mechanical distress, premature rupture of membranes (PROM), preterm labor, abruptio placentae, cord prolapse, inadequate uterine contraction, increased operative interference, and postpartum hemorrhage (PPH)
- *Fetal:* Prematurity, intrauterine fetal death (IUD), fetal distress, and increased perinatal mortality.

Management (Flowchart 1)

Depends largely on possible underlying etiology. Referral to maternal–fetal medicine specialists in cases of:
- Suspected fetal anomaly
- Small for gestational age fetus
- Concerns with fetal movements
- Persistent or worsening polyhydramnios.

Medical Management

Prostaglandin synthetase inhibitors: Such as indomethacin (COX1 and 2 inhibitor) and sulindac (COX-2) have been used. These drugs reduce AFV by decreasing fetal urinary output and by enhancing resorption of lung fluid secondary to increased fetal breathing. Dose of indomethacin 25 mg orally 6 hourly to 2–3 mg/kg/day orally or per rectally. Maternal complications include gastrointestinal tract (GIT) intolerance, transient cholestatic jaundice, transient renal insufficiency, and pulmonary edema.

Fetal complications: Oligohydramnios and ductal constriction.

Neonatal complications: Renal insufficiency, persistent fetal circulation, ileal perforation, and necrotizing enterocolitis (NEC).

Monitoring during drug therapy:
- Weekly assessment of AFI
- Fetal echocardiography within 24 hours then weekly.

Discontinuation of therapy: If AFI reduced >2/3rds of initial volume or echocardiography shows tricuspid regurgitation (TR).

Some fetal medicine units in the UK use sulindac as it is a selective COX-2 inhibitor and has a better adverse-effect profile. Sulindac at the dose of 200 mg 12 hourly has been shown to be most effective in unexplained polyhydramnios or polyhydramnios associated with distal gastrointestinal (GI) obstruction. As these medications are associated with significant fetal adverse effects such as dose and gestational-age-dependent constriction of ductus arteriosus and impaired renal function, these drugs are to be used only under strict specialist supervision.

Amnioreduction

Therapeutic amniocentesis is reserved to treat polyhydramnios with significant maternal discomfort and impending PTL. Complications such as PTL, PROM, chorioamnionitis, and placental abruption are relatively small (~1.5%). However, there is a high likelihood of recurrence, thus requiring repeated procedures. Serial amniodrainage can be technically difficult and the risk of the aforementioned complications increases with each procedure. Once the cause is ascertained, treat accordingly and follow-up these patients with serial ultrasound scans to monitor liquor volume and fetal growth. Mild polyhydramnios resolves frequently without any intervention.

Timing of Delivery and Management of Labor

There is insufficient evidence in literature for induction of labor for polyhydramnios alone. Mild polyhydramnios can be simply monitored and treated conservatively. Usual recommendations are induction of labor by controlled artificial rupture of the membranes (ARM), performed by an obstetrician and with consent to proceed to lower-segment cesarean section (C/S) if required, as there is increased risk of cord prolapse/abruptio placentae with such procedure.

There is no absolute contraindication to use of oxytocin or prostaglandins, these agents should be used with caution. Elective preterm delivery is not indicated even in severe polyhydramnios, consideration should be given to deliver at 39 weeks because of maternal discomfort. There is a marked increase in the incidence of postpartum hemorrhage related to atony, preparation for such complications as well as shoulder dystocia and PPH, are advisable. In case of unexplained polyhydramnios, a thorough neonatal examination, with a minimum of checking the patency of upper GIT using a nasogastric tube, is recommended.

Prognosis

Polyhydramnios is associated with a higher fetal loss rate of up to 4%, which increases to 60% if fetus has coexistent structural anomalies. Long-term outcome for infants following a prenatal diagnosis of polyhydramnios depends on the gestational age at delivery and on the presence of associated structural malformations. In cases of additional malformations, the long-term outcome will

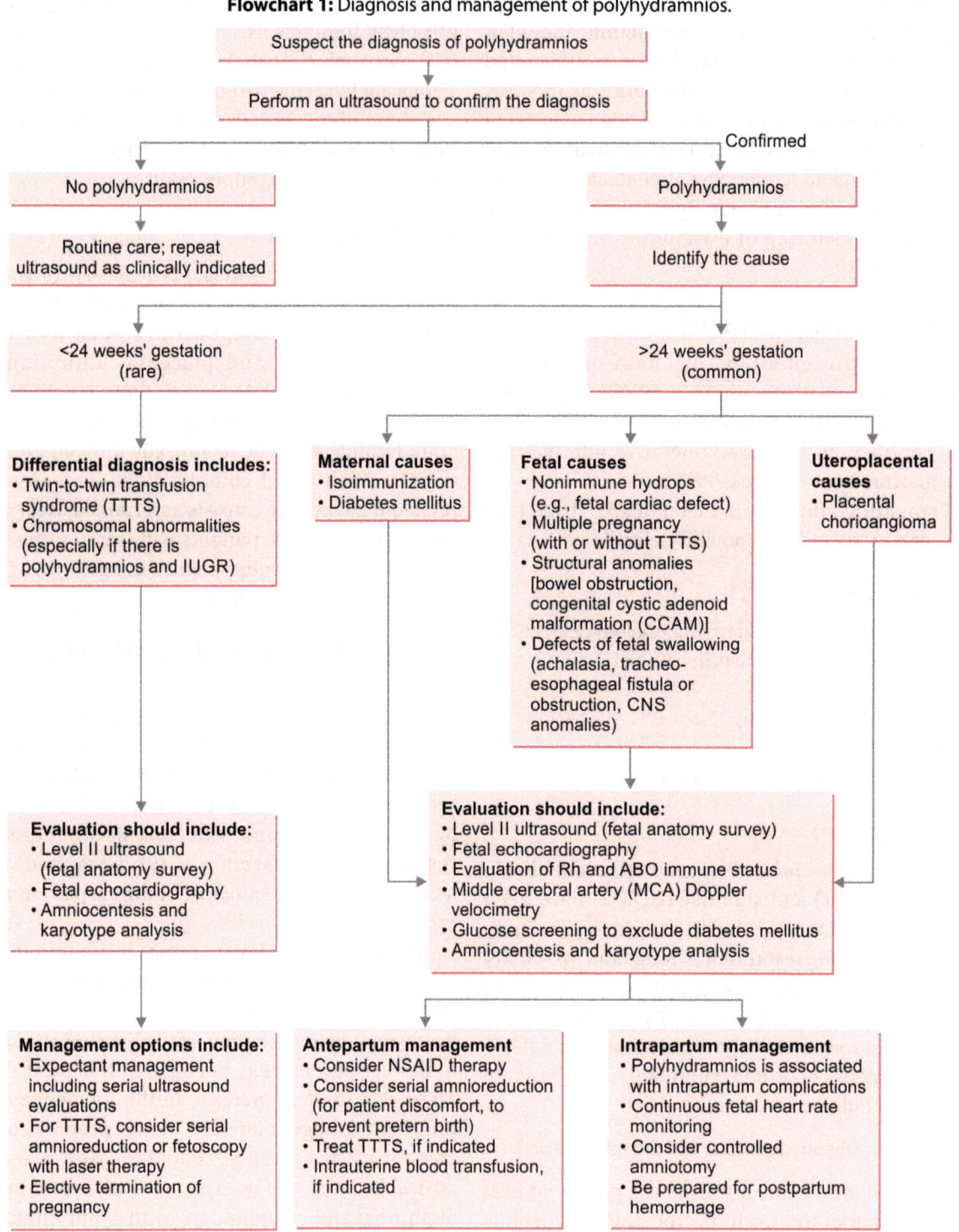

Flowchart 1: Diagnosis and management of polyhydramnios.

(CNS: central nervous system; IUGR: intrauterine growth restriction; NSAID: nonsteroidal anti-inflammatory drug)

primarily be dictated by the nature of the abnormality rather than by the existence of polyhydramnios.

Genetics and Recurrence Risk

Recurrence of idiopathic polyhydramnios is uncommon. Risks associated with recurrent polyhydramnios include the risk of fetal malformations and premature delivery. Polyhydramnios attributable to a specific genetic diagnosis may recur based on the pattern of inheritance of the condition.

Practice Recommendations

- Polyhydramnios means an excessive accumulation of the AF; it can be associated with an increased risk of adverse pregnancy outcomes, such as preterm birth, placental abruption, and fetal anomalies.

- The AFV depends on a balance between its production (mainly by fetal kidneys and lungs) and its uptake or removal (by fetal swallowing or absorption into the fetal surface).
- Polyhydramnios can be idiopathic, or due to fetal or maternal causes. Severe polyhydramnios (AFI >30 cm) in the second trimester being associated with significant perinatal morbidity due to prematurity or aneuploidy.
- The current main modality of diagnosing polyhydramnios is ultrasound assessment of AFV whether subjectively or quantitative assessment using either the single MVP ≥8 cm or AFI ≥25 cm. A quantitative estimation should be performed to differentiate between mild, moderate, or severe polyhydramnios (AFI < 30, between 30 and 35, and >35 cm, respectively).
- A comprehensive maternal and fetal evaluation including detailed fetal anatomic ultrasound evaluation to identify the cause of polyhydramnios (whether fetal, or maternal, or idiopathic cause) is essential to guide the further management.
- Management depends mainly on the treatment of the underlying cause and the relief of the maternal symptoms caused by the excessive AF.
- Treatment should be individualized and in a multidisciplinary team with involvement of a fetal medicine specialist and may require amnioreduction to control symptoms in severe cases and to prolong pregnancy in preterm cases.
- There is no clear evidence or guidelines regarding timing of delivery or management of labor, but labor should be managed with continuously monitored fetal heart rate by cardiotocography (CTG) and rupture of membranes should be managed considering the risk of cord prolapse.

■ OLIGOHYDRAMNIOS

Introduction

Low AF, or oligohydramnios, is usually defined as a MVP <2 cm or an AFI <5 cm. Oligohydramnios also defined as a decrease in the volume of AFV below 5th centile for the gestational age. If AFI is <5 cm or MVP <1 cm, it falls into the category of severe oligohydramnios.

Oligohydramnios is associated with an increased risk for fetal or neonatal death, which may be related to the underlying cause of the reduced AFV or due to sequelae of the reduced AFV. The pregnancy outcome principally depends on the underlying cause of the low AFV and the gestation at recognition. Oligohydramnios in early mid-pregnancy typically has a different cause to that diagnosed in the late second or the third trimester, reflecting different perinatal outcomes.

Epidemiology

Oligohydramnios complicates approximately 4.5% of all pregnancies and severe oligohydramnios affects approximately 0.7% of pregnancies. It is more common in pregnancies beyond term, complicates as many as 12% of pregnancies beyond 41 weeks.

Etiology

Oligohydramnios is secondary to either an excess loss of fluid, or a decrease in fetal urine production or excretion. The three main underlying causes of oligohydramnios are:

1. Preterm premature rupture of the membranes (pPROM)
2. Congenital renal abnormalities
3. Intrauterine growth restriction.

Congenital malformations of the fetal renal tract with absence of functioning renal tissue or lower urinary tract obstruction are recognized causes of second trimester oligohydramnios. These severe fetal conditions are readily recognized by ultrasound with absence of renal tissue bilaterally, abnormal renal appearances or megacystis. The outcome for these fetuses tends to be universally dismal.

Causes of Oligohydramnios

Fetal Causes

- Premature rupture of the membranes
- Chromosomal abnormalities such as trisomy 13 and triploidy
- Congenital anomalies (particularly renal anomaly)
- Intrauterine infection
- IUGR, IUD, postdated pregnancy.

Maternal Causes

- Preeclampsia
- Antiphospholipid syndrome and systemic lupus erythematosus (SLE)
- Chronic hypertension (HTN)
- Chronic renal disease.

Placental Causes

- Placental insufficiency
- TTTS
- Amnion nodosum.

Iatrogenic

Amniocentesis.

Drug induced

- Angiotensin-converting enzyme (ACE) inhibitor
- Prostaglandin synthetase inhibitor.

Idiopathic/unexplained: The majority of oligohydramnios cases, 50.7% diagnosed in the third trimester, are of unexplained etiology and, typically, associated with better outcome.

Fetal Congenital Anomalies and Oligohydramnios

- Bilateral renal agenesis (Potter syndrome)
- Nonfunctioning fetal kidneys, e.g., bilateral multicystic dysplastic kidneys, infantile polycystic kidney diseases
- Obstructive uropathy (posterior urethral valves, urethral atresia, bilateral ureteropelvic junction obstruction)
- Chromosomal anomalies (trisomy 13 and aneuploidy)
- Viral infections [cytomegalovirus (CMV)]

Diagnosis

In most of the cases, patients do not give any specific symptom of oligohydramnios. They may complaint of less fetal movement, or per vaginal watery discharge.

History

Detailed history of the patient includes H/O per vaginal watery discharge, history of chronic HTN, antiphospholipid antibody (APLA) syndrome, SLE, pregnancy-induced hypertension in current pregnancy, drug history (COX-2 inhibitor), history of anomalous baby in previous pregnancy, any evidence of recent maternal viral infection.

Examination

Measurement of blood pressure (BP) is of utmost importance. On abdominal examination, symphysial fundal height (SFH) is usually found less than gestational age, abdominal girth is also less than gestational age, uterus is full of fetus, IUGR may be found. Per speculum examination with aseptic precaution must be carried out if patient complaints of escape of liquor.

Confirmation of Diagnosis

Amniotic fluid volume changes with gestational age and ways of accurately estimating it have changed over the years. Transabdominal USG is the gold standard for the detection of liquor volume. Suspicion of oligohydramnios may be prompted by discrepancies in sequential fundal height measurements, or by easily palpable fetal parts through maternal abdomen. During ultrasound, normal-appearing fetal kidneys and fluid-filled bladder may be observed to rule out renal agenesis, cystic dysplasia, and ureteral obstruction.

Fetal growth should be checked to exclude intrauterine growth restriction leading to oliguria. Doppler ultrasound could be used to assess placental insufficiency, in suspected cases.

Amniotic Fluid Index and Maximal Vertical Pocket

The two most commonly used objective methods of determining AFV include measurement of the MVP depth and the summation of the depths of the largest vertical pocket in each quadrant, or the AFI. (The pregnant abdomen is divided into four quadrants by using the umbilicus as a reference point to divide the uterus into upper and lower halves, and by using the linea nigra to divide the uterus into left and right halves.) The four measurements are summed to obtain the AFI in centimeter. Pockets should be free of fetal limbs and the umbilical cord **(Figs. 4A and B)**.

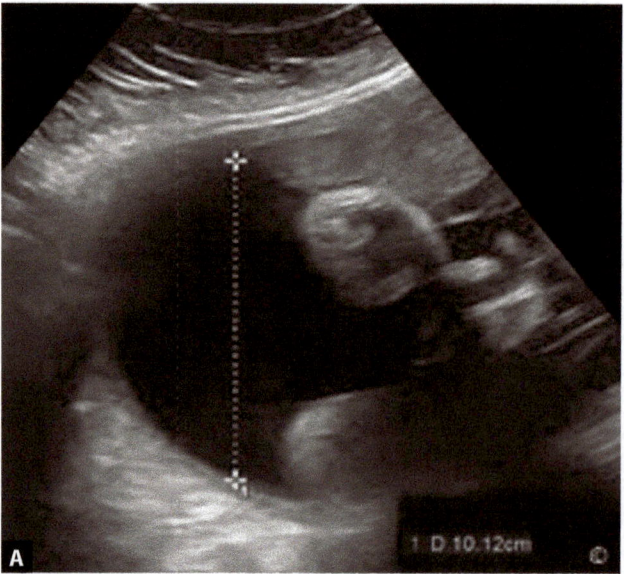
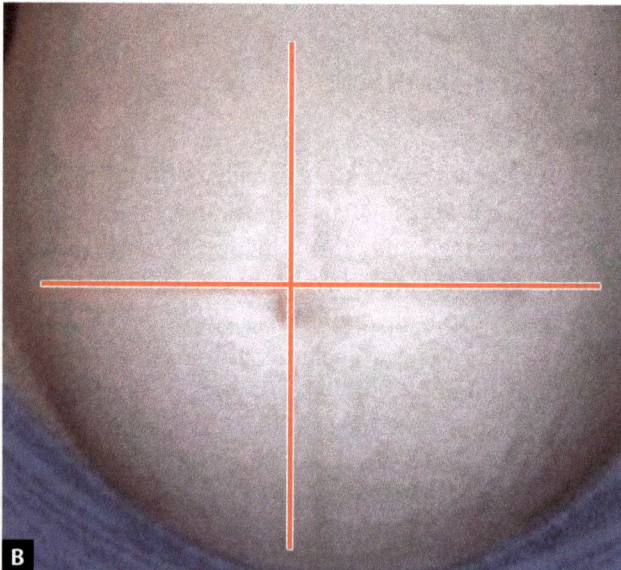

Figs. 4A and B: Measurement of single vertical pocket and amniotic fluid index.

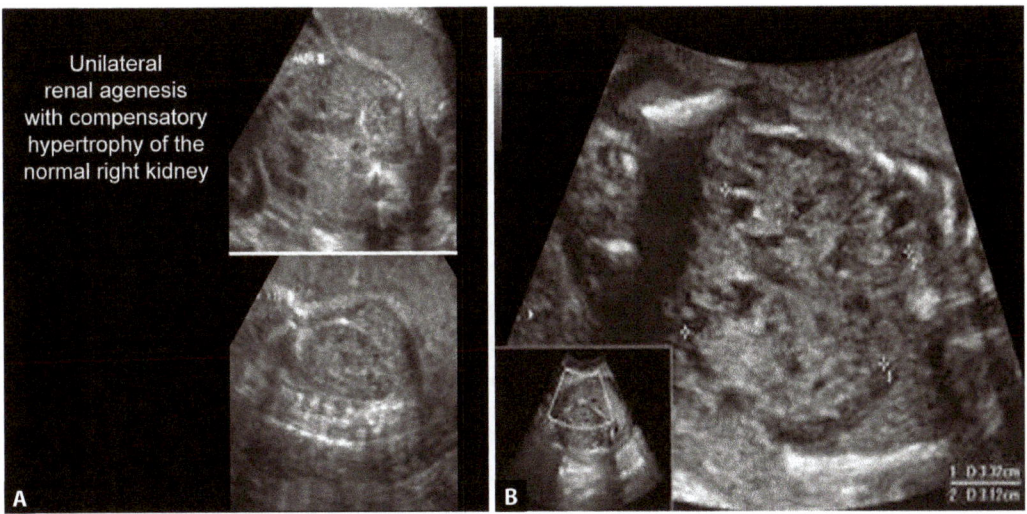

Figs. 5A and B: (A) Unilateral renal agenesis; (B) Polycystic kidney disease.

Amniotic fluid volume may be artificially increased if the transducer is not maintained perpendicular to the floor. Excessive pressure on the maternal abdomen with the transducer may lead to an artificially reduced measurement.

A meta-analysis of randomized controlled trials concluded that MVP measurement during fetal surveillance is a better choice. The use of the AFI increases the rate of diagnosis of oligohydramnios and the rate of induction of labor without any improvement in peripartum outcomes. In a systematic review, Nabhan and Abdelmoula assessed four randomized controlled trials in singleton pregnancies comparing AFI and MVP as components of antepartum fetal surveillance to prevent adverse pregnancy outcome. Use of AFI to determine oligohydramnios compared with MVP was associated with an increase in the diagnosis of oligohydramnios [relative risk (RR), 2.33; 95% confidence interval (CI), 1.67–3.24], an increase in labor induction (RR, 2.10; 95% CI, 1.60–2.76), and an increase in cesarean delivery for fetal compromise (RR, 1.45; 95% CI, 1.07–1.97). There was no difference in adverse perinatal outcomes using either measurement technique (admission to neonatal intensive care unit, cord arterial pH < 7.1, Apgar score < 7 at 5 minutes or meconium). The authors concluded that MVP is the preferred measurement method for AFV, with AFI overestimating the presence of oligohydramnios and leading to increased obstetric intervention with no improvement in pregnancy outcomes.

In a recent review, Moise found that the MVP was superior to the AFI in diagnosing oligohydramnios using an MVP < 2 cm. Although the MVP appears to be the preferred method to diagnose oligohydramnios near term, the vast majority of research on ultrasound measurement of AFV utilizes the AFI.

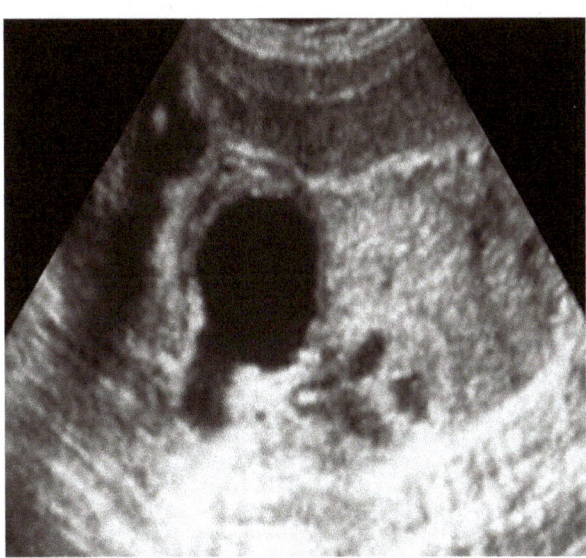

Fig. 6: Keyhole sign with outlet obstruction.

Detailed Anatomic Survey (Figs. 5 and 6)

A targeted ultrasound may help to identify a cause. Assessment includes structural abnormalities especially fetal kidney and bladder, size, shape, position, number and echogenicity of fetal kidney, corticomedullary differentiation, presence of renal cysts, any dilatation in renal pelvis, ureter, any obstruction, and key hole sign (suggestive of bladder outlet obstruction). Absence of bladder filling following a 1-hour period of observation suggests urinary tract abnormality. Thorough examination of other system including any evidence of trisomy, evidence of intrauterine infection, IUGR, placental insufficiency, or evidence of pulmonary hypoplasia should also be noted.

With oligohydramnios diagnosed before 24 weeks of gestation, possibility of pulmonary hypoplasia should be ruled out. Normal values for fetal thoracic circumference to abdominal circumference remain constant throughout gestation at 0.89. A ratio < 0.8 in the setting of severe oligohydramnios along with bell-shaped chest and flattened diaphragm in the second trimester is suspicious for pulmonary hypoplasia.

Other Investigations

Amniocentesis for detection of chromosomal anomalies—it is particularly indicated in cases of early-onset oligohydramnios with structural anomalies and/or if fetus shows evidence of symmetrical IUGR. Tests for APLA syndrome and for fetal infection in suspected cases.

Complications

The risks associated with oligohydramnios depend on the gestational age at which it is diagnosed. Early-onset oligohydramnios is often associated with more serious complications.

Fetal Complications

- Pulmonary hypoplasia
- Fetal compression syndrome. Deformity due to intra-amniotic adhesion or compression: Limb contractures or amputation, dolichocephaly, club feet, and Potter syndrome
- Amniotic band syndrome and fetal infection (in prolonged rupture of membrane)
- Cord compression and meconium staining
- An increased chance of stillbirth.

Maternal Complications

- Prolonged labor due to uterine inertia
- Iatrogenic preterm birth
- Increased operative interference—cesarean delivery.

Management

Management depends on underlying cause of oligohydramnios, gestational age at diagnosis, severity, progression of the condition, fetal status, and well-being.

Treatment Options

Presence of fetal congenital malformation needs referral to a fetal medicine unit. A team approach, including a medical geneticist, should be ideal to discuss about possible fetal outcome, available postnatal treatment options, mode, and timing of delivery. The finding of significant oligohydramnios in the second trimester is associated with very high perinatal mortality.

A combination of oligohydramnios and fetal growth restriction is associated with significantly increased perinatal mortality and morbidity and close fetal surveillance is indicated. In cases of severe oligohydramnios prior to 24 weeks' gestation, termination of pregnancy should be discussed with the patient.

Treatment Strategies for Isolated Oligohydramnios

Occasionally oligohydramnios in mid-pregnancy may not have an identifiable etiology and is termed "isolated oligohydramnios." The pathophysiology of isolated oligohydramnios itself is not clearly understood, but it reflects chronic or late-onset placental insufficiency. In term pregnancies with isolated oligohydramnios, baby should be delivered and in preterm with isolated oligohydramnios, conservative management is advisable to minimize perinatal morbidity due to prematurity.

Oral Hydration Therapy

The mother's fluid balance (and also therefore the fetus') has a major effect on the AFV. Increased maternal fluid intake has been shown to increase the AFV in women with oligohydramnios. The treatment of maternal dehydration with oral or intravenous rehydration has been shown to increase the AFV by 30%.

Rapid oral hydration in women with no other high-risk factor has been found to be effective in increasing AFV. Intake of 250 mL of water (or hypotonic solution) in 15 minutes, total of 2 L of water or hypotonic solution in 2 hours can lead to an increase in fluid volume in both oligohydramnios and normohydramnios, with minimal risks to the mother and the baby.

Hydration with water reduces maternal plasma osmolality and increased uteroplacental perfusion. It has the advantages over others as it is cheap, easily available, noninvasive, and does not require hospitalization or extensive monitoring. However, it requires consistent and long-term therapy.

Intravenous Hydration Therapy

Several studies on maternal hydration by IV fluids over a short duration found an increase in AFI. Better results were achieved by IV *hypotonic solution of 2 L administered within a single day*. However, significant improvements were not reported by isotonic hydration. Mechanism of action was similar to oral hydration, but increase in fluid volume was transitory.

Drug Treatment

L-arginine is a promising drug for the treatment of oligohydramnios. Nitric oxide (NO) synthesized from L-arginine is a potent vasodilator, which improves uteroplacental perfusion by reducing viscosity of blood. Several studies have reported an improvement in AFV after *L-arginine* intake of 3 g as sachet daily for 2-4 weeks. It is noninvasive and does not require monitoring and has an added advantage that its administration does not require hospitalization. However, most of these studies had small sample size and no meta-analysis found in literature.

Management Based on Gestational Age

Planned birth in an obstetric unit is recommended. Transfer to a tertiary referral center may be appropriate if oligohydramnios is severe.

Before Term

Expectant management is often the most appropriate course of action, depending on maternal and fetal condition. Ongoing antepartum surveillance including assessment of fetal growth and follow-up monitoring of AFV is necessary. Continuous fetal heart rate monitoring during labor has been advocated for all pregnancies complicated by oligohydramnios. Emergency delivery anytime when fetal compromise is suggested on CTG or on Doppler.

At Term

Delivery is often the most appropriate management. With reassuring fetal testing, delivery may be safely delayed on the basis of the parity, gestational age, inducibility of the mother's cervix, and the severity of the oligohydramnios.

Observational studies have reported that prolonging pregnancy till 37 completed weeks in patients with isolated mild oligohydramnios and no other comorbid condition resulted in a good perinatal outcome. To prevent antepartum stillbirth, American College of Obstetricians and Gynecologists (ACOG) recommends labor induction between $36^{0/7}$ and $37^{6/7}$ weeks in pregnancies with isolated or otherwise uncomplicated oligohydramnios (MVP < 2 cm).

After Term

Timing of delivery in patients with isolated oligohydramnios is controversial. Isolated oligohydramnios in the post-term patient has no greater risk for caesarean delivery and there is insufficient evidence to support induction for women with oligohydramnios.

Mode of Delivery

Based on usual obstetric practices, there is no indication to alter mode of delivery based solely on the presence of oligohydramnios. Elective C/S for significant oligohydramnios with unfavorable cervix.

Fetal Intervention

Amnioinfusion

Amnioinfusion has been described to reduce incidence of pulmonary hypoplasia in patients with severe oligohydramnios remote from term. In this process, sodium chloride or Ringer lactate is infused under ultrasound guidance via a needle inserted through the uterine wall. The current evidence on the safety and efficacy of this procedure means it is only undertaken in the UK under special arrangements that include audit and research.

Vesicoamniotic Shunts

Vesicoamniotic shunts may be used to divert fetal urine to the amniotic cavity where fetal obstructive uropathy is determined to be the cause of oligohydramnios. The procedure though effective in reversing oligohydramnios, its ability to achieve sustainable good renal function in infancy is variable. Pulmonary function cannot be guaranteed with restoration of AFV. Although an established procedure, there are limited safety and efficacy data and it is only undertaken in the UK under special arrangements for research.

Prognosis

The earlier in pregnancy that oligohydramnios occurs, the poorer the prognosis. Fetal mortality rates as high as 80-90% have been reported with oligohydramnios diagnosed in the second trimester. Most of this mortality is a result of major congenital malformations and pulmonary hypoplasia secondary to PROM before 22 weeks of gestation. The inspiration of AF at regular intervals is probably needed for terminal alveolar development.

Pregnancies complicated by severe oligohydramnios have been shown to be at increased risk of fetal morbidity. Mid-trimester PROM often leads to pulmonary hypoplasia, fetal compression syndrome, and amniotic band syndrome.

Genetics and Recurrence Risk

If the underlying cause is due to bilateral renal agenesis, recurrence risk is approximately 3-4% with negative family history. The recurrence risk for PROM occurring in a future pregnancy is uncertain, but may be as high as 32%. Such patients should therefore be considered at high risk for this complication in all future pregnancies.

■ SUGGESTED READING

1. Abhyankar S, Salvi V. Indomethacin therapy in hydramnios. J Postgrad Med. 2000;46(3):176-8.
2. ACOG committee opinion no. 764: Medically indicated late-preterm and early-term deliveries. American College of Obstetricians and Gynecologists. Obstet Gynecol. 2019;133(2):e151-5.

3. Aref A, Napolitano R. Common Obstetric Conditions, Polyhydramnios. GLOWN. 2021. [online] Available from: https://www.glowm.com/article/heading/vol-10—common-obstetric-conditions—polyhydramnios/id/409583#.YmaaXNpByUk. [Last accessed April 2022].
4. Beloosesky R, Ross MG. Oligohydramnios: etiology, diagnosis, and management. Up To Date. 2021.
5. Bianchi DW, Crombleholme TM, Mary D'Alton ME, Malone F. Fetology: diagnosis and management of the fetal patient, 2nd edition. New York: Mc Grew-Hill, Medical Pub Division; 2010.
6. Chauhan NS, Namdeo P, Modi JN. Evidence based management of oligohydramnios. J Gynecol. 2018;3(3):2-7.
7. Hamza A, Herr D. Polyhydramnios: causes, diagnosis and therapy. Geburtshilfe Frauenheilkd. 2013;73(12):1241-6.
8. Hwang DS, Bordoni B. Polyhydramnios. Treasure Island (FL): StatPearls. 2021.
9. Jones J. Polyhydramnios. Radiopedia. 2021. [online] Available from: https://radiopaedia.org/articles/polyhydramnios. [Last accessed April 2022].
10. Karkhanis P, Patni S. Polyhydramnios in singleton pregnancies: perinatal outcomes and management. Obstet Gynaecol. 2014;16:207-13.
11. Keilman C, Shanks AL. Oligohydramnios. Treasure Island (FL): StatPearls. 2021.
12. Lockwood CJ, Moore T, Copel J, Silver RM, Resnik R. Creasy and Resnik's maternal-fetal medicine: principles and practice, 8th edition. Amsterdam: Elsevier; 2019.
13. Nabhan AF, Abdelmoula YA. AFI versus single deepest vertical pocket as a screening test for preventing adverse pregnancy outcome. Cochrane Database Syst Rev. 2008(3): CD006593.
14. OBGYN Key. (2019). Amniotic fluid disorders. [online] Available from: https://obgynkey.com/disorders-of-amniotic-fluid. [Last accessed April 2022].
15. The Fetal Medicine Foundation. (2021). Polyhydramnios. [online] Available from: https://fetalmedicine.org/education/fetal-abnormalities/amniotic-fluid/polyhydramnios. [Last accessed April 2022].

CHAPTER 21

Congenital TORCH Infections

INTRODUCTION

TORCH infections are a group of congenitally acquired infections that cause significant morbidity and mortality in the neonates. The infections that comprise to form acronym of *TORCH* include T = toxoplasmosis, O = others (syphilis, varicella zoster, parvovirus B19), R = rubella, C = cytomegalovirus (CMV), and H = herpes simplex virus (HSV) infection. These pathogens are most commonly transmitted from the mother to the child either transplacentally or during the birth process, through contact with blood and vaginal secretions or from breast milk (for few infections). While each infection is distinct, there are many similarities in how these infections present. The infected fetus may show abnormal growth, developmental anomalies, or multiple clinical and laboratory abnormalities; many of the clinical syndromes in the immediate neonatal period overlap, while some pathogens show distinct classic physical stigmata.

The epidemiology of these infections varies; but the burden of the disease is maximum in low to middle-income countries (LMIC). In these countries, TORCH infections are major contributors to prenatal, perinatal, and postnatal morbidity and mortality including miscarriages, stillbirths, and a constellation of severe birth defects in infants; evidence of infection may be seen at birth, in infancy, or years later.

Most of the TORCH infections cause mild maternal morbidity, also treatment of maternal infection frequently has no impact on fetal outcome. Recognition of maternal disease and fetal monitoring once the disease is recognized are important. For many of these pathogens, treatment or preventive strategies are available; knowledge of these diseases will help the clinicians appropriately counsel mothers on preventive measures to avoid these infections and will aid in counseling on the potential for adverse fetal outcomes when these infections are present.

SCREENING FOR TORCH INFECTIONS

- There is significant controversy regarding the benefits and cost-effectiveness of routine screening of TORCH infections in pregnancy. According to American College of Obstetricians and Gynecologists (ACOG) and Federation of Obstetric and Gynaecological Societies of India (FOGSI), routine full "TORCH PANEL" screening is not recommended in low-risk asymptomatic pregnant women and should not be done for investigation of recurrent miscarriage (FOGSI, 2014).
- "TORCH Panel screening" is done in a pregnant woman in the following conditions: When congenital infections are suspected in pregnancies; such as those with:
  - Unexplained intrauterine growth restriction (IUGR)
  - Unexplained intrauterine death (IUD)/stillbirth
  - Fetal brain lesions (intracranial calcifications, microcephaly, and hydrocephalus)
  - Fetal hydrops
  - Other sonographic markers (hepatosplenomegaly and echogenic bowel) of fetal infection
- Pregnant women with nonvesicular rash with other signs and symptoms suggestive of systemic infection
- Pregnant women with significant contact with a person of such illness.

INTERPRETATION OF TORCH SEROLOGY

Screening of TORCH infections in the pregnant women is most commonly done by enzyme-linked immunoassay (ELISA). Paired serological tests are to be done 3–4 weeks apart and are most helpful only when the first sample has been drawn during clinical illness. Rise in titer in the second sample is indicative of recent infection.

- Immunoglobulin M (IgM) and IgG both –ve would mean woman is unexposed to infection or is unvaccinated (in case of Rubella).
- IgM +ve and IgG –ve would mean an acute or primary infection.
- IgM –ve and IgG +ve usually mean past infection.
- IgM +ve and IgG +ve would mean that the mother has faced the pathogen sometime in the past. IgM may be present due to cross reactivity with other microbes. And IgG may be present due to nonspecific polyclonal stimulation of the immune system.

When serology cannot give the conclusive result about when infection has occurred, IgG avidity test is indicated. Avidity assay measures the maturity of the IgG antibody, which helps to identify a primary infection with greater accuracy than simple IgG and IgM titers.

A high avidity means an infection before 3 months and a low avidity means an infection within 3 months. Knowing when infection has occurred during pregnancy is important:
- To evaluate the risk of fetal transmission
- To ensure appropriate prenatal counseling
- To initiate appropriate therapy.

DIAGNOSIS OF TORCH INFECTIONS IN THE FETUS

Fetal infection is suspected when maternal infection is diagnosed during the pregnancy or fetal ultrasound is suggestive of infection. Definitive diagnosis of fetal infection is done by amniotic fluid polymerase chain reaction (PCR), culture, or cordocentesis. The amniotic fluid PCR will become positive only after 4 weeks from the time of maternal infection. So, amniocentesis needs to be timed accordingly. Evidence of maternal infection does not necessarily mean fetal affection, on the contrary, the fetus may not have structural anomalies in spite of getting infected. So, serial monthly sonography should be done. Long-term fetal squeal is not predictable.

TOXOPLASMOSIS

Toxoplasma gondii is a parasitic infection that can be acquired by ingestion of toxoplasma tissue cysts in raw or undercooked meat or from infectious oocysts which are excreted by cats or which are present in contaminated soil/water or unpasteurized goat milk.

Incidence

Seroprevalence in pregnant women varies greatly among countries; the highest prevalence is noted in regions with tropical climates, where the oocysts can survive in soil, as well as countries with dietary customs of raw meat consumption. Seroprevalence among Brazilian, French women, and women in the United States (US) at childbearing age is approximately 77, 44, and 11%, respectively. Prevalence of maternal infection ranges from 0.5 to 1:10,000 live births per year in the US.

Symptoms and Transmission (Fig. 1)

Primary infection is often asymptomatic (60–70%) but some women may suffer from malaise, fever, or lymphadenopathy. Overall risk of symptomatic infection is 10%. Fetal infection occurs only when there is primary maternal infection. Fetal transmission risk increases with gestational age at seroconversion (from 1% before 4 weeks, between 4 and 15% at 13 weeks, to 60% at 36 weeks), but the severity is

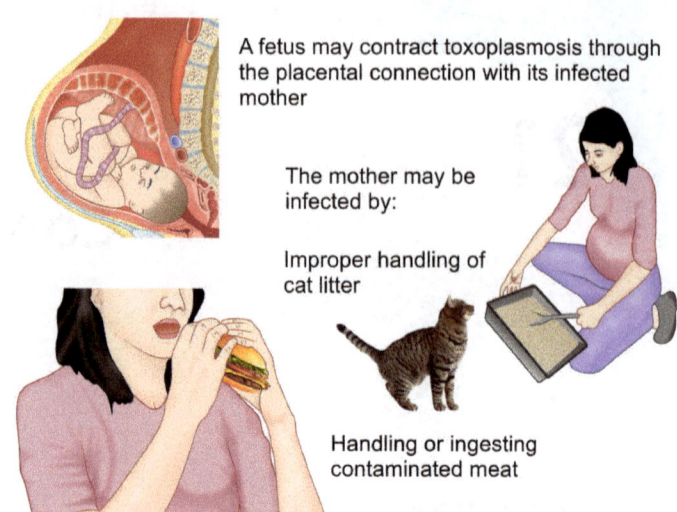

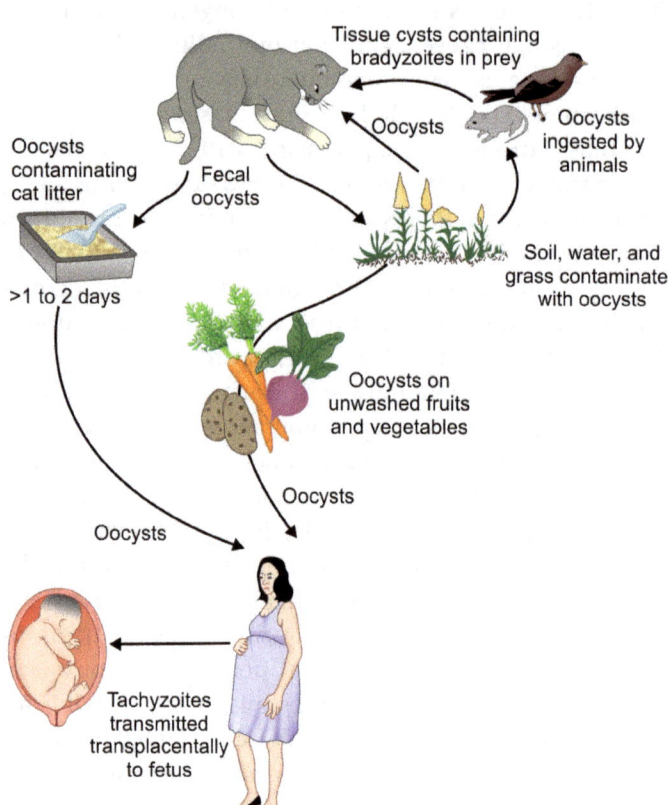

Fig. 1: Transmission of toxoplasmosis in pregnancy.
Source: Slideplayer.com

greatest when infection occurs during the first trimester. The combined risk of having an affected fetus, with proven maternal primary infection, is highest in the middle of pregnancy, at 13–28 weeks.

Diagnosis of Maternal Infection

Mainly based on serological testing for toxoplasma-specific IgG and IgM. IgM usually appears within 2 weeks of exposure and can persist up to 18 months but varies between individuals and method of assay used. The false positive rate is around 2%, therefore a positive test on a sample should be

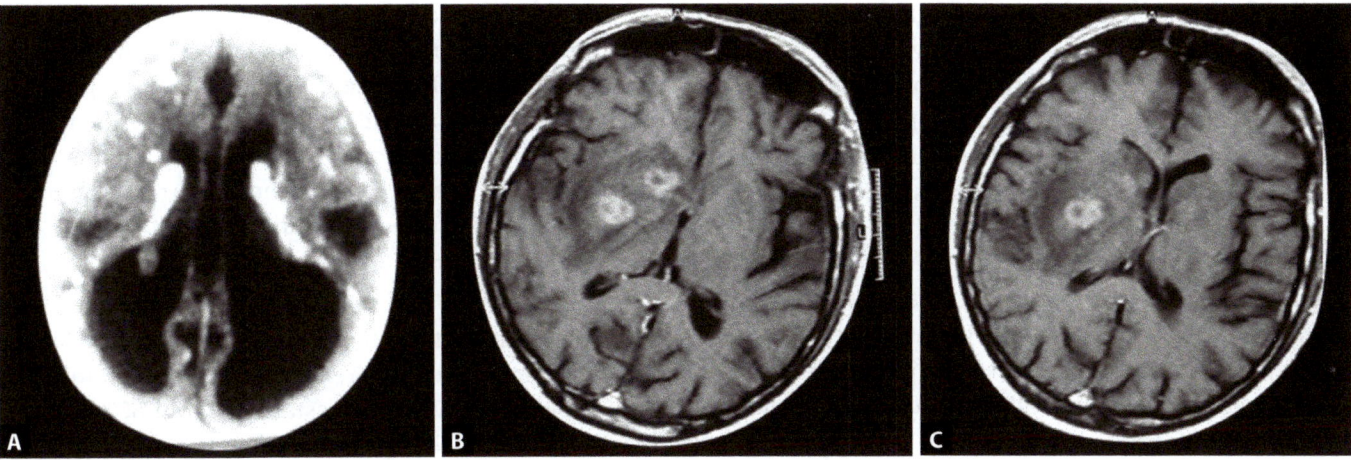

Figs. 2A to C: MRI brain. Diffuse intracerebral calcifications and hydrocephalus in neonatal toxoplasmosis.

repeated [Royal College of Obstetricians and Gynaecologists (RCOG)]. IgG usually appears approximately 2 weeks after the exposure and persists lifelong. Measurement of IgG reactivity on sequential samples is informative. IgG measurement using enzyme immunoassay (EIA)/Latex is moderately sensitive and specific but dye test is very sensitive and specific. If both IgG and IgM are positive, the infection may be acute and serologic testing should be repeated in 2–3 weeks. If on subsequent testing IgG is increased, the infection is most likely acute.

Avidity Test

Avidity 30% indicates infection within the preceding 3 months, while 40% indicates infection 6 months previously.

Diagnosis of Fetal Infection

If there is confirmed primary maternal infection or if fetal infection is suspected from ultrasonography (USG), the patient should be referred to a fetal medicine unit. Fetal diagnosis is based on the detection of *T. gondii* DNA in amniotic fluid. Amniocentesis should be considered after 18 weeks of gestation, since fetal diuresis is not fully established until 18–20 weeks of gestation and accumulation of toxoplasma to detectable levels may not occur for up to 6 weeks after maternal seroconversion; a negative result prior to this may necessitate a repeat procedure, and a positive result would lead to a change from treatment with spiramycin to a pyrimethamine/sulfadiazine regimen. Cordocentesis to detect toxoplasma IgM has been used but has significantly lower sensitivity for detection of fetal infection.

Ultrasound features of fetal infection include ventriculomegaly, hydrocephalus, microcephaly, intracerebral calcification, cataract formation, and ascites. Magnetic resonance imaging (MRI) of the fetal brain when the ultrasound is inconclusive or incomplete, or to rule out definitive brain lesions in the presence of a normal ultrasound.

Detection of Neonatal Infection (Figs. 2A to C)

- Computed tomography (CT)/MRI will show intracranial calcification, hydrocephalus, ring-enhancing lesion
- *T. gondii*-specific IgM antibody in serum/cerebrospinal fluid (CSF)
- PCR for *T. gondii* DNA in CSF/serum
- *Ophthalmological examination:* Chorioretinitis.

Congenital Toxoplasmosis

Although any organ can be affected by *T. gondii*, toxoplasmosis mainly affects the central nervous system (CNS) and eyes.

Classic triad of congenital toxoplasmosis includes: Microcephaly or hydrocephalus, intracranial calcification, and chorioretinitis.

Nonspecific signs:
- Blueberry muffin' rash—cutaneous erythropoiesis
- Hepatosplenomegaly and jaundice
- Thrombocytopenia
- Growth restriction.

Sequelae of Subclinical Congenital Toxoplasmosis

Infants with subclinical congenital toxoplasmosis who do not receive treatment have an increased risk of long-term sequelae. The most common late finding is chorioretinitis which can result in vision loss. Intellectual disability, deafness, seizures, and spasticity can be seen in a minority of untreated children.

Management of Infected Fetus

Spiramycin administered to the mother reduces the risk of fetal infection by 60–70%; however, no good evidence that it reduces the severity of the disease. Spiramycin therapy does not appear to have any maternal or fetal toxicity. Therefore, where primary maternal infection is confirmed before 16 weeks of gestation, it is sensible to begin treatment empirically rather than delay starting until after amniocentesis is undertaken, as longer the interval between maternal seroconversion and the start of treatment, the greater the likelihood of fetal transmission. If amniocentesis is not possible, spiramycin should be started and continued throughout pregnancy with the aim of reducing transmission to the fetus.

In cases where the amniotic fluid is positive for toxoplasma DNA, transmission to the fetus is assumed. Since the negative predictive value of PCR is not 100%, monthly ultrasound follow-up should be initiated even in cases of negative amniocentesis. The risk of an affected fetus should be assessed in conjunction with timing of maternal infection. In cases of confirmed fetal infection, the options include maternal drug therapy with a pyrimethamine/sulfadiazine regimen throughout pregnancy, with ultrasound surveillance for evidence of fetal damage, or termination of pregnancy.

Treatment
- *Confirmed maternal infection:* Spiramycin 1 g three times daily
- *Confirmed fetal infection:* Pyrimethamine 50 mg once daily, sulfadiazine 1 g three times daily, folinic acid 50 mg weekly. This regimen is alternated weekly with spiramycin regimen.

Note: Infants diagnosed prenatally with toxoplasmosis, either symptomatic or asymptomatic, as well as infants diagnosed postnatally 12 months, treatment with pyrimethamine and sulfadiazine is indicated. Weekly full blood count (FBC) is necessary in mothers and babies taking pyrimethamine as this drug is a folate antagonist.

Prevention of Toxoplasmosis During Pregnancy
- Avoid raw meat and cured meat, such as Parma ham, eat meat that has been thoroughly cooked (i.e., with no trace of blood or pinkness).
- Wash hands, chopping boards, and utensils thoroughly after preparing raw meat.
- Wash all fruit and vegetables thoroughly before cooking/eating to remove all traces of soil.
- Avoid unpasteurized goats' milk and dairy products made from it.
- Avoid handling cat litter.

■ RUBELLA

Rubella also called "German measles" is caused by an RNA virus. Maternal infection occurs through airborne infection as respiratory droplets. The proportion of women of childbearing age thought to be susceptible to the rubella virus is in the region of 1–2%. Infection in pregnancy is rare since the introduction of routine measles/mumps/rubella (MMR) vaccine.

Incubation period for rubella is 14–21 days and women are infectious from 7 days before until 7 days after the onset of the rash. Maternal rubella infection is generally asymptomatic or a mild illness of malaise, headache, coryza, and lymphadenopathy, followed by a diffuse, fine, maculopapular rash. In contrast, the effects on the fetus can be devastating if infected in the first trimester.

Fetal Infection

Transplacental vertical transmission from infected mother occurs during maternal viremia; the risk of fetal infection is 90% before 12 weeks of gestation, about 55% at 12–16 weeks, and it declines to 45% after 16 weeks. The risk of congenital defects in infected fetuses is 90% before 12 weeks, 20% between 12 and 16 weeks and, thereafter, deafness is a risk, until 20 weeks. Reinfection can occur and is more likely after prolonged or intense exposure and with vaccine-induced, rather than natural, immunity. It is usually subclinical, however, the risk to the fetus is thought to be 5%.

Diagnosis of Maternal Infection

Diagnosis is serological, accurate interpretation of results is dependent on appropriate timing of testing in relation to the onset of the rash. Commonly used tests are:
- *Rubella-specific IgM:* Diagnosis must be made with caution and with reference to history of rash, exposure, history of vaccination, and previous rubella testing. In the UK, women are screened for rubella IgG antibody in the beginning of pregnancy and those with IgG 10 IU/mL are considered susceptible to infection (IgG usually appears 1 week after the onset of the rash).
- *Rubella avidity test:* It may help distinguish between recent and distant infection. Presence of high avidity indicates infection at least 6 months ago, low avidity means recent infection.

Screening Recommendation

Vaccination when both IgG and IgM negative before planning pregnancy. Only IgM positive—recent infection and patient advised to delay pregnancy by 3 months. IgM negative with positive IgG would suggest immunity against rubella either due to past infection or vaccination and no action is required.

Diagnosis of Fetal Infection

The need for prenatal diagnosis is to determine the gestation at which the infection is likely to have occurred. There is no "gold standard" for prenatal diagnosis of rubella infection but most commonly reverse transcriptase polymerase chain reaction (RT-PCR) is used for the detection of viral nucleic acid in amniotic fluid. Fetal blood can also be tested

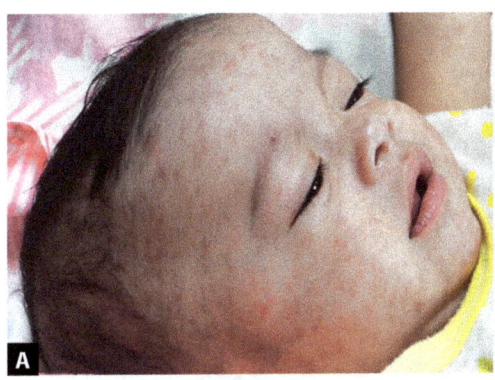
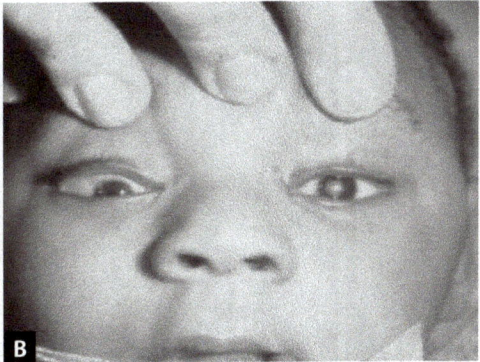

Figs. 3A and B: (A) Rash in Rubella infection; (B) Congenital cataract.

for viral RNA or rubella-specific IgM. Some studies have shown improved sensitivities where testing was delayed for >6 weeks after maternal infection. A negative result may warrant further amniocentesis or fetal blood sampling at a later gestation. The fetus should also be monitored with serial monthly ultrasound scans.

Sequelae of Fetal Infection

Congenital rubella syndrome (CRS) involves a wide spectrum of clinical features. In order of decreasing frequency, manifestations include hearing loss, learning disability, cardiac malformations, and ocular defects. Multiple defects and those affecting the CNS, eye, and heart appear only to occur when transmission takes place before 16 weeks. Other consequences include fetal growth restriction, hepatosplenomegaly, jaundice, thrombocytopenic purpura, anemia, and rash.

Management of Fetal Infection

Given the high risk of congenital infection and severe malformation in the first 12 weeks, it would be reasonable to consider termination of pregnancy/ultrasound surveillance to identify features of CRS. After 16 weeks of gestation, the risks to the fetus are negligible and the value of prenatal testing is questionable. Prenatal diagnosis is probably best reserved for infections occurring between 12 and 16 weeks, when there is a 55% risk of transmission and a 20% risk of CRS (RCOG).

Congenital Rubella Syndrome

The triad of CRS includes:
- *Cardiac defect:* Most common defect is patent ductus arteriosus, pulmonary artery stenosis
- Congenital cataract **(Fig. 3B)**, other eye defects may appear later on, e.g., "Salt and Pepper" retinopathy and glaucoma
- *Cochlear defect:* Bilateral sensory neural hearing loss.

Diagnosis of Neonatal Infection

- From typical triads of CRS
- Culture of rubella-specific RNA from blood, urine, CSF, oral/nasal secretions/OR, IgM antibody testing.

Neonatal Sequelae

Neonatal manifestations may include growth restriction, radiolucent bone disease (not pathognomonic of congenital rubella), hepatosplenomegaly, thrombocytopenia, purpuric skin lesions (classically described as "blueberry muffin" lesion representing extramedullary hematopoiesis), hepatosplenomegaly, hyperbilirubinemia, and interstitial pneumonitis.

Late Manifestations

Many infants with CRS experience late manifestations, including diabetes, thyroid disease, hearing defect, glaucoma, arterial hypertension (HTN), progressive mental retardation, autism, and subacute sclerosing panencephalitis.

Prevention of Congenital Rubella Syndrome

No specific treatment is available, prophylactic rubella vaccine to susceptible population, especially young female population may prevent rubella infection. MMR vaccination in childhood:
- Antibody induced in 95% cases after one dose
- One dose confers lifelong immunity in 90%
- Two doses MMR schedule captures primary vaccine failures.

Health Education

Vaccination is the best way of prevention of infection in women, give at least 28 days before conception, however, vaccine is not recommended for pregnant women. Breastfeeding women may be vaccinated. Those women who are nonimmune to rubella should avoid the infected person.

CYTOMEGALOVIRUS

Cytomegalovirus has emerged as the most common congenital viral infection and the most common cause of

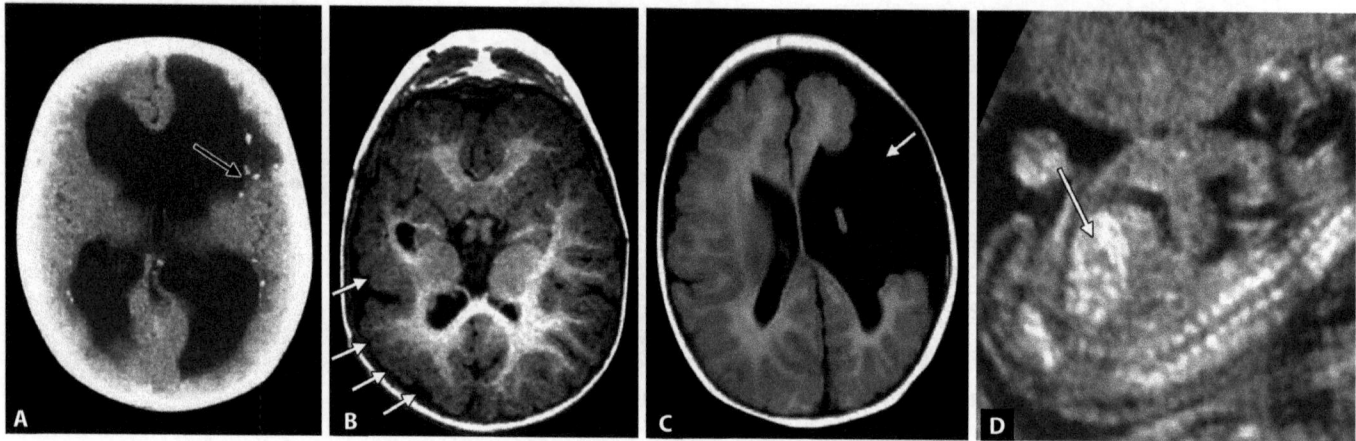

Figs. 4A to D: (A to C) Ventriculomegaly and cerebral calcification in fetal cytomegalovirus (CMV) infection; (D) USG image of fetal echogenic bowel in CMV infection.

congenital infective brain damage, occurring in 0.2–2.4% of live births. It is one of the leading causes of childhood deafness. Maternal CMV infection during pregnancy most often results from close contact with young children, particularly children attending daycare centers. Approximately 50–70% of women in Europe and in the USA have evidence of previous CMV infection **(Figs. 4A to D)**.

Primary infection is usually asymptomatic or a mild illness characterized by fever, lethargy, and malaise. Congenital CMV is mainly related to primary maternal infection **(Flowchart 1)**. The risk of vertical transmission is 40% in the first and second trimesters; fetal damage occurs in about 10% of these cases. Transmission occurs in about 80% of cases in the third trimester. In recurrent infection (reactivation of an existing infection or reinfection with a different strain), the transmission rate is in the region of 0.15–2%.

Sequelae of Fetal Infection

Congenital CMV infection is the leading cause of nonhereditary sensorineural hearing loss and can cause other long-term neurodevelopmental disabilities, including cerebral palsy, intellectual disability, vision impairment, and seizures. Vast majority (90%) of infected babies are asymptomatic at birth, but some may go on to develop symptoms after 6–9 months.

The spectrum of problems associated with congenital CMV comprises the following: Ocular defects, including chorioretinitis, microphthalmos, cataracts, and optic atrophy; sensorineural deafness; hepatosplenomegaly; jaundice; thrombocytopenic purpura; pneumonitis; fetal growth restriction; microcephaly; and neurodevelopmental consequences such as cerebral palsy, learning disability, and epilepsy.

The overall risk of damage as a result of primary maternal infection is about 25%. Approximately 10% of infected fetuses are clinically symptomatic at birth and a further 10–15% of those asymptomatic at birth will develop some long-term sequelae, primarily sensorineural hearing loss. The expression of disease tends to be worse the earlier the fetus is affected.

A recent study suggested that children with congenital CMV infection following first trimester maternal infection are more likely to have CNS sequelae, especially sensorineural hearing loss, than those affected later in gestation (RCOG).

Diagnosis of Maternal Infection

Diagnosis is traditionally based on serological testing for CMV-specific IgM and IgG. It is most helpful if paired samples are available, particularly if the woman's serostatus can be confirmed prior to conception or at the time of booking. Results must be interpreted in conjunction with an accurate record of maternal history and consultation with a virologist.

- *CMV IgM EIA:* Positive in primary infection and in reinfection. Usually positive within 2 weeks, IgM persists for 3–4 months after primary infection, may persist at low level for many years. The false positive rate of IgM is around 2%.
- *CMV IgG EIA:* IgG usually appears within 2–3 weeks of primary infection. IgG may be boosted by reinfection/reactivation, a fourfold rise would be considered significant.
- *CMV IgG avidity test:* It is based on the fact that antibodies bind less avidly to antigen in early infection compared to chronic infection. Avidity 30% means infection within the preceding 3 months, while avidity 40% indicates infection >6 months back. This test may differentiate primary infection from reactivation/reinfection where there is a low or equivocal IgM response and a positive IgG. In case of suspicion, check maternal IgM and IgG with avidity testing.

Diagnosis of Fetal Infection

If CMV infection of the fetus is suspected, the maternal infection status should be confirmed. Once primary infection or reactivation of maternal CMV is confirmed, prenatal diagnosis is offered to determine the risk of fetal infection. Fetal diagnosis is based on the detection of CMV in amniotic fluid:

Flowchart 1: Algorithm for the diagnosis and management of congenital CMV infection.

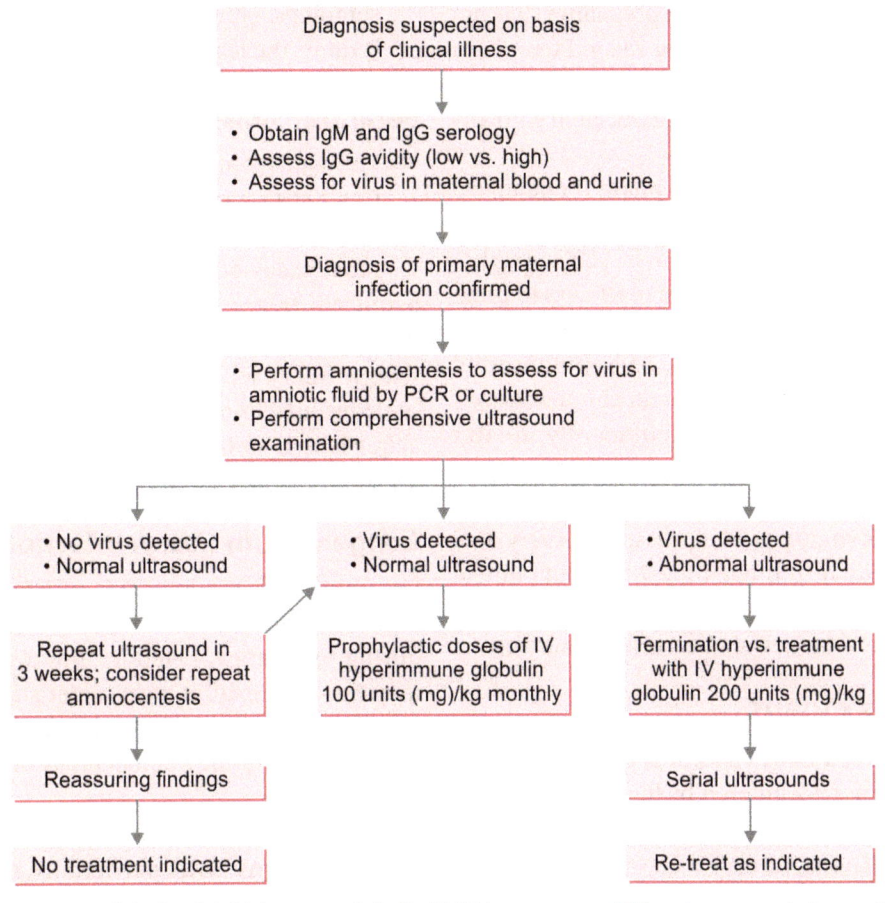

(IgG: immunoglobulin G; IgM: immunoglobulin M; IV: intravenous; PCR: polymerase chain reaction)

- *CMV DNA by PCR:* A highly sensitive technique for detection of viral genome and is now recommended for diagnosis of fetal CMV infection. PCR on amniotic fluid for CMV is more sensitive after 21 weeks' gestation (ACOG, 2015).
- *Immunofluorescence test:* Designed to detect CMV after limited growth in cell culture, not very sensitive but highly specific for transplacental infection.

Amniocentesis should be delayed for a minimum of 6 weeks after maternal seropositivity is confirmed to allow accumulation of CMV to detectable levels in amniotic fluid. Since fetal diuresis is not established until approximately 18–20 weeks of gestation, amniocentesis may be negative before this time, so, a repeat procedure and laboratory diagnosis are considered. Fetal blood sampling can be used for the detection of CMV or CMV-specific IgM but it appears to have lower sensitivity in the detection of fetal infection compared to detection from amniotic fluid.

Management of the Infected Fetus

If CMV is detected in amniotic fluid, transmission to the fetus is assumed. Patients should be counseled about the risk of fetal damage in relation to the gestational age at which infection has occurred and a detailed ultrasound examination of the fetus should be carried out. The sonographic features include microcephaly, cerebral atrophy, ventriculomegaly, intracerebral calcification, periventricular cyst formation, leukomalacia, fetal growth restriction, echogenic bowel, and hepatic calcifications. Further fetal surveillance using serial ultrasound scanning should be arranged, as some of these features may manifest later in pregnancy. It is important to note that, whilst the absence of sonographic findings is reassuring, it cannot exclude the presence of neurological abnormalities at birth.

There are no licensed antiviral agents and none proven to be effective for use in pregnancy; however, a recent nonrandomized study suggested that CMV-specific hyperimmune globulin (HIG 200 U/kg of maternal weight/day) may be effective in the treatment and prevention of congenital CMV infection (RCOG). In immunocompromised (nonpregnant) women, the antiviral drugs which are licensed for use for CMV infection include ganciclovir, valganciclovir, cidofovir, foscarnet, and valaciclovir, but, with the exception of valaciclovir, their teratogenic and toxic effects preclude their use in pregnancy.

Valaciclovir is a prodrug that is converted in vivo by esterases into the active drug aciclovir in the liver during first-pass metabolism. Valaciclovir is favored because it has greater oral bioavailability than aciclovir (55% vs. 10-20%). Aciclovir has an excellent safety profile in pregnancy. It is not genotoxic and in animal studies no drug-related neoplasia has been observed. There is considerable evidence that its use in humans in the first trimester is not associated with any increase in the rate of birth defects.

Oral valaciclovir 8 g/day studied in a phase II open label trial entitled "In Utero Treatment of Cytomegalovirus Congenital Infection with Valacyclovir (CYMEVAL)". High-dose valaciclovir given for a median of 89 days to pregnant women carrying a moderately-infected fetus, presenting with nonsevere ultrasound features (extracerebral ultrasound abnormalities and/or mild ultrasound brain abnormalities). Valaciclovir was associated with a significantly greater proportion of neonates born asymptomatic with treatment (82% with treatment vs. 43% without treatment from a historical cohort). This study provided reassuring safety data for the use of valaciclovir in pregnancy: Maternal clinical and laboratory tolerances to this high-dose regimen were excellent, and no adverse neonatal effects were observed.

■ HERPES SIMPLEX VIRUS

Herpes simplex virus is a DNA virus. It is one of the most prevalent viral infection encountered by humans. The virus primarily infects the mother and the newborn but rarely the fetus. Estimated rate of neonatal HSV is between 1/1,000 and 1/5,000.

Causative Organism

The causative organism is human herpesvirus types 1 and 2.

Clinical Manifestations

Both type 1 and type 2 viruses can cause either genital or oropharyngeal lesion. Genital HSV infection during pregnancy poses a significant risk to the developing fetus and the newborn.

Type 1 infection typically produces less severe symptoms and relatively little local manifestations compared to type 2 infection. In adult, typical lesion is vesicular or ulcerative involving only the skin and the mucous membrane, lasting for 3-6 weeks and cause regional lymphadenopathy, fever, and other constitutional symptoms. Primary infection poses a higher risk of vertical transmission than does recurrent infection. Recurrent genital herpes is much milder and shorter in duration (3-10 days), recurs in 50% of patients in 6 months.

Diagnosis of Maternal Infection

- The gold standard for diagnosis is PCR for HSV DNA. Swab for viral culture may be taken from throat, nasal pharynx, and vaginal lesion; vesicular fluid is commonly used.
- HSV IgM in maternal serum
- *Immunologic assays:* To detect HSV antigen in lesion scrapings, either ELISA or fluorescent microscopy assay is done, the test is very specific and 80-90% sensitive.

Fetal Transmission

- Perinatal (contact with vaginal secretion during delivery)
- Contact after rupture of membranes
- Direct contact with affected areas.

Most cases of neonatal HSV infection are perinatally acquired, transmitted during birth through an infected maternal genital tract. The risk of transmission is greater with primary HSV infection compared to reactivation of previous infection. Among mothers with primary infection, acquisition near the time of labor is the major risk factor for transmission to the neonate.

Congenital (In Utero) Infection

Intrauterine HSV infection is rare and usually results from maternal viremia associated with primary HSV infection during pregnancy. Liveborn infants with congenital HSV infection may exhibit a characteristic triad of skin vesicles, ulcerations, or scarring, eye damage; and severe CNS manifestations, including microcephaly or hydranencephaly.

Neonatal Infection

Most newborns with perinatally acquired HSV appear normal at birth, many are born prematurely. HSV infection in newborns usually develops one of the three patterns, occurs roughly with equal frequency.

- *SEM (skin, eyes, and mouth) disease (localized to skin, eyes, and mucosa) (42%):*
  - Vesicular lesions on an erythematous base
  - Keratoconjunctivitis, cataracts, and chorioretinitis
  - Ulcerative lesions of the mouth, palate, and tongue
- *CNS disease (35%):* Seizure, lethargy, irritability, tremor, poor feeding, temperature instability, and full anterior fontanelle.
- *Disseminated disease (23%):*
  - Multiple organ involvement (CNS, skin, eye, mouth, lung, liver, and adrenal glands)
  - May appear septic—fever/hypothermia, apnea, irritability, lethargy, and respiratory distress
  - Hepatitis, ascites, direct hyperbilirubinemia, neutropenia, disseminated intravascular coagulation, pneumonia, hemorrhagic pneumonitis, necrotizing enterocolitis, meningoencephalitis, and skin vesicles.

Diagnosis of Neonatal Infection

For diagnosis of neonatal infection PCR from CSF, HSV culture of a lesion, IgM titer should be done.

Treatment of mother

- Oral analgesic

TABLE 1: Antiviral treatment for herpes simplex virus.			
Indication	Valacyclovir	Acyclovir	Famciclovir
First clinical episode	1,000 mg twice a day for 7–14 days	200 mg five times a day or 400 mg three times a day for 7–14 days	250 mg three times a day for 7–14 days
Recurrent episodes	500 mg twice a day for 5 days	200 mg five times a day or 400 mg three times a day for 5 days	125 mg twice a day for 5 days
Daily suppressive therapy	500 mg once a day (≤9 recurrences per year) or 1,000 mg once a day or 250 mg twice a day (>9 recurrences per year)	400 mg twice a day	250 mg twice a day

- *Drug treatment:* Many antiviral compounds are available for the treatment of HSV infection **(Table 1)**; however, none has received approval from the US Food and Drug Administration (FDA) for use in pregnancy.
- Antiviral therapy is recommended for women with primary HSV infection during pregnancy to reduce viral shedding and help in the healing of lesions. Oral acyclovir reduces viral shedding, reduces pain, and heals lesions faster. The drug is safe and has minimal side effects, only 20% of each oral dose is absorbed. Dose: Oral acyclovir (400 mg) thrice daily for 10–14 days, highly effective for primary and recurrent infection.
- Valacyclovir is better absorbed and has a longer half-life than acyclovir but expensive.
- *Third trimester acquisition:* Following first or second trimester acquisition, daily suppressive acyclovir 400 mg three times daily from 36 weeks of gestation reduces HSV lesions at term and hence reduces the need for cesarean section.
- *Recurrent genital herpes:* Women with recurrent genital herpes should be informed that risk of neonatal herpes is low, even if lesions are present at the time of delivery (0–3% for vaginal delivery). Daily suppressive acyclovir 400 mg three times daily from 36 weeks. A randomized trial of acyclovir given after 36 weeks of gestation in women with recurrent genital herpes infection has shown significant decrease in clinical recurrences.
- Valacyclovir and famciclovir have been approved by the FDA for the treatment of primary genital herpes, recurrent disease, and suppression of recurrent outbreaks.

Indications of Cesarean Section in Women with Herpes Simplex Virus Infection (ACOG Recommendations)

- Women with active genital lesions or symptoms of vulvar pain or burning should be delivered by cesarean section. While the incidence of infection in infants whose mothers have recurrent infection is low, cesarean delivery is recommended because of the potentially serious nature of the disease. Cesarean delivery is not necessary in women with a history of HSV but no active genital disease during labor.
- For women at or beyond 36 weeks of gestation with a first episode of HSV infection occurring during the current pregnancy, antiviral therapy should be considered.
- Cesarean delivery should be performed on women with recurrent HSV infection who have active genital lesions or prodromal symptoms at delivery.
- Expectant management of patients with preterm labor or preterm premature rupture of membranes and active HSV infection may be warranted.
- For women at or beyond 36 weeks of gestation who are at risk for recurrent HSV infection, antiviral therapy may also be considered, although such therapy may not reduce the likelihood of cesarean delivery.
- In women with no active lesions or prodromal symptoms during labor, cesarean delivery should not be performed on the basis of a history of recurrent disease.

Treatment of Neonate

- Acyclovir intravenous (IV) at a dose of 60 mg/kg per day in three divided doses.
- Treatment for localized SEM disease should be for a minimum of 14 days if disseminated and CNS disease have been excluded.
- Treatment for disseminated and CNS disease should be for a minimum of 21 days and repeat lumbar puncture is recommended to make sure the HSV DNA PCR is negative and all CSF parameters have returned to normal before discontinuing therapy.

Outcome

- With antiviral treatment, mortality from local CNS disease is around 6% and neurological morbidity (which may be lifelong) is 70%.
- Disseminated disease carries the worst prognosis; with appropriate antiviral treatment, mortality is around 30% and 17% have long-term neurological sequelae.
- The poor outcomes of disseminated and local CNS disease have been attributed to delay between symptom onset and treatment.

HUMAN PARVOVIRUS B19

Incidence

Incidence is 1/400 pregnancies.

Transmission of Infection

Infection is transmitted through air and contaminated blood. Mothers usually gets infected from contact with children having erythema infectiosum infection. The incubation period is 5–7 days following exposure and women are infectious for 3–10 days postexposure or until the rash appears. Symptoms peak around day 9 and the rash may appear up to 18 days after exposure.

Adult infections are frequently subclinical but may present as erythema infectiosum, which consists of transient fever, malaise, and arthralgia. In children, it is a mild illness characterized by fever and a typical facial rash ("slapped cheek") with a pruritic, laticiform macular rash on the trunk, which spreads to the extremities and may be accompanied by a polyarthritis. Approximately 60% of adults have serological evidence of prior infection.

Sequelae of Maternal Infection

Transplacental transmission occurs in 15% of cases before 15 weeks and 25% between 15 and 20 weeks, this rises to 70% toward term. Human parvovirus B19 has a predilection for rapidly dividing cells, mainly the erythroid cell precursors, thereby interrupting red cell production, can cause profound fetal hemolytic anemia, leading to high-output cardiac failure from anemia, hydrops, and intrauterine death. Maternal infection can also lead to miscarriage. The risk of hydrops is low (3%) but it has a fatality rate of 50%. Hydrops usually occurs about 5 weeks after maternal infection (range 2–12 weeks) and spontaneous resolution may occur 1–7 weeks after diagnosis. The risk of intrauterine fetal death in parvovirus B19 IgM positive mothers is 10% and most deaths occur 4–6 weeks following the onset of maternal symptoms but they can occur up to 3 months later. Most intrauterine infections do not result in fetal developmental defects. There is no reliable epidemiological evidence of adverse long-term effects in babies who were hydropic and mothers should be reassured that, following resolution, no long-term problems are expected.

Diagnosis of Maternal Infection

- Serologic assays by EIA for virus-specific IgG and IgM. IgM is detected 10 days after infection peaks and may be very short lived—only 4 weeks. If rash is present, IgM should be tested because rash is immune-mediated. Human parvovirus IgG appears to confer lasting immunity.
- *Parvovirus DNA by PCR:* Sensitivity reported up to 96%, this is useful where there is high clinical suspicion, but there is no rash or where IgM is negative and IgG seroconversion not demonstrable.

Diagnosis of Fetal Infection

Testing for parvovirus B19 during pregnancy is most commonly done with the history of recent maternal exposure or the finding of fetal hydrops during sonographic examination. Fetal infection can be diagnosed by detection of human parvovirus B19 IgM or viral DNA, using amniotic fluid or fetal blood. In the absence of signs of fetal anemia, however, the value of testing is of uncertain clinical importance.

Once maternal infection has been confirmed, monitoring of the fetus using serial ultrasound examinations should be undertaken. These should start 4 weeks after the onset of illness or date of seroconversion and then be done at 1- to 2-weekly intervals for up to 12 weeks. The aim of monitoring is to identify signs of potential fetal anemia, which include ascites and hydrops and placentomegaly. Measurement of fetal middle cerebral artery peak systolic velocity (MCA-PSV) has been shown to be useful in identifying cases of moderate or severe anemia. One study showed MCA-PSV had 100% sensitivity for moderate and severe anemia, with a false positive rate of 12%.

Management of the Infected Fetus (Figs. 5A and B)

Fetal hydrops secondary to parvovirus B19 infection can resolve spontaneously in up to one-third of cases. Fetal blood sampling may be indicated when the MCA-PSV is 1.5 multiples of the median or where there is ascites or hydrops. Intrauterine blood transfusion may be indicated if the fetal hemoglobin is below the gestational age mean, there is evidence to suggest that this is associated with a reduction in the risk of fetal death.

Potential Benefits of Fetal Transfusion

Firstly, mature erythrocytes are not susceptible to parvovirus infection and, therefore, the oxygen-carrying capacity of the fetal circulation can be restored and stabilized to improve the fetal heart function. Secondly, the half-life of formed erythrocytes is approximately 120 days, which should provide sufficient cover for the intrinsic fetal immune system to develop or for maternal antibodies to cross the placenta and assist in the resolution of viral infection. Finally, some passive transfer of antiparvovirus antibody can be expected along with the red cells from a seropositive donor, which could further aid recovery of the fetus.

Fetal blood sampling and transfusion can be carried out from 18 weeks but ideally are performed after 22 weeks. Cordocentesis is associated with a 1% procedure-related loss rate. The risks of intrauterine therapy at later gestation carry risk of premature delivery and extrauterine transfusion. Resolution of hydrops should occur following transfusion, although the time taken for this varies, in one study, 94% had resolved within 6 weeks of intrauterine blood transfusion.

VARICELLA ZOSTER

Causative Organism

Varicella virus is a member of the herpes virus family.

Varicella-zoster virus is endemic in the UK and 90% of the antenatal population are seropositive for varicella-zoster

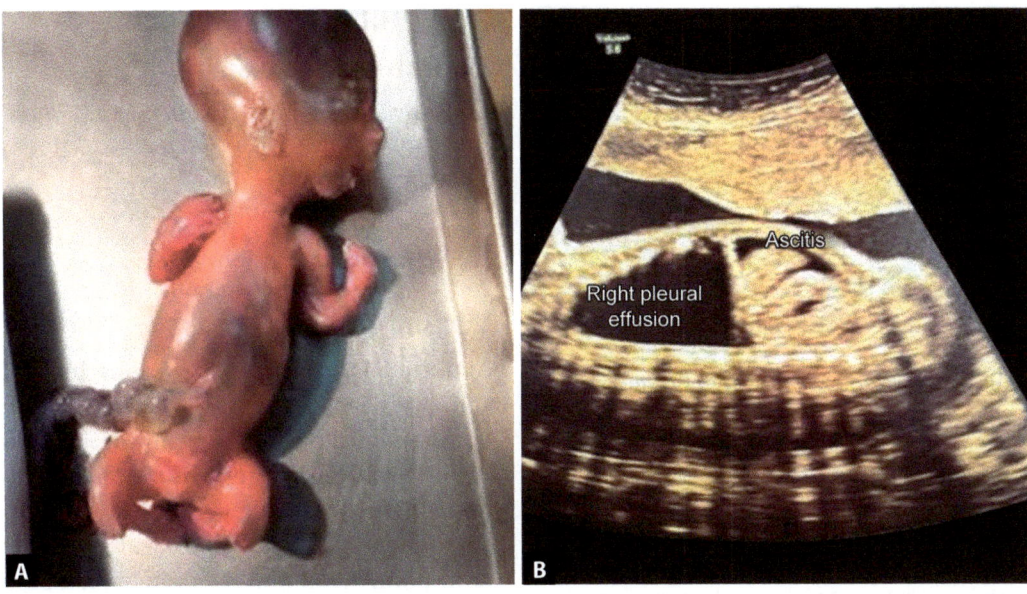

Figs. 5A and B: (A) Non-immune hydrops with skin edema; (B) Fetal pleural effusion and ascitis in Parvovirus B infection.

virus IgG. For this reason, primary infection is uncommon in pregnancy and is estimated to occur in 3 per 1,000 pregnancies.

Maternal Infection

Primary infection is characterized by fever, malaise, and a distinctive pruritic maculopapular rash that becomes vesicular and then crusts before it heals over. The incubation period is 10–21 days and patients are infectious from 48 hours prior to the onset of the rash until the vesicles crust over.

Maternal symptoms include "shingles," rash, hemorrhagic chickenpox, viral pneumonia, meningitis, and encephalitis. 10–20% of pregnant women who contract a primary varicella infection may develop pneumonia that can cause serious maternal morbidity and death in a minority. Thus, these patients should be treated with oral acyclovir and varicella-zoster immune globulin (VZIG).

Fetal Infection

Risk of fetal congenital infection is low (0.4–2.0%). Only 2% of fetuses whose mother have infected with this virus in first 20 weeks of pregnancy will develop varicella-zoster virus embryopathy. Fetal varicella syndrome does not occur at the time of initial fetal infection. A prospective study shown women who had primary varicella during the first 36 weeks of pregnancy, the risk of fetal varicella syndrome was 0.4% prior to 13 weeks of gestation and 2% between 13 and 20 weeks, there does not appear to be any risk of fetal infection when maternal infection occurs between 20 and 36 weeks. In utero, infection may present as shingles in the first few years of life. After 36 weeks or when delivery occurs within 4 weeks of maternal infection, up to 50% of babies are infected and about a quarter of neonates develop clinical varicella.

Diagnosis of Maternal Infection

Testing in pregnancy is most commonly done after maternal contact with a known case of chickenpox. The distinctive nature of the rash makes clinical diagnosis reliable and therefore, where there is a definite history of previous varicella infection, protection can be assumed and testing need not be undertaken. When there is no such history and in the presence of significant contact (face-to-face for 5 minutes or in the same room for 15 minutes or more), the woman's susceptibility may be determined by testing for varicella-zoster virus IgG. Maternal chickenpox is usually diagnosed by immunofluorescence detection of viral antigens from lesion scrapings. Where the infection is suspected to have occurred some time ago, it can be confirmed by seroconversion.

- *Varicella-zoster IgM EIA:* IgM appears toward the end of rash but persists 3–4 months.
- *Varicella-zoster IgG EIA:* IgG usually appears within 10 days but provides lifelong immunity.
- *Immunofluorescence:* Basal epithelial cells are scraped from a vesicle, fixed on slide, and stained with antibody to varicella zoster virus labeled with fluorescence dye.
- PCR for varicella zoster virus DNA has high sensitivity and specificity.

Diagnosis of Fetal Infection

Polymerase chain reaction can be used to detect varicella-zoster virus DNA in amniotic fluid; however, its presence does not necessarily imply progression to fetal varicella syndrome.

The mainstay of diagnosis of fetal varicella syndrome is detailed ultrasound scanning. The key findings include microcephaly, hydrocephalus, microphthalmia, limb deformities, fetal growth restriction, and soft tissue calcifications.

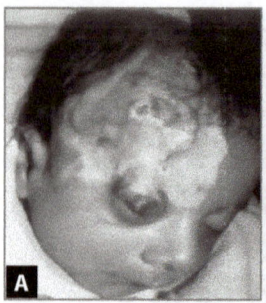 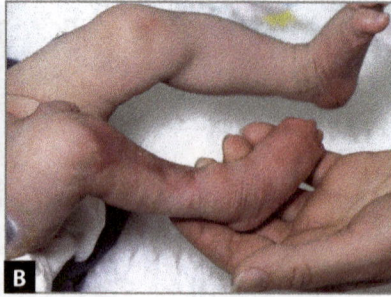

Figs. 6A and B: Cicatricial lesions of skin with fetal varicella infection.

Prenatal ultrasound appears to have reasonably good correlation with fetal outcome at birth. Hoffmeyer et al. suggested that sonographic examination at 5 or more weeks after the initial infection should identify most cases of varicella embryopathy. Abnormalities appear to be collective, although one author reported a case of skin lesions as the sole manifestation. Serial ultrasound examinations should be carried out from 5 weeks after infection or 16 weeks of gestation.

Sequelae of Fetal Infection

Fetal varicella syndrome is characterized by cicatricial lesions **(Figs. 6A and B)** of skin/hypoplasia of tissues in a dermatomal distribution, limb defects, and damage to the eyes and CNS including cataracts, chorioretinitis, and seizure. In a literature review, skin lesions (scars and skin loss) were the most common symptoms (76%), neurological defects (cortical atrophy, spinal cord atrophy, limb paresis, seizures, microcephaly, Horner syndrome, encephalitis, and dysphagia) in 60%, eye diseases (microphthalmia, chorioretinitis, cataracts, and optic atrophy) in 51%, and limb hypoplasia in 49% cases. Other abnormalities include fetal growth restriction, muscle hypoplasia, gastrointestinal and genitourinary defects, developmental delay, and, more rarely, cardiac defects. Congenitally infected fetuses with no varicella-associated anatomic abnormalities have normal neurodevelopment (ACOG).

Management of Infected Fetus

In the presence of ultrasound abnormalities in a pattern consistent with fetal varicella syndrome, termination of pregnancy may be offered. In the absence of ultrasound abnormalities on serial ultrasound scans performed by a fetal medicine specialist, reassurance may be provided.

No conclusive evidence that fetal varicella syndrome can be prevented or ameliorated by maternal administration of varicella immunoglobulin or antiviral chemotherapy. Specific VZIG administered within 96 hours of exposure will usually modify illness, administered up to 9 days there may be attenuation of symptoms. If mother has chickenpox in the time period 2 days before to 5 days after delivery, the infant should be given VZIG and carefully observed; if any lesions develop, IV acyclovir should be given.

SYPHILIS

Causative Organism

Causative organism is *Treponema pallidum*.

Transmission

- Sexual activity
- Vertical transmission.

Transmission

Maternal infection with syphilis has three stages. The primary stage (3-6 weeks) infection presents as a painless, spontaneously resolving papule. The secondary stage occurs 6-8 weeks later, with diffuse inflammation and a disseminated rash (often on the palms and soles). The latent stage then occurs, in which women are characteristically asymptomatic. If untreated, may then progress to the final or tertiary stage of the disease, which is characterized by granulomas affecting the bones and the joints as well as the cardiovascular and neurologic systems.

Treponemas are able to cross the placenta at any time during pregnancy, can cause: Abortion/fetal death, hydrops fetalis, preterm labor, IUGR, congenital infection—depending on the stage of maternal infection and duration of fetal infection prior to delivery. Infection of the neonate occurs when maternal infection is active, inadequately treated, or untreated. Untreated infection in the first and second trimesters often leads to significant fetal morbidity, while in the third trimester infection, many infants are asymptomatic. Diagnosis of syphilis can be performed using dark-field microscopy or using direct immune—fluorescence assay of the collected sample taken from placenta or umbilicus.

Manifestations of Congenital Syphilis

Women with primary and secondary stages of the disease rather than in the tertiary stage transmit the spirochaete to her children. Congenital syphilis can be divided into two phases: Early disease (before 2 years) and late disease (after 2 years).

- Majority of newborns are asymptomatic at birth, do not have signs of primary syphilis from in utero acquired infection.
- *Early congenital syphilis* (symptoms at 1-2 months of age), includes "snuffles" (hemorrhagic nasal discharge), maculopapular rash, lymphadenopathy, hepatomegaly, thrombocytopenia, anemia, meningitis, chorioretinitis, osteochondritis, fulminant sepsis, and bullous/desquamating rash on back, legs, palm, and soles.
- *Late congenital syphilis* (symptoms after 2 years of age):
  - Hutchinson teeth
  - Mulberry molars
  - Perforated hard palate

- Rhagades (cracks or fissures in the skin around the mouth)
- Saber shins
- Sensorineural hearing loss [cranial nerve (CN) VIII]
- Interstitial keratitis
- Saddle nose.

Diagnosis of Maternal Infection

- Diagnosis of syphilis can be performed using dark-field microscopy or using direct immune-fluorescence assay of the collected sample taken from lesions.
- A presumptive diagnosis is made using nontreponemal and treponemal tests. Nontreponemal tests included the venereal disease research laboratory (VDRL) and rapid plasma reagin (RPR) tests; and the treponemal tests, included the fluorescent treponemal antibody absorption (FTA-ABS) assay and the chronic periostitis microhemagglutination assay for *T. pallidum* antibody (MHA-TP).
- New diagnostic methods such as EIA, PCR, and immunoblotting have greater sensitivity and specificity. EIA based on the antibody capture method utilizing (recombinant) treponemal antigen is commercially available which detects treponemal IgG, has sensitivity of 100% and a specificity of 99%.

Treatment of Infected Women

In general, treatment of congenital syphilis requires a 10-day course of penicillin (aqueous penicillin-G 100,000 to 150,000 units/kg/24 hours). Proper treatment of the mother can eliminate the risk of infection of infants. The infected infant should be followed up routinely until nontreponemal test reported negative. In a study involving 204 pregnant women with primary, secondary, or early latent syphilis, a single intramuscular dose of benzathine penicillin, 2.4 million units prevented fetal infection in 98% of the cases.

Treatment of Neonates/Child

Penicillin Treatment

- For infants <1 month, either as a single dose of benzathine penicillin G (50,000 units/kg intramuscularly) or as a 10-day course [aqueous penicillin G 50,000 units/kg intravenously every 12 hours (for infants ≤7 days of age) and every 8 hours (for infants >7 days of age)], or Procaine penicillin G 50,000 units/kg intramuscularly as a single daily dose for 10 days.
- Single-dose therapy is *contraindicated* for asymptomatic infants born to women with inadequate/suboptimal treatment unless the infant has undergone appropriate evaluation [CSF, quantitative VDRL, cell count, and protein; complete blood count (CBC) with differential and platelet count; and long-bone radiographs] and has completely normal results.
- For children diagnosed with congenital syphilis after 1 month of age (including those with late congenital syphilis) and children with acquired syphilis should be treated with aqueous penicillin G (50,000 units/kg intravenously every 4–6 hours for 10 days), some experts suggest that the 10-day course of aqueous penicillin be followed with a single dose of benzathine penicillin (50,000 units/kg intramuscularly).

SUGGESTED READING

1. ACOG Guidelines at a Glance: Key points about 4 perinatal infections. Obstet Gynecol Women Health. 2015.
2. American College of Obstetricians and Gynecologists. Practice bulletin no. 151: Cytomegalovirus, parvovirus B19, varicella zoster, and toxoplasmosis in pregnancy. Obstet Gynecol. 2015;125:1510-25.
3. Centers for Disease Control and Prevention. Toxoplasmosis. DPDx - laboratory identification of parasitic diseases of public health concern. [online] Available from http://www.cdc.gov/dpdx/toxoplasmosis/dx.html. [Last accessed April 2022].
4. Centers for Disease Control and Prevention. Updated recommendations for use of VariZIG--United States, 2013. MMWR Morb Mortal Wkly Rep. 2013;62:574-6.
5. Creasy RK, Resnik R, Lams JD, Lockwood CJ, Moore TR, Greene MF. Maternal-Fetal Medicine: principles and practice. Part 3, 7th edition. Amsterdam: Elsevier; 2013.
6. De Jong EP, Lindenburg IT, van Klink JM, Oepkes D, van Kamp IL, Walther FJ, et al. Intrauterine transfusion for parvovirus B19 infection: long-term neurodevelopmental outcome. Am J Obstet Gynecol. 2012;206:204 e1–5.
7. de Jong EP, Vossen AC, Walther FJ, Lopriore E. How to use... neonatal TORCH testing. Arch Dis Child Educ Pract Ed/ 2013;98:93.
8. FOGSI Guideline development Group. (2014). Screening and management of TORCH in pregnancy. [online] Available from fogsi.org/wp-content/uploads/2015/11/smtp.pdf. [Last accessed April 2022].
9. International Journal of Obstetrics and Gynaecology. Congenital Cytomegalovirus Infection: Update on Treatment. BJOG. 2017;125(1):e1-11.
10. Johnson KE. Overview of TORCH infections. UpToDate. 2021.
11. Khan NA, Kazzi SN. Yield and costs of screening growth-retarded infants for torch infections. Am J Perinatol. 2000;17:131.
12. Neu N, Duchon J, Zachariah P. TORCH infections. Clin Perinatol. 2015;42:77.
13. Neu N, Duchon J. TORCH Infections Clin Perinatol. 2015;42:77-103.
14. Practice Bulletin on Management of Herpes in Pregnancy. Am Fam Physician. 2000;61(2):556-61.
15. Reef SE, Plotkin S, Cordero JF, Katz M, Cooper L, Schwartz B, et al. Preparing for elimination of congenital Rubella syndrome (CRS): summary of a workshop on CRS elimination in the United States. Clin Infect Dis 2000; 31:85.
16. The University of Chicago. Paediatrics Clerkship. [online] Available from https://pedclerk.uchicagoACOG. [Last accessed April 2022].
17. To M, Kidd M, Maxwell D. Review prenatal diagnosis and management of fetal infection. Obstetr Gynaecol. 2009;11:108-16.

CHAPTER 22

Fetal Congenital Malformation

INTRODUCTION

Congenital anomalies are also known as birth defects, congenital disorders, or congenital malformations. Congenital anomalies are defined as structural or functional anomalies (for example, metabolic disorders) that occur during intrauterine life and can be identified prenatally, at birth, or sometimes may only be detected later in infancy, such as hearing defects. Some are major structural anomalies, while others are minor defects. Major defects are defined as structural changes that have significant medical, social, or cosmetic consequences for the affected individual, and typically require medical intervention. The most common, severe congenital anomalies are heart defects, neural tube defects (NTDs), and Down syndrome. Major structural anomalies account for most of the deaths, morbidity, and disability. In contrast, minor congenital anomalies, although more prevalent among the population, are structural changes that pose no significant health problem in the neonatal period and tend to have limited social or cosmetic consequences for the affected individual, for example, preauricular tags and clinodactyly.

An estimated 295,000 newborns die, within 28 days of birth every year worldwide, due to congenital anomalies. According to March of Dimes (MOD) global report on birth defects, 7.9 million births (6% of total birth) occur annually with serious birth defect and 94% of these births occur in low- and middle-income countries (LMIC). According to World Health Organization (WHO) and MOD joint meeting report, birth defects account for 7% of all neonatal mortality and 3.3 million under five deaths. Additionally, congenital anomalies can contribute to long-term disability, which may have significant impacts on individuals, families, healthcare systems, and societies. Although congenital anomalies may be the result of one or more genetic, infectious, nutritional, or environmental factors, it is often difficult to identify the exact cause. Some congenital anomalies can be prevented, while others are not preventable. Vaccination, adequate intake of folic acid or iodine through fortification of staple foods or supplementation, and adequate antenatal care are three examples of prevention methods.

RISK FACTORS

Although approximately 50% of all congenital anomalies cannot be linked to a specific cause, there are some known genetic, environmental, and other causes or risk factors. Congenital malformations may be caused by chromosomal defect, single gene defect, may be of multifactorial inheritance and micronutrient deficiency.

Genetic Factors

Genes play an important role in many congenital anomalies. This might be through inherited genes that code for an anomaly or resulting from genetic mutations during fertilization. Some ethnic communities, such as Ashkenazi Jews or Finns, have a higher prevalence of rare genetic mutations for cystic fibrosis and hemophilia C. Consanguinity increases the risks of rare genetic congenital anomalies, nearly doubles neonatal and childhood death as well as intellectual disability.

Socioeconomic and Demographic Factors

Low income may be an indirect determinant of congenital anomalies, with a higher frequency among resource-constrained families and countries. It is estimated that about 94% of severe congenital anomalies occur in LMIC. This higher risk relates to a possible lack of access to sufficient nutritious foods by pregnant women, an increased exposure to agents or factors such as infection and alcohol, or poorer access to healthcare and screening.

Maternal Age

Advanced maternal age (35 years) increases the risk of chromosomal abnormalities, including Down syndrome. Fetal chromosomal abnormalities may be caused by a non-disjunction phenomenon that occurs in the period of meiosis during maternal oogenesis, which has been reported to have a direct association with maternal age. Currently, fetal chromosomal abnormalities due to maternal age have been reported to include not only trisomy 21 but also trisomy 18, trisomy 13, triple X syndrome, and Klinefelter syndrome.

Environmental Factors

Maternal exposure to pesticides and other chemicals, as well as certain medications, alcohol, tobacco, and radiation during pregnancy, may increase the risk of having a fetus or neonate affected by congenital anomalies. Working or living near waste sites, smelters, or mines may be a risk factor, particularly if the mother is also exposed to other environmental risk factors or nutritional deficiencies.

Infections

Maternal infections such as Zika virus infection during pregnancy cause microcephaly and other congenital abnormalities in the developing fetus and newborn. Zika infection also causes fetal loss, stillbirth, and preterm birth. Rubella or German measles and cytomegalovirus (CMV) infection can result in miscarriage, deafness, intellectual disability, heart defects, and blindness in the newborn. Congenital toxoplasmosis cause hearing loss, vision problems, and intellectual disability. Sexually transmitted infections (STIs) such as syphilis also cause serious birth defects.

Maternal Nutritional Status

Maternal folate insufficiency increases the risk of having a baby with a NTD, while excessive vitamin A intake and iodine deficiency may affect the normal development of an embryo or fetus.

■ DIAGNOSIS

For the detection of congenital anomalies, screening can be done during preconception period, during pregnancy, and after child birth.

Preconception Screening

Inherited disorders tend to cluster within families, preconception screening is useful to identify those at risk for specific disorders or at risk of passing a disorder onto their children. Screening includes obtaining family histories and carrier screening (e.g., thalassemia and sickle cell disorders) and is particularly valuable in countries where consanguineous marriage is common.

Periconception Screening

Young or advanced maternal age as well as maternal obesity increases the risk of congenital anomaly. Screening should include women with known risk factors as well as those exposed to alcohol, tobacco, teratogens, and offer appropriate care according to risks identified from screening results.

Ultrasound can be used to screen for Down syndrome and major structural abnormalities during the first trimester, and for severe fetal anomalies during the second trimester. Maternal blood can be screened for placental biomarkers to aid in prediction of risk of chromosomal abnormalities or NTDs, or cell free fetal DNA to screen for many chromosomal abnormalities. Diagnostic tests such as chorionic villus sampling and amniocentesis can be used to diagnose chromosomal abnormalities and infections in women at high risk.

Neonatal Screening

Neonatal screening includes clinical examination and screening for disorders of the blood, metabolism, and hormone production. Screening for deafness, congenital hypothyroidism as well as early detection of heart defects can facilitate life-saving treatments. In some countries, babies are routinely screened for abnormalities of the thyroid or adrenal glands before discharge from the maternity unit. Many structural congenital anomalies can be corrected with pediatric surgery and early treatment can be administered to children with some functional problems such as thalassemia and sickle cell disorders.

■ PREVENTION

Preventive public health measures work to decrease the frequency of certain congenital anomalies through the removal of risk factors or the reinforcement of protective factors. Important interventions and efforts include:
- Ensuring adolescent girls and mothers have a healthy diet including a wide variety of vegetables and fruit, and maintain a healthy weight
- Ensuring an adequate dietary intake of vitamins and minerals, and particularly folic acid in adolescent girls and mothers
- Ensuring mothers avoid harmful substances, particularly alcohol and tobacco
- Avoidance of travel by pregnant women (and sometimes women of childbearing age) to regions experiencing outbreaks of infections known to be associated with congenital anomalies
- Reducing or eliminating environmental exposure to hazardous substances (such as heavy metals or pesticides)
- Controlling diabetes prior to and during pregnancy through weight management, diet, and administration of insulin when required
- Ensuring that any exposure of pregnant women to medications or medical radiation (such as imaging rays) is justified and based on careful health risk–benefit analysis

- Vaccination, especially against rubella for children and reproductive aged women
- Screening for infections, especially rubella, varicella, and syphilis, and consideration of treatment
- Strengthening education of health staff and others involved in promoting prevention of congenital anomalies

Common Congenital Abnormalities (Table 1)

TABLE 1: Common anomalies affecting different organ system.

CNS abnormalities: • Anencephaly • Spina bifida • Encephalocele • Ventriculomegaly • Hydrocephaly • Iniencephaly • Holoprosencephaly • Agenesis of corpus callosum	*Thoracic abnormalities:* • Congenital diaphragmatic hernia (CDH) • Congenital cystic adenoid malformation (CCAM) • Hydrothorax *Abdominal abnormalities:* • Gastroschisis • Omphalocele • Esophageal atresia/tracheoesophageal fistula • Large intestinal atresia/stenosis • Anorectal atresia/stenosis
Abnormality of neck: Cystic hygroma *Orofacial clefts:* • Cleft lip only • Cleft palate only • Cleft lip and palate	*Skeletal anomaly:* • Achondroplasia • Osteogenesis imperfect *Limb defects:* • Reduction defects of upper and lower limbs • Talipes equinovarus/club foot
Cardiac abnormalities: • VSD • ASD • Hypoplastic left heart syndrome • Ebstein anomaly • Common truncus • Interrupted aortic arch • Transposition of great arteries • Tetralogy of Fallot • Pulmonary valve atresia • Tricuspid valve atresia • Fetal arrhythmia • Fetal cardiomyopathy	*Abnormalities of urinary tract:* • Hydronephrosis • Obstructive uropathy • Polycystic kidney disease • Multicystic dysplastic kidney *Defects of genitalia:* • Hypospadias, epispadias • Ambiguous genitals • Congenital adrenal hyperplasia

(ASD: atrial septal defect; CNS: central nervous system; VSD: ventricular septal defect)

Central Nervous System Abnormalities

Congenital abnormalities of the central nervous system (CNS) are defects of the physical structure of the brain or the spinal cord that encompasses a broad range of disorders and medical conditions, from minor abnormalities to severe ones. CNS anomalies are one of the most common group of congenital malformations and are second only to cardiac malformations in their frequency of occurrence. Nearly 200 congenital malformations of the CNS have been identified. Almost 1% of all live births and an estimated 2% of all conceived pregnancies have CNS anomalies. Forty percent of infant deaths and 75% of fetal deaths are attributed to CNS malformations.

A wide range of factors may contribute to congenital CNS abnormalities. Some are caused by genetic factors, in other cases, it is multifactorial resulting from a complex interaction between several genes and poorly understood environmental factors. Exposure to one or more of alcohol, smoking, drugs, vitamins, medications, environmental toxins, prenatal infection or irradiation, obesity, poorly controlled diabetes, and maternal medication (antiepileptic drugs and thalidomide), all have been implicated as etiologic factors in these malformations. In many cases, no known or identifiable cause is found.

Prenatal ultrasonography (USG) has been shown to be an effective primary imaging modality for depiction of these anomalies. Prenatal USG has a sensitivity and specificity of 72.2% and 100%, respectively, indicating that USG offers a relatively accurate, safe, and cost-effective means of screening in pregnancy.

■ NEURAL TUBE DEFECT

Neural tube defects are birth defects of the brain, spine, or spinal cord. Anencephaly, encephalocele/meningocele, and spina bifida are the most common NTDs. The neural tube usually fuses 18–26 days after ovulation. Failure of closure may lead to NTD.

■ EPIDEMIOLOGY

Prevalence of NTDs varies between countries and races, with noted hot spots in Guatemala, northern China, Mexico, and parts of the United Kingdom. Hispanic and non-Hispanic whites are affected more frequently than women of African descent, and females are affected more frequently than males. In the United States, estimated incidence of NTD is as high as 1 in 1,000 pregnancies. The prevalence in England and Wales has fell from the 1970s onward to just under 0.8/1,000 total births by 1994. Some of the decline was due to antenatal diagnosis but some is unexplained. In the UK, anencephaly and spina bifida are approximately equal in prevalence and together make up 95% of all NTDs.

Anencephaly

Anencephaly is the most frequent open NTD and is the second most common type of congenital malformations. This is a serious developmental defect characterized by a total (holo) or partial (mero) absence of the brain with absence of the cranial vault (calvaria) and covering skin. The cerebrum is reduced or absent, but the hindbrain (cerebellum, brainstem, and spinal cord) is intact.

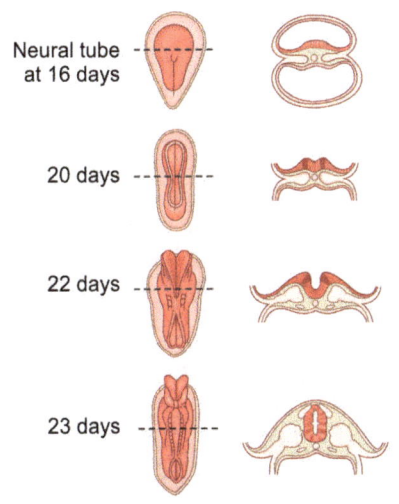

Fig. 1: Development of the central nervous system.
Source: Visual Search

Development of CNS (Fig. 1)

In the normal human embryo, the neural plate arises approximately 18 days after fertilization. During the fourth week of development, the neural plate invaginates along the embryonic midline to form the neural groove. The neural tube is formed as closure of the neural groove progresses from the middle toward the ends in both directions, with completion between day 24 for the cranial end and day 26 for the caudal end, failure of the neural tube to close gives rise to NTDs. Anencephaly results from failure of neural tube closure at the cranial end of the developing embryo.

Types

Absence of the brain and calvaria may be partial or complete, *accordingly* anencephaly is divided into two subcategories:
1. Acrania, there is small defect in cranial vault with extensive disorganization of the remaining tissue
2. Holocrania, the more severe form, in which brain is completely absent

Associated anomaly includes congenital heart disease, hypoplastic lungs, congenital diaphragmatic hernia, malrotation of gut, renal malformation, omphalocele, single umbilical artery (UA), patent ductus arteriosus, and patent foramen ovale. When additional malformations are present, the likelihood of cytogenetic abnormality is increased.

Etiology

Most cases of anencephaly follow a multifactorial pattern of inheritance, with interaction of multiple genes as well as environmental factors. A variety of environmental factors appear to influence the closure of the neural tube. Folate antimetabolites including sodium valproate, folic acid antagonists, maternal diabetes, obesity, mycotoxins in contaminated corn meal, arsenic, and hyperthermia in early development or disruption of the amniotic membrane have been identified as stressors that increase the risk of NTDs.

Genetics

Anencephaly is often an isolated, nonsyndromic anomaly. Chromosomal abnormality associated with anencephaly includes trisomy 13 and 18, Turner syndrome, triploidy, or it may be part of a more complex process involving single-gene defect. Over a hundred candidate genes have been examined for risk association to human NTD; yet, very few studies have identified candidate genes that confer even a minor effect on NTD risk, genes involved in folate metabolism are believed to be important. One such gene, methylenetetrahydrofolate reductase (*MTHFR*), has been shown to be associated with the risk of NTDs. In 2007, a second gene, a membrane-associated signaling complex protein called *VANGL1*, was also shown to be associated with the risk of NTDs.

Inadequate Folic Acid

Folic acid deficiency is by far the most identifiable cause of NTD. It has been estimated that up to 70% of NTD are preventable by adequate preconceptional supplementation of folic acid. Since the United States began fortifying grains with folic acid, there has been a 28% decline in pregnancies affected by NTDs (spina bifida and anencephaly). Folic acid antagonists such as trimethoprim, triamterene, carbamazepine, phenytoin, phenobarbitone, and primidone, that interfere with normal folate metabolism during the critical period of neural tube development (up to 6 weeks after last menstrual period) increase the likelihood of NTD. Valproic acid has been shown to increase the chance of NTD when exposure occurs in early development.

Insulin-dependent Diabetes Mellitus

Maternal type 1, or pregestational insulin-dependent diabetes mellitus (IDDM), confers a significant increase in the risk for NTDs. IDDM delays the production of alpha-fetoprotein (AFP) during pregnancy, therefore, for risk calculation, adjustment of the expected values for AFP in maternal serum must be made if the patient is known to have IDDM. Well-controlled IDDM confers a lower risk for NTDs, while gestational diabetes does not appear to be associated with any significant increase in NTD risk.

Obesity

There is ample evidence that overweight and obesity, both of which are detected in increasing prevalence in developed countries, more than doubles the risk of NTD.

Maternal Hyperthermia

Maternal hyperthermia has been associated with an increased risk for NTD; therefore, pregnant women should

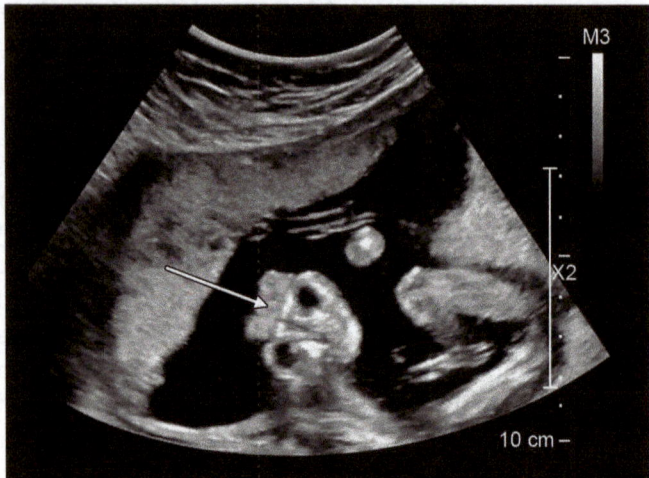

Fig. 2: Two-dimensional (2D) image of anencephalic fetus.

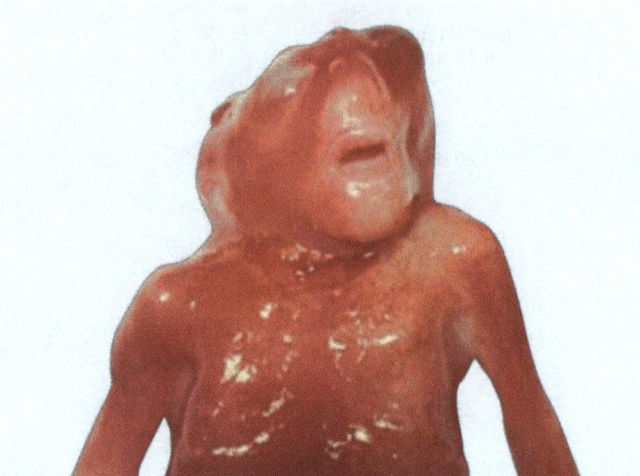

Fig. 4: Anencephalic baby.

The absence of cranial vault and presence of some brain tissue give the head a Mickey Mouse shape, accuracy of diagnosis is 100% in expert hand. Maternal serum alpha-fetoprotein (MSAFP) screening during the second trimester of pregnancy (15–18 weeks) is an effective screening tool. False positives from amniotic fluid alpha-fetoprotein (AFAFP) can be excluded based on the results of testing for acetylcholinesterase (ACHE), which should be clearly positive for open anencephaly. Amniocentesis to detect raised AFAFP has been largely superseded by detailed ultrasound imaging **(Figs. 2 and 3)**.

Management
Approximately one-fourth of all pregnancies are complicated by polyhydramnios. Because of polyhydramnios, labor and delivery are frequently associated with complications such as an unstable lie, dysfunctional labor, increased incidence of placental abruption, and postpartum hemorrhage.

Anencephaly is lethal because of the severe brain malformation that is present. A significant proportion of all anencephalic fetuses are stillborn or are aborted spontaneously. Liveborn anencephalic babies usually die in hours or days **(Fig. 4)**. Once a diagnosis of anencephaly is made, pregnancy management varies according to the gestational age at diagnosis. If diagnosis is made before 24 weeks, the option of pregnancy termination is offered.

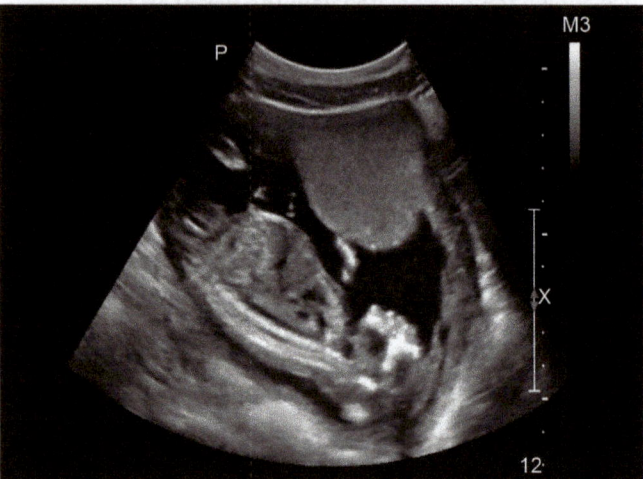

Fig. 3: Ultrasonographic (USG) image of anencephalic fetus.

avoid hot tubs and other environments that may induce transient hyperthermia. Similarly, maternal fever in early gestation also has been reported as a risk factor for anencephaly and other NTDs.

Amniotic Band Disruption Sequence
Amniotic band disruption sequence is a condition resulting from rupture of the amniotic membranes. This can cause disruption of normally formed tissues during development, including the structures of the head and the brain. Anencephaly caused by amniotic band disruption sequence is frequently distinguishable by the presence of remnants of the amniotic membrane. Recurrence risk for anencephaly caused by this mechanism is lower, and the risk is not modified by the use of folic acid.

Diagnosis
Diagnosis of anencephaly is made sonologically by the absence of cerebral tissue and cranial vault, as early as 14 weeks.

Prevention
Every couple who has/had anencephaly fetus should consult with a geneticist and/or a genetic counselor to obtain information regarding recurrence risks, prevention, screening, and diagnostic testing options in future pregnancies. Folic acid supplementation and/or a folate-enriched diet prior to and during future pregnancies are recommended.

The recurrence risk for NTDs, in general, is 2–4% in subsequent pregnancies. Folic acid supplementation has been shown to be an effective means of lowering recurrence risks for future pregnancies. Recommended that women having had a previous pregnancy with a NTD and women with family history of NTD planning pregnancy take 4 mg of folic acid daily before conception and during the first 12 weeks of pregnancy. All women of childbearing age should consume 0.4 mg of folic acid daily, especially those attempting to conceive regardless of family history; this amount of folic acid is found in most over-the-counter multivitamins. Supplementation at these levels is estimated to prevent two-thirds of both recurrent and new cases of NTD, and may result in 30–40% reduction in the prevalence. Increased folate intake may also be achieved through food fortification; however, the bioavailability of natural folates in foods is often lower than that of folic acid.

Cephaloceles

Cephaloceles are cranial defects with a sac-like protrusion or herniation of brain, meninges, or both along bony sutures, which can be occipital, parietal, or frontal. In 80% cases, it is occipital, parietal cephalocele occurs in up to 37% cases, frontal cephalocele/frontoethmoidal cephalocele ~10%. In Caucasian population, the most common location is occipital, while in South East Asians, frontal is common.

If the sac contains only brain tissue, it is called *encephalocele*; if it contains only cerebrospinal fluid (CSF), it is called *meningocele*. The condition is usually isolated, but in a small percentage of cases, may be a part of chromosomal or nonchromosomal defect. There is a genetic (inherited) component to the condition, occurs in families that have other family members with NTD.

Incidence

The estimated incidence is 0.8–4:10,000 live births with a well-recognized geographical variation between types. There is no recognized gender predilection.

Diagnostic Features

Cephalocele is a sac-like structure adjacent to or posterior to the fetal head. Brain tissue in the sac is covered by skin and a skull defect. Hydrocephalus is present in 80% cases of occipital encephalocele; associated anomaly presents in up to 50% of cases and includes ventricular septal defect (VSD), coarctation of aorta, single UA, pyelectasis, ureteral agenesis, talipes, abnormality of thorax, and abdominal wall.

Occipital encephaloceles may be associated with a number of additional malformations—Chiari malformations, Dandy-Walker malformations, and Meckel-Gruber syndrome. Other anomalies include cleft lip and palate, hypertelorism, and amniotic band syndrome. Chromosomal abnormalities most commonly seen with encephalocele are trisomy 13 and 18, mosaic 20, unbalanced translocation, and inversion.

Detailed ultrasound examination will make the diagnosis in most cases. Sonographically, these lesions may appear as a cyst protruding from the fetal calvarium representing a meningocele or cyst within cyst appearance, a solid mass protruding from the calvarium representing a herniated brain; either or both of the above associated with a defect in the calvarium **(Figs. 5 and 6)**. Sometimes a small encephalocele can go undetected, diagnosed after birth. Magnetic resonance imaging (MRI) may help in better delineating fetal CNS abnormality. Invasive testing is required for confirmation of chromosomal abnormality and incudes karyotyping and chromosome microarray.

Sign Symptoms

Sign symptoms include hydrocephalus, microcephaly, complete loss of strength in the arms and the legs, developmental delay, intellectual disability, vision problems, and seizure. An encephalocele at the back of the skull is more likely to cause nervous system problems, as well as other brain and facial defects.

Obstetric Management

Obstetric management is dictated by the size of the defect, gestational age, and presence or absence of associated anomaly. Termination of pregnancy should be discussed with parents, if continuation is decided, consultation with medical geneticist and pediatric neurosurgeon is obtained.

Treatment

Surgical treatment includes to place the protruding part of the brain and the membranes covering it back into the skull and close the opening in the skull. However, neurologic problems caused by the encephalocele will still be present. Long-term treatment depends on the child's condition. Multiple surgery may be needed, depending on the location of the encephalocele and the parts of the head and the face that were affected by the encephalocele.

Prognosis

Prognosis depends on the size, content, and location of the encephalocele, prognosis is better in meningocele. Prognosis also depends on presence or absence of associated anomalies. Mortality for posterior encephalocele is >50% and for posterior meningocele and anterior encephalocele is about 20%. Neurological handicap is present in >50% of survivors, the presence of microcephaly carries a much poorer prognosis. Among the survivors, normal development occurs in 48% cases, mild developmental delay in 11% cases, moderate developmental delay in 16% case, and severe developmental delay occurs in 25% cases. Normal intelligence has also been reported. Chromosome analysis should be done either prenatally or postnatally.

Recurrence

In isolated encephalocele, recurrence risk is 3–5%, when it occurs as a part of trisomy, recurrence is 1% and as part

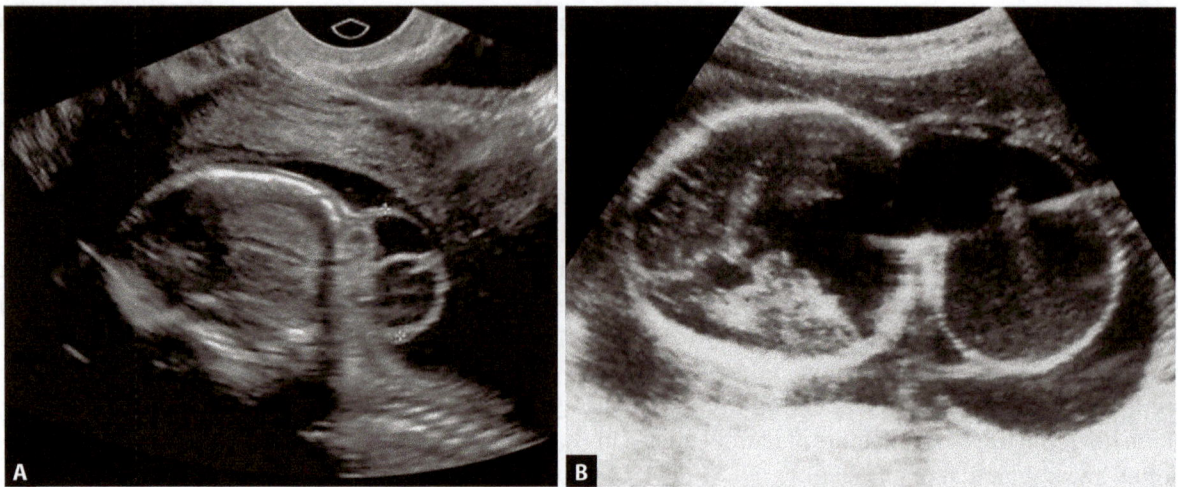

Figs. 5A and B: Ultrasonographic (USG) images of occipital encephalocele.

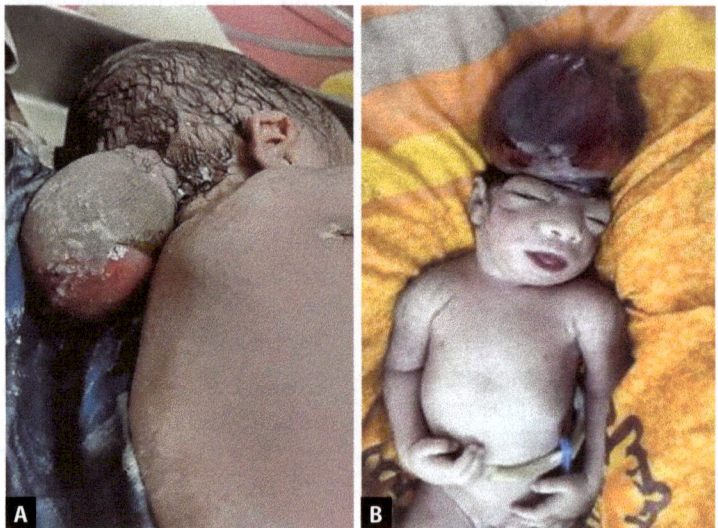

Figs. 6A and B: (A) Occipital encephalocele; (B) Frontal encephalocele.

of an autosomal recessive condition, there is 25% risk of recurrence.

Spina Bifida

Spina bifida is the most common, permanently disabling birth defect, which results from failure of fusion in the spinal region of the neural tube with exposure of the contents of the neural channel.

Classically, there are two types of spina bifida—spina bifida aperta (open) and occulta (closed) **(Fig. 7)**:
1. In *open spina bifida*, the defect is usually covered by a thin meningeal membrane, giving the appearance of a cystic tumor. If the mass contains spinal fluid and meningeal tissue, it is known as *meningocele* and if it contains spinal fluid and neural tissue, it is called *myelomeningocele (MMC)*. MMC is the most common lesion (80–90% cases), which occurs in the lumbosacral in region in 80% cases. Rachischisis/myeloschisis is the rarest type of defect, the neural tube is completely open, no meninges, or skin covering.
2. *Spina bifida occulta* is usually a small, clinically asymptomatic defect, covered by skin, with no protrusion in about 12% of the population. Most people are not aware that they have spina bifida occulta, unless it is discovered on an X-ray performed for an unrelated reason. However, one in 1,000 individuals will have an occult structural finding that leads to neurological deficits or disabilities such as bowel or bladder dysfunction, back pain, leg weakness, or scoliosis.

Incidence

In USA, about 1,500–2,000 of the 4 million babies born every year have spina bifida. The prevalence appears to have decreased in the recent years due in part to preventative measures and follow-up of at-risk expectant mothers prior to and during pregnancy as well as prenatal testing. After having one child with the condition, or if

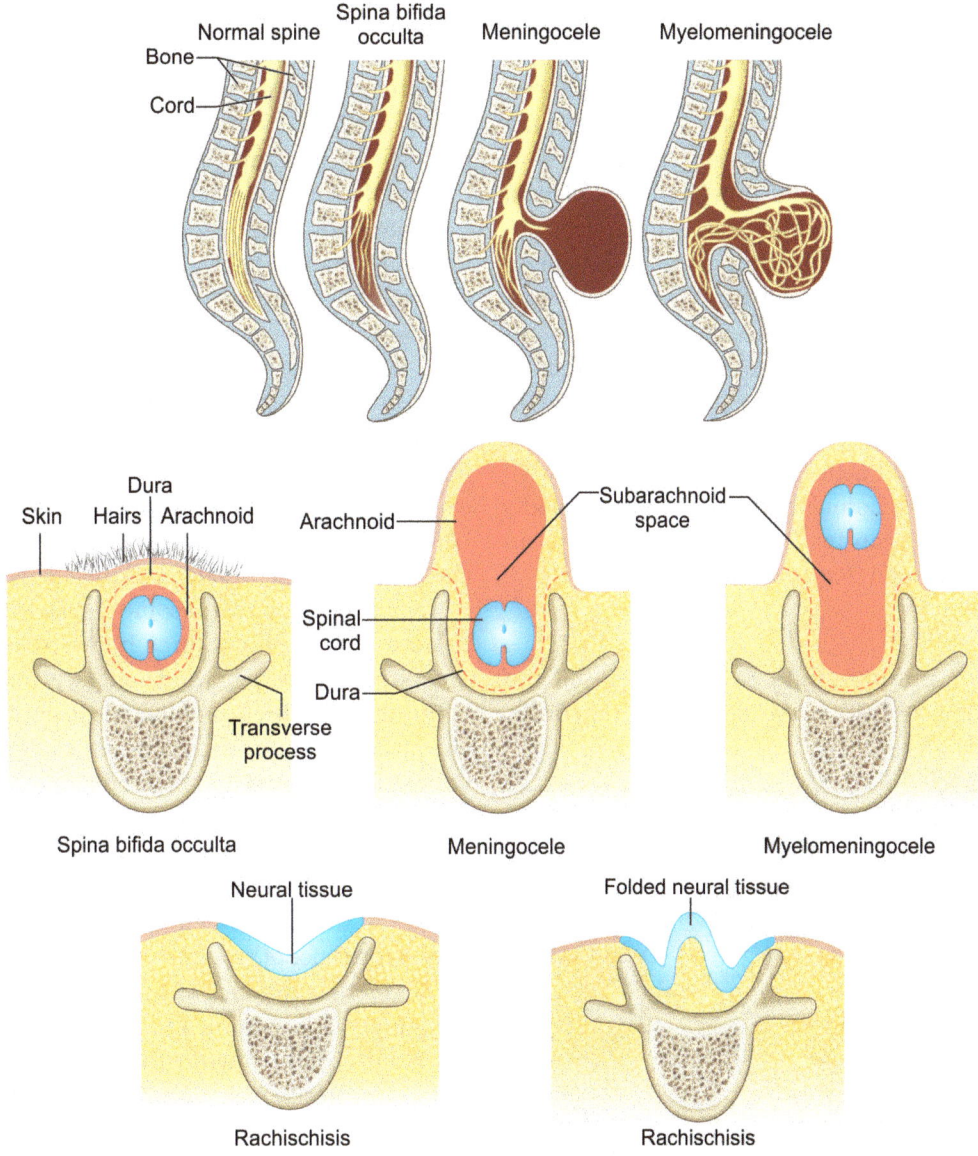

Fig. 7: Types of spina bifida.

one of the parents has the condition, there is a 4% chance that the next child will also be affected and 10% risk for a third child.

Etiology

Normally, the neural tube forms early in pregnancy and it closes by the 28th day after conception. In spina bifida, a portion of the neural tube does not close or develop properly, causing defects in the spinal cord and in the bones of the spine, believed to be due to a combination of *genetic and environmental factors* (multifactorial inheritance). Some of these factors have been identified, many remain unknown.

Genes involved in folate metabolism are believed to be important. Mutation in the *gene* for the enzymes, *MTHFR*, has been shown to be associated with the risk of NTDs, a second gene, a membrane-associated signaling complex protein called *VANGL1*, was also shown to be associated with the risk of NTDs. Variation in the gene for another enzyme methionine synthetase (MTRR) also carries an increased risk when present in combination with decreased vitamin B_{12}.

Some cases of spina bifida may be associated with chromosome abnormalities, or fetal exposure to teratogens. Other possible risk factors include poorly controlled diabetes mellitus, maternal obesity, exposure to high heat (such as a fever or use of a hot tub or sauna) in early pregnancy, and the use of certain antiseizure medications (valproic acid and carbamazepine) during pregnancy. However, it is unclear how these factors may influence the risk of spina bifida.

Symptoms

The signs and symptoms of spina bifida can range from mild to severe. There is usually a mixture of upper and lower motor neuron signs depending on the location and extent of spinal cord involvement and there is always disturbance of bladder and bowel function. Generally, the higher the defect located on the spine, the more severe the complications. Surviving infants require complex orthopedic and urological support, including surgery. Possible symptoms include a loss of feeling below the level of the opening, weakness or paralysis of the feet or legs, problems with bladder and bowel control, sexual dysfunction, hydrocephalus, and learning problems.

About 5% of cases of spina bifida cystica are meningoceles in which there is no neural tissue in the cyst wall, there is no associated hydrocephalus, and neurological examination may be normal. In many cases, the brain develops an Arnold–Chiari II malformation, in this anomaly, the cerebellar vermis is herniated through the foramen magnum, displacing the 4th ventricle inside the neural canal and causing obstructive hydrocephalus. This herniation of the hindbrain blocks the circulation of CSF, causing hydrocephalus which can injure the developing brain **(Fig. 8)**.

Diagnosis

Determination of amniotic fluid ACHE is helpful, but direct visualization by USG is the method of diagnosis.

High-resolution USG can diagnose the defect as early as 16 weeks. CNS lesion frequently associated with spina bifida is hydrocephalus secondary to presence of an *Arnold–Chiari malformation*. Other associated anomaly includes holoprosencephaly, agenesis of corpus callosum, limb deformity, e.g., clubfoot and dislocation of hip.

Sonographic appearance includes cerebral ventriculomegaly, microcephaly, abnormalities of the frontal bone, obliteration of the cisterna magna with absent or abnormal concavity of cerebellum referred as *lemon and banana sign*. Lemon sign is present in 98% fetuses at or before 24 weeks. Lemon sign is due to decreased intracranial pressure because of caudal herniation of hindbrain contents. Banana sign is more typical before 24 weeks, and is due to caudal herniation of cerebellum through foramen magnum. Lemon sign may be seen in 1% of normal fetus, whereas banana sign is not present in normal fetus **(Figs. 9A and B)**.

Ultrasonography of the spine on transverse plane **(Fig. 10)** in normal fetus shows three bony structures—two lateral processes of the vertebra and midline vertebral body. In spina bifida, there is absence of the postlamina and lateral vertebral processes are set apart. Spina bifida can be demonstrated in both longitudinal and coronal plane. In the longitudinal plane, the spine should appear like a railroad track (the distal part of the spine may not be ossified in normal fetuses up to 22 weeks). In the coronal plane, widening of the ossification centers in the neural arch gives a U-shaped configuration. There is presence of kyphosis or scoliosis associated with NTD.

Magnetic resonance imaging provides additional complimentary information and is superior to USG in case of maternal obesity, oligohydramnios, low position of fetal head, or posterior position of fetal spine **(Figs. 12A and B)**.

Pathological Changes

Pathological changes in spina bifida occur in two stages, the two-hit hypothesis:
1. The first hit is the failure of neurulation early in gestation.

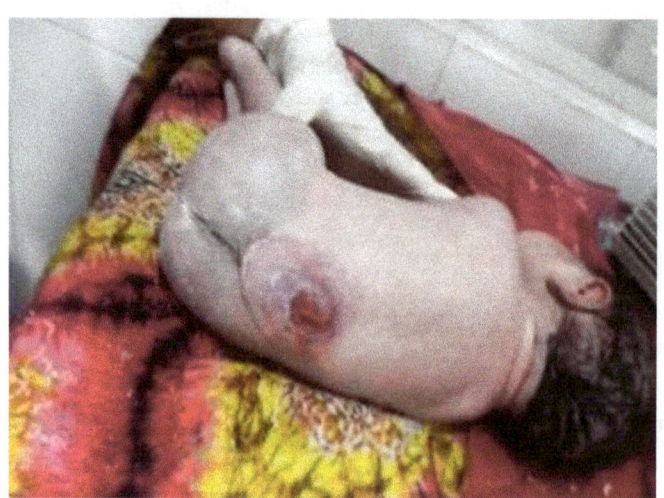

Fig. 8: Neonate with meningocele.

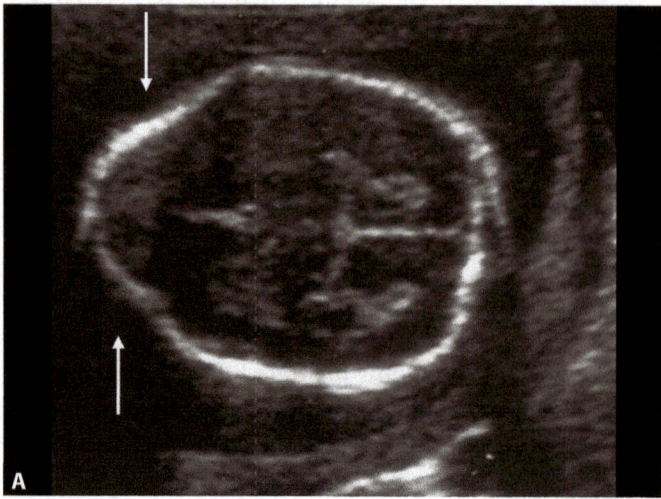

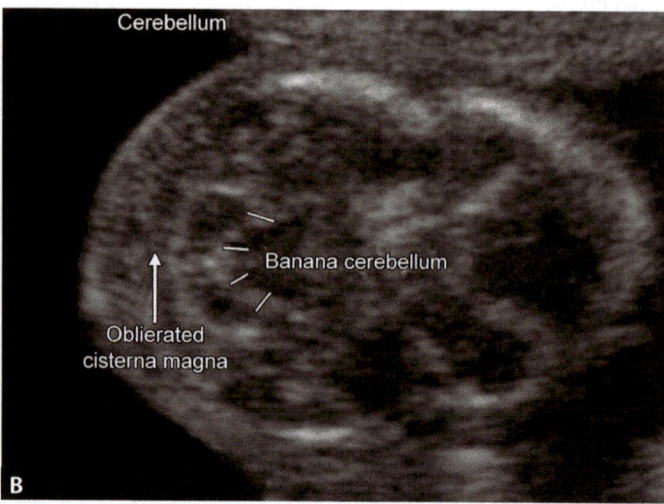

Figs. 9A and B: Cranial changes in spina bifida lemon and banana sign.

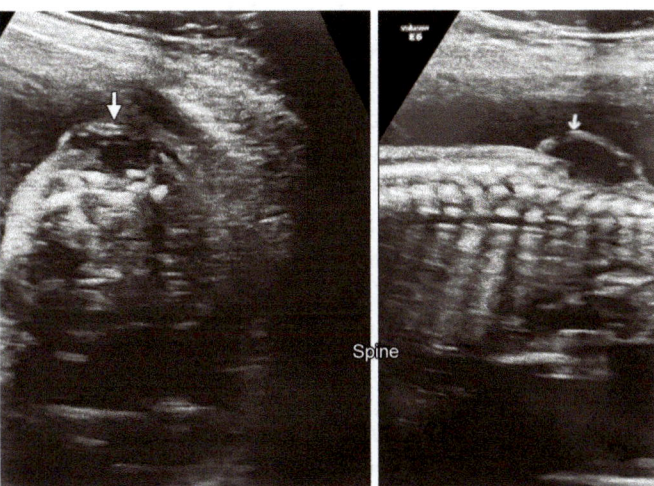

Fig. 10: USG image of spina bifida (Longitudinal and transverse views).

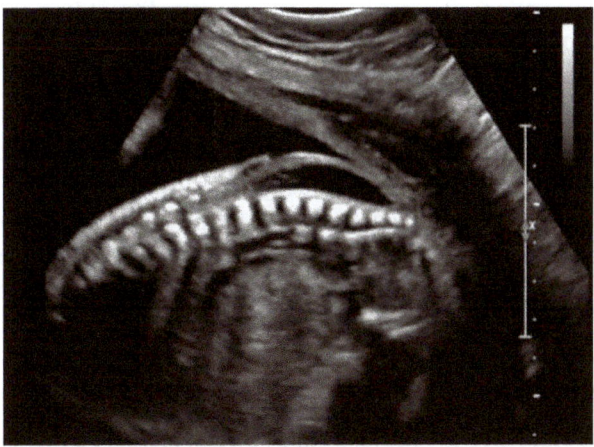

Fig. 11: Ultrasonographic (USG) image of spina bifida in longitudinal view.

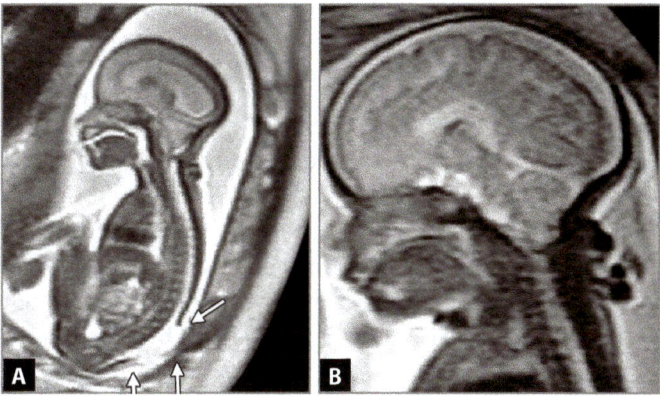

Figs. 12A and B: Magnetic resonance imaging (MRI)—myelomeningocele (MMC) hydrocephalus and cerebellar tonsillar herniation.

2. The second hit is the spinal cord injury resulting from prolonged exposure of the neural tissue to the intrauterine environment—partly due to chronic mechanical injury and chemical trauma induced by exposure to amniotic fluid.

The second hit can be prevented if adequate prenatal covering of the exposed neural tube can be provided, repair must be done before the onset of irreversible damage.

Management

Long-term prognosis is related to location of MMC. Lower the location of the defect, the better is the prognosis. Termination may be offered if spina bifida is diagnosed before 24 weeks. Diagnosis after 24 weeks and if parents want to continue pregnancy—delivery by cesarean section (C/S), particularly if fetus shows movement of the knees and the ankles and MMC sac is seen beyond plane of fetal back.

Surgical Treatment

Treatment for spina bifida typically involves surgery to repair the opening in the spine. Surgery can be done before or shortly after birth. Surgery before birth (fetal surgery) is an option depending on the severity of the spina bifida and the health of the mother. Fetal surgery showed better than predicted lower extremity function compared to postnatal repair. While surgery may prevent symptoms from getting worse, it cannot correct any damage to the nerves that is already present.

A randomized study (MOMS Trial) compared in-utero repair versus repair after birth and had encouraging, but mixed, results. Patients who underwent fetal repair were less likely to need a ventriculoperitoneal shunt (44 vs. 84%) and more likely to be able to walk (44 vs. 24%). The fetal surgery group also had many more maternal and infant complications. Given the higher risk of complications as well as the lack of long-term follow-up, the current recommendation of the American College of Obstetricians and Gynecologists (ACOG) is that fetal surgery only be considered at specialty centers with teams experienced in fetal surgery.

Postnatal Treatment

Postnatal treatment typically involves antibiotics, sac closure, and ventriculoperitoneal shunting, usually performed shortly after birth (within the first 48 hours of baby's life). Long-term physical, occupational, and/or speech therapy may be needed. In some cases, the condition is not treatable.

Long-term outcome: To stand erect, motor function is needed up to 3rd lumber level. To walk, motor function is needed from 4th to 5th lumber vertebra and to have sexual function must have motor function to at least 2nd to 4th sacral level. The degree of handicap and survival rate depends on the level and severity of the lesion. The lower the spinal lesion, the better is the prognosis. Lifelong disability accompanying MMC includes paraplegia (with lesion above L2), hydrocephalus, pulmonary dysfunction, sexual dysfunction, skeletal and spinal deformity, incontinence, and cognitive impairment. Long-term consequences include low intelligence quotient (IQ), renal failure in adulthood, 25% of survivors have IQ below 50, one-fourth have IQ above 100.

Despite postnatal intervention, approximately 14% do not survive beyond 5 years.

Recurrence Risk
Recurrence risk is 1.5–3%. Women who have given birth to one affected baby should take 4 mg folic acid daily at least 3 months prior to next pregnancy and continue till 12 weeks of gestation. Research has shown that if all women of childbearing age took a multivitamin with folic acid (0.4 mg), the risk of NTDs could be reduced by up to 70%.

Ventriculomegaly

Definition
Ventriculomegaly is defined as dilatation of the lateral ventricle measuring [>4 standard deviation (SD) above mean] at the level of posterior horn with normal intracranial pressure. The ventricle is measured from inner margin of the medial ventricular wall to inner margin of the lateral wall. Normal ventricular diameter remains constant between 14 and 38 weeks of gestation and is 7.6 ± 0.6 mm and a measurement of 10 mm is 2.5-4 SD above the mean. An appropriately obtained sonographic measurement of <10 mm should be considered normal. Although mild fetal ventriculomegaly is often incidental and benign, it can be associated with genetic, structural, and neurocognitive disorders. In the setting of isolated mild ventriculomegaly (10–12 mm), the likelihood of survival with normal neurodevelopment is >90%.

Types
Ventriculomegaly can be classified as: *Mild/borderline* ventriculomegaly: When lateral ventricular diameter is between 10 and 12 mm, *moderate* fetal ventriculomegaly: 12.1–15 mm, and *severe* fetal ventriculomegaly (also sometimes classified as fetal hydrocephalus): lateral ventricular diameter >15 mm **(Figs. 13 and 14)**.

It is important that the lateral ventricle be measured correctly, as small differences in technique can result in false-positive or false-negative results. Substantial interobserver variability in interpretation can occur, particularly at borderline ventricular diameters (i.e., about 10 mm). Measurement technique: Head in the axial plane, image is magnified appropriately, so that fetal head fills majority of image. The atrium of the lateral ventricle should be measured in the transventricular (axial) plane at the level demonstrating the frontal horns and cavum septum pellucidum, in which the cerebral hemispheres are symmetric in appearance. The calipers should be positioned on the internal margin of the medial and lateral walls of the atria, at the level of the parietal-occipital groove and glomus of the choroid plexus, on an axis perpendicular to the long axis of the lateral ventricle.

The diagnosis of ventriculomegaly can also be made using ventricular to hemisphere ratio [lateral ventricle width/hemispheric width (LVW/HW)]. The ratio is approximately 0.71 at 15 weeks which decreases to 0.37 at 24 weeks. Any value above 0.5 after 24 weeks is abnormal. When ventriculomegaly is pronounced, the choroid plexus will no longer lie in an almost parallel fashion against the lateral ventricular wall, tethered at the foramen of Monro the free hanging choroid will "hang down" and appear to "dangle" within the dilated ventricle. This appearance is often termed as the dangling choroid sign.

Incidence
The incidence is 1 in 1,000–2,000 births, increased incidence in male fetuses. Unilateral ventriculomegaly is present in approximately 50–60% of cases, and bilateral ventriculomegaly occurs in approximately 40–50% cases.

Etiology
The most common causes of ventriculomegaly are aqueduct stenosis, Chiari II malformation, Dandy-Walker

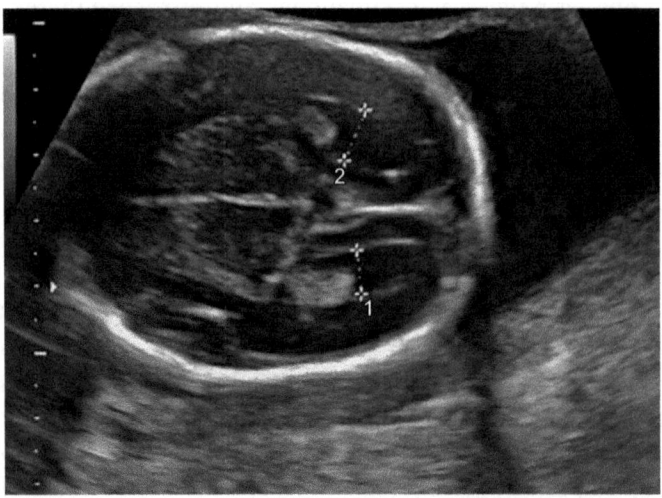

Fig. 13: Ultrasonographic (USG) appearance of fetal ventriculomegaly.

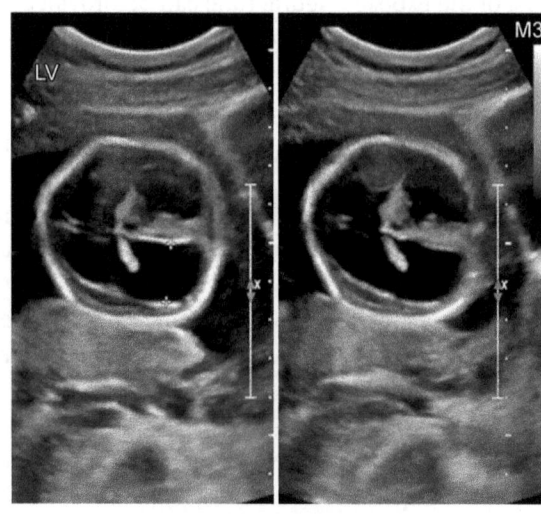

Fig. 14: Fetal hydrocephalus.

malformation, agenesis of corpus callosum, and chromosomal aneuploidy. Ventriculomegaly is considered *"isolated"* when the fetus does not present any other structural anomalies and possess normal karyotyping.

Pathogenesis

The pathogenesis of mild ventriculomegaly is not clearly elucidated, it is most likely multifactorial, frequently associated with other brain abnormality, chromosomal abnormality is present in 10–15% cases, fetal infection may be present in 0.4% cases.

Diagnosis

A detailed fetal anatomic survey is necessary as additional CNS and non-CNS defects and genetic syndromes are found in 50% of cases. Chromosomal defects, mainly trisomy 21, 18, or 13, balanced translocation, and mosaicism, are found in 10% of cases. In isolated ventriculomegaly, there is a fourfold increase in risk for trisomy 21. The risk is inversely related to the severity of ventriculomegaly. Associated anomaly includes hydronephrosis, dysplastic kidney, VSD, tetralogy of Fallot (TOF), gastrointestinal (GI) abnormalities including omphalocele, gastroschisis, and tracheoesophageal (TE) fistula. The fetal heart should be carefully examined, and fetal biometry should be assessed for evidence of growth restriction. Finally, a thorough inspection should be performed for signs of fetal infection, including intracranial or extracranial calcifications, hepatosplenomegaly, ascites, and fetal growth restriction.

Investigations

Amniocentesis with chromosome microarray analysis should be offered when ventriculomegaly is detected. Testing for CMV and toxoplasmosis by maternal serology or polymerase chain reaction (PCR) on amniotic fluid regardless of known exposure or symptoms. The most common modality of diagnosis is USG which may miss fetal agenesis of the corpus callosum.

Magnetic resonance imaging is most useful before 22–24 weeks of gestation, milestones of CNS development become more evident with advancing gestation. MRI can be considered in cases of mild or moderate fetal ventriculomegaly when this modality and expert radiologic interpretation are available. It is also beneficial in assessing the extent of destructive injury in fetuses with known infection, hemorrhage, or ischemia, and when other sonographic evidence of CNS malformation is present, such as agenesis of the corpus callosum or Dandy-Walker malformation.

Follow-up: Ultrasound scans every 4 weeks to assess for progression of the ventricular dilation.

Delivery

No evidence that preterm or cesarean delivery improves maternal or neonatal outcomes in the setting of mild-to-moderate ventriculomegaly. Timing and mode of delivery should therefore be based on standard obstetric indications. Given the potential for mild-to-moderate ventriculomegaly to be associated with long-term adverse neurodevelopmental outcomes, the primary pediatrician should be made aware of this prenatal finding.

Prognosis

Prognosis depends on specific cause and presence of associated anomaly. In fetuses with mild isolated ventriculomegaly, prognosis is good but there is an increased risk of neurodevelopmental disabilities. In a recent meta-analysis, the rate of neurodevelopmental delay in truly isolated mild ventriculomegaly was 7.9%. In the setting of mild-to-moderate ventriculomegaly with associated abnormalities, the prognosis primarily depends on the specific abnormality rather than the degree of ventricular dilation. Isolated mild/moderate ventriculomegaly: Neurodevelopmental delay in 10% of cases, this may not be higher than in the general population. In cases in which ventriculomegaly progresses, the rate of adverse outcomes is reported to be as high as 44%, while outcomes are normal in >90% of cases in which ventriculomegaly improves. If the ventriculomegaly is mild and isolated, the outcome is most commonly normal.

Risk of Recurrence

Risk of recurrence of isolated ventriculomegaly in future pregnancies is low (<1%), which increases to 5% if there is a history of affected fetus or sibling. In cases with an underlying cause, such as a chromosomal or genetic condition, risk of recurrence will depend on the specific diagnosis. X-linked hydrocephaly with severe ventriculomegaly has poorest prognosis. When ventriculomegaly occurs as part of infection, there is no increased risk, if it occurs as part of trisomy recurrence risk is ~1%.

Hydrocephalus

Definition

The term hydrocephalus is derived from the Greek word, "hydro" meaning water and "cephalus" meaning the head. An abnormal increase in the amount of CSF within the cranial cavity with increased CSF pressure accompanied by expansion of the cerebral ventricles, enlargement of the skull and especially the forehead, and atrophy of the brain. Prenatally, a common convention is to use the term hydrocephalus when the lateral ventricles measure >15 mm or an obstructive etiology associated with increased CSF pressure is evident.

Cerebrospinal Fluid (CSF) Formation and Circulation

The CSF is a clear, colorless body fluid found in the brain and the spinal cord. It is produced by specialized ependymal cells in the choroid plexuses of the ventricles of the brain, and absorbed in the arachnoid granulations. There is about 125 mL of CSF at any one time, and about 500 mL is generated every day. CSF acts as a cushion or buffer, providing basic mechanical and immunological protection to the brain, also serves a vital function in the autoregulation of cerebral blood flow. It occupies the subarachnoid space and the ventricular system around and inside the brain and the spinal cord, fills the ventricles of the brain, cisterns, and sulci, as well as the central canal of the spinal cord **(Fig. 15)**.

The majority of CSF is produced from within the two lateral ventricles. From the lateral ventricles, CSF reaches the 3rd ventricle through foramen of Monro. From 3rd ventricle, it reaches through cerebral aqueduct or aqueduct of Sylvius to 4th ventricle. From 4th ventricle, it reaches spinal canal through foramen of Magendie and into subarachnoid spaces throughout CNS through foramina of Luschka. CSF formed gets absorbed after its function is over. Most CSF gets absorbed into arachnoid villi and granulations which dip into subdural venous sinuses.

Under normal conditions, a delicate balance exists between the amount of CSF produced and the rate at which it is absorbed. Hydrocephalus develops when this balance is altered and is characterized by an abnormal accumulation of CSF within the ventricles. This accumulation of CSF increases the pressure in the brain causing the ventricles to enlarge and the brain to be pressed against the skull. When CSF absorption is blocked or reduced, hydrocephalus can develop. This is often referred to as communicating hydrocephalus because there is no obvious blockage within the ventricular system.

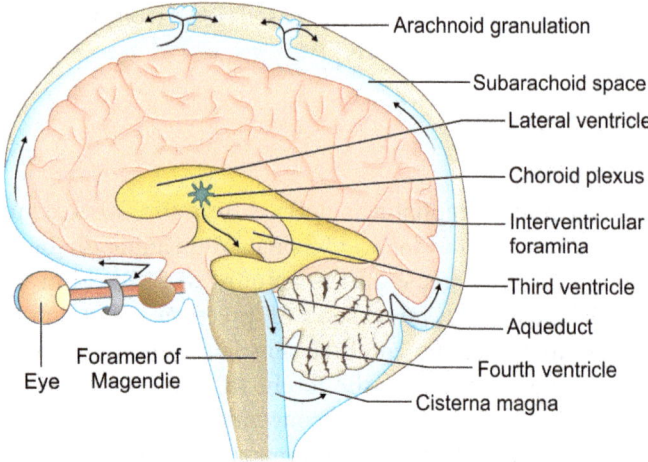

Fig. 15: Cerebrospinal fluid, its formation and circulation.
Source: thescienceinfo.com

Cause of Fetal Hydrocephalus

Hydrocephalus may be caused by genetic or nongenetic factors. The most common genetic cause is mutations in the *L1CAM* gene. It is estimated that about 40% of hydrocephalus have a possible genetic etiology. Inherited genetic abnormalities, which cause aqueductal stenosis (AS), are the most common form of fetal hydrocephalus. Blockage of the aqueduct can also be caused by a tumor, or swelling due to infection such as CMV, toxoplasma, syphilis, or intraventricular bleeding.

It can also be caused by developmental disorders, such as those associated with NTDs including spina bifida, encephalocele, and Dandy-Walker malformation. Exposition to certain drugs (teratogens), maternal alcohol use can also cause fetal hydrocephalus. Other possible causes include complications of premature birth such as intraventricular hemorrhage, and diseases such as meningitis, tumors, traumatic head injury, or subarachnoid hemorrhage, which block the exit of CSF from the ventricles to the cisterns or eliminate the passageway for CSF within the cisterns. Hydrocephalus may result from reduced flow and absorption of CSF into specialized blood vessels (arachnoid villi), which results in buildup of CSF in the ventricles and cause communicating hydrocephalus.

Congenital hydrocephalus can be an isolated malformation or be part of a syndrome where there are other associated malformations. Approximately 40% of cases of ventriculomegaly have associated CNS or extra CNS abnormality and 12% have abnormal karyotype.

Diagnosis of Fetal Hydrocephaly

Antenatal ultrasound will demonstrate enlarged ventricles with variable degrees of parenchymal thinning. The choroid may be seen floating within the ventricle giving a dangling choroid sign. Often a separation of >3 mm between the choroid plexus and the margin of the ventricle is considered abnormal. In some cases, there may also be evidence of macrocephaly **(Fig. 16)**.

Associated anomaly includes:
- *Central nervous system anomalies* (more common and reported in >80% of cases):
  - *AS:* One of the most common causative associations
  - Chiari malformations
  - NTDs
  - Dandy-Walker malformation
  - Encephalocele
  - Alobar holoprosencephaly
  - Posterior fossa cysts
  - Craniosynostosis
- *Noncentral nervous system anomalies:*
  - Craniofacial-cleft lip +/− palate, low set ears, bilateral optic atrophy, and facial bone anomalies
  - Congenital cardiovascular anomalies

Fetal Congenital Malformation

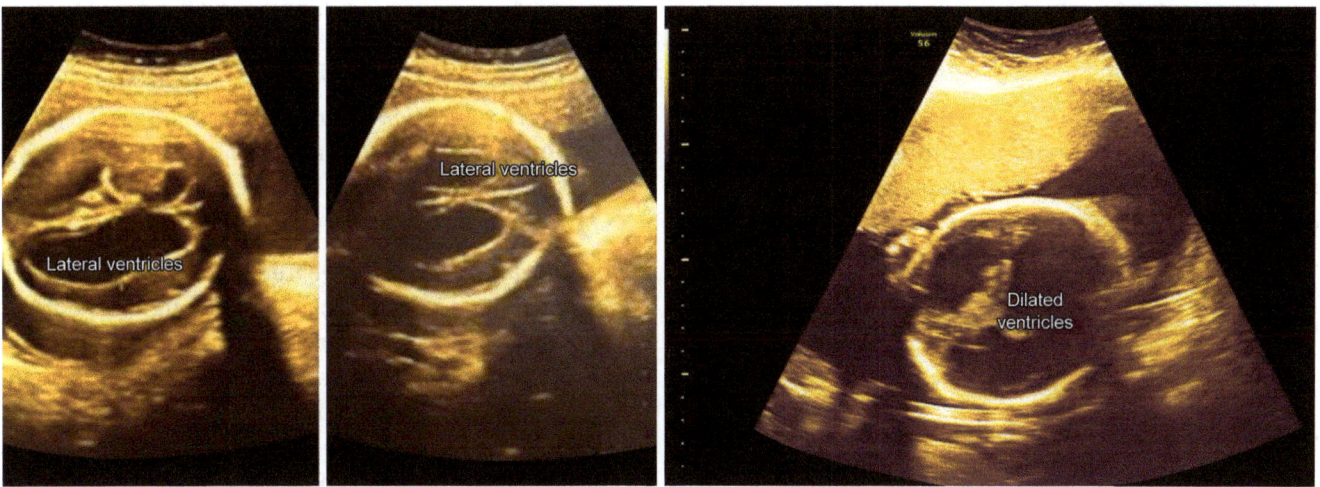

Fig. 16: USG appearance of fetal severe ventriculomegaly.

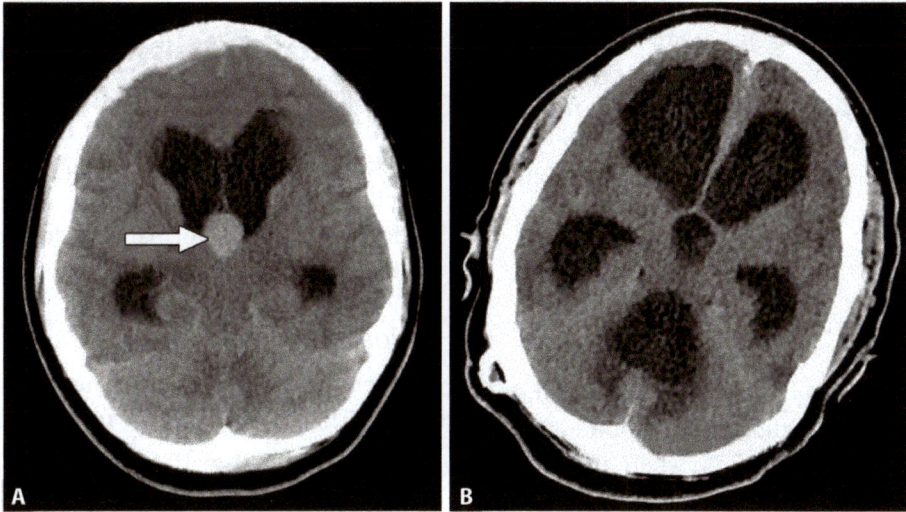

Figs. 17A and B: (A) CT scan of colloid cyst (large white arrow) of the third ventricle with associated non-communicating hydrocephalus; (B) Communicating hydrocephalus. (CT: computed tomography)
Source: radiopaedia.org

- GI anomalies
- Genitourinary anomalies—congenital renal fusion
- Skeletal anomalies—clubfeet
- *Syndromes:*
  - Meckel–Gruber syndrome and Miller–Dieker syndrome
  - Chromosomal anomalies: May be present in ~20% of cases

Incidence

The estimated incidence is 0.5–3 cases per 1,000 live births. There may be a very slight increase in female predilection.

Types (Figs. 17A and B)

There are two types of hydrocephalus:
1. *Communicating hydrocephalus:* When flow of CSF is blocked after it exits the ventricles. This form is called communicating because the CSF can still flow between the ventricles, the passages between the ventricles remain open.
2. *Noncommunicating hydrocephalus (or obstructive):* Happens when the flow of CSF is blocked in one or more of the narrow passages that connect the ventricles, e.g., aqueduct stenosis.

Diagnostic study includes detailed fetal anatomic survey, fetal echocardiography to exclude associated anomaly. For X-linked hydrocephalus, *L1CAM* gene-microarray, infection work-up for CMV and toxoplasmosis, karyotype to exclude most common chromosomal abnormality—trisomy 9, 13, and 18 as well as triploidy.

An antenatal USG examination will demonstrate enlarged ventricles with variable degrees of parenchymal thinning as well as secondary macrocephaly. MRI better delineates the extent of obstructive hydrocephalus with an enlargement (often marked) of the lateral and third ventricles. In aqueduct stenosis, the aqueduct will show funneling superiorly, the fourth ventricle is not dilated. In cases of secondary obstruction, the underlying abnormality may also be evident (e.g., web and tumor). Serial follow-up USG to see the progression.

Symptoms

Symptoms in neonates and children may include an unusually large head with thin, transparent scalp, bulging forehead with dilated fontanelles, and a downward gaze. Other symptoms may include seizures, abnormal reflexes, slow heartbeat and respiratory rate, headaches, vomiting, irritability, weakness, and visual problems.

Management in Pregnancy

Serial sonography to see whether the condition is stable, progressive, or regressive, fetal MRI in significant ventriculomegaly. Decision on management options depends on gestational age at diagnosis and associated anomaly. Regardless of etiology, early detection and early interention of this condition are very important to prevent brain insult and normal development of children. Decrease of volume accumulation and decrease in intracranial pressure maintain normal chemical balance and normal function of blood–brain barrier. At the present time, there is no fetal treatment for this disorder.

Treatment

After birth, hydrocephalus is treated with one of *three surgical options*:

1. *Shunt:* Device that allows the pressure in the brain to normalize by draining the fluid into the abdominal cavity, right atrium, or pleural cavity from where the fluid can be reabsorbed. Complications of shunt include infection and blockage, rare complications like upward herniation. Overall failure rate of different shunt is approximately 40% in the first year after surgery.
2. *Endoscopic third ventriculostomy (ETV):* This method is a selective surgical management in patients with congenital aqueduct stenosis. Ventriculostomy is also useful for patients with intracranial cysts and local CSF collection.
3. *Combined endoscopic third ventriculostomy/choroid plexus cauterization (ETV/CPC):* It is used as the primary treatment for most infants with hydrocephalus. ETV/CPC is known to reduce the rate of CSF production and provide a new pathway for the fluid to escape.

Outcome and recurrence: Degree of ventricular dilatation does not appear to be associated with long-term outcome, approximately 40–50% survivors have normal IQ, and others may have seizure disorder, borderline intelligence, and significant motor impairment. *L1CAM* gene mutations account for up to 50% male cases of isolated congenital hydrocephalus. Recurrence risk in the absence of positive family history or absence of L1CAM mutation is low (4%).

Aqueductal Stenosis (Figs. 18 and 19)

Aqueductal stenosis is narrowing of the aqueduct of Sylvius which blocks the flow of CSF in the ventricular system. Blockage of the aqueduct can lead to hydrocephalus, specifically a common cause of congenital and/or obstructive hydrocephalus. The normal aqueduct measures about 1 mm in diameter, and is about 11 mm in length.

Incidence

Congenital aqueduct stenosis has an estimated incidence of ~1:5,000 births, although the reported range varies.

Causes of Aqueductal Stenosis (AS)

In 75% cases, etiology of AS is not known (idiopathic AS), may be due to a mass or congenital tumor leading to compression of the aqueduct from outside or from intrinsic pathology. Chromosomal abnormality is seen in 10–15% cases, AS may be inherited in an X-linked recessive manner (Becker Adams Edwards syndrome) or L1 syndrome

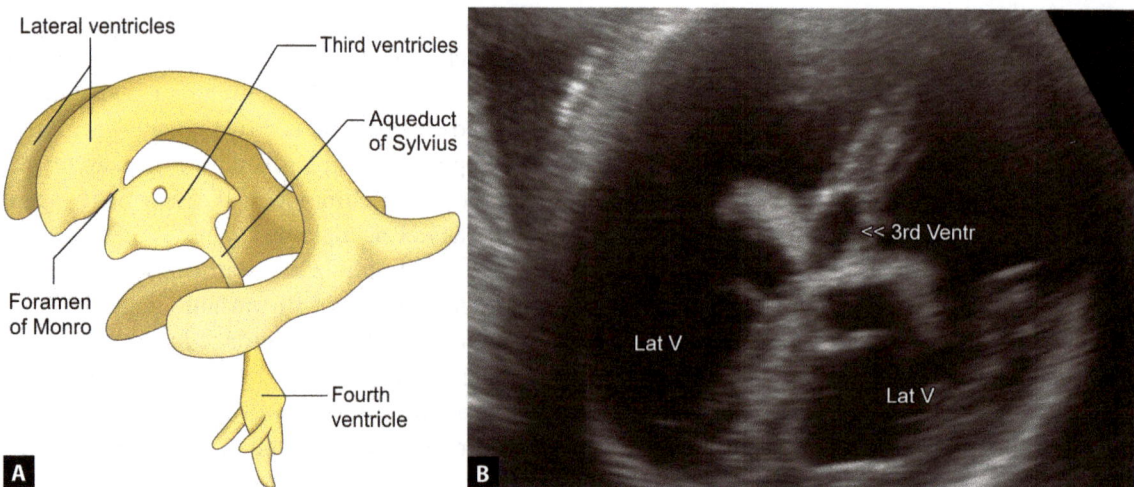

Figs. 18A and B: Aqueduct stenosis with dilated third and lateral ventricles.

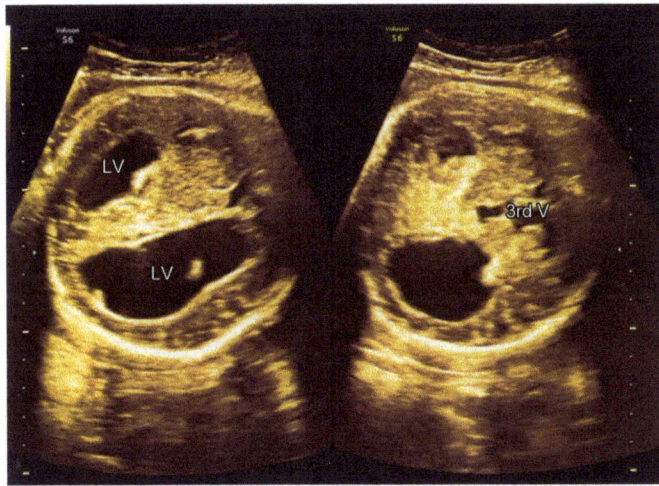

Fig. 19: Aqueductal stenosis with dilated lateral and 3rd ventricle.

(occurs in 1 in 30,000 male—L1CAM mutation on Xq28), which causes familial X-linked hydrocephalus. X-linked AS accounts for approximately 5–15% of the congenital case.

Aqueductal stenosis may also be part of a syndrome, e.g., MASA syndrome (mental retardation, aphasia, shuffling gait, adducted thumbs), spastic paraplegia syndrome (SPG1). Bacterial and viral infections, such as CMV, toxoplasmosis, or Zika virus, intraventricular hemorrhage leading to obstruction of aqueduct and CNS anomaly such as Chiari 11 and Dandy–Walker malformation, are other causes of aqueduct stenosis.

Symptoms

The clinical presentation depends on the severity and age of presentation as well as whether or not it is X-linked. In the infant enlarged head size, bulging fontanelles and gaping cranial sutures are seen. Setting Sun phenomenon may also be present. In X-linked form (Bickers Adams Edwards syndrome), which is associated with profound intellectual disability, clinical assessment would reveal bilateral adducted thumbs.

Management

- Fetal anatomic survey
- Fetal echocardiography
- Genetic counseling and prenatal karyotype (L1CAM mutation)
- PCR—for virus
- Serial follow-up of the brain anatomy to see progression
- Neonatal surgery in progressive ventriculomegaly

Treatment of AS is surgical; ventriculoperitoneal or ventriculoatrial shunt and ETV.

Arnold–Chiari Malformation

Type 1 happens when the lower part of the cerebellum (called the cerebellar tonsils) extends into the foramen magnum. Normally, only the spinal cord passes through this opening. Type 1—which may not cause symptoms—is the most common form of Chiari malformations. Chiari malformation affects females more often than males.

Chiari malformation type II is a complex congenital anomaly resulting from presence of open spinal defect (MMC) with herniation of cerebral vermis and brainstem through foramen magnum. Noncommunicating hydrocephalus develops in most of the cases.

Incidence

Incidence is 1.9/10,000 live births.

Inheritance

Chiari malformation type 2 usually occurs sporadically (in people with no family history of the condition). However, the exact cause is not known. Genes may play a role in predisposing a person to the condition, but environmental factors (such as lack of proper vitamins or nutrients in the maternal diet during pregnancy) may also contribute to the condition.

Diagnosis

Diagnosis is based on high MSAFP, prenatal USG will show U-shaped spine, bulging mass, or irregularities of posterior contour of spine in sagittal section. Classical cranial findings include lemon and banana sign between 16 and 24 weeks in 95% cases. In the first trimester, there will be lack of visualization of intracranial translucency.

Associated anomaly includes small post fossa, low lying tentorium, and enlarged foramen magnum. Other abnormality, for example, posterior fossa abnormality including descent of cerebellar vermis through foramen magnum, hydrocephaly in 80–90% cases, spinal anomaly-kyphosis or scoliosis, hip deformity, and club foot. Chromosomal defect is present in 10% cases, include trisomy 13 or 18 and 22q deletion.

Treatment

Fetuses only with isolated progressive ventriculomegaly are most likely to be benefitted from in utero treatment, as they represent only minority of cases, in utero treatment is not recommended at present. Treatment in the newborn includes placement of a shunt within first 4 days of life.

Dandy–Walker Malformation (Figs. 20A and B)

Dandy–Walker malformation is the most common *posterior fossa malformation*, characterized by the triad of: *hypoplasia of the vermis* and cephalad rotation of the vermian remnant, cystic dilatation of the fourth ventricle extending posteriorly.

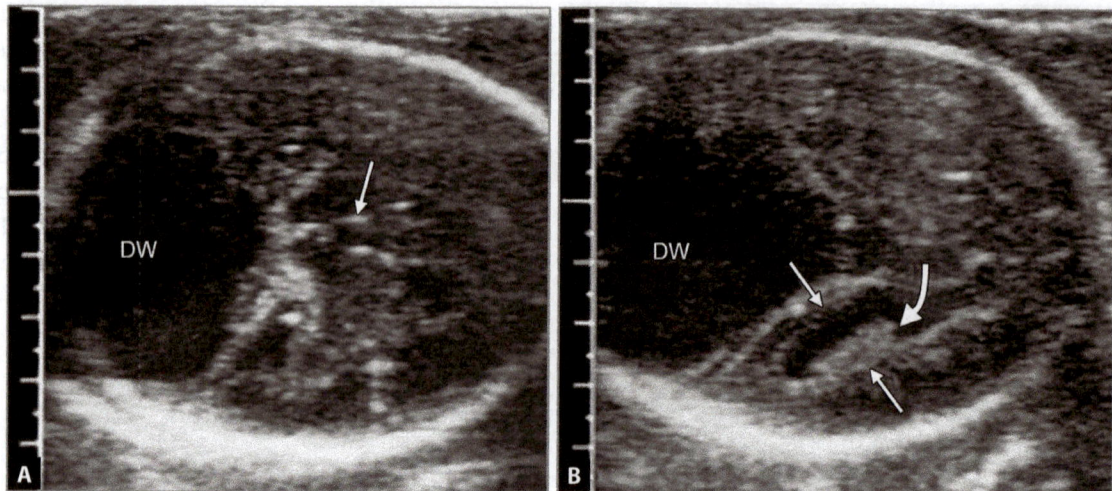

Figs. 20A and B: Dandy-Walker Malformation with posterior fossa cyst and absent cerebellar vermis.

Epidemiology

The estimated prevalence of a Dandy-Walker malformation and related variants is about 1 per 30,000 live births and accounts for ~7.5% (range 4–12%) of the cases of infantile hydrocephalus. It is known as the most common posterior fossa malformation.

Dandy-Walker malformation is a nonspecific CNS abnormality, which can occur as single gene disorder or chromosomal abnormality. It may be environmentally induced, e.g., exposure to CMV, toxoplasmosis, rubella infection, exposure to coumadin and alcohol; may exist as isolated malformation or exist in conjunction with other abnormality. Chromosomal abnormality includes trisomy 9, 13, and 18 and presents in 20–50% cases with increased incidence of both mental retardation and perinatal mortality.

Diagnosis

Antenatal sonographic features that would suggest the diagnosis include the combination of:
- Marked enlargement of the cisterna magna (≥10 mm)
- Complete aplasia of the vermis
- A trapezoid-shaped gap between the cerebellar hemispheres.

Antenatal ultrasound may falsely overdiagnose the condition if performed before 18 weeks, as the vermis has not properly formed.

Magnetic resonance imaging: MRI is the modality of choice for the assessment of Dandy-Walker malformation, although both computed tomography (CT) and ultrasound will demonstrate the pertinent features.

Long-term Outcome and Recurrence

When acquired as Mendelian disorder, recurrence chance is of that specific disorder. When associated with chromosomal disorder, recurrence risk includes maternal age or those of family with unbalanced chromosomal abnormality. In case of multifactorial origin (cleft lip or palate or cardiac abnormality), additional 5% recurrence risk for those disorders, in isolated variety 1–5% risk of recurrence. Mortality is 30–70% in prenatally detected cases and 10–25% in postnatal detection.

COMMON FETAL ABDOMINAL WALL DEFECT

Overview

Abdominal wall defects (AWDs) form a wide spectrum of congenital abnormalities and have an overall prevalence of six cases per 10,000 births. The most common fetal GI and abdominal wall abnormalities detected antenatally are omphalocele and gastroschisis. They may be detected either during a second trimester scan for anomalies or by chance during an examination for an unrelated indication.

They may be isolated or have associated abnormalities. Following detection, the abnormality should be managed in consultation with a multidisciplinary team.

Embryologic Features

By the end of the second week of embryonic life, a bilaminar embryo has developed with an epiblast (the layer facing the amniotic cavity) and a hypoblast (the layer facing the yolk sac). Gastrulation, the major event during the third week of embryonic life, transforms this bilaminar disk into a trilaminar embryo. Cells proliferate and migrate from the primitive streak (a thickened band of cells on the epiblast) between the two layers, creating an embryo with three definitive germ layers. The disk is then a mesoderm "sandwich" bordered above by ectoderm and below by endoderm, except for two small areas on both ends where the embryonic ectoderm and endoderm are in contact. These contact points are the oropharyngeal membrane (the future mouth) at the cranial end and the cloacal membrane (the future urogenital and anal orifices) at the audal end **(Fig. 21)**.

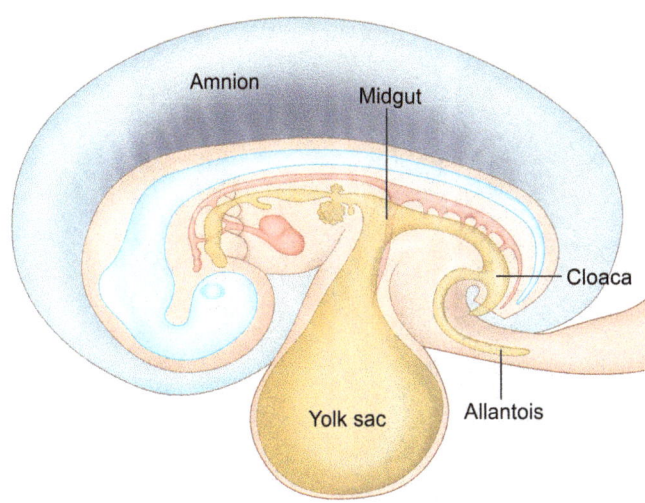

Fig. 21: Development of fetal abdominal wall.

During the fourth week, the embryo undergoes a combination of craniocaudal and lateral folding that converts the flat trilaminar embryonic disk into the basic tube (gut tube) within a tube (body tube) design. Craniocaudal folding creates the typical C-shaped appearance seen at USG; lateral folding closes the abdominal wall. The lateral edges (somatic mesoderm) move ventrally toward each other, constricting the yolk sac and creating a coelomic space (future peritoneal cavity) that separates the gut tube (GI tract) from the body tube (primary abdominal wall). Myoblasts then migrate into the primary abdominal wall and form the muscles and connective tissue.

Omphalocele

Omphalocele is a common AWD, with an estimated prevalence of two to three cases per 10,000 live births. Omphalocele is a midline ventral wall defect, results from herniation of abdominal viscera through an enlarged umbilical ring to the base of the umbilical cord. Possible causes include failure of the bowel to return to the abdominal cavity after normal physiologic herniation and failure of the abdominal wall to close with bowel or liver (or both) herniating through the base of the umbilicus and covered by a membrane consisting of amnion on the outside and peritoneum on the inside. Size of the defect varies from few centimeters to most of the ventral abdominal wall and sac contents are variable which may include bowel, liver, and other viscera. The umbilical cord inserts on the covering membrane, not directly on the abdominal wall.

Risk and Association

Up to 75% of cases of omphalocele have associated chromosomal and nonchromosomal congenital abnormalities. A study by Barisic et al. showed that 25% of cases were associated with chromosomal abnormalities (most commonly, trisomy 18), 10% were part of a syndrome, and 21% were associated with other major malformations. Cardiac, CNS, and urogenital abnormalities are the most common associated malformations. Cardiac abnormality (in up to 50% cases) includes atrial septal defect (ASD), VSD, patent ductus arteriosus (PDA), and pulmonary stenosis. GI anomaly (40%) includes atresia, Meckel's diverticulum, and imperforated anus. Omphalocele may also be a component of the more complex *OEIS complex*—including omphalocele, bladder or cloacal exstrophy, imperforated anus, or may be a component of a syndrome—pentalogy of Cantrell, and Beckwith-Wiedemann syndrome.

Fetal growth restriction is commonly associated and may be associated with polyhydramnios. There is increased risk of in utero and neonatal demise regardless of defect size or liver position with omphalocele.

Risk Factors

Risk factors are advanced maternal age and high parity.

Diagnosis

Antenatal detection is done either at a routine ultrasound examination, because of raised MSAFP or during USG examination for polyhydramnios. The diagnosis of AWD is suspected if herniation continues after 12 weeks. Second trimester MSAFP screening (at 15–20 weeks) with a cut-off value of 2 MoMs (multiples of medians) has a diagnostic accuracy range between 60 and 86.9%.

Sonographic Findings (Figs. 22A to D)

- Midline mass seen at the base of the umbilical cord, with the liver and bowel herniating from the abdominal cavity (not free-flowing), usually seen as hyperechogenic content (nonfluid-filled bowel)
- The umbilical cord insertion is directly into the omphalocele. The defect is covered by a smooth, limiting membrane.
- Size of the defect may extend from few centimeters to most of ventral abdominal wall.
- Abdominal circumference may be smaller, there may be evidence of polyhydramnios, an allantoic cyst is often present.

Prenatal Management

Before doing the management plan, we have to know about the *prognostic variables*.

Fetal mortality is most strongly associated with concurrent malformation or chromosomal abnormalities, absence of liver in the omphalocele correlates with fetal karyotypic abnormalities and increased perinatal mortality. Giant omphalocele (base >6 cm and most of the liver extracorporeal) often associated with small thoracic cage and

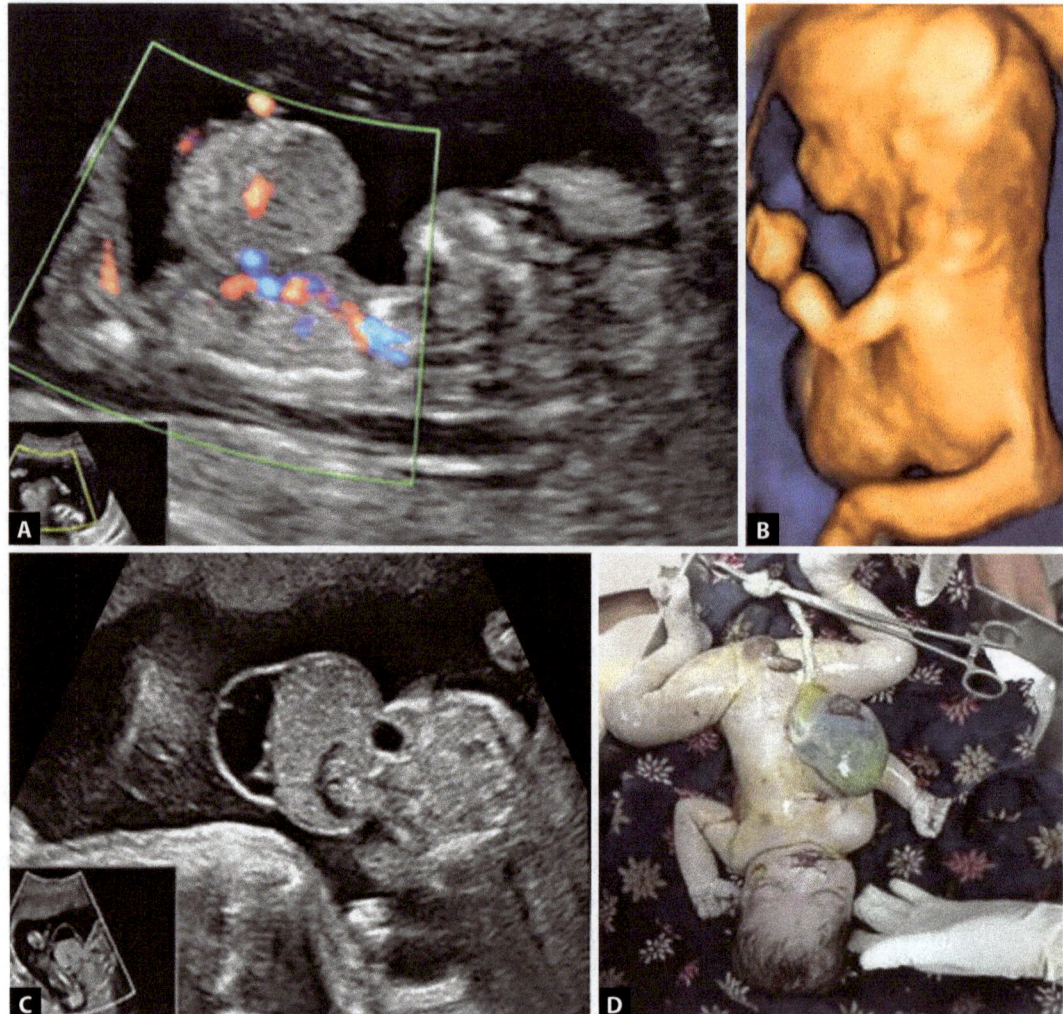

Figs. 22A to D: Omphalocele. (A) First trimester; (B) three-dimensional (3D) image; (C) second trimester; (D) Neonate with omphalocele.

lead to pulmonary hypoplasia and postnatal respiratory complications.

After Diagnosis of Omphalocele

- *Detailed ultrasonographic* examination at 18–22 weeks to estimate the size and content of sac, presence of an amnioperitoneal membrane, to search for other fetal anomalies
- *Fetal echocardiography* at 24 weeks to confirm normal cardiac anatomy
- *Amniocentesis* to exclude aneuploidy
- *Comprehensive counseling* of parents by fetomaternal medicine specialist, pediatric surgeon, geneticist, neonatologist, and pediatric cardiologist as required regarding prognosis, postnatal surgery, postoperative care, and long-term outcome. Large AWD can pose particular problems for both neonatal respiratory management and surgical closure.
- *Option for termination of pregnancy:* If there is chromosomal abnormality, associated anomalies or a particular syndrome is suspected.

- *Continuation of pregnancy:* If decision for continuation of pregnancy, then attention is focused on antepartum surveillance for development of preterm labor and intrauterine growth restriction (IUGR):
  - Goal of the management is to delivery as close to term as possible
  - Serial USG to monitor fetal growth, amniotic fluid volume
  - Fetal nonstress test or biophysical profile (BPP) test (or both) twice weekly beginning at 32–34 weeks
  - Delivery at a tertiary care center providing optimal immediate care for the newborn and with neonatal surgical facilities.

Management in Labor and Delivery

Mode of delivery does not affect outcome. Monitoring should be done for intrapartum fetal distress. Respiratory distress may occur with ruptured or giant omphalocele. Neonatal morbidity in all recent series relates to associated anomalies and prematurity. There is no evidence that elective caesarean delivery confers any benefit to the neonate with omphalocele, whether or not the sac is ruptured and irrespective of the contents of the sac. Theoretical concerns for vaginal delivery (visceral trauma, dystocia, and infection) are unsupported. There are untested scenarios in which cesarean delivery might be considered, such as extracorporeal liver when torsion with obstruction and cardiac return is a theoretical concern.

Neonatal Management
- Prevention of heat, fliud loss and infection prevention are the initial goals after delivery while the neonatal evaluation is completed and the surgery planned
- Intravenous fluid hydration
- Nasogastric decompression
- Protection of omphalocele sac with saline socked gauze dressing

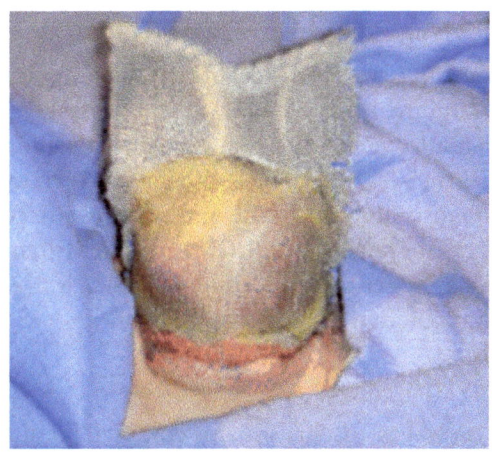

Fig. 23: Primary closure of a large omphalocele with placement of mesh.

Surgical Repair (Fig. 23)

Immediate primary closure: The management approach for infants with an omphalocele depends on the defect size, gestational age at delivery, weight of the baby, and the existence of associated anomalies. In a stable patient with a small defect, primary repair with surgical closure may be possible. Done in cases of small defect <4 cm. The sac may be removed or inverted before fascial closure. If the sac is adherent to the liver, some defects may need to be left in place to avoid liver injury and hemorrhage. However, more commonly, because of the size of the defect, loss of domain of the peritoneal cavity, or instability of the infant, primary closure is not possible, and various techniques are used for coverage and closure—staged or delayed closure.

Delayed staged closure: Omphalocele sac is excised. Silastic sheet is sewn to rectus fascia or to full thickness of abdominal wall.

Conservative (scarification treatment): Done when defect is too large for primary repair and if neonate has significant cardiac or respiratory issue. Staged or delayed closure of the defect is typically used. "Paint and wait" technique, is often used, in which a topical agent, most commonly silver sulfadiazine, is applied to the sac daily. It creates a gradual eschar with subsequent epithelization, leaving a ventral hernia. This process takes weeks to months to complete and may be combined with compressive dressings once the sac is thick enough to slowly reduce the contents into the abdomen. Secondary scar formation and epithelization may take 4-10 weeks and repair as ventral hernia at 1-5 years of age. Later closure may involve mobilization of skin flaps, component separation, use of tissue expanders, or a patch.

Prognosis

The main determinant of prognosis for infants with an omphalocele is the association with structural or chromosomal anomalies that may occur in as many as 80% of affected patients. Major cardiac anomalies are seen in approximately one-third of patients with omphaloceles. Survival rates range from 70 to 95%, with most of the mortality arising from associated anomalies. In addition, a number of long-term medical problems have been found in patients with large omphaloceles, including gastroesophageal reflux disease, pulmonary insufficiency, asthma, and feeding difficulties. Patients with giant omphaloceles have increased morbidity because of an increased visceral abdominal disproportion leading to prolonged mechanical ventilation and a longer hospital stay, half have neurodevelopmental delay.

Recurrence Risk
- Depends on cause of omphalocele. If there is associated aneuploidy—recurrence risk is 1%.
- If a syndrome is diagnosed, the recurrence risk is that of the syndrome, e.g., in Beckwith–Wiedemann syndrome—recurrent risk is 50%.
- Isolated omphalocele—sporadic.

Gastroschisis

Definition

The name gastroschisis is derived from two words. Gastro meaning related to the stomach, Schisis, is a Greek term, meaning separation. The International Clearinghouse for Birth Defects Surveillance and Research defines gastroschisis as "a congenital malformation characterized by visceral herniation usually through a right-sided abdominal wall defect to an intact umbilical cord and not covered by a membrane." The defect usually contains small bowel and has no surrounding membrane.

Incidence

Incidence is 5/10,000 live birth.

Risk and Association

About 85% of gastroschisis occurs as isolation, rarely associated with other birth defects (most commonly CNS and cardiac anomaly). It is seldom associated with chromosomal abnormality (1–3% trisomy 18). Other abnormalities such as bowel stenosis and/or atresia, and volvulus are complications of gastroschisis itself. IUGR and oligohydramnios are common. Presence of polyhydramnios is suggestive of bowel atresia. Intrauterine demise is uncommon.

Pathogenesis

The cause of gastroschisis is not completely understood; at one time, a vascular insult to the abdominal wall was hypothesized, but the cause is now thought to more likely involve an abnormality of lateral body wall folding with deficient mesenchyme. Recent human evidence appears to support the theory that gastroschisis is not a defect of the abdominal wall, but an abnormality of the rudimentary umbilical ring, resulting in a separation of the fetal ectoderm from the amnion's epithelium on the right side.

Risk Factors

The exact cause of a gastroschisis is not known, but more common in babies born to young mothers, or to mothers who may use alcohol or tobacco during their pregnancies or having low socioeconomic status. The incidence among teenage mothers is more than seven times higher than that of mothers aged at least 25 years. Use of periconceptional recreational drug, e.g., methamphetamine (Yabba), cocaine, amphetamine, use of pseudoephedrine, salicylate, and acetaminophen is other risk factor. The defect is more common in fetuses in non-Hispanic white women, and there is no sex predilection.

Diagnosis

Second trimester MSAFP screening (at 15–20 weeks) has diagnostic accuracy range between 60 and 86.9% (cut-off value is 2 MoM).

The diagnosis of gastroschisis can be facilitated by using USG as early as 12 weeks' gestation. The umbilical cord insertion site is normal, but free-floating extra-abdominal loops of bowel protrude through the paramedian defect. The stomach is usually positioned abnormally, with the gastric fundus pulled toward the defect. Inflammation and direct trauma may cause wall thickening in the herniated bowel, and subsequent bowel atresia is a complication. Twisting (malrotation) of the bowel is present and the exposed bowel is at risk for obstruction leading to decay and interruption of the blood supply due to the small size of the defect. Intestinal atresia may manifest as dilatation of either intra- or extra-abdominal loops of bowel at prenatal USG.

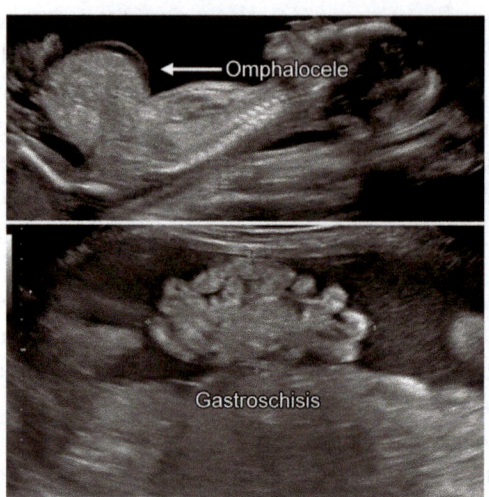

Fig. 24: Ultrasonographic (USG) image of omphalocele and gastroschisis.

Ultrasonography Findings (Fig. 24)

- Multiple loops of bowel are seen floating freely in the amniotic fluid, with a typical cauliflower appearance with no surrounding membrane.
- AWD is typically located to the right of the umbilical cord insertion.
- Size of the defect is about 2–3 cm in diameter and typically, umbilical cord is on one side of the mass.
- The intestines may look swollen, inflamed, thickened, short, and covered with a thick fibrous peel due to exposure to amniotic fluid.

Prenatal Management

Once the diagnosis of gastroschisis is made, a multidisciplinary team, including the obstetrician, neonatologist, pediatric surgeon, and social worker, should provide initial counseling and be involved in the ongoing care of the patient and her fetus. Prenatal USG may be helpful in identification of reliable predictors of postnatal outcome. A recent meta-analysis of 26 studies involving over 2,000 fetuses found significant positive associations between intra-abdominal bowel dilatation and bowel atresia [odds ratio (OR), 5.48; 95% confidence interval (CI), 3.1–9.8], polyhydramnios and bowel atresia (OR, 3.76; 95% CI, 1.7–8.3), and gastric dilatation and neonatal death (OR, 5.58; 95% CI, 1.3–24.1). Serial USG to assess fetal growth, amniotic fluid volume and bowel appearance for mural thickening, bowel dilatation (>17 mm), and to exclude dilated stomach. If sonographic evidence of bowel damage is detected, consideration can be given to delivery as soon as the lungs mature to prevent ongoing injury. Fetal echocardiography should be done at 24 weeks to confirm normal cardiac anatomy, karyotyping is not recommended. A significant number of newborns with gastroschisis are small for gestational age (SGA), with approximately 47–61% neonates weighing at or below the 10th percentile at birth.

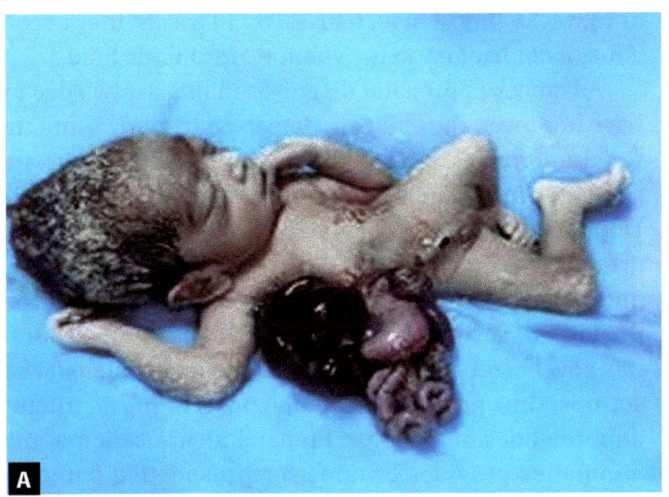 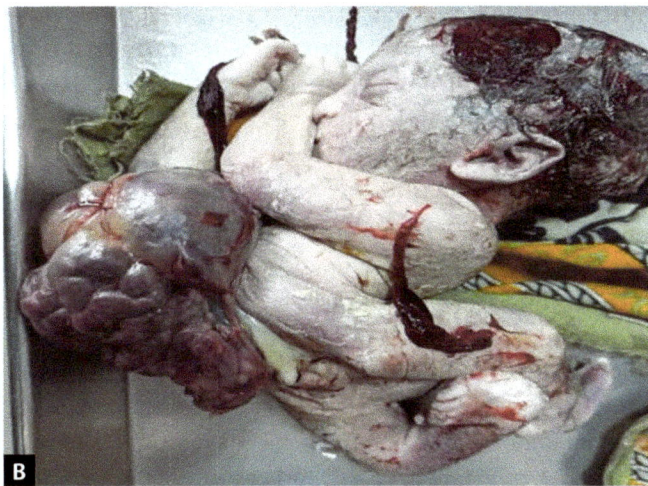

Figs. 25A and B: (A) Neonate with gastroschisis most of the intestine outside abdomen; (B) Big omphalocele with scoliosis fetal liver is outside.

As there is high incidence of stillborn in late third trimester, weekly BPP testing should begin at 30–32 weeks.

Prenatal counseling is emphasized. The presence of intestinal atresia does not have a significant effect on the survival rate, which has been reported to be as high as 91–94%, *primary closure* rate is nearly *80%*, repeated admission is common in those with short bowel syndromes. In the long term, additional surgery may be needed and up to 41% children may need hospitalization for abdominal pain.

Timing and Mode of Delivery

Approximately 30–40% of pregnancies with gastroschisis go into spontaneous preterm labor and delivery. The higher rates of preterm labor in these patients have been attributed to the presence of increased levels of proinflammatory cytokines (including interleukin-6 and interleukin-8) in the amniotic fluid. It has been observed that spontaneous preterm labor is associated with more severely damaged bowel loops, bowel occlusion, and stained amniotic fluid, possibly related to repeated fetal vomiting of the GI contents into the amniotic fluid, increasing the inflammatory mediators. The incidence of intrauterine fetal death (IUFD) in pregnancies complicated by gastroschisis is approximately 5%, may be related to umbilical cord compression due to acute extra-abdominal bowel dilatation, oligohydramnios, cytokine-mediated inflammation, or volvulus and vascular compromise.

The optimal mode of delivery of prenatally diagnosed gastroschisis has been a subject of several observational studies, systematic reviews, and meta-analyses. The mode of delivery was not significantly associated with overall mortality, necrotizing enterocolitis (NEC), secondary repair, sepsis, short gut syndrome, time until full enteral feeding, or length of stay (LOS). In one study, C/S was identified as an independent risk factor for the development of respiratory distress at birth (OR, 7.11; 95% CI, 1.06–47.7). Therefore, planned C/S in the absence of the usual obstetric indications is not generally recommended.

Neonatal Management

Intravenous fluid hydration, orogastric, or nasogastric decompression. Protection of herniated bowel from heat loss and dehydration by immediately placing the baby in a sterile plastic bag (or Vi-Drap isolation bag) containing warmed electrolyte and antibiotic solution (1 L lactated Ringer's solution + 500 mL stable plasma protein + 1 million unit of penicillin) to protect the bowel and retain heat and moisture. In an emergency, any sterile covering that will prevent drying of bowel and neonatal fluid loss would suffice (covering in warm, saline-soaked gauze).

Surgical Repair

- Primary closure with reduction of bowel into peritoneal cavity
- *Staged silo closure to gradually replace bowel into abdomen:* A silastic pouch is first placed over the baby's exposed bowel and anchored to the surrounding muscle. Each day, the pouch is tightened to push the intestine back into the abdominal cavity followed by delayed sutured or suture-less closure.

Prognosis

The prognosis of infants with gastroschisis is largely dependent on the condition of the bowel at birth. In patients with simple gastroschisis, with the mean length of hospital stay (LOS) 41 ± 32 days and mortality rate is 3.4%, while patients with complex gastroschisis have a mean LOS of 85 ± 60 days and a mortality rate of 9.3%. Approximately 25% of infants with simple gastroschisis and over 70% of infants with complex gastroschisis will develop subsequent bowel obstruction resulting from adhesions, anastomotic stricture, or volvulus, requiring repeat surgical interventions, with

mortality rate 17%, most deaths occur as a result of premature delivery, sepsis, and bowel infarction. Poor prognosis when evidence of bowel damage such as atresia; necrosis or inability to close the abdominal defect.

Long-term Complications

Long-term complications include dysfunctional bowel (50%) and short gut syndrome (5%). At a median age of 9 years, Harris et al. found that 41% of children with history of gastroschisis were suffering from weekly bouts of abdominal pain. Recurrent abdominal complaints (more than once a week) during the teenage years and beyond included abdominal pain (14%), gas bloat (36%), difficulty with completing a meal (21%), and gastroesophageal reflux symptoms (43%).

Recurrence Risk

Recurrence risk is low.

FETAL RENAL DISORDERS

Introduction

Congenital anomalies of the kidney, urinary tract, and genitalia are among the most frequent types of congenital malformation. Renal anomalies constitute about 20% of all congenital abnormalities, include a range of anatomic abnormalities with a wide spectrum of severity, many are diagnosed by ultrasound examination during anomaly scan, some discovered after birth. It is important to diagnose and differentiate between abnormalities incompatible with life and those asymptomatic in the newborn and remaining asymptomatic for a long time, even up to until adulthood. This variation creates challenge and often dilemma in the diagnosis, prognosis, and treatment of fetal renal anomalies.

There are many genetic disorders associated with failure or abnormal renal development. Prenatal diagnosis of obstructive and renal agenesis/dysgenesis disorders are important for early reproductive decisions by the parents. For example, bilateral renal agenesis is not compatible with fetal/neonatal survival.

The fetal kidneys can first be visualized by transabdominal ultrasound at 9 weeks and can be seen in all cases from 12 weeks onward. In early pregnancy, the echogenicity of the fetal kidneys is high, decreases in the course of gestation when they become hypoechoic. At about 28 weeks, the renal pyramids can be detected and also the borders of the kidneys can be seen more clearly, since fat tissue is developing around the kidneys from that moment on. The fetal bladder can be visualized from the onset of urine production, at about 10 weeks of gestation. At 11 weeks, the bladder can be visualized, both transvaginally and transabdominally in 80% of fetuses and at 13 weeks almost in all fetuses. By 14 weeks, they become a major contributor to the volume of amniotic fluid.

Advances in prenatal diagnosis in the last two decades have improved the ability to detect, characterize, and treat renal anomalies. Although newer diagnostic tests such as fetal urinary chemical analysis, genetic mapping, and Doppler flow studies have been added to the diagnostic armamentarium, renal USG remains the most important antenatal diagnostic tool. Assessment of fetal anatomy during the second trimester using ultrasound scanning has now become standard practice in most antenatal care set-ups, thus permitting the diagnosis of most structural abnormalities in the fetus. Prenatal identification of renal anomalies provides options for prospective parents to take decision early, as they significantly affect perinatal morbidity and mortality, which may otherwise present itself later on in life, conceivably with more advanced sequelae.

Embryology of Human Kidney Development (Fig. 26)

The urogenital system develops from the mesodermal ridge (intermediate mesoderm) in the posterior wall of the abdominal cavity. During intrauterine life, three renal systems develop; namely the pronephros, mesonephros, and metanephros. The pronephros and mesonephros are transient excretory systems, and disappear without contributing to the permanent renal system. The mesonephric duct gives rise to some reproductive organs in male fetuses while degenerating in female fetuses.

The metanephros appears in the 5th week of development and contributes to the metanephric mesoderm, forming the nephron units of the kidney. The ureteric bud arises from the mesonephric bud and forms the collecting system of the kidney, including the ureter, the renal pelvis, the major and minor calyces, and about 1–3 million collecting tubules. The cranial end of the ureteric bud comes into contact with the metanephric cell mass, and this induces the development of the metanephric mesoderm into the future nephron and the ureteric bud into the collecting system. The definitive kidney develops in the sacral region and ascends up into the renal fossa in the lumbar region as the embryo matures, and demonstrates differential growth of the abdominal wall.

The definitive kidney becomes functional by week 12, although they do not have any major excretory function. Nephrons continue to be formed up until the time of birth when they are about 1 million in number. The number of nephrons remains static while they grow in size during infancy.

During weeks 4–7, the cloaca develops into the urogenital sinus anteriorly and the anal canal posteriorly. The developing mesonephric ducts drain into the upper

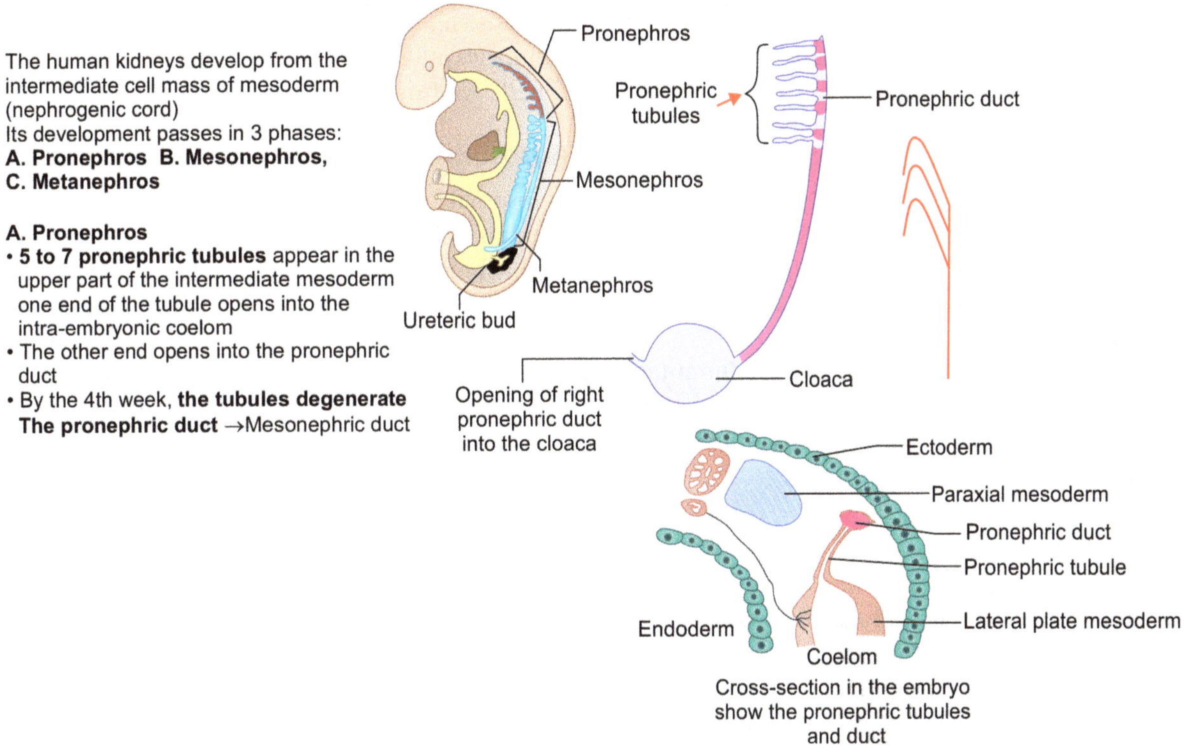

The human kidneys develop from the intermediate cell mass of mesoderm (nephrogenic cord)
Its development passes in 3 phases:
A. Pronephros B. Mesonephros,
C. Metanephros

A. Pronephros
- **5 to 7 pronephric tubules** appear in the upper part of the intermediate mesoderm one end of the tubule opens into the intra-embryonic coelom
- The other end opens into the pronephric duct
- By the 4th week, **the tubules degenerate** The pronephric duct →Mesonephric duct

Fig. 26: Development of the kidney.
Source: You Tube, Professor (Dr) Ahmed M Kamal

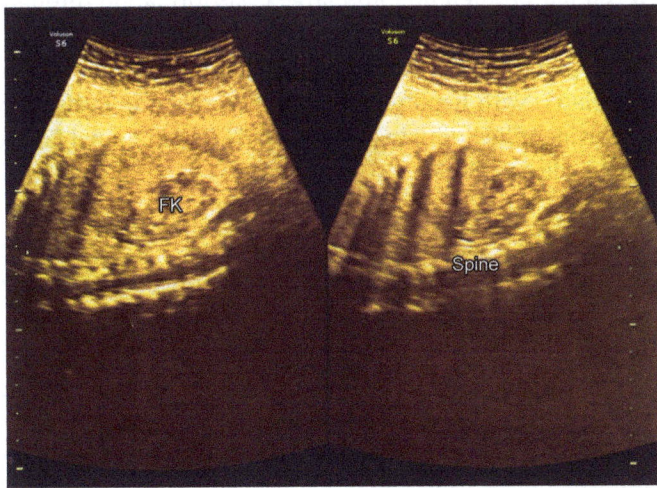

Fig. 27: Normal fetal kidney.

part of the urogenital sinus, laying the foundation for the future bladder. This developing bladder is initially in communication with the allantois, but with progressive development of the anterior abdominal wall, the allantois disappears, leaving behind an obliterated thick fibrous tissue called the urachus, which connects the bladder apex to the umbilicus. It forms the medial umbilicus ligament in the adult. The developing bladder incorporates the mesonephric duct into its trigone, and posteriorly spaces out the two ureteric orifices appropriately. The lower part of the urogenital sinus develops into the prostatic and membranous urethra in the male.

Etiology and Types of Congenital Renal Anomaly

Congenital anomalies of kidney and urinary tract (CAKUT) is a group of abnormalities affecting the kidneys or other structures of the urinary tract including the bladder, the ureters, and the urethra. The causes of CAKUT are complex. It is likely that a combination of genetic and environmental factors may contribute to the development of the abnormalities.

Congenital anomalies of kidney and urinary tract includes renal hypoplasia or agenesis, dysplasia [multicystic dysplastic kidney (MCDK)], hydronephrosis, autosomal dominant polycystic kidney disease (ADPKD), autosomal recessive polycystic kidney disease (ARPKD), duplex kidney or duplicated collecting system, ureteropelvic junction obstruction (UPJO), megaureter, vesicoureteral reflux (VUR), and posterior urethral valve (PUV).

Inheritance of CAKUT is complex and not completely understood. About 10–20% of cases are thought to occur in families. When inherited, CAKUT most commonly follows an autosomal dominant pattern, less commonly follows an autosomal recessive pattern. In many cases, the inheritance pattern is unknown or the condition is not inherited. In some of these cases, a new (de novo) mutation in the gene that occurs during the embryonic development may underlie the urinary system abnormality.

Syndromic CAKUT is caused by mutations in the genes associated with the particular syndrome as in

Fraser syndrome, the branchiootorenal syndrome, Kallmann syndrome, Ehlers–Danlos syndrome. The genes most commonly associated with isolated CAKUT are *PAX2*, which is also associated with renal coloboma syndrome, and *HNF1B*, which is involved in 17q12 deletion syndrome and RCAD syndrome. These two genes play critical roles in the formation of the kidneys, urinary tract, and other tissues and organs during embryonic development. Mutations in these genes are thought to disrupt development of the kidneys or other parts of the urinary tract.

Environmental factors (maternal diabetes or intrauterine exposure to angiotensin-converting enzyme inhibitors) may lead to disturbance of normal nephrogenesis and anomalies of the renourinary tract.

Renal Agenesis

Renal agenesis or congenital absence of kidneys can be bilateral or unilateral. Bilateral renal agenesis is incompatible with life, and occurs in 0.1–0.3 per 1,000 births. Isolated unilateral agenesis accounts for 1 in 1,000 births, and is three times more common in males. Renal agenesis can be an isolated finding, but is more commonly part of a syndrome and warrants a detailed anomaly scan to look for associated anomalies. Various inheritance patterns exist in families with renal agenesis. The risk of bilateral renal agenesis in the fetus is thought to be around 1% if one parent has unilateral agenesis. If renal agenesis is detected in the fetus, it warrants renal imaging in parents.

The most common presentation in bilateral renal agenesis is anhydramnios, generally identified at the time of a routine mid-trimester anomaly scan. The fetal kidneys are not visualized in the renal fossa, and the bladder does not fill during the scan, with noticeably reduced or absent liquor from 16 weeks. If the fetal bladder is not visualized during the scan, it is recommended to repeat the scan after 30 minutes to allow for an empty bladder to refill. Persistence of an empty bladder in the absence of demonstrable renal tissue and anhydramnios strongly points to bilateral renal agenesis. The lack of recognizable renal arteries on color Doppler would strongly support the suspicion of bilateral renal agenesis. The adrenal will show a linear appearance but can sometimes appear ovoid in certain scans.

Unilateral agenesis is three to four times more common than bilateral agenesis, and carries a better prognosis. On an ultrasound examination, the fetal bladder is usually seen to fill and empty normally with normal liquor volume. The contralateral kidney may appear hypertrophied, and usually functions normally. Cho et al. showed that the ratio of anteroposterior to transverse renal diameter gives a better guide to the size of the contralateral kidney. If the ratio is >0.9, it is highly suggestive of absence of the other kidney, and has a sensitivity, specificity, and accuracy of 100%. The identification or suspicion of unilateral or bilateral renal agenesis should always prompt a thorough search for other anomalies in the fetus, as the risk of associated anomalies or genetic syndrome may be as high as 30%.

Autosomal Dominant Polycystic Kidney Disease

Autosomal dominant polycystic kidney disease also known as adult polycystic kidney disease is the (formerly Potter type III) most common lethal genetic disease inherited as a dominant Mendelian trait characterized by bilaterally enlarged echogenic kidney, (smaller than in autosomal recessive disease), kidneys are moderately enlarged with increased corticomedullary differentiation and hyperechogenic. Renal pelvises can be visualized, with normal bladder and normal amniotic fluid.

Incidence

Incidence is 1/400–1,000 live births.

Genetics

Autosomal dominant polycystic kidney disease results from mutation in *PKD1* gene (85%) or *PKD2* (15%) gene, which encode abnormal protein, polycystin. Abnormal polycystin-1 or polycystin-2 affects the physiologic mechanisms of differentiation and repair of renal tubules leading to upregulation of cellular proliferation and large cysts formation throughout the nephrons with concurrent interstitial fibrosis. Cysts develop in localized segments anywhere along the nephron associated with hepatic, pancreatic, or ovarian cysts. May not be identified until hypertension (HTN) and renal failure appears in adulthood.

Symptoms

Symptoms vary in severity and age of onset, but usually develop between the ages of 30 and 40 years. ADPKD is a progressive disease and symptoms tend to get worse over time. The most common symptoms are kidney cysts, pain in the back and the sides, and headaches. Other symptoms include liver and pancreatic cysts, urinary tract infections (UTIs), abnormal heart valves, high blood pressure, kidney stones, and brain aneurysms. Hyperechoic renal parenchyma is associated with abnormal renal function in 80% cases.

Prenatal Diagnosis

The prenatal diagnosis of ADPKD is now being reported with increasing frequency. Increased echogenicity and renal enlargement are the main ultrasonographic signs of ADPKD, renal cysts are uncommon. The disease is caused by mutations in the *PKD1* gene (85% of cases) on chromosome 16p13.13 and *PKD2* gene (15% of cases) on chromosome 4q13.23, detected by microarray. In an affected family, prenatal diagnosis can be carried out by first-trimester chorion villous sampling or amniocentesis if there is associated anomaly. Risk of recurrence: 50%.

Autosomal Recessive Polycystic Kidney Disease (Figs. 28A and B)

Autosomal recessive polycystic kidney disease is also known as infantile polycystic kidney disease. A fetus or baby with ARPKD has fluid-filled kidney cysts that may make the kidneys too big, or enlarged. The signs of ARPKD frequently begin before birth, so it is often called "infantile PKD", some people do not develop symptoms until later in childhood or even adulthood. Children born with ARPKD often, but not always, develop kidney failure before reaching adulthood; babies with the worst cases die hours or days after birth due to respiratory difficulties or respiratory failure.

Frequency

Frequency is 1/40,000 live births.

Results from mutation of *PKHD1* gene, an affected individual has alterations in two genes, with one mutation inherited from each parent. Mutation in *PKHD1* gene which encodes abnormal protein fibrocystin, causing innumerable corticomedullary microcyst formation in the collecting tubule, with subsequent interstitial fibrosis. Over 300 mutations in PKHD1 gene have been identified. Carrier rate of recessive *PKHD1* gene is 1:70, most cases result from heterogenous mutation.

Prenatal Diagnosis of Autosomal Recessive Polycystic Kidney Disease

Autosomal recessive polycystic kidney disease is often first suspected based on routine prenatal ultrasound. Suggestive fetal features include symmetrically enlarged, echogenic kidneys (due to multiple microscopic cysts) with loss of corticomedullary differentiation due to medullary hyperechogenicity. Discrete cysts are sometimes observed. Oligohydramnios may be present due to poor fetal urine output.

Prenatal genetic testing in families at risk can be carried out by first-trimester chorion villous sampling by using next-generation sequencing (NGS) to detect *PKHD1* mutation on chromosome 6p21 to differentiate ARPKD from other phenotypically similar entities.

Ultrasonography will show massively enlarged echogenic kidney (>5 SD above mean), small or absent bladder, renal pelvises cannot be visualized.

Gradual onset of *oligohydramnios* from the second trimester/anhydramnios (80% cases), liver appearances are normal despite the presence of cysts, portal fibrosis, and proliferation of bile ducts. The more severe the renal disease, the less severe is the hepatic fibrosis. Fetal MRI may be warranted to better delineate renal anatomy in the presence of severe oligohydramnios.

Syndromes associated with echogenic kidney are Beckwith–Wiedemann, Meckel–Gruber, Finish-type nephrotic syndrome, Pearlman syndrome, *VACTERL association* (vertebral abnormality, anal atresia, cardiac defect, tracheoesophageal fistula, renal and radial limb abnormality), as well as aneuploidy.

Management

Detailed ultrasound examination. Genetic testing to exclude mutations in the *PKHD1* gene. Consider *termination if anhydramnios*, which is lethal either in utero or in the neonatal period due to pulmonary hypoplasia.

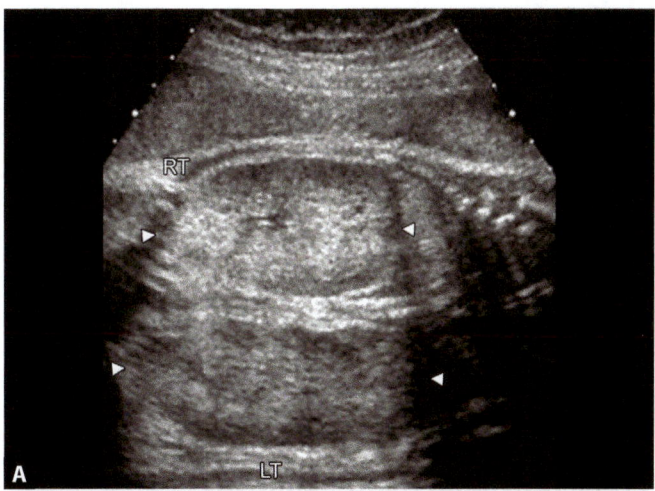
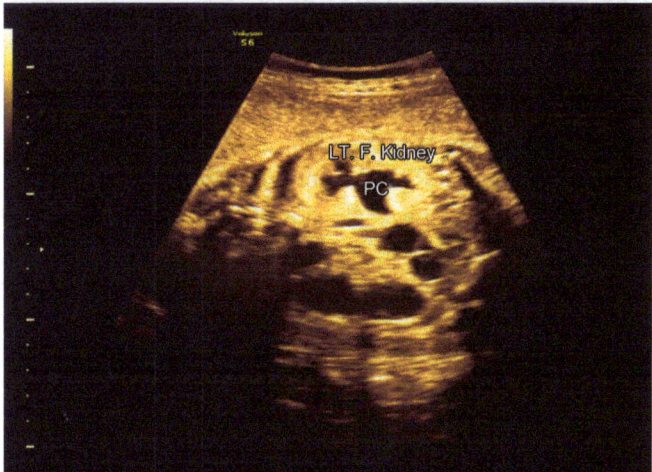
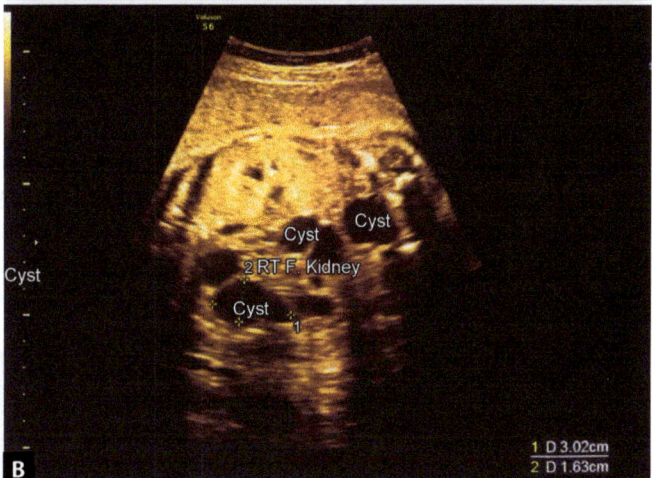

Figs. 28A and B: (A) Autosomal recessive polycystic kidney disease (ARPKD) ultrasonography (USG); (B) Bilateral polycystic kidney.

Prognosis

Short-term outcome depends on amniotic fluid. Oligo- or anhydramnios in the second trimester with large echogenic kidney (>4 SD above mean) is associated with poor prognosis with neonatal mortality due to pulmonary hypoplasia or renal failure. 1 year survival rate for those surviving neonatal period is 95%, 60% require dialysis or renal transplantation by 10 years of age, 7% need liver transplant due to concomitant hepatic fibrosis and portal HTN.

Recurrence

Risk of recurrence is 25%

Pyelectasis/Mild Hydronephrosis (Figs. 29A and B)

Pyelectasis/mild hydronephrosis is fluid collection causing dilation of the renal pelvis, the vast majority are mild and called physiological hydronephrosis, but there is risk of persistent postnatal renal impairment and/or need for surgical intervention. Pyelectasis is the *most common abnormality* reported in prenatal USG.

Renal pelvis diameter varies from 3 to 11 mm in 18% of normal fetus. Caliectasis is dilatation of renal calyx; while hydronephrosis is combination of pyelectasis with caliectasis, being bilateral in 17–54% cases.

Incidence

The reported incidence of fetal hydronephrosis ranges from 0.6 to 4.5% of pregnancies.

Cause

Potential causes of mild dilatation of fetal urinary tract include transient obstruction, e.g., compression by fetal vessels crossing the ureter, VUR, natural kinks, and folds in the ureter that may occur during development, hyperfiltration of fetal kidney; influence of metabolic or hormonal factor. Progesterone is a smooth muscle relaxant, may be responsible for mild fetal upper urinary tract dilatation.

Congenital anomalies of the kidney and urinary tract is the *cause of fetal hydronephrosis* in one-third of the patients. UPJO is the most *common* diagnosis and increased in frequency with the severity of hydronephrosis. VUR, the second most common diagnosis, is not associated with the severity of fetal hydronephrosis. Moderate-to-severe reflux (grades III through V) appears to be associated with a greater degree of renal pelvic dilation [renal pelvic diameter (RPD) >10 mm] both in utero and postnatally.

Other less common causes include megaureter, MCDK, ureterocele, PUVs, ectopic ureter, prune-belly syndrome, urachal cyst, duplex collecting system, and urethral atresia.

Classification of Urinary Tract Dilation

Different classification system of urinary tract dilation (UTD) is used based upon the ultrasound criteria.
- *Renal pelvis diameter:* Based on gestational age, *minimal hydronephrosis* is defined as renal pelvis diameter 4–7 mm between 15 and 20 weeks, after 30 weeks mild, moderate, and severe hydronephrosis is defined as 5–8 mm, 9–15 mm, and >15 mm. Significant fetal hydronephrosis can be defined as a ratio of the RPD to AP renal diameter >0.5.
- Society of urology has defined a grading system based on two parameters—central renal complex and renal parenchymal thickness to classify hydronephrosis.

Society of Fetal Urology Grading System

The Society of Fetal Urology (SFU) focuses on the degree of hydronephrosis in the kidney without directly assessing the state of the ureter and the bladder:
- *Grade 0:* Normal examination with no dilation of the renal pelvis

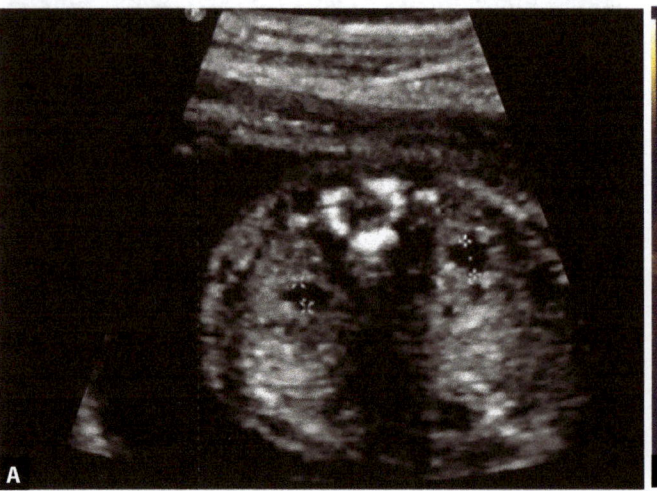
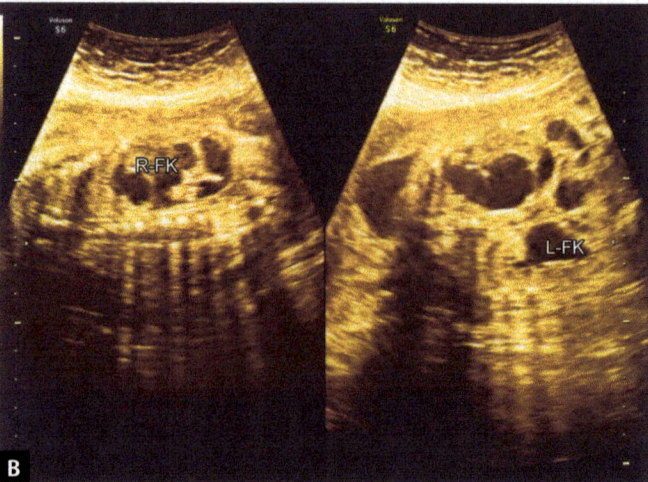

Figs. 29A and B: (A) Bilateral pyelactasis; (B) Bilateral hydronephrotic kidney.

- *Grade I:* Mild dilation of the renal pelvis only
- *Grade II:* Moderate dilation of the renal pelvis including a few calyces
- *Grade III:* Dilation of the renal pelvis with visualization of all the calyces, which are uniformly dilated, and normal renal parenchyma
- *Grade IV:* Similar appearance of the renal pelvis and calyces as grade III, plus thinning of the renal parenchyma

MULTIDISCIPLINARY PANEL CLASSIFICATION SYSTEM

A multidisciplinary panel consisting of radiologists, nephrologists, and urologists has proposed a classification system that applies to UTD that presents either antenatally or postnatally based on six ultrasound findings:

1. Anterior and posterior RPD
2. Calyceal dilation
3. Renal parenchymal thickness
4. Renal parenchymal appearance
5. Bladder abnormalities
6. Ureteral abnormalities.

The severity of findings is denoted by a numerical system (1 through 3, with 3 being the most severe grade).

Factors Predictive of Congenital Anomalies of Kidney and Urinary Tract

Several factors are predictive of CAKUT including severity of fetal hydronephrosis, whether it is bilateral or unilateral, abnormally low amniotic fluid volume (severity of oligohydramnios), the presence of other anomalies (both renal and nonrenal abnormalities), maternal risk factors, and whether progression occurred or not. Presence of these findings directly impacts management decisions, including need for further prenatal evaluation (e.g., genetic testing and the timing and frequency of repeat ultrasound) and postnatal evaluation (e.g., imaging studies) and, in some cases, surgical intervention.

Antenatal Management

All fetuses with minimal hydronephrosis should have repeat USG between 32 and 34 weeks to determine progression or regression. Fetuses with bilateral hydronephrosis should be monitored frequently, frequency of monitoring varies from 4 to 6 weeks, depending on gestation at which it was detected, its severity, and presence of oligohydramnios.

Ultrasonography should include assessment of overall growth and development of fetus, amniotic fluid index (AFI), evaluation for lower urinary tract obstruction, renal dysplasia, renal parenchymal appearance, extent of dilatation of collecting system, whether involvement is unilateral or bilateral, as well as bladder size, thickness and emptying, extrarenal structural malformations, and genitalia. The risk of aneuploidy is increased in fetuses with antenatal hydronephrosis and those with a major structural anomaly.

Minimal hydronephrosis before 24 weeks: There is 90% chance of complete resolution with no postnatal sequelae, among fetuses with renal pelvis diameter >7 mm—40% will resolve, 50% will remain unchanged, and 10% will have worsening of hydronephrosis.

Hydronephrosis may be associated with trisomy, several syndromes, and VACTERL; discussion regarding amniocentesis if sonographic minor marker of trisomy present.

Renal parenchyma: Thinning of the parenchyma and/or cortical cysts indicate injury or impaired development of renal cortex. An echogenic cortex may indicate abnormal renal parenchymal development (dysplasia), which may be associated with VUR or obstruction. Abnormalities of the bladder, such as increased thickness and trabeculation of the bladder wall, are consistent with obstructive uropathy distal to the bladder (e.g., PUV).

Management of Newborn

At birth, complete physical examination including urethral orifice should be checked. Causes of failure to void within 48 hours may be due to normal fluid shift or may be due to urologic abnormality including obstructive uropathy, renal failure, neurogenic bladder, or effects of maternal medication.

Examination of abdomen: To detect presence of a mass that could represent an enlarged kidney due to obstructive uropathy or MCDK.

A palpable bladder in a male infant, especially after voiding, may suggest bladder outlet obstruction such as the presence of PUVs. A male infant with prune belly syndrome will have deficient abdominal wall musculature and undescended nonpalpable testes.

Investigations

Serum electrolytes, blood urea nitrogen, and creatinine measured after 24 hours, to avoid overestimation of creatinine that may be high and reflective of maternal creatinine values.

Ultrasonography of the abdomen and the pelvis including scan of bladder usually after 3–7 days, if severe hydronephrosis detected prenatally evaluation should be done within 1–2 days. If initial evaluation is normal, repeat scan after 3–4 weeks. If postnatal USG shows cortical thinning or upper tract dilatation with normal bladder, voiding cystourethrography (VCUG) is the definitive method for assessment of the lower urinary tract to exclude VUR. Cystourethrogram is indicated in patients with unilateral or bilateral hydronephrosis with renal pelvic anteroposterior diameter (APD) >10 mm, SFU grade 3–4 or ureteric dilatation.

Diuretic renography is performed after 6–8 weeks. The procedure may be repeated after 3–6 months if ultrasound shows worsening of pelvicalyceal dilatation. Diuretic renography allows differentiation between obstructive and nonobstructive hydronephrosis and estimating relative renal function. In case of severe UPJO and if kidney shows 35% or less function—pyeloplasty.

Prophylactic antibiotic (penicillin derivative): In infants with postnatally confirmed moderate or severe hydronephrosis (SFU 3-4; renal APD >10 mm) or dilated ureter while awaiting evaluation, patients with VUR receive antibiotic prophylaxis through the first year of life. Follow-up USG every 3 months.

Prognosis

Although antenatal hydronephrosis resolves by birth or during infancy in 41–88% patients, urological abnormalities requiring intervention are identified in 4.1–15.4% and rates of VUR and UTIs are several-fold higher. Long-term prognosis depends on presence of coexisting anomalies or aneuploidy and whether unilateral or bilateral kidneys are affected.

Approximately 90% of pyelectasis seen in mid-trimester resolve spontaneously during antenatal or early postnatal period, one-third of fetuses with persistent moderate-to-severe hydronephrosis or with associated caliectasis will require postnatal urologic surgery. Untreated VUR can lead to recurrent renal infection, parenchymal scarring, and ultimately renal failure.

Posterior Urethral Valves

Posterior urethral valves are membranes in the posterior urethra causing bladder outlet obstruction with subsequent hydronephrosis and pressure-induced renal dysplasia.

Incidence

Incidence is 3/10,000 live births. Occurs almost exclusively in *male fetuses*, and in females, a complete urethral atresia may cause similar syndrome.

Diagnostic Features

Signs of lower urinary tract obstruction: Oligohydramnios and thick-walled or dilated bladder, marked and persistent dilatation of bladder with thickened often trabeculated bladder, thickness >3 mm. The posterior urethra is dilated: The dilated proximal urethra resembles a "key hole" **(Fig. 30)**. The dilated bladder can become quite large filling fetal pelvis and abdomen—megacystis.

Severe bladder obstruction can lead to ureterectasis and caliectasis, the end stage is often bilateral renal dysplasia. There is abundant fibrous tissue which increases renal parenchymal echogenicity. USG shows increased renal parenchymal echogenicity with loss of corticomedullary

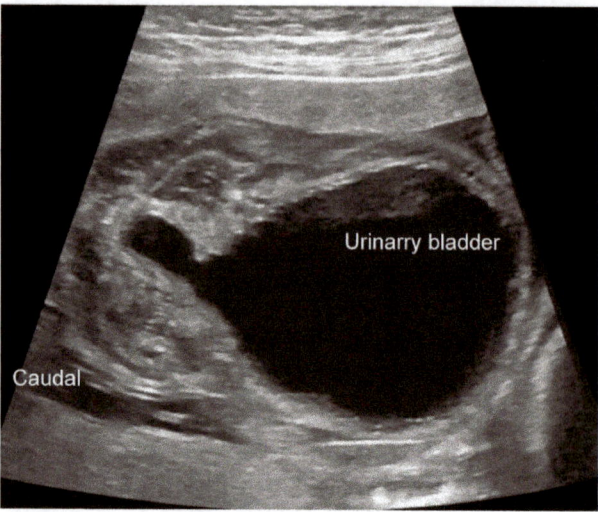

Fig. 30: Keyhole sign.

differentiation and presence of subcortical cysts, which reliably predicts end-stage renal disease. Lack of caliectasis in presence of obstructed urinary tract may suggest renal dysplasia and lack of urine production by severely damaged kidney. Oligohydramnios indicates high-grade obstruction and in long-standing cases may show Potter facies and club foot.

Fetal MRI is useful as adjunctive imaging modality.

Antenatal Management

Sonographic features of trisomy 13, 18, and 21 ruled out, as chromosomal abnormality is present in 12% cases. Oligohydramnios in first trimester may indicate aneuploidy, consider amniocentesis with microarray testing. Echocardiography to rule out cardiac abnormality.

Fetal intervention: In utero decompression appears to prevent neonatal death from pulmonary hypoplasia. Because renal development or maldevelopment is complete at birth, relief of obstruction in infancy or childhood may not prevent the progression to end-stage renal failure. Relief of obstruction during 20–30 weeks (most active phase of nephrogenesis) may obviate further damage and allow normal nephrogenesis.

Investigations

Because amniotic fluid is predominantly composed of fetal urine, measurement of biochemical markers (i.e., sodium and β_2-microglobulin) contained in fetal urine can be used to assess fetal renal function. Urinary levels of sodium and β_2-microglobulin decrease with increasing gestational age, while urine osmolality increases. Impaired resorption is seen in fetuses with bilateral renal dysplasia or severe bilateral obstructive uropathy resulting in abnormal urinary levels of electrolytes, β_2-microglobulin, and osmolality.

In general, high urinary electrolyte excretion, sodium, and chloride concentration >90 mEq/L (90 mmol/L), and

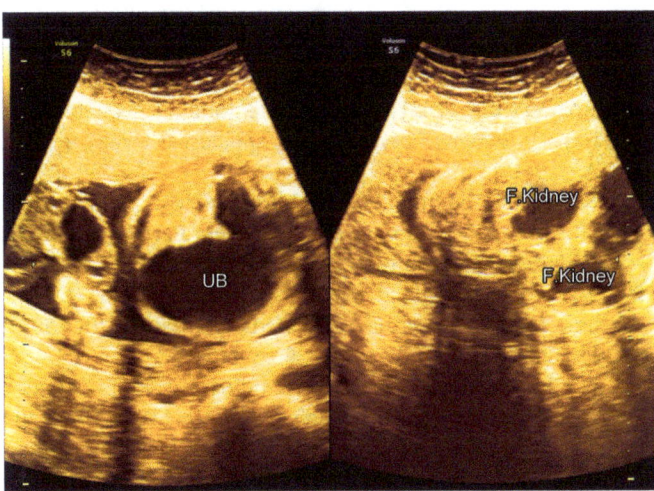

Fig. 31: Posterior urethral valve with dilated renal pelvis.

urinary osmolality <210 mOsm/kg H_2O in the amniotic fluid are indicative of fetal renal tubular impairment and poor renal prognosis. Amniocentesis can be used to detect chromosomal abnormalities often associated with renal defects such as trisomy.

In Utero Treatment

Fetal vesicocentesis on 2 occasions allows estimation of urinary electrolytes, β_2-macroglobulin, and osmolality to predict renal maturity and function. Decreasing levels of sodium (<100 mg/dL), calcium (<8 mg/dL), osmolality (<200 mOsm/kg), β_2-microglobulin (<4 mg/L), and protein (<20 mg/dL) identify fetuses that are likely to benefit from therapeutic interventions.

In fetuses with suspected lower urinary obstruction and favorable indices, parents should be counseled regarding the role of vesicoamniotic shunting or in utero endoscopic ablation of valves. In utero decompression using a Harrison double pigtail catheter (with its distal and proximal tips within the fetal urinary bladder and amniotic cavity, respectively) was introduced in 1981. Percutaneous vesicoamniotic shunt is used since 1986. In one study, the survival rate was 48% with 3% procedure-related mortality.

Severe oligohydramnios with bilateral hydramnios due to bladder outlet obstruction need open fetal surgery with fetal vesicostomy. Owing to the inherently highly invasive nature and high frequency of maternal and fetal complications, these procedures are performed at only a few specialized centers. Vesicocentesis remaining widely controversial and debated in the literature. Fetal cystoscopy can be used to disrupt the valves by hydroablation guidewire passage or laser ablation.

Neonatal Management

Monitoring urinary output, failure to void in first 24–48 hours may be the first sign of significant urologic abnormality. Prenatal severe dilatation of renal pelvis needs early USG evaluation for early intervention, otherwise USG is delayed for 3–7 days.

Mild cases of hydronephrosis needs careful watch. Signs that predict postnatal pathology or need for surgery include bilateral hydroureteronephrosis, dilated posterior urethra, perinephric urinoma, and progressive calyceal or ureteric dilatation. Cases with cortical thinning, upper tract dilatation, and normal bladder need cystourethrography. In severe PUJ obstruction (35% or less function), need pyeloplasty.

Prognosis

Despite restoring amniotic fluid volume, genitourinary shunts do not protect developing kidney, fetal mortality approximately 50% even with fetal intervention, associated with oligohydramnios and pulmonary hypoplasia. Short-term prognosis depends on sonographic appearance of kidney, fetal urine concentration, and amniotic fluid volume.

Good prognosis (10% mortality)—with nondysplastic kidney and normal urine, poor prognosis (70% mortality)—if kidney appears abnormal and abnormal urine parameter, and worst prognosis (95% mortality) with severe oligohydramnios or anhydramnios. Long-term prognosis in survivors includes renal insufficiency (>50% cases), necessitating renal dialysis or transplantation; recurrent infection and VUR. PUV is a sporadic event, no risk of recurrence.

■ SUGGESTED READING

1. American Association of Neurological Surgeons. spina bifida. types and treatment options. [online] Available from: https://www.aans.org/Patients/Neurosurgical-Conditions-and-Treatments/Spina-Bifida. [Last accessed April 2022].
2. American International Medical University. (2016). Congenital anomalies (birth defects) Diagnosis and management. [online] Available from: https://www.aimu.us/2016/12/05/congenital-anomalies-birth-defects-diagnosis-and-management/. [Last accessed April 2022].
3. Best RG. Anencephaly. [online] Available from: https://emedicine.medscape.com/article/1181570-overview. [Last accessed April 2022].
4. Bhat V, Moront M, Bhandari V. Gastroschisis: A state-of-the-art review. Children (Basel). 2020;7(12):302.
5. Bianchi DW. Abdominal wall defects. Gasrtoschisis. Fetology, Part 1, 2nd edition. New York: McGraw Hill/Medical; 2010. pp. 435-43.
6. Bianchi DW. Abdominal wall defects. Omphalocele. Fetology, Part 1, 2nd edition. New York: McGraw Hill/Medical; 2010. pp. 426-34.
7. Center for Disease Control and Prevention (CDC). Facts about encephalocele. [online] Available from: https://www.cdc.gov/ncbddd/birthdefects/encephalocele.htm. [Last accessed April 2022].
8. Center for Disease Control and Prevention. Congenital anomalies-definitions. [online] Available from: https://www.cdc.gov/ncbddd/birthdefects/surveillancemanual/

chapters/chapter-1/chapter1-4.html#:~:text=Congenital%20 anomalies%20comprise%20a%20wide,commonly%20on%20 major%20structural%20anomalies. [Last accessed April 2022].
9. El-Feky M. (2021) [online] Available from: https://radiopaedia. org/articles/dandy-walker-malformation-1. [Last accessed April 2022].
10. Erős FR, Beke A. (2017). Congenital fetal anomaly and role of prenatal ultrasound. Intechopen. [online] Available from: https://www.intechopen.com/chapters/57858. [Last accessed April 2022].
11. Greene S, Ellenbogen RG. Congenital malformations of the brain and spinal cord. In: Fuhrman BP, Zimmerman JJ (Eds). Pediatric Critical Care Medicine. Missouri: Mosby-Year Book; 2005.
12. Intechopen. (2012). Management of hydrocephalus. [online] Available from: https://cdn.intechopen.com/pdfs/29502/ InTech. [Last accessed April 2022].
13. James D, Steer PJ. Fetal gastro-intestinal and abdominal abnormality. High-risk Pregnancy, Volume 1, 5th edition. Cambridge: Cambridge University Press; 2018. pp. 433-42.
14. Medline Plus. Congenital anomalies of kidney and urinary tract. [online] Available from: https://medlineplus.gov/ genetics/condition/congenital-anomalies-of-kidney-and-urinary-tract/. [Last accessed April 2022].
15. Mileto A, Itani M, Katz DS. Fetal urinary tract anomalies: Review of pathophysiology, imaging and management. Am J Roentgenol. 2018;210(5):1010-21.
16. National Center for Advancing Translational Sciences. Congenital hydrocephalus. Genetic and rare disease. [online] Available from: https://rarediseases.info.nih.gov/diseases/6682/ congenital-hydrocephalus. [Last accessed April 2022].
17. Norton ME. Fetal cerebral ventriculomegaly. UpToDate. [online] Available from: https://www.uptodate.com/contents/ fetal-cerebral-ventriculomegaly. [Last accessed April 2022].
18. Radiopaedia. (2021). Cephalocele. [online] Available from: https://radiopaedia.org/articles/cephalocele-1. [Last accessed April 2022].
19. Richard B. Abdominal imaging. Gasrtoschisis. Wolf in Creasy and Resnik's Maternal-Fetal Medicine, Part 1, 7th edition. Philadelphia: Saunders; 2013. Pp. 334-6.
20. Richard B. Abdominal imaging. Omphalocele. Wolf in Creasy and Resnik's Maternal-Fetal Medicine, Part 1, 7th edition. Philadelphia: Saunders; 2013. Pp. 340-2.
21. Society for Maternal-Fetal Medicine (SMFM). Nathan S, Monteagudo A, Kuller JA, Craigo S, Norton ME. Fox mild fetal ventriculomegaly: diagnosis, evaluation, and management. Am J Obstetr Gynecol. 2018;219(1):B2-9.
22. The Fetal Medicine Foundation. Encephalocele. [online] Available from: https://fetalmedicine.org/education/fetal-abnormalities/brain/encephalocele. [Last accessed April 2022].
23. The Fetal Medicine Foundation. Ventriculomegaly. [online] Available from: https://fetalmedicine.org/education/fetal-abnormalities/brain/ventriculomegaly. [Last accessed April 2022].
24. The Genetic and Rare Diseases Information Center (GARD). Spina bifida. [online] Available from: https://rarediseases.info. nih.gov/diseases/7673/spina-bifida. [Last accessed April 2022].
25. Verity C, Firth H, ffrench-Constant C. Congenital abnormalities of the central nervous system. J Neurol Neurosurg Psychiatry. 2003;74(Suppl 1):i3-8.
26. World Health Organization. Congenital anomalies. [online] Available from: https://www.who.int/health-topics/ congenital-anomalies#tab=tab_1. [Last accessed April 2022].

Index

Page numbers followed by *f* refer to figure, *fc* refer to flowchart, and *t* refer to table

A

ABO
  blood group status 203
  incompatibility 203
Abortion
  induced 208
  spontaneous 208
  threatened 207
Acanthosis nigricans 74
Acardiac mass 197
Acardiac twin 198*f*
Acquired immunodeficiency syndrome 72
Activated partial thromboplastin time 44, 96, 97, 200
Acute cutaneous lupus erythematosus 165
Acute respiratory distress syndrome 28
Acyclovir 257
Adenosine 93
Adrenal disease 22
Adrenocorticotropic hormone 218
Adult respiratory distress syndrome 45
Affronti endouterine hemostatic square 140
Air pollution 48
Airway malformation, congenital pulmonary 238
Alanine aminotransferase 23, 41
  serum 111
Albumin, low serum 168
Alcohol 180
Aldosteronism, primary 22
Alkaline
  phosphatase 102
  transaminase 102
Alloimmune factors 179, 184
Alloimmunization 202
Alobar holoprosencephaly 274
Alpha-fetoprotein 50, 102, 144, 265
  serum 62
Alpha-thalassemia 10
American Association for Study of Liver Diseases 109
American Association of Clinical Endocrinologist 77*t*, 156
American College of Cardiology 98
American College of Endocrinology 77*t*
American College of Obstetricians and Gynaecologists 22, 31, 32, 58, 73, 74, 147, 157, 181, 206, 223, 247, 249, 271
American College of Rheumatology Classification 166
American Diabetes Association Classification 72-74
American Fertility Society 178
American Heart Association Guidelines 98
American Institute of Ultrasound in Medicine 132
American Society for Reproductive Medicine 176
American Thyroid Association Guidelines 153, 155, 158
Amiodarone 93, 156
Ammonia 113
  elevated 43
Amniocentesis 243, 251, 280
Amnioinfusion 234, 247
Amnion nodosum 243
Amnioreduction 241
Amniotic band
  disruption sequence 266
  syndrome 246
Amniotic fluid 211, 237
  disorder 237
  dynamics 238*f*
  embolism 117, 119
  index 237, 240*f*, 244, 244*f*
    centile chart for 240
  synthesis, physiology of 237
  ultrasound evaluation of 240*f*
  volume 23, 56, 237, 245
    subjective assessment of 239
AmniSure rupture of membranes test 231
Anemia 1-3, 7, 10, 43, 48, 93, 156, 165, 190, 204
  aplastic 2
  autoimmune hemolytic 3
  chronic
    disease 3
    disorders 2
  classification of 2, 3
  correction of 136
  deficiency 2
  hemolytic 2, 43
  impact of 2
  microangiopathic hemolytic 2, 117
  mild 10
  moderate 10
  pregnancy 1
  renal 2
  severity of 5
  sideroblastic 2
Anencephalic fetus
  two-dimensional image of 266*f*
  ultrasonographic image of 266*f*
Anencephaly 264
Anesthesia 45, 139, 148
  general 36
  regional 36
Aneuploidy 244
Angiogenic factors 50
Angiotensin-converting enzyme inhibitor 15, 23, 39, 93, 243
Angiotensin-receptor blockers 23, 39, 93
Anhydramnios 287
Antenatal anti-D prophylaxis 207
Antenatal care 81, 94
Antenatal management 190, 289, 290
Antenatal visit 23, 191
Antepartum management 15, 197
Antepartum period 7
Antibiotics 226, 233
Antibody 167
  mediated immune suppression 207
    mechanism of 207
  screening 206
Anticardiolipin 178
  antibody 167
Anticholinergics 102
Anticoagulant 117
  regimen 95, 96*t*
Anticoagulation 97*fc*, 126
  regimens 95
Anti-D
  dose calculation 209
  immune globulin 136, 202
  prophylaxis 208*fc*
Antiemetics 102
Antigenic stimulus 203
Antihemophilic factor 118
Antihypertensives 23, 39
  therapy 37, 44
  treatment 23, 36
Antinuclear antibody 23, 166, 167
Antioxidant therapy 33
Antiphospholipid antibody 126, 165, 167, 173
  presence of 173
  syndrome 118, 178, 182, 244
Antiphospholipid syndrome 43, 52, 62, 118, 173, 176, 178, 243
Antiproliferative drugs 172
Antishock garments 138
Antithrombin 115
  deficiency 125
Antithyroid drugs 155, 160
  side effects of 160
Aorta, coarctation of 22, 86
Apex beat, shifting of 89
Apgar scores, low 46
Appendicitis 217
Aqueductal stenosis 276, 276*f*, 277*f*
  causes of 276
Arnold-Chiari malformation 270, 277
Arrhythmia
  rapid and irregular pulse 89
  treatment of 93
Arterial embolization 141

Arterial stiffness index 92
Arthritis 167
Ascites 106
Aspartate
  aminotransferase 23, 41, 111
  transaminase 102
Aspirin 23, 58, 117, 172
  low-dose 95
  role of 33
Assisted reproduction technology 132, 176, 218
Asthma, cardiac 89
Atenolol 38
Atosiban 225
Atrial contraction 67
Atrial fibrillation 94
Atrial septal defect 86, 89, 264, 279
Atrioventricular septal defect 86
Autoimmune 156
  disease 62
Autotransfusion 98
Avidity test 251
Azathioprine 172

B

Bacteriuria, asymptomatic 217, 226
Bacteroides 229
Ballantyne's syndrome 196
Bayes Theorem-based method 30
B-cell activating factor 172
Belimumab 172
Beta-blockers 38, 161
Beta-human chorionic gonadotropin 63
Betamethasone 222, 223, 233
  antenatal 222
Beta-thalassemia 10, 12, 12t, 19
  major 13f
  trait 12, 13f
Bile acids
  maternal 104
  serum 103
Biliary diseases 101
Bilirubin 43, 106
  elevated 43
  estimation of 211
Biochemical
  changes 102, 103
  indices 102
  markers 31
  monitoring 36
  tests 35
Biophysical profile 23, 55, 56, 82, 95, 199, 214
  modified 78
Biopsy 106
  renal 168
Bipolar coagulation 201
Birth
  control pills 22
  defects 262
  spacing 226
  timing of 25, 35
  weight, low 1, 156
Bladder
  abnormalities 289
  invasion of 144f
Bleeding
  disorders 117
    acquired 117

fetomaternal 209
gastrointestinal 121
piles 2
placenta previa, acute care of 137
prediction of 134
recurrent 209
reduce risk of 134
time 117
Blood
  bank 148
  components 138
  glucose 71, 77t
    fasting 72
    monitoring 81
    self-monitoring 77
    target capillary 77
  loss 2, 3, 137
    acute 136
    anemia 3
    assessment of severity of 138t
    massive 134
    quantify 138
  pressure 21, 34, 35
    measurement of 21, 244
    systolic 21, 122
  products 123
    transfusion of 138
  tests 34
  transfusion
    indications of 7
    place of 7
  urea nitrogen 168
  volume 1f
Blueberry muffin rash 251
Blunt abdominal trauma 209
B-lynch suture, application of 141f
Body mass index 31, 49, 216
Bone
  density scan 14
  marrow
    examination 4
    failure 2, 3
Brain
  magnetic resonance imaging of 251f
  sparing effect 47
Branchiootorenal syndrome 286
Breastfeeding 36, 82, 99, 112
Bridging vessels 146
British Committee for Standards in
  Hematology 7, 183
Budd-Chiari syndrome 101

C

Caffeine 180
Calcium supplementation 33
Calyceal dilation 289
Canadian Diabetic Association 75
Carbimazole 156
Carcinoma, hepatocellular 108
Cardiac arrest 39
Cardiac chamber diameter 89
Cardiac defect 253
Cardiac disease 86, 91-93
  types of 86
Cardiac magnetic resonance imaging 14
Cardiac output 87, 88
Cardiac strain 66

Cardiac team 90f
Cardiomyopathy 86
Cardiomyopathy, peripartum 86, 99
Cardiotocography 23, 35, 56, 59, 82, 98, 138,
  191, 213, 231, 243
Cardiovascular disease 74, 86, 99
Cardiovascular drugs 93
Cardiovascular system 86
Cataract, congenital 253, 253f
Cell salvage 148
Cell-free deoxyribonucleic acid 203, 208, 214
  testing, benefits of 206
Centers for Disease Control and Prevention
  72, 233
Central nervous system 28, 166, 239, 242, 264
  abnormalities 264
  congenital abnormalities of 264
  development of 265, 265f
Cephaloceles 267
Cerebellar tonsillar herniation 271f
Cerebellar vermis 278f
Cerebral artery, middle 47, 48, 53, 55f, 61, 67,
  191, 214
Cerebral palsy 229
Cerebroplacental ratio 48, 54, 67
Cerebrospinal fluid 267, 274, 274f
Cerebrovascular accident 28
Cervical cerclage 136, 227, 236
Cervical dilation 220, 221
Cervical length 220, 221, 226
  measurement 134
Cervical weakness 178
Cesarean
  delivery 139
  hysterectomy 148
  procedure 139
  section 71, 82, 97, 104, 131, 190
    indications of 257
    lower segment 173
Chemicals 180
Chemotherapeutic agents 180
Chest pain 89
Chiari malformations 267, 274
Chlamydia 179, 230
  trachomatis 229
Chloramphenicol 2
Chlorothiazide 93
Chlorpromazine 102
Cholangitis 44
  primary sclerosing 101
Cholecystitis 44
Cholelithiasis 101, 103
Cholestasis 101, 107
  obstetric 102, 190
Cholestyramine 104
Chorioamnionitis 49, 233, 234
Chorioangioma, placental 238
Choriodecidual inflammation 230
Chorionic villus sampling 13
Chorionicity, diagnosis of 188
Chorioretinitis 251
Choroid plexus cauterization 276
Chromosomal abnormality 177, 181
Chromosomal defect 177f
Chromosomal microarray 59
  analysis 49, 181
Chromosome microdeletion 48
Chronic cutaneous lupus erythematosus 165

Chronic obstructive pulmonary disease 3
Circulatory fibrinolysis test 122
Cirrhosis 101
Clot observation test 121
Clotting mechanism, activated 127
Clotting system 116
Coagulation
    disorders, assessment of 116
    inhibitors, reduction of 116
Coagulopathy, acquired 119
Cocaine 48
Cochlear defect 253
Collagen vascular disorders 3
Colloid cyst, computed tomography scan of 275*f*
Color Doppler 145
Combined medical therapy 185
Complete blood count 43, 116, 170
Computed tomography 275*f*
    scan 106, 275*f*
Conduction defects 86
Congenital anomalies 190, 262
Congenital cytomegalovirus infection
    diagnosis of 255*fc*
    management of 255*fc*
Congenital malformations 84, 200
Congenital renal anomaly
    etiology of 285
    types of 285
Congenital toxoplasmosis 251
    classic triad of 251
    rubella cytomegalovirus, herpes simplex infections 249
Conjoined triplets 192
Conjoined twin 188, 189*f*, 190, 192
Connective tissue disease 22
Conservative surgery 149
    one-step 150
Contraception 82, 83, 99, 99*f*
    emergency 99
Contraction, assessment of 219
Cooley's anemia 11
Coombs' test
    direct 205, 211
    indirect 205, 211
Copper intrauterine contraceptive device 83, 100
Cord
    blood acidemia 46
    entanglement 190
    prolapse 190
Coronary artery disease 86
Corticosteroid, antenatal 57, 135, 222, 233
Corticotropin-releasing hormone 218
Craniosynostosis 274
C-reactive protein 231
    elevated 168
Crown-rump length 81
Crystalloid 137
Cushing syndrome 22
Cyanosis 89
Cyclooxygenase 2 71
Cyclophosphamide 172
Cystic fibrosis 72
Cystoscopy 148
Cytokines 179
Cytomegalovirus 14, 49, 52, 107, 239, 244, 249, 253, 263
    immunoglobulin G avidity test 254

D

Dandy-Walker malformation 267, 274, 277, 278, 278*f*
D-dimer 43
De Quervain thyroiditis 156
Death, maternal 86, 150
Deep venous thrombosis 115
Dehydroepiandrosterones 218
Delivery 7, 57, 78, 82, 109, 137, 139, 147, 158, 161, 173, 201, 232
    emergency 95
    mode of 135, 247, 283
    route of 35
    timing of 23, 57, 78, 104, 135, 147, 192, 241, 213, 283
Deoxyribonucleic acid 11, 12, 118
    analysis 12
Depression, respiratory 39
Desferrioxamine 14
Desmopressin-1-deamino-8-D-arginine vasopressin 124
Dexamethasone 223, 233
Diabetes mellitus 14, 22, 71, 73, 81, 178
    gestational 71-73, 75, 77-79, 172, 190
    insulin dependent 265
    maternal 62
    pathophysiology of 72
    pregestational 94
    type 1 80
    type 2 80
Diabetic ketoacidosis 71, 83
    diagnosis of 83
    therapeutic management of 83
Diabetic pregnancies, intrauterine milieu of 71
Dichorionic diamniotic 188, 190*f*
    triplets 192
    twin 191
Dichorionic twin 200, 201
    pregnancies 192, 199
Dicycloverine 102
Diet 17
    modification 93
Dietary iodine deficiency, maternal 154
Digital cervical examination 220, 230
Diiodotyrosine 153
Dipstick proteinuria testing 34
Direct surgical scar 143
Discoid lupus erythematosus 165
Disseminated intravascular coagulation 25, 28, 42, 43, 105, 115, 120, 127, 139, 199
    pathogenesis of 121*fc*
    prevention of 113
    types of 120*f*
Distended jugular veins 89
Diuretics 93
Dizygotic twin 187, 189*f*
Dizziness 89
Dopamine antagonists 102
Doppler
    ultrasonography 61
    velocimetry 52, 53, 197
Double outlet right ventricle 86
Down syndrome 177, 262, 263
    translocation 177
Drugs 2
    treatment 160, 171, 246

Ductus venosus 61
    Doppler 54, 62, 63, 66, 68*f*
    flow 67
Duodenal atresia 238
Duplex kidney 285
Duplicated collecting system 285
Dysplasia, bronchopulmonary 216
Dyspnea 89
    paroxysmal nocturnal 89
    severe 89

E

Ebstein anomaly 86
Eclampsia 101, 117, 190
Edema, pulmonary 45, 98
Ehlers-Danlos syndrome 217, 286
Eisenmenger syndrome 86, 94
Electrocardiography 89
Electrophoresis, capillary 13*f*
Elevated serum glutamic pyruvic transaminase 168
Elliptocytosis 2
Embolism, pulmonary 171
Encephalocele 267, 274
    frontal 268*f*
    occipital 268*f*
Encephalopathy 106
    hepatic 113
    portosystemic 113
    prevention of 113
End-diastolic flow 61
End-diastolic velocity 48, 59
    absent 56
Endocarditis
    infective 86
    subacute bacterial 98, 98*t*
Endocrine disease 83
Endocrine Society Guideline 157
Endoplasmic reticulum 153
Endothelial colony forming cells 71
Endothelial dysfunction 29
Enterocolitis, necrotizing 216
Environmental toxins 48, 50
Enzyme
    defect 2
    inhibitor, nonspecific 125
    linked immunoassay 249
Epigenetic disorders 48
Epsilon amino caproic acid 125
Epstein-Barr virus 164
Erythrocyte sedimentation rate 168
Erythropoiesis
    cutaneous 251
    isolated secondary failure of 2
Escherichia coli 229
European Association for Study of Liver 112
European League against Rheumatism 166, 171
European Society for Gynecological Endoscopy Classification 178
European Society of Cardiology 98
European Society of Human Reproduction and Embryology 176, 178
European Working Group on Abnormally Invasive Placenta 145
Exercise 33
Expectant management 136, 197, 234

External cephalic version 209
Extirpative technique 149
Extravillous trophoblast 28

F

Factor V leiden 117, 125
Fallot tetralogy 86, 89, 239
Famciclovir 257
Fatigue 93
Fatty liver 101
    acute 42, 43, 101, 105, 107, 120, 190
    disease, nonalcoholic 101, 103
Federation of Obstetric and Gynaecological Societies of India 249
Fern test 230
Ferric carboxymaltose 6
Ferritin, serum 3
Fetal abdominal wall
    defect, common 278
    development of 279f
Fetal anatomic survey 277
Fetal anemia 67
Fetal aneuploidy screening 62
Fetal assessment 17, 34, 35t, 136
Fetal behavior biophysical profile 52
Fetal blood
    detection of 205
    estimation of 205
Fetal brain
    lesions 249
    magnetic resonance imaging of 251
Fetal complications 83, 174, 241, 246
Fetal compression syndrome 246
Fetal congenital
    anomalies 244
    malformation 262
Fetal cytomegalovirus infection, cerebral calcification in 254f
Fetal death 209
Fetal demise 193
Fetal deoxyribonucleic acid analysis 13
Fetal disorders 48
Fetal Doppler indications 62
Fetal echocardiography 94, 277, 280
Fetal fatty acid oxidation disorders 105
Fetal fibronectin 216, 220, 223, 229
    test 220, 230
Fetal genetic studies, indications of 52
Fetal growth 95
    restriction 13, 22, 46-49, 52, 58, 59, 62, 63, 174, 190, 191
        diagnosis of 191
        late-onset 47
        management of 59fc, 191
        prevention of 58
        screening of 191
    velocity 52
Fetal heart rate 57, 98, 173, 230
    continuous monitoring of 82
Fetal hemoglobin, hereditary persistence of 10
Fetal hydrocephalus 272f
    cause of 274
Fetal hydrocephaly, diagnosis of 274
Fetal hydronephrosis, cause of 288
Fetal hypoxia 69f
Fetal infection 250, 252, 259

diagnosis of 251, 252, 254, 258, 259
management of 253
sequelae of 253, 254, 260
Fetal intervention 200, 247, 290
Fetal kidney, normal 285f
Fetal medicine foundation algorithm 30
Fetal membranes, rupture of 229
Fetal monitoring 25, 94, 98, 138
Fetal morbidity 95
Fetal movement 62
Fetal outcomes 112
Fetal perfusion concerns 7
Fetal renal disorders 284
Fetal Rh disease, risk of development of 203
Fetal risk 22, 79, 91, 104, 156, 174, 189, 196
Fetal sex 203
Fetal surveillance 23, 78, 195
Fetal survey 52
Fetal swallowing 238
Fetal thyroid development 155
Fetal transfusion, potential benefits of 258
Fetal transmission 256
Fetal urination 238
Fetal varicella
    infection 260f
    syndrome 260
Fetal ventriculomegaly, ultrasonographic appearance of 272f
Fetal weight
    discordance 192
    estimated 46-48, 59, 191
Fetofetal transfusion, acute 193
Fetomaternal hemorrhage 208, 211
    screening for 210
    volume of 203
Fetoplacental circulation 62, 62f
Fetoscopic laser ablation 196
Fibrin 149
    degradation products 117, 119, 121
    glue 140
Fibrinogen 43, 117, 122, 149
    concentrations 123fc
    replacement 44
    therapy 149
Fibrinolysis 115f
    inhibition, reduction of 116
Fibrinolytic inhibitors 125
First-line therapy 225
Flow cytometry 206, 207f
Fluid management 35, 97
Fluorescent treponemal antibody absorption assay 261
Focal exophytic mass 145
Folic acid 265
    deficiency 2, 3
Food and Drug Administration 76, 172, 225
Fossa cyst, posterior 274, 278f
Fossa malformation, posterior 277
Foul smelling vaginal discharge 235
Free thyroxine 156
Free triiodothyronine 156
Fresh frozen plasma 106, 119, 123, 124, 139
Full blood count 3

G

Gallbladder 14
Gamma-aminobutyric acid 113

Gamma-glutamyl transpeptidase 103
Gardnerella vaginalis 216, 229
Gastric ulcer 44
Gastritis 44
Gastrointestinal tract 38, 239
Gastroschisis 48, 281, 283f
    ultrasonographic image of 282f
Genetic 202, 265, 286
    aberration 49
    analysis 240
    counseling 181, 277
    disorders 48
    factors 30, 48, 163, 262
    hypercoagulable states 117
    ultrasonography test 94
Genital herpes, recurrent early 257
Genital infection 217, 227
German measles 252, 263
Gestational age 221, 247
    large for 79, 239
    small for 22, 46-48, 65, 126, 282
Gestational diabetes mellitus 71-73, 75, 77-79, 172, 190
    diagnosis of 74
    pathophysiology of 72fc
    risk factors for 74
    screening of 74
Gestational hypertension 24, 24t
    management of 24
Glargine 76
Glasgow coma scale 28
Globin chains 10
Glomerular filtration rate 32, 154
Glomerulonephritis 22
    diffuse proliferative 166
    focal proliferative 166
Glucocorticoids 128, 172
Glucose
    6-phosphate dehydrogenase 2
    capillary 82
    tolerance test 74
Gonorrhea 230
Granulocyte colony-stimulating factor 184
Graves' disease 155, 159, 161
Great arteries, transposition of 86
Group B *Streptococcus* prophylaxis 217, 222, 233
Growth
    chart 47f
    discordant 190
    restriction 46, 48t, 190, 251
        management of 200
    symmetric 52
    scan 78
Guillain-Barré syndrome 166

H

Haemophilus influenzae 14
Haptoglobin, low serum 42
Harsh systolic murmur 89
Hashimoto's disease 156
Hashimoto's thyroiditis 155-157
Health education 253
Heart 14
    block, congenital complete 167
    defects 262
    disease 89, 89t

acyanotic 86
congenital 48, 86, 94
coronary 86
cyanotic 62, 86, 89
diagnosis of 89
ischemic 86
rheumatic 86
failure
congestive 98
early prevention of 93
features of 89
treatment of 93
rate 88, 89
Helicobacter pylori infection 102
Hematinic deficiency 7
Hematocrit 214
Hematological tests 35
Hematoma, subcapsular 45
Hemoglobin 1, 9, 12, 73
E 11, 18, 19
disease, genetics of 18f
trait, electrophoresis in 18f
F 13
glycosylated 240
H 11
Hemoglobinopathy 2, 3
Hemoglobinuria, paroxysmal nocturnal 2
Hemolysis, elevated liver enzymes, and low platelets syndrome 41, 43-45, 101, 115, 117-119, 127
pathogenesis of 41
Hemolytic disease 202
Hemolytic uremic syndrome 43, 120
Hemophilia 118, 119
A 117
B 117
Hemoptysis 89
Hemorrhage 190
acute 7
antepartum 2, 49, 115, 190
decidual 218
intracranial 216
intrapartum 2
intraventricular 229, 277
life-threatening 149
major obstetric 137
massive obstetric 7
postpartum 45, 87, 104, 115, 123, 132, 140, 156, 190, 230, 241
Heparin 117, 125
unfractionated 96, 97, 127, 173, 182
Hepatic rupture 45
Hepatitis
A 107
virus 107
acute viral 101, 107
B 101, 107, 108
immunoglobulin 109, 110
virus 14, 108
C 101, 107, 110
virus 110, 127
E 101, 107, 111
virus 107, 111, 112f
viral 44, 107, 107t
Hepatorenal syndrome, prevention of 113
Hepatosplenomegaly 174, 251
Heritable thoracic aortic diseases 92
Hernia, congenital diaphragmatic 239

Herpes simplex virus 249, 256
antiviral treatment for 257t
infection 257
Homocysteine 126
Homocysteinemia 184
Hookworm infestation 2
Hormonal fluctuations 72
Hormone 164
luteinizing 183
Human chorionic gonadotropin 102, 144, 152, 154
Human immunodeficiency virus 1, 72
Human kidney development, embryology of 284
Human leukocyte antigen 164, 179
Human parvovirus B19 14, 257
Human umbilical vein endothelial cells 71
Hutchinson teeth 260
Hydatidiform mole 209
Hydralazine 38
Hydramnios 194, 237, 238
Hydration 246
Hydrocephalus 251f, 271f, 273, 275, 275f
noncommunicating 275
Hydronephrosis 285, 289
mild 288
minimal 289
Hydronephrotic kidney, bilateral 288f
Hydroxychloroquine 171, 172
Hydroxyprogesterone caproate 226
Hydroxyprostaglandin dehydrogenase 219
Hyperbilirubinemia, neonatal 204
Hyperemesis gravidarum 101, 102, 190
Hyperglycemia 74, 82
intrauterine 71f
maternal 79
Hyperhomocysteinemia 118, 126
Hyperprolactinemia 178, 183
Hypertension 21, 24, 28, 34, 46, 74, 83, 166, 190, 286
chronic 22-24, 101, 243
control of 35
gestational 24, 24t
pregnancy-induced 93, 244
pulmonary 86, 94
renovascular 22
secondary 22
severe 24, 34, 38
gestational 25
pulmonary 119
Hypertensive disorders 21, 37, 62, 86
classification of 21
Hyperthermia, maternal 265
Hyperthyroidism 159
causes of 159
subclinical 162
Hypofibrinolysis 116
Hypogastric artery ligation 149
Hypoglycemia 43, 106
neonatal 84
Hypogonadism, hypogonadotropic 12
Hypoplasia, pulmonary 246
Hypoprothrombinemia 119
Hypothalamic-pituitary
adrenal axis 218
thyroid axis 152
Hypothesis 164
Hypothyroidism 155

congenital 156
subclinical 156, 158
Hypothyroxinemia, isolated 156
Hypoxemia 46, 48, 67
chronic 62
effects of 67
Hypoxia 67
Hysterectomy 141
subtotal 149
total 149
Hysterosalpingography 182
Hysterotomy, transverse 148

I

Iatrogenic membrane defect 196
Iatrogenic twin anemia polycythemia sequence 196
Ibuprofen 172
Idiopathic thrombocytopenia 128
pathophysiology of 128f
Immune maladaptation 29
Immunofluorescence test 255, 259
Immunoglobulin
G 255
types of 203
intravenous 129, 171, 172
M 255
Immunomodulatory therapies 213
Immunotherapy 184
Impaired glucose tolerance 74
In utero
infection 256
treatment 291
In vitro fertilization 31, 49, 144, 180
Indian Society for Pediatric and Adolescent Endocrinology 158
Indigo-carmine dye 231
Indomethacin 138, 172
Induced hepatotoxicity, drug 101
Infections 2, 14, 93, 179, 183, 218, 263
acute viral 107
congenital 48, 256
control 94
extragenital 217
maternal 252, 259
prevention of 98
transmission of 257
viral 244
Infectious disease 49
Inflammation 218
Insulin 80, 81
choice of 81
regimens 76
treatment 76
types of 76
Intensive care unit 131, 147, 232
Interferon regulatory factor 5 164
Interleukin 27, 164, 219
International Association of Diabetes and Pregnancy Study Group 73
International Committee for Monitoring Assisted Reproductive Technology 176
International Diabetes Federation 73
International Federation of Gynecology and Obstetrics 47, 75, 143, 191
International normalized ratio 96, 97, 116

International Society for Abnormally Invasive Placenta 150
International Society for Study of Hypertension in Pregnancy 21, 31, 33
International Society of Ultrasound in Obstetrics and Gynecology 193
International Society on Thrombosis and Hemostasis 121
Intrapartum management 35, 58, 97, 192
Intraperitoneal transfusion 213
Intrauterine fetal
    death 2, 82, 99, 249, 283
    demise 125, 196, 198, 204
Intrauterine growth
    intervention trial, disproportionate 57
    restriction 16, 47-49, 62, 125, 171, 193, 200, 240, 242, 249, 280
Intrauterine infection, pathophysiology of 218, 218*fc*
Intrauterine transfusion 212
Intravascular transfusion, direct 212
Iodine 154
    deficiency 156
Iron 2, 6
    binding capacity, total 4, 11, 12
    carboxymaltose 6
    deficiency 2
        anemia 1, 3, 4, 7, 12, 12*t*
    deficit, calculation of 7
    dextran 6
    profile
        analysis 11
        serum 4
    study 12
    sucrose 6
Isophane insulin 80
Isovolumetric relaxation 66

J

Jaundice 43, 251

K

Kallmann syndrome 286
Keyhole sign 245*f*, 290*f*
Kidney
    congenital anomalies of 285, 289
    development of 285*f*
    injury, acute 28, 36, 45
Kleihauer-Betke test 205, 206*f*, 240
Klinefelter syndrome 263

L

Labetalol 37, 38
Labor 78, 82, 158, 161, 173
    analgesia 82
    first stage of 97
    induction of 96, 234
    management of 241
    prodromal signs symptoms of 219
    second stage of 35, 98
    third stage of 98
Lactate dehydrogenase 23, 41, 106
Laser ablation 195, 201
Lead 48
    poisoning 2

Lethal quad 123
Leukocytosis 235
Leukomalacia, periventricular 216
Leukopenia 165, 169
Levothyroxine, dose of 157
Liley's chart 211, 212*f*
Liley's curve 212
Lipoprotein, high-density 74
Listeria monocytogenes 179
Lithium 156
Liver 14, 113
    biopsy 103
    disease 2, 3, 101, 107, 117
        autoimmune 101
        pregnancy-associated 101
    disorders, pregnancy-associated 101
    enzymes 106
    function test 4, 42, 43, 101, 106, 168, 170
    injury, severe 112*f*
    transaminases, elevated 42
    tumor 101
Long-chain 3-hydroxyacyl-coenzyme A dehydrogenase deficiency 41, 105
Loop electrosurgical excision procedure 217
Loud first heart sound 89
Low-molecular weight heparin 58, 96, 97, 127, 173, 182
Lung disease
    chronic 48
    severe restrictive 170
Lupus erythematosus 22
    neonatal 174
    subacute cutaneous 165
Lupus flare 43
Lupus nephritis 165, 166
    exacerbation 174
Luteal phase defect 179

M

Macrocytosis, physiologic 2
Macrosomia 84
Magnesium
    sulfate 39, 222, 225, 234
        administration of 138
    toxicity, treatment of 39
Magnetic resonance imaging 89, 106, 133*f*, 134, 146, 195, 270, 271*f*, 273, 278
    role of 146
Major histocompatibility complexes 30
Malabsorption 48
Malar rash 165*f*, 167
Malaria 2, 48
Malignancy 3
Marfan syndrome 94
Marrow suppression 118, 127
Maternal fetal monitoring 171
Maternal infection 252, 259
    diagnosis of 110, 250, 252-254, 256, 258, 259, 261
    sequelae of 258
Maternal monitoring 94, 138, 200
Maternal serum alpha-fetoprotein 266
Matrix metalloproteinase 218, 219
Maturity-onset diabetes of young 72
Maximum vertical pocket technique 238, 240*f*
Mean arterial pressure 30, 32, 65, 88

Mean corpuscular
    hemoglobin 3, 11, 12
        concentration 11, 12
    volume 2, 11, 12
Mean uterine arteries pulsatility index 48
Measles, mumps, rubella 252
Mechanical prosthetic heart valve 95
Mechanical valve
    anticoagulation in 97*fc*
    replacement 94
Meckel-Gruber syndrome 267
Medical nutrition therapy 75
Membrane
    bacterial degradation of 218
    defect, acquired 2
Meningocele 267, 268, 270*f*
Mercury 48
Messenger ribonucleic acid 144
Metformin 75
Methamphetamine 48
Methimazole 156, 160
Methotrexate 150, 172
Methyldopa 37
Methylenetetrahydrofolate reductase 111, 126, 265
Methyltetrahydrofolate 126, 179
Metoclopramide 102
Middle cerebral artery 47, 48, 53, 55*f*, 61, 67, 191, 214
    Doppler of 212
    normal 68*f*, 69*f*
    peak systolic velocity 67
    pulsatility index 54
Mini pill 83
Miscarriage 190
    recurrent 176, 179, 183, 185
    spontaneous 177
Mississippi classification 42
Mitral regurgitation 86
Mitral stenosis 86, 92
Monitoring, frequency of 77
Monoamniotic twin 192
Monochorionic diamniotic 188, 190*f*
    triplets 192
    twin pregnancies 192
Monochorionic monoamniotic 190*f*
    triplets 192
    twin 188, 192
Monochorionic twin 192, 193*f*, 197*f*, 200, 201
    complications of 193
Monoiodotyrosine 153
Monozygotic twin 187, 189*f*
Mortality
    maternal 83, 190
    perinatal 83, 190, 237
Mucous membrane lesion 169
Mulberry molars 260
Müllerian duct anomaly 217
Müllerian tract malformations, congenital 178
Multicystic dysplastic kidney 285
    bilateral 244
Multicystic encephalomalacia 198, 199*f*
    pathophysiology of 199
Multidisciplinary panel classification system 289
Multidrug resistance protein 3 103
Multifetal gestation 187
Multiple births 187

Multiple daily insulin injection therapy 76
Multiple gestation 49, 187, 218, 219
Multiple pregnancy 93
    fetal risks of 189
    management of 189
    maternal risk of 189
Murmur, continuous 89
Mycophenolate mofetil 172
Mycoplasma 226, 227
    hominis 179, 216, 229
Myelodysplasia 3
Myelodysplastic syndrome 3
Myelomeningocele 268, 271*f*
Myeloschisis 268
Myocardial infarction 100
Myosin light chain kinase 218
Myxedema 3

N

Nasal ulcers 165
National High Blood Pressure Education Program Working Group on High Blood Pressure in Pregnancy 21
National Institute for Health and Care Excellence 3, 31, 32, 76, 191, 192, 220, 227, 231, 233
National Institute of Cardiovascular Disease 86
National Institute of Child Health and Human Development 50
National Institutes of Health 235
Natural killer cell function 179
Necrosis 29
Nefidipine 37
Neisseria gonorrhoeae 229
Neonatal infection 256
    detection of 251
    prevention of 109
Neonatal intensive care unit 232
Nephropathy 71
Neural tube defect 262, 264
Neutral protamine Hagedorn 76, 77
New York Heart Association 90-93, 95
Next-generation sequencing 287
Nifedipine 37, 38
Nitric oxide 71
Nitrazine paper test 230
Nitric oxide 27, 29
Nocturnal cough 89
Noncentral nervous system anomalies 274
Nonsteroidal anti-inflammatory drugs 36, 171, 172, 242
Nonstress test 23, 53, 55, 199, 214
    frequency of 56
    reactive 137
Nuchal translucency 63, 81
Nutritional status, maternal 263

O

Obesity 265
    morbid 74
Obstetrical hemorrhage, treatment of 123*fc*
Obstetrics, Doppler in 61
Oligohydramnios 62, 237, 243-245, 287
    causes of 243
    isolated 246

Omphalocele 279, 280*f*
    ultrasonographic image of 282*f*
Oral contraceptive pill 100, 126
    low-dose 83
Oral desogestrel 99
Oral glucose tolerance test 73, 74, 240
Oral hydration therapy 246
Oral iron 6
    therapy 5
Oral medications 75
Oral ulcers 165, 167
Organ
    system 264*t*
    transplantation 72
Orthopnea 89, 93
Overt hypothyroidism 156
    management of 157
Oxygen saturation 89, 98
Oxytocin 140
    receptor 218

P

Packed red blood cells 123
Pain
    abdominal 106
    relief 97
Palmar erythema 101
Palpation, abdominal 51
Palpitation 89
Pancreatitis
    acute 44
    chronic maternal 72, 104
Paralysis, respiratory 39
Parenchyma, renal 289
Parenteral iron therapy 6
    types of 6, 6*t*
Partial thromboplastin time 43, 117
Partograph 82
Parvovirus B
    infection 259*f*
    testing for 258
Patellar reflexes 39
Patent ductus arteriosus 86, 216
Peak systolic velocity 69, 191, 214
Pedal edema 89
Pelvic diameter, renal 288
Pelvis, renal 288, 291*f*
Penicillin derivative 290
Penicillin treatment 261
Peptic ulcer disease 2
Periarteritis nodosa 22
Pericarditis 169
Perinatal hepatitis B prevention program 110*f*
Periodontal diseases 217
Peripheral blood smear 4, 11, 43, 122
Peripheral nervous systems 166
Peripheral vascular resistance 37
Persistent twin-to-twin transfusion syndrome 196
Pessary 227
Phenothiazines 102
Pheochromocytoma 22
Phosphorylated insulin-like growth factor binding protein-1 220
Photosensitivity 167
Placenta accreta 144
    spectrum 131, 137, 143, 145
        disorder 143, 144, 151

Placenta creta 144
Placenta increta 144
Placenta percreta 144, 144*f*
    color Doppler of 146*f*
    post-hysterectomy specimen of 148*f*
Placenta previa 131, 132, 132*f*, 133, 133*f*, 134, 135*f*, 136, 141, 143, 146*f*
    color Doppler of 133*f*
    gray scale of 145*f*
    management of 136, 137*fc*
    types of 131*f*
Placenta, low-lying 132*f*, 134
Placental abruption 45, 117, 119
Placental growth factor 24, 27, 29, 62
Placental removal 148
Plasma
    glucose, fasting 73
    protein-A 29, 30, 49, 144
    volume 1*f*
Plasmapheresis 213
Plasmin 125, 149
Plasminogen 125
    activator inhibitor-1 116
Platelet 122
    abnormalities 127
    count 117
    disorders 118
    effects on 116
    function
        analyzer 117
        poor 118
    production 118, 127
    target 124
    transfusion 129
Pleurisy 169
Poiseuille law 68
Polycystic kidney disease 22, 245*f*
    autosomal
        dominant 285, 286
        recessive 285, 287, 287*f*
    infantile 244
Polycystic ovarian syndrome 74, 179, 182
Polycythemia sequence 194
Polydipsia 106
Polyhydramnios 190, 219, 237, 241-243
    causes of 238, 239*t*
    complications of 241
    diagnosis of 242*fc*
    management of 242*fc*
    sequence 193, 195*f*
    subacute 238
Polymerase chain reaction 206, 250, 255, 273
Polyuria 106
Postliver transplantation state 101
Postnatal management 7, 36, 104, 158, 173
Postpartum 78, 82, 161
    monitoring 99, 99*f*
    period 7
    transmission 110
Postreversible encephalopathy syndrome 28
Potter syndrome 244
Prazosin 38
Preconception 39
    screening 263
Preeclampsia 21, 24-27, 28*f*, 29, 31-33, 43, 101, 119, 173, 190, 243
    classification of 30
    etiopathology of 26

fetal consequences of 36
first-trimester prediction of 63
long-term prognosis of 36
management of 34, 34t
maternal consequences of 36
prediction of 30
prevention of 33
severe 30, 35
symptoms of 26
Pregnancy 1, 7, 21, 39, 95, 108, 159, 170, 221
   abnormal placentation in 26
   acute fatty liver of 43, 101, 105, 107, 120, 190
   cardiac disease in 86, 91, 93
   cardiovascular changes in 87
   cholestasis of 101
   classification of
      anemia in 2
      liver diseases in 101, 101t
   coagulation disorders in 115
   complications of 101
   continuation of 280
   current 216
   diabetes mellitus in 71, 73
   diagnosis of
      heart disease in 89
      thyroid disorders in 155
   disorders promoting thrombosis in 117
   Doppler interpretation in 61f
   duration of 5
   ectopic 209
   effects of 88, 116
   etiology of anemia in 1
   hypertension in 21
   hypertensive disorders of 21, 37, 62
   interval 217
   intrahepatic cholestasis of 101, 102
   iodine requirement in 154
   liver disease in 101
   loss 177
      mechanism of 178
      recurrent 176, 176f, 177
      spontaneous 176
   management of 24, 24t, 33, 118, 170, 199, 276
   medical termination of 94
   molar 41, 117
   monochorionic 199
   normal physiological changes in 101
   placental remodeling in 62
   systemic lupus erythematosus in 163
   termination of 280
   thalassemia in 9
   thrombocytopenia in 127
   thyroid
      disorders in 152
      dysfunction in 158fc
   transmission of toxoplasmosis in 250f
   triplet 192
Premature rupture of membranes 190, 229, 234, 235, 241
   diagnosis of 230
   prevention of 235
Prenatal management 91, 282
Prepregnancy 157
   body mass index 216
   evaluation 22
Preterm birth 174, 190, 196, 216, 226

prevention of 226
risk factors for 217f
spontaneous 226
Preterm labor 190, 216, 222t, 223
   management of 223fc, 226fc
   pathophysiology of 218
Preterm premature rupture of membranes 129, 194, 195, 229, 235fc
   risk factors of 229
Prochlorperazine 102
Progesterone 83, 179, 183, 236
   choice of 227
   only pill 83
   prophylactic 227
   supplementation 226, 233
   therapy 183
Progestin
   implants 99
   only pills 99
Prophylactic endovascular balloon catheters 149
Propranolol 38
Propylthiouracil 156, 160
Prostaglandin 27, 218
   E 219
   imbalance 29
   synthetase inhibitor 241, 243
Protein
   C deficiency 117, 125
   placental 29
   S deficiency 117, 125
Proteinuria 169
   measurement of 22
Prothrombin
   gene mutation 125, 126
   time 43, 116, 117, 200
Pulsatility index 53, 61, 69
Puncture, site of 212
Pyelactasis 288, 288f
Pyelonephritis 217
Pyrimethamine 251
Pyruvate kinase deficiency 2

Q

Qualitative disorders 118
Queenan curve 211, 212, 212f
Quinidine 93
Quintero staging 194

R

Rachischisis 268
Radiofrequency 201
Random plasma glucose 73
Randomized controlled trial 33, 76, 179
Rash, discoid 167
Raynaud's phenomenon 165f
Reactive oxygen species 12, 28
Rectovaginal swab 220
Red blood cell 1, 11, 12, 68, 139, 168, 202
   count 12
   membrane defects 2
Red cell
   concentrates 139
   distribution width 3, 4, 12
   mass 1f
   morphology 2

Regurgitation, aortic 86
Renal agenesis 286
   bilateral 244
   unilateral 245f
Renal disease
   active 169
   chronic maternal 62, 243
Renal failure, acute 22, 45
Renal function test 4, 106, 168
Renal insufficiency, chronic 22
Renal parenchymal
   appearance 289
   thickness 289
Respiratory distress syndrome 84, 216, 229
Respiratory problems, neonatal 84
Resuscitation 123
Reticulocyte count 3
Retinopathy 71, 83
   of prematurity 216
Reversed end-diastolic velocity 56
Reversible ischemic neurological deficit 28
Rhesus
   alloimmunization 202
   immunoglobulin 129
Ribonucleic acid 14
Ribonucleoprotein 167
Rifampicin 104
Ringer's solution 123
Rituximab 172
Robertsonian translocation 177
Rosette screening test 205, 205f
Routine antenatal anti-D prophylaxis 207, 208
Royal College of Obstetricians and Gynaecologists 10, 22, 47, 65, 145, 176, 181, 206, 232, 251
Rubella 252, 263
   avidity test 252
   infection 253f
   syndrome, congenital 253
Rupture of membranes
   artificial 98, 241
   test, limitations in 231

S

Sacrococcygeal teratoma 238
S-adenosyl methionine 104
Scleroderma 22
Scoliosis 283f
Second-line therapy 225
Sedation, maternal 212
Sepsis 2, 118, 119, 127
Sequelae, neonatal 253
Serosa bladder interface, hypervascularity of 146
Serositis 167
Serum glutamic-oxaloacetic transaminase 168
Sexually transmitted disease 217
Shock 136, 137
   index 122
Sickle cell hemoglobinopathies 2
Single fetal demise 190, 199
   maternal risk of 199
Single nucleotide polymorphisms 206
Singleton pregnancy 49, 131
Sitagliptin 184

Skin
    active 169
    cicatricial lesions of 260f
    edema 259f
Small bowel obstruction 238
Society for Maternal Fetal Medicine 56, 59, 110, 147, 223
Society of Fetal Urology Grading System 288
Society of Obstetric Medicine 22
Society of Obstetricians and Gynaecologists of Canada 22
Sonographic fetal biometry 51
Sonography
    transabdominal 131, 221
    transvaginal 133, 133f, 221
Sonohysterography 182
Spastic paraplegia syndrome 277
Spherocytosis, hereditary 2, 3
Spina bifida 268, 270f, 271f
    occulta 268
    open 268
    types of 269f
Spiramycin 251
Splenectomy 129
Steatohepatitis, nonalcoholic 74
Stenosis
    aortic 86, 97
    pulmonary 86
Sterile speculum examination 230
Sterilization 100
Stillbirth 62, 190
Streptococcus agalactiae 222
Stress
    maternal 218fc
    psychosocial 218
Stroke volume 88
Sulfadiazine 251
Supportive therapy 106
Surgery, cardiac 94
Swansea criteria 106
Symphysio fundal height 49, 230
Syncope 89
Synovitis, acute 169
Syphilis 48, 260
    congenital 260
    early congenital 260
    late congenital 260
Systemic arterial oxygen saturation 98
Systemic lupus erythematosus 31, 50, 118, 163, 164, 166, 171, 243
    activity 170
    diagnosis of 166
    flare 169
        mild 169
        risk of 174
        severe 169
    moderate 169
    pathophysiology of 164f
    symptoms of 165
Systolic ejection murmur 89

T

Tachycardia 89
Tacrolimus 172
Tennessee classification 42
Tenofovir disoproxil fumarate 109
Teratogens 48, 50
Terbutaline 225
Thalassemia 2, 9, 10, 10t, 12, 13, 15f
    diagnosis of 11
    fertility in 12
    genetic basis of 10
    intermedia 10
    major 10
        pathophysiology of 11
    minor 10
    trait, blood parameter of 12t
Thrombin time 117
Thrombocytopenia 42, 43, 127, 129t, 169, 251
    autoimmune 127
    drug-induced 118, 129
    features suggestive of 128
    gestational 118, 127
    idiopathic 128
    mild 42
    neonatal 129
    severe 42
Thromboelastography 116, 124
Thromboembolism, venous 125
Thrombophilia 125
    acquired 118, 126
    high-risk 126
    inherited 125, 179, 183
    low-risk 126, 127
Thromboprophylaxis 39, 94, 95
Thrombotic thrombocytopenia purpura 42, 43, 115, 118, 130
Thyroid
    binding globulin 152, 154
    disease 183
    disorders 152, 155
        diagnosis of 155
    dysfunction 158fc, 178
        management of 161
    function tests 14, 152
    hormone 152
        formation of 152, 153f
        level, trimester specific 156t
        metabolism of 154f
        production 152
        secretion of 152, 153f
    peroxidase 178
        antibody 156, 158
    physiology, normal 152
    releasing hormone 152, 154
    status 152
    stimulating hormone 102, 152, 154, 156, 158, 161
    storm 161
Thyroiditis
    postpartum 156
    subacute 156, 159
    transient 156
Thyrotoxicosis 22, 86
    effects of 159
    gestational transient 159
Thyroxine 153, 154, 161
Tissue
    factor 119
    plasminogen activator 115
    sealants 234
Tocolysis 138, 232, 233
    contraindications of 224
    mechanism of action of 224
Tocolytic 222, 224
    choice of 224
    drugs 222
Toxic
    adenoma 159
    nodular goiter 159
Toxoplasma gondii 179, 250
Toxoplasmosis
    congenital 251
    neonatal 251f
    prevention of 252
    subclinical congenital 251
Toxoplasmosis, rubella cytomegalovirus, herpes simplex 48
    infections 249
        diagnosis of 250
        screening for 249
    serology, interpretation of 249
Tranexamic acid 118, 140, 149
Transfusion 138
    maternal 16
Transient ischemic attack 28
Transvaginal ultrasound 220, 223, 226
    examination 220
Trauma, surgical 143
Treponema pallidum 260
Tricuspid
    atresia 86
    flow pattern 63
    regurgitation 63, 241
Triiodothyronine 153, 154, 161
Triple P procedure 150
Triple X syndrome 263
Triploidy 48
Trisomy 21, 48, 177, 244, 263
Trophoblast
    apoptosis 29
    invasion 27
Trophoblastic disease 159
Tuberculosis 1
Tumor necrosis factor alpha 27, 28, 102, 164, 184, 218
Turbulent lacunar blood flow 145, 146
Twin
    anemia 194
        polycythemia sequence 190, 196, 200
    classification of 187, 188f
    entrapment 190
    malformations in 200
    oligohydramnios 193, 195f
    pregnancy 131
    reversed arterial perfusion sequence 190, 193, 197
    to-twin transfusion 50
        syndrome 61, 190, 193-195, 238

U

Ultrasonography 34, 188, 240, 251
    assessment 193
    prenatal 264
    test 106
Ultrasound, transvaginal 220, 223, 226
Ultraviolet 164
Umbilical artery 48, 58, 59, 61, 66, 66f, 265
    abnormal 47
    Doppler 53, 65, 67
        normal 58
    pulsatility index 48, 195

Umbilical cord factors 48
Umbilical vein 61
    Doppler flow 69*f*
Upper segment transverse uterine incision 148
Ureaplasma 226, 227
    urealyticum 179, 229
Ureteral abnormalities 289
Ureteric stents, preoperative 148
Ureteropelvic junction obstruction 285
    bilateral 244
Urethral atresia 244
Urethral valve, posterior 244, 285, 290, 291*f*
Uric acid 43
Urinary iodine concentration 154
Urinary tract 289
    congenital anomalies of 285
    dilation 288
        classification of 288
    infection 44, 83, 190, 229, 286
    obstruction, lower 290
Urine analysis 168
    abnormal 169
Urine culture 220
Uropathy, obstructive 244
Ursodeoxycholic acid 104
Uterine
    anomalies 217
    artery 61, 64
        Doppler 31, 31*f*, 53, 53*f*, 64, 64*f*
        Doppler, normal 64*f*
    compression sutures 141
    contraction 220
    distention 218, 219
    factors 177
    incision 148
    pathology 144
Uterotonic agents 149

V

Vaccination 108
Vaginal bleeding, painless 134
Vaginal delivery, operative 190
Vaginal progesterone 227
Vaginosis, bacterial 216
Valacyclovir 256, 257
Valsalva maneuvers 98
Valvular disease, rheumatic 86
Varicella zoster 258, 259
Vasa previa 133
Vascular dysfunction, programming of 71
Vascular endothelial growth factor 27-29
Vasculopathy, decidual 29
Vasopressin 139
Venereal disease research laboratory 261
Ventricular septal defect 86, 89, 264, 267
Ventriculostomy, endoscopic third 276
Vermis, hypoplasia of 277
Vesicoamniotic shunts 247
Vesicoureteral reflux 285
Virus, types of 107
Vitamin
    B_{12} 2
        deficiency 3
    D 33, 184
    K deficiency 119
Vomiting 106
von Willebrand
    disease 117, 118
    factor 116

W

Weakness 93
Weight
    gain
        gestational 75
        poor 48
    management 23
Wernicke's encephalopathy 102
White cell count 231
Whole blood transfusion 123
Wilson disease 101
World Health Organization 1, 2, 51, 92, 176, 222
Wright's stain 122

X

X-ray irradiation 180

Z

Zidovudine 2
Zika virus 48, 49, 277
    infection 263
Zinc protoporphyrin 4